Cardiomyopathy - Disease of the Heart Muscle

Edited by Gustav Mattsson and Peter Magnusson

Published in London, United Kingdom

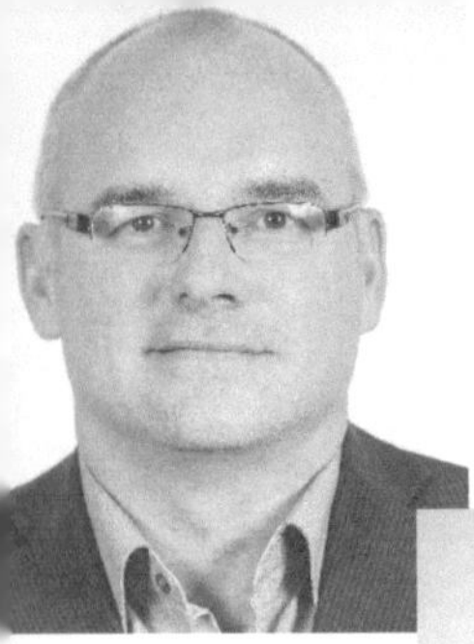
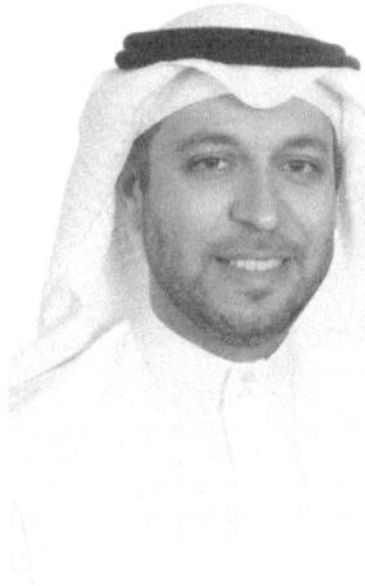
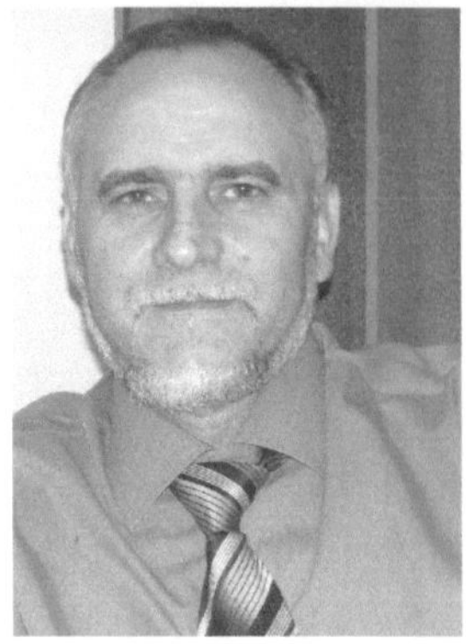
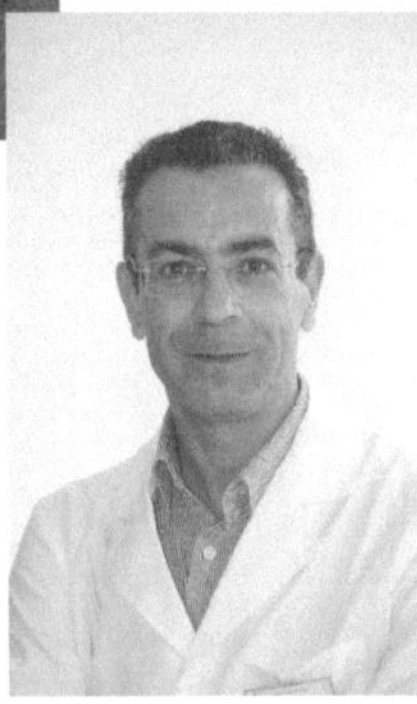
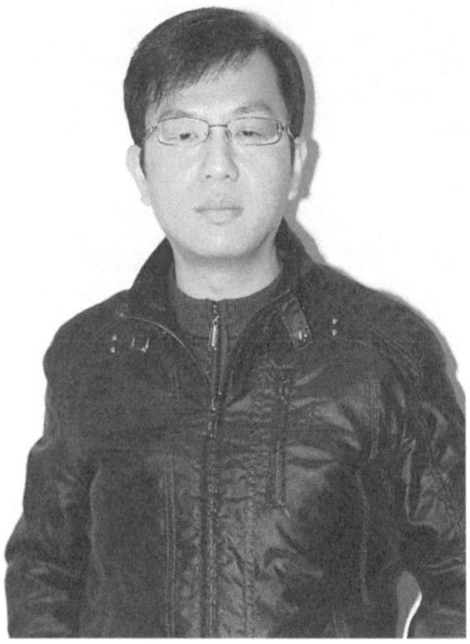
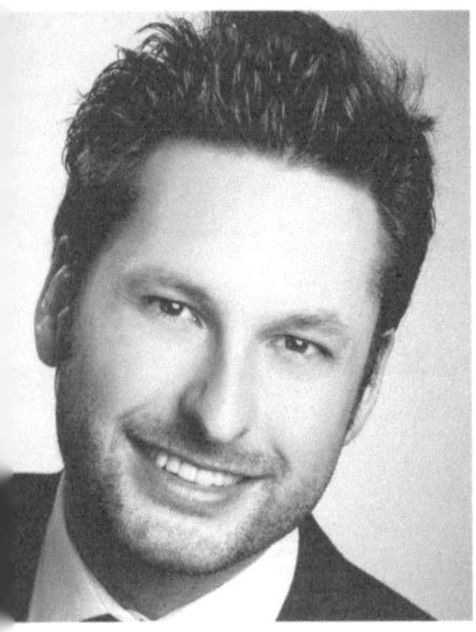
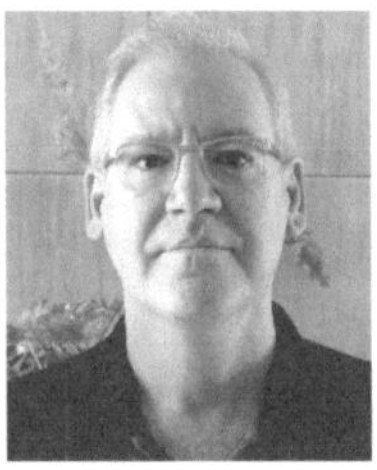

IntechOpen

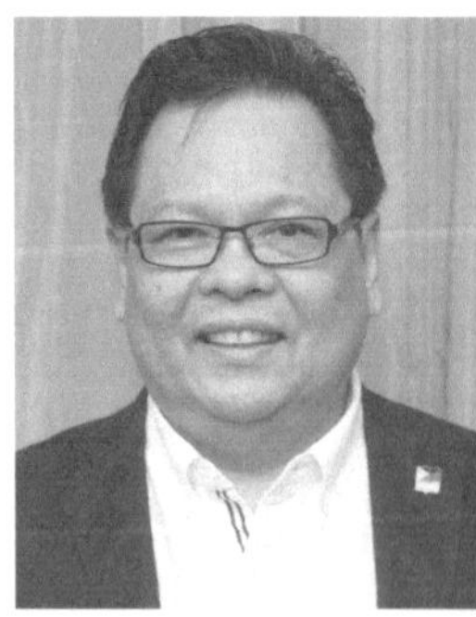
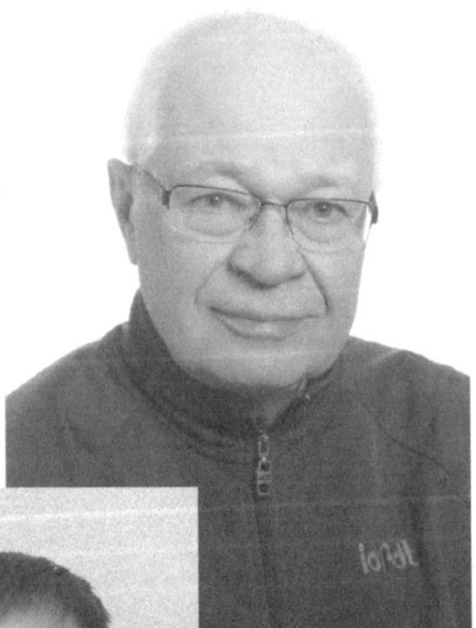
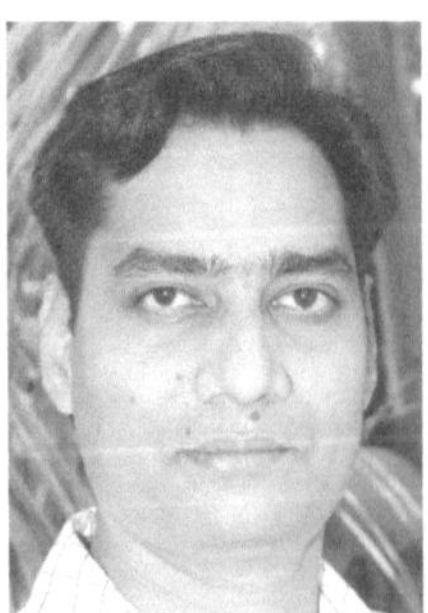
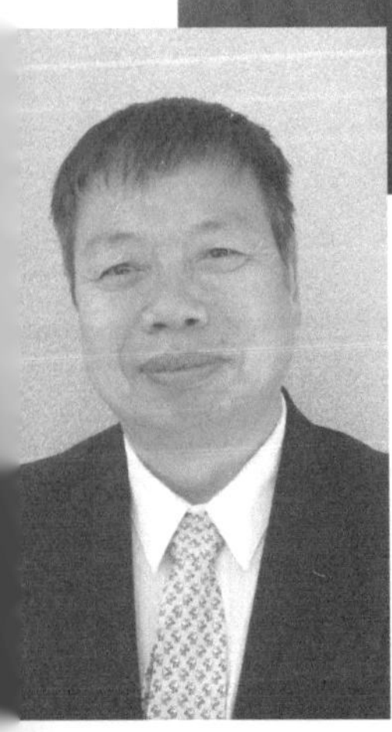
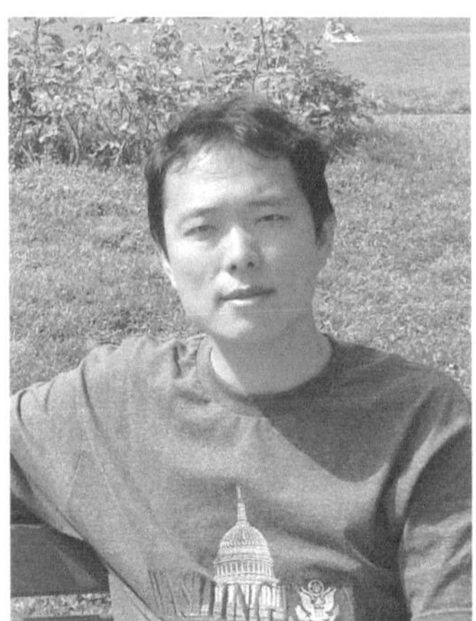
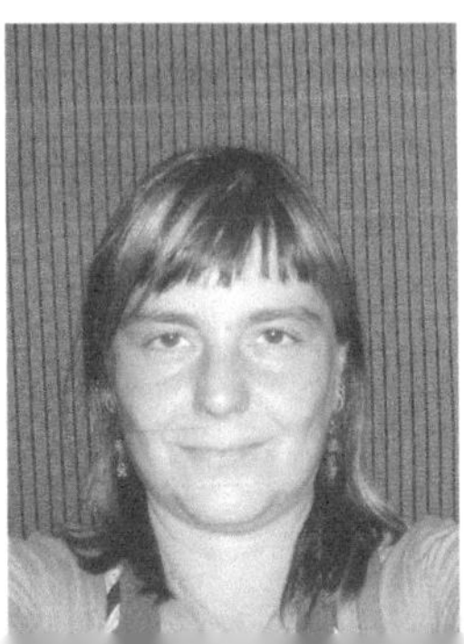

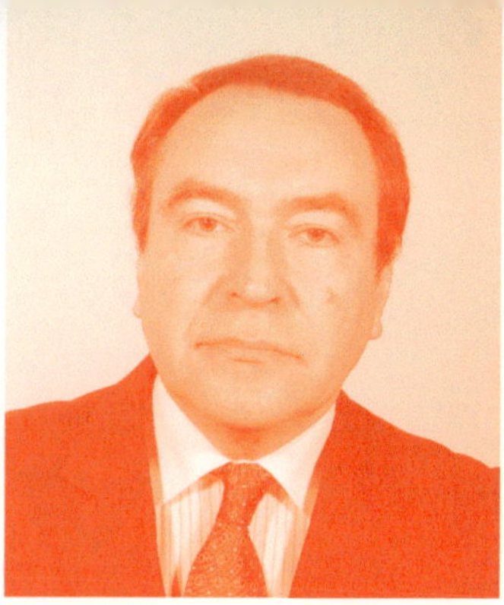

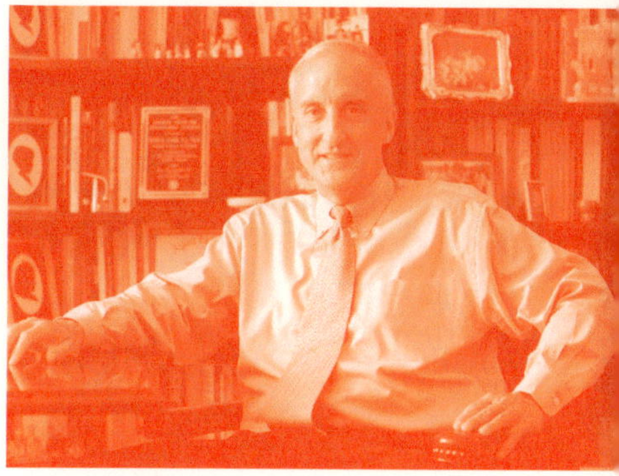

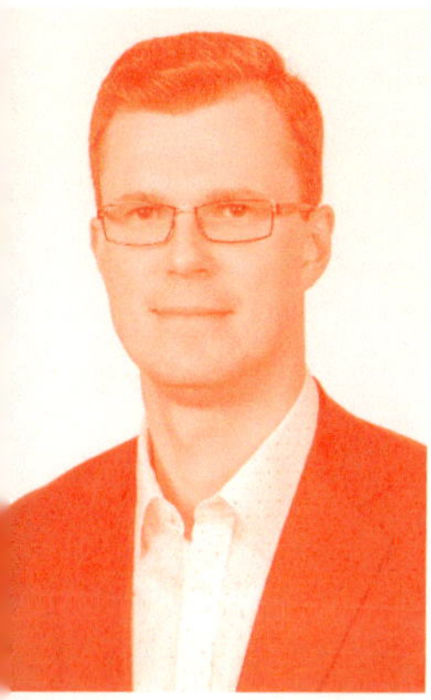

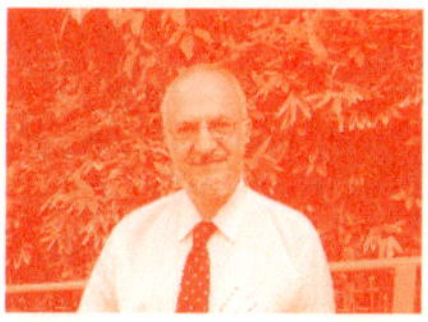

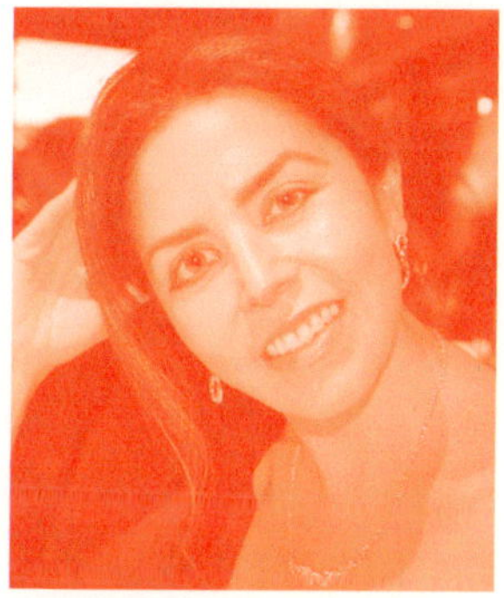

Supporting open minds since 2005

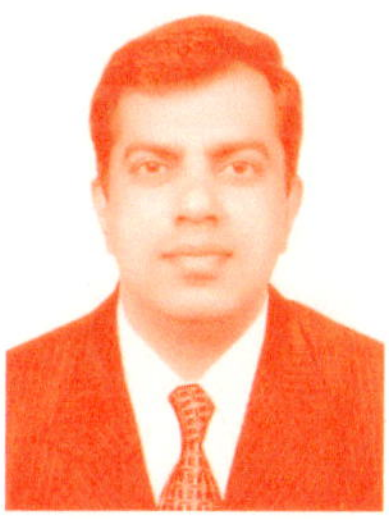

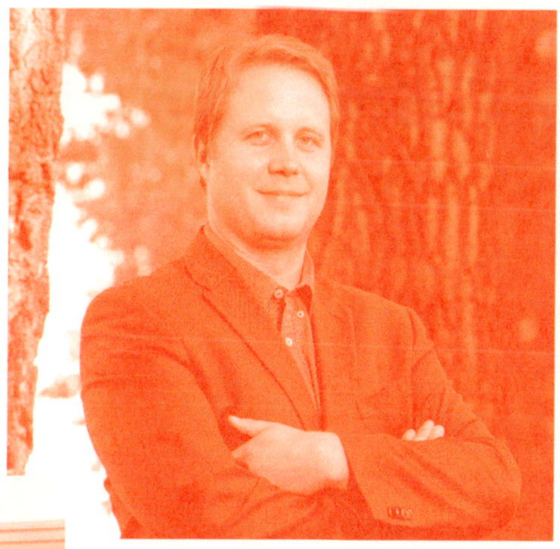

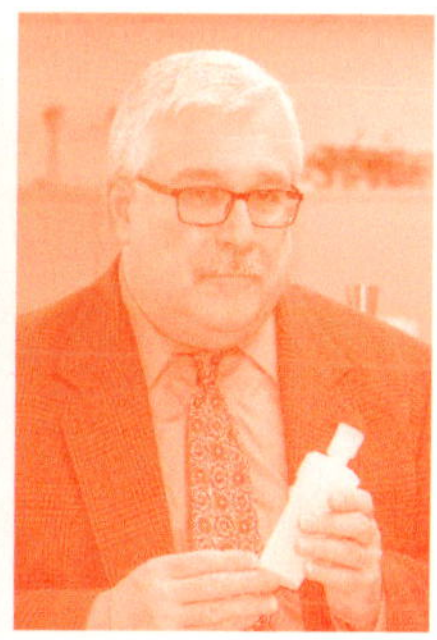

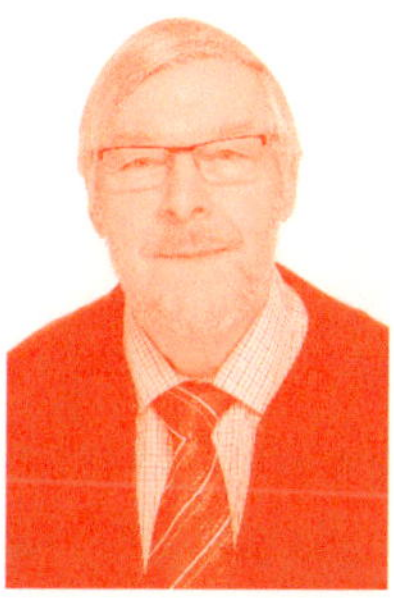

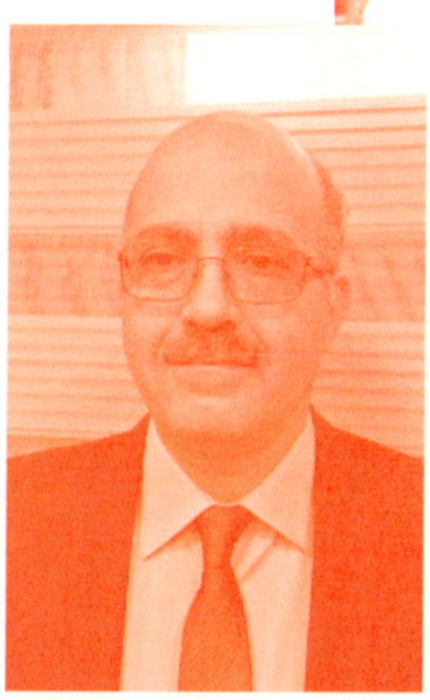

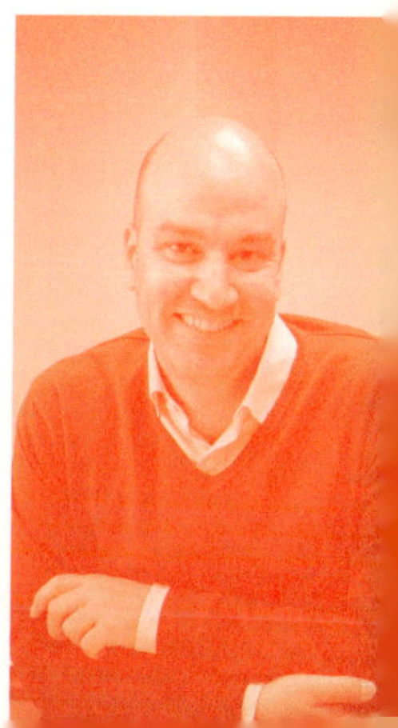

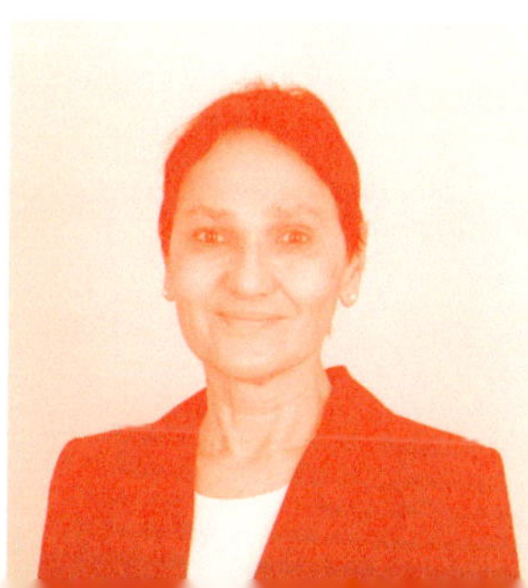

Cardiomyopathy - Disease of the Heart Muscle
http://dx.doi.org/10.5772/intechopen.91489
Edited by Gustav Mattsson and Peter Magnusson

Contributors
Ida Kåks, Gustav Mattsson, Peter Magnusson, Marianna Leopoulou, Sukanya Ghosh, Oscar Campuzano, Marta Vallverdú-Prats, Mireia Alcalde, Georgia Sarquella-Brugada, Sergi Cesar, Josep Brugada, Ramon Brugada, Elena Arbelo, Enkhsaikhan Purevjav, Jeffrey A. Towbin, Hugo R. R. Martinez, Evan M. Harvey, Murad Almasri, Timothy Vittorio, Niel Shah, Miguel Rodriguez-Guerra, Muhammad Saad, Anthony Kang, Kristjan Karason, Emanuele Bobbio, Shingo Sasaki, Davide Lazzeroni, Claudio Stefano Centorbi, Marco Antonio López Hernández, Saraí López De Lucio, David F. Wieczorek, Ronald Zolty, Luis Oscar Vernengo, Haluk Topaloglu, Takaaki Senbonmatsu, Yoshihiro Yamada, Keiki Sugi, Hiroyuki Nakajima, Pradeep P.A. Mammen, Theo Lee-Gannon, Rahul Sheth, Hannah Lehrenbaum, Keerat Kaur, Lior Zangi, Ravinder K. K. Kaundal, Waleed Kian, Melanie Zemel, Emily H. Kestenbaum, Wafeek Alguayn, Boris Shvarts, Adam A.Sharb, Yousef Kian, Nir Peled, Alexander Yakobson, Dina Levitas, Rachele Adorisio, Erica Mencarelli, Nicoletta Cantarutti, Maria Grandinetti, Sara Oualim, Fatima Zahra Merzouk, Mohammed Sabry, Dan Blendea, Sorin Pop, Cerasela Mihaela Goidescu, Iulia Zehan, Giorgia Pastiu, Csilla Andrea Eötvös, Roxana Chiorescu, Roxana Lazar, Florina Fringu, Raluca Tomoaia, Adrian Molnar, Monica Pop

First published in London, United Kingdom, 2021 by IntechOpen
IntechOpen is the global imprint of INTECHOPEN LIMITED, registered in England and Wales, registration number: 11086078, 5 Princes Gate Court, London, SW7 2QJ, United Kingdom
Printed in Croatia

British Library Cataloguing-in-Publication Data
A catalogue record for this book is available from the British Library

Additional hard and PDF copies can be obtained from orders@intechopen.com

Cardiomyopathy - Disease of the Heart Muscle
Edited by Gustav Mattsson and Peter Magnusson
p. cm.
Print ISBN 978-1-78985-223-3
Online ISBN 978-1-78985-224-0
eBook (PDF) ISBN 978-1-78985-923-2

Meet the editors

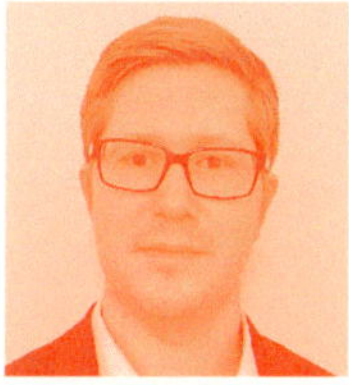

Gustav Mattsson, MD, graduated from Uppsala University, Sweden, and is currently working in internal medicine at Gävle Hospital, Sweden. He is active in research at the Centre for Research and Development, Gävleborg, Uppsala University, and has a strong interest in research and scientific writing in the field of cardiology. He is an author of thirty peer-reviewed articles, twenty-four articles with an editorial review, six book chapters, and ten scientific posters. His research interests include cardiomyopathies, arrhythmia, and device therapy.

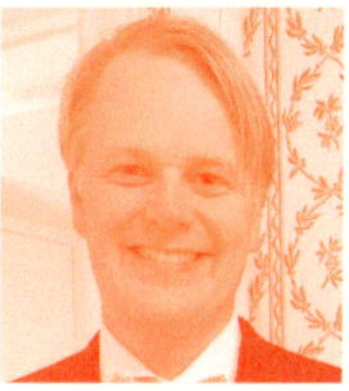

Dr. Peter Magnusson earned his MD from Lund University, Sweden, and his Ph.D. from the Karolinska Institute, Sweden. He is currently working as a senior consultant at Gävle Hospital, Sweden. His clinical work mainly involves the management of patients with cardiac arrhythmias, heart failure, cardiomyopathies, and implantable cardiac devices. His research overlaps with these clinical areas but also covers broad aspects of medicine and innovation. Dr. Magnusson is a renowned speaker and leader of educational activities for diverse groups of professionals.

Contents

Preface

Heart failure places a considerable burden on both patients and healthcare systems. It causes increased morbidity and mortality and is a risk factor for arrhythmia and sudden cardiac death. Heart failure is commonly caused by ischemic heart disease, abnormal loading, or cardiomyopathies. Cardiomyopathies are diseases of the heart muscle with diverse etiologies ranging from myocarditis to gene mutations. Definitions of cardiomyopathies differ over time and between clinical traditions. While in the future cardiomyopathies might be classified after causative mutations, they have traditionally been classified by phenotype and cardiac morphology. This system of classification has the advantage that the phenotype is most often known prior to the genotype. Originally, cardiomyopathies were considered distinct primary myocardial disorders of unknown etiology, whereas heart muscle disorders of known etiology or caused by systemic disease were classified as secondary or specific heart muscle disease. In 2006, the American Heart Association proposed a classification that defined cardiomyopathies as either primary or secondary, referring either to a disease where the heart is the sole or primarily affected organ or where myocardial involvement is part of a systemic disease. In 2008, the European Society of Cardiology proposed an alternate classification in which cardiomyopathy is defined as "a myocardial disorder in which the heart muscle is structurally and functionally abnormal in the absence of coronary artery disease, hypertension, valvular disease, and congenital heart disease sufficient to cause the observed myocardial abnormality." Furthermore, the European Society of Cardiology subdivides cardiomyopathies depending on morphology and function, that is, dilated cardiomyopathy, hypertrophic cardiomyopathy, arrhythmogenic cardiomyopathy, restrictive cardiomyopathy, and unclassified cardiomyopathies (e.g., left-ventricular non-compaction cardiomyopathy). They are then further categorized based on inheritance pattern, distinguishing between familial or genetic forms versus non-familial or non-genetic forms of cardiomyopathy and based on specific etiologies.

This book is divided into seven sections. The "Overview" section introduces the topic, and the "Genetics" section provides information on the genetic basis of many of the cardiomyopathies. "Arrhythmogenic Cardiomyopathy," "Hypertrophic Cardiomyopathy," and "Dilated Cardiomyopathy" include chapters sorted by category of cardiomyopathy. The book ends with sections on "Miscellaneous Cardiomyopathies" and "Treatment and Future Perspectives."

We wish to thank the chapter authors, all of whom are expert clinicians and researchers in the fields of cardiology, cardiomyopathies, and cardiogenetics.

Gustav Mattsson and Peter Magnusson
Centre for Research and Development Region Gävleborg/Uppsala University,
Gävle, Sweden

Section 1

Overview

Chapter 1

An Overview of the Cardiomyopathies

Ida Kåks, Marianna Leopoulou, Gustav Mattsson and Peter Magnusson

Abstract

Cardiomyopathies constitute a heterogeneous group of heart diseases. In fact, cardiomyopathies is a major cause of death either as end-stage heart failure or sudden cardiac death. Even though prognosis is, in many cases, poor there are several approaches to optimal disease management, which improves outcome and implies better quality of life including reduced risk of hospitalization. Differentiation of underlying etiology in individual cases of cardiomyopathies requires careful clinical evaluation. Echocardiography is the cornerstone in initial evaluation and follow-up but cardiac magnetic resonance provides additional value. ECG, biomarkers, detailed history taking and extracardiac features may provide clues to less common entities. While forty years ago cardiomyopathy was defined as heart muscle disease of unknown origin, the underlying pathophysiology has now been elucidated. Indeed, the last decades the genetic explanations have evolved. Advanced treatment with pacemakers, including cardiac resynchronization, implantable defibrillators, and mechanical devices in the most severe cases are nowadays available for many patients. The evidence-based pharmacological approach to heart failure provides multiple interaction of pathophysiological pathways and has improved outcome. In selected cases specific agents are indicated why differential diagnosis is crucial and the genetic link imply cascade screening. This chapter aims to present a comprehensive overview of the cardiomyopathies, categorized into: dilated-, hypertrophic-, restrictive-, arrhythmogenic and unclassified cardiomyopathy.

Keywords: arrhythmogenic cardiomyopathy, cardiomyopathy, dilated cardiomyopathy, heart failure, hypertrophic cardiomyopathy, left ventricular non-compaction, restrictive cardiomyopathy, sudden cardiac death, takotsubo cardiomyopathy

1. Introduction

The term cardiomyopathy was introduced by Brigden in 1957, to describe isolated noncoronary myocardial disease [1]. In 1980 the World Health Organization (WHO) released a document defining cardiomyopathies as "heart muscle diseases of unknown cause" [2]. Since then the understanding of these entities has grown considerably, and although some are deemed idiopathic, the underlying etiology of other cardiomyopathies have been elucidated. In 2008, the European Society of Cardiology (ESC) used the following definition of cardiomyopathy in their position statement:

"A myocardial disorder in which the heart muscle is structurally and functionally abnormal, in the absence of coronary artery disease, hypertension, valvular disease and congenital heart disease sufficient to cause the observed myocardial abnormality [3]."

Many cardiomyopathies are of genetic origin [4], and the inheritance pattern is most often autosomal dominant, although autosomal recessive and X-linked inheritance patterns are encountered [5]. Non-familial forms include, among others, cardiomyopathy secondary to myocarditis caused by toxic or infectious agents [3, 6].

Terminology has historically been a challenge for many of the cardiomyopathies; takotsubo cardiomyopathy has acquired at least 75 different names [7] and for hypertrophic cardiomyopathy (HCM) that number exceeds 80 [8]. The goal of this chapter is to use the most established nomenclature, while in cases when the preferred term is less clear, it will be addressed.

2. Classification

Several attempts have been made to classify the cardiomyopathies. One classification was suggested by Goodwin in 1961 [9], which described three clinical types, according to the effect the disease has on the heart's function: congestive, obstructive, and constrictive. These categories are still in use, but are now termed dilated, hypertrophic, and restrictive, respectively [10]. In the 1980 report by the WHO [2], three distinct conditions were described: dilated-, hypertrophic- and restrictive cardiomyopathy. In addition to these forms WHO included unclassified cardiomyopathy, covering the cases that did not fit in any of the other groups. Specific heart muscle disease, including, among others, conditions with infectious and metabolic etiology, was not considered to belong to the concept of cardiomyopathy. As the understanding of the pathogenesis and etiology grew, this classification was updated 15 years later - now with the addition of arrhythmogenic cardiomyopathy (ACM), at the time called arrhythmogenic right ventricular cardiomyopathy (ARVC), and the term specific cardiomyopathies replacing specific heart muscle disease [11].

In 2006 the American Heart Association (AHA) proposed a new classification, stating that the identification of several new diseases, diagnostic advancements and precise knowledge of causation called for an updated version [6]. The dilated-hypertrophic-restrictive classification, was considered limited in several regards. For example, mixing anatomical descriptions (hypertrophic and dilated) with one that is merely functional (restrictive), can result in one disease belonging in two categories. Furthermore, remodeling can cause a disease to develop from one category into another during its natural course. Instead, they propose a division of cardiomyopathies into two groups: primary and secondary. Primary cardiomyopathies include those that solely, or predominantly, affect the myocardium. Secondary cardiomyopathies replace the term specific cardiomyopathies, hence including pathology of the heart muscle caused by systemic disorders. The two groups are further divided into categories based on etiology. The AHA also includes ion channelopathies as a cardiomyopathy, contrary to former classifications.

The ESC also suggested a classification two years later, aiming for a more clinically oriented system based on morphology and function [3]. This position statement proposes five categories: dilated-, hypertrophic-, restrictive-, arrhythmogenic- and unclassified cardiomyopathy. Each category is then sub-classified as familial or non-familial (**Figure 1**). As opposed to the AHA, channelopathies and

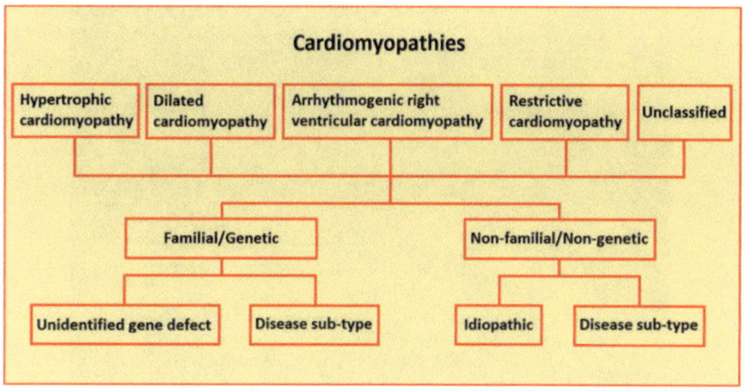

Figure 1.
Classification of cardiomyopathies as proposed by the European Society of Cardiology [3]. Cardiomyopathies are first classified according to morphology and function, then based on whether the disease is familial or non-familial, and lastly depending on either known disease causing mutation or pathophysiological mechanism. Image from Mattsson et al. [12]. Published by IntechOpen under open access https://creativecommons.org/licenses/by/3.0/.

conduction disorders were not considered cardiomyopathies. Neither in the classification system developed by the AHA nor the ESC, myocardial dysfunction caused by valvular, coronary, hypertensive or congenital heart disease, is considered as cardiomyopathy [4].

Lastly, a phenotype–genotype nomenclature, the MOGE(S) classification was suggested [4]. The letters each describe a feature of the cardiomyopathic condition where M stands for morphofunctional characteristic, O for organ involvement, G for genetic or familial inheritance pattern, and E for etiology. The S is optional, and refers to functional status.

For educative reasons, this book chapter will employ the classification suggested by the ESC.

3. Dilated cardiomyopathy

3.1 Definition

Dilated cardiomyopathy (DCM) involves a dilated left ventricle with impaired left ventricular systolic function not solely explained by abnormal loading conditions or coronary artery disease [13] (**Figure 2**). Left ventricular dilatation is defined as left ventricular end-diastolic volume or diameter that is >2 standard deviations from normal according to nomograms corrected for body surface area, age, and sex [13]. In some cases, dilatation and dysfunction of the right ventricle may occur as well [13]. It can be of genetic origin or can be attributed to non-genetic factors. To be categorized as familial, DCM has to be diagnosed in the proband and in at least on first- or second-degree relative [13].

3.2 Clinical features

DCM can lead to progressive heart failure and arrhythmias, and is associated with an increased risk of sudden cardiac death (SCD) [10]. Besides ventricular arrhythmias that may be fatal, atrioventricular block, atrial fibrillation and supraventricular tachycardia (both with and without preexcitation) may also occur [15]. Idiopathic or familial DCM is usually first diagnosed in patients between 20 and 50 years of age [16]. The most common presentation at diagnosis is related to congestive heart failure symptoms [17].

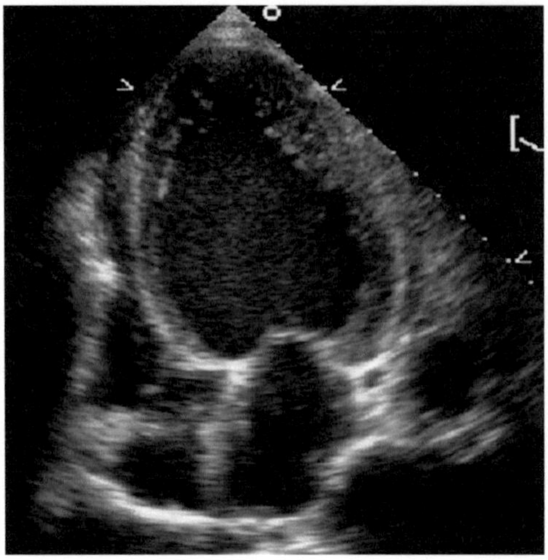

Figure 2.
Echocardiography that shows dilatation of the left ventricle and signs of diastolic dysfunction. Image adapted from Jamil et al. [14]. Published by IntechOpen under open access https://creativecommons.org/licenses/by/3.0/.

3.3 Epidemiology

DCM is the leading cause of heart transplantation and the third most common reason for heart failure [6]. The estimated prevalence is 1:2500 [6], and it more commonly affects men than women [18].

3.4 Etiology

There are several known causes for the sporadic form of DCM; toxins (for example ethanol, lead and cocaine), metabolic abnormalities (including hypothyroidism and thiamine deficiency), neuromuscular disorders (for example Duchenne muscular dystrophy) and inflammatory or infectious (viral, bacterial, fungal) conditions are all among them [16]. Chagas' disease, caused by the protozoan parasite *Trypanosoma cruzi*, is an example of an infectious disease that can lead to DCM [19]. WHO estimated that 10 million people were infected in 2009, and the cardiac form affects up to 30% [20]. Peripartum cardiomyopathy is a form of acquired DCM [15].

Approximately 20–35% of DCM cases are familial, while the most common inheritance pattern is autosomal dominant; X-linked, autosomal recessive and mitochondrial patterns occur seldom [6]. Mutations in genes coding cytoskeletal and sarcomeric proteins are the most common. Mutations in the gene coding for the protein titin is the most common, accounting for up to a quarter of known mutations [21]. Mutations in most genes result in similar phenotypes, thus broad gene panels are required. However, among patients who have atrioventricular block, mutations in the gene coding for lamin A/C (LMNA) are the most common [15]. Between 5 and 10% of patients with DCM have disease-causing LMNA mutation [18]. When no etiology is identified, DCM is categorized as idiopathic [16].

3.5 Treatment

DCM is treated similarly to other forms of heart failure with reduced ejection fraction (EF) [10]. Initial medical treatment consists of angiotensin-converting enzyme (ACE)-inhibitors or angiotensin receptor blockers (ARB), beta-blockers, and mineralocorticoid receptor antagonists (MRA). In patients who are still symptomatic and have an EF ≤35% or, the ACE-inhibitor or ARB should be replaced by an angiotensin receptor neprilysin inhibitor. Cardiac resynchronization therapy should be considered in patients who have a QRS duration ≥150 ms, or QRS duration ≥130 ms and left bundle branch block. Ivabradine should be considered for patients in sinus rhythm with pulse above 70 beats per minute. Heart transplantation may be considered in end-stage heart failure, and left ventricular assist devices can be used a bridge to transplantation, or as a permanent treatment [22]. The sodium-glucose transporter protein 2 inhibitor dapaglifozin has been associated with a reduced cardiovascular mortality and a reduced risk of worsening heart failure in patients with heart failure with reduced EF, in both patients with diabetes type 2 [23] and non-diabetics [24].

In patients who have experienced a hemodynamically not tolerated ventricular arrhythmia, implantable cardioverter defibrillator (ICD) therapy is recommended. Furthermore, an ICD is recommended for those with symptomatic heart failure (New York Heart Association [NYHA] class II-III) with reduced EF of ≤35%, following at least three months of optimal medical therapy. These recommendations apply if the expected survival exceeds one year with good functional status. In the case of an established disease-causing LMNA mutation and clinical risk factors, an ICD should also be considered [18].

4. Hypertrophic cardiomyopathy

4.1 Definition

The ESC defines HCM as "presence of increased left ventricular wall thickness that is not solely explained by abnormal loading conditions" [25]. More precisely, a wall thickness of ≥15 mm in at least one left ventricular myocardial segment is required for the diagnosis of HCM in adults (**Figure 3**). In borderline cases with 13–14 mm, careful evaluation, including family history, is needed; if a first-degree relative had definite HCM the diagnosis is made [25]. Notably, the American guidelines from 2011 hold another position. They recognize HCM as a clinical entity "... characterized by unexplained left ventricular hypertrophy associated with nondilated ventricular chambers in the absence of another cardiac or systematic disease that itself would be capable of producing the magnitude of hypertrophy ..." [26]. There are several diseases, especially in children and young adults, which mimic

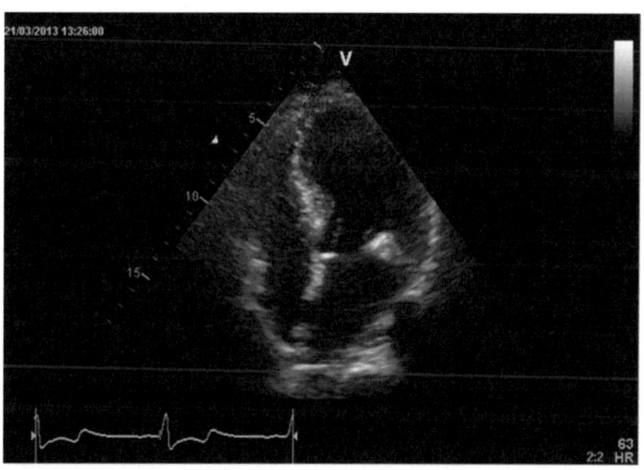

Figure 3.
Echocardiography showing septal hypertrophy in a patient with HCM. Image used with permission from the author Peter Magnusson.

hypertrophy caused by sarcomeric protein mutations. The American guidelines emphasize that these conditions, so-called phenocopies, should not be included in the term HCM [26].

In the American definition of HCM, there are other groups of diseases and conditions that present with hypertrophy, that are not included in the term HCM. These can be categorized based on cellular mechanisms, i.e. neuromuscular, mitochondrial, and metabolic disorders (glycogen storage, carnitine, lysosomal storage). Among the metabolic disorders are glycogen storage diseases such as Danon disease, Pompe disease, and Anderson-Fabry disease. Malformation syndromes are typically diagnosed in pediatric settings; LEOPARD (lentiges, ECG abnormalities, ocular hypertelorism, pulmonary stenosis, abnormal genitalia, retardation of growth, and sensorineural deafness), Noonan syndrome (facial features, short height, congenital heart disease, bleeding problems, and skeletal malformations), and others.

4.2 Clinical features

Typical symptoms include dyspnea, palpitations, syncope and chest discomfort, but many patients lack specific symptoms altogether [25]. Indeed, the majority are likely never diagnosed [27]. Chest discomfort sometimes occurs at rest or during exertion, postprandial or following alcohol consumption. It is uncommon for people with HCM to present with decompensated heart failure, but symptoms of chronic heart failure are often present. The pathology varies, from diastolic dysfunction with preserved EF to systolic left ventricular dysfunction or left ventricular outflow tract obstruction. Among those with left ventricular outflow tract obstruction, a systolic murmur can sometimes be auscultated at the left sternal edge [25].

As for syncope as a symptom of HCM, the cause can be, among others, complete heart block, sinus node dysfunction, or ventricular tachycardia [25]. Causes that are not directly related to the conduction system include left ventricular outflow obstruction, diastolic dysfunction and altered baroreflex mechanisms [28].

According to U.K. data on 357 sudden death cases in athletes the mean age was 29 years and the vast majority males (92%) [29]. Sudden arrhythmic death was the most common cause of death, and HCM accounted for 6% of all deaths. Interestingly, 40% of these athletes died during resting conditions. An Italian sample of 54 fatal cases (mean age 27 years; 76% men) revealed HCM in 9.2% [30].

4.3 Epidemiology

In adults, the prevalence of HCM is frequently reported as 1:500 [31], but a recent Icelandic study reported 1:1600 [32]. On the other hand an extremely high prevalence (about 1:200) was claimed when both phenotypes and genotypes were included based on cohorts from expert centers [33]. Moreover, misclassifications are common in HCM [34].

4.4 Etiology

HCM is often explained by a genetic disease (in approximately half of the cases); a mutation in cardiac sarcomeric protein genes, with an autosomal dominant pattern of inheritance. X-linked inheritance is less common, and autosomal recessive is the most uncommon pattern. Other genetic disorders, such as inherited neuromuscular diseases or chromosome abnormalities, are the underlying reason for 5–10% of adult cases. Non-genetic causes of HCM include amyloidosis and drug toxicity. The etiology of the remaining 25–30% is unknown [25].

4.5 Treatment

Patients with symptomatic left ventricular outflow tract obstruction should initially receive beta-blockers in the highest tolerated dose. If symptoms persist, the next step is adding disopyramide. For those who cannot tolerate beta-blockers or when they are ineffective, verapamil is an option. Loop- or thiazide diuretics may be used in low doses to improve dyspnea. For patients with a left ventricle outflow tract obstruction gradient exceeding 50 mmHg, persistent symptoms (moderate to severe) and/or repeated syncope upon exertion, despite medical therapy, invasive treatment with septal myectomy or alcohol septal ablation should be considered. For symptomatic elderly patients who are not candidates for invasive treatment, permanent pacing with short atrioventricular interval may be considered [25].

For those without left ventricle outflow tract obstruction who have symptoms of heart failure but a normal EF, beta-blockers, verapamil (or diltiazem) and careful administration of diuretics is indicated. Renin-angiotensin-aldosterone system inhibition is not extensively studied in HCM patients, but the ESC recommends the use of beta-blockers, ACE-inhibitors, ARB, MRA and diuretics for HCM patients with symptoms of heart failure and reduced EF, in line with their general recommendations for management of chronic heart failure [25].

Pacemaker therapy in bradycardia is recommended according to the general ESC guidelines [25]. When it comes to ICD treatment, patients with HCM who have not experienced ventricular fibrillation or ventricular tachycardia with hemodynamic compromise, may be candidates for ICD based on the 5-year risk, determined by the validated ESC calculator HCM Risk-SCD [18, 35].

5. Restrictive cardiomyopathy

5.1 Definition

Restrictive cardiomyopathy (RCM) is defined as the presence of restrictive filling in combination with normal or decreased diastolic ventricular volume in one or both ventricles. The systolic function is normal or only slightly impaired [11]. Different underlying causes may result in normal or increased wall thickness [36].

5.2 Clinical features

Since either one or both ventricles can be affected, both left and right ventricular failure may occur. Symptoms of right ventricular failure generally predominate (ascites, peripheral edema), but breathlessness as a symptom of left-sided heart failure occurs as well [36]. In an advanced stage of the disease all signs of heart failure, except cardiomegaly, develop [36]. Certain findings are more common with specific etiologies, such as conduction disturbances in amyloidosis [37] and sarcoidosis, and atrial fibrillation in idiopathic RCM and amyloidosis [36]. Overall, conduction disturbances as well as arrhythmias occur frequently [38]. Distinguishing RCM from constrictive pericarditis (which presents with similar findings) can be challenging, but is important due to the differences in prognosis and management [36, 39].

5.3 Epidemiology

Epidemiologic data is scarce, but RCM has been described as the least common cardiomyopathy [36].

5.4 Etiology

RCM can be idiopathic or familial. Furthermore, there are a number of different local or systemic disorders that can cause RCM [36]. Endomyocardial fibrosis is believed to be the most common cause of RCM [40]. It is endemic to parts of Africa, Asia, South and Central America, but can occur elsewhere sporadically [36]. It predominantly affects children and adolescents. The etiology is not known [40]. Other endomyocardial causes of RCM include radiation and metastatic cancers. Infiltrative diseases causing RCM include cardiac amyloidosis and sarcoidosis. Finally, RCM can develop due to storage diseases, such as hemochromatosis [36].

5.5 Treatment

Prognosis is poor, especially in children, where the 2-year survival rate is less than 50% [41]. Treatment serves to manage heart failure and, if possible, treat the underlying disease [38]. Venous congestion is treated with diuretics, used with caution as to avoid reducing filling pressures and decrease cardiac output [36]. Since atrial fibrillation can increase diastolic dysfunction, maintaining sinus rhythm is of importance and antiarrhythmic agents may be indicated [36]. Beta-blockers and calcium channel blockers are sometimes not tolerated, and should be carefully introduced if needed. Regarding ACE-inhibitors and ARB, there is not much proof of benefit and they are not always tolerated, but can be considered [38]. Due to the propensity for thrombus to form in the left atrial appendage, anticoagulation may benefit most patients [36, 38]. Selected patients may be candidates for heart transplantation or left ventricular assist device [38].

6. Arrhythmogenic cardiomyopathy

6.1 Definition

In ACM, the ventricular myocytes are replaced by fibrofatty tissue [42]. The myocardial atrophy is progressive, starting in the epicardium, it becomes transmural with time and leads to wall thinning [42]. ACM was previously known as ARVC or ARVD where the D stands for dysplasia, which it was originally characterized as [42]. With time it has become apparent that there are variants where the left ventricle is more severely involved than the right, which is the reason some have suggested an updated terminology [42]. Notwithstanding, the fibrofatty tissue replacement often occurs in a "triangle of dysplasia", involving the right ventricular inflow, outflow and apex [3]. In the 2008 classification by the ESC, the term ARVC is used. In 2019 the Heart Rhythm Society published a consensus statement on ACM, where ARVC and arrhythmogenic left ventricular cardiomyopathy were considered to be separate cardiomyopathies with specific phenotypes, under the umbrella of the term ACM [43].

In their 2008 classification, the ESC defines ARVC as dysfunction of the right ventricle, with or without left ventricular involvement, in the presence of histological evidence and/or ECG abnormalities in accordance with published criteria [3]. These include, but are not limited to, epsilon waves in leads V_1-V_3, inverted T-waves in leads V_1-V_3 or beyond in people above 14 years of age in the absence of right bundle branch block and sustained or nonsustained ventricular tachycardia of left bundle-branch morphology with superior axis [44]. The diagnostic criteria for ARVC are subdivided into major and minor criteria, where diagnosis requires two major criteria, or one major criterion in combination with two minor criteria, or four minor criteria from different categories. The categories are global or regional dysfunction and structural alterations, tissue characterization of walls, repolarization abnormalities, depolarization or conduction abnormalities, arrhythmias, and family history [44]. Variants of the disease, such as Naxos disease and Carvajal syndrome, albeit rare, present with a specific phenotype and are considered cardiocutaneous entities; they share the presentation and risk of common ARVC [45, 46].

6.2 Clinical features

The presentation of ACM varies greatly; while some patients are asymptomatic, others suffer from supraventricular arrhythmias, ventricular tachycardia, right-heart failure [47], or even biventricular heart failure [48]. In addition to this, ACM is one of the most common causes for SCD among young people [42], and one study has reported that 10% of SCDs (in people between 1 and 65 years of age) can be attributed to ARVC [47]. A retrospective study found that among 130 patients with ARVC, overall mortality was primarily of cardiovascular origin, where heart failure accounted for two thirds of the cardiac deaths and SCD for the remaining one third [49].

6.3 Epidemiology

The prevalence of ARVC has been estimated to range between 1:1000 and 1:5000 in adults [50, 51].

6.4 Etiology

ACM is usually familial, with an autosomal dominant pattern of inheritance. The majority of patients have at least one disease-causing variant of a gene coding for a desmosomal protein [43]. The protein plakoglobin is reported to be implicated in ACM, most notably in the autosomal recessive form Naxos disease [52]. Another autosomal recessive variant of ACM is Carvajal syndrome [46].

6.5 Treatment

Competitive exercise has been shown to increase the risk of SCD in adolescents and young adults five-fold [53], and frequent exercise increases the risk of ARVC diagnosis, ventricular arrhythmias and heart failure among carriers of desmosomal mutations [54]. Consequently, it is a class I recommendation from the ECS that patients with ARVC must refrain from competitive- and endurance sports, and a class IIa recommendation that they do not participate in any athletic activities (with the possible exception of recreational low-intensity sports) [48].

Regarding medical therapy, beta-blockers should be considered in all ARVC patients, and are specifically recommended for those with recurrent ventricular tachycardia or ICD shocks (either appropriate, or inappropriate shocks due to supraventricular tachycardias). Antiarrhythmic drugs can be used to prevent ventricular arrhythmias. Amiodarone, by itself or combined with beta-blockers, has been suggested by available evidence as the most effective alternative. It has not been proven to prevent SCD [48]. Patients who develop heart failure should receive standard medical treatment [48].

There is no proof that catheter ablation prevents SCD in ARVC, but it can reduce the recurrence of ventricular tachycardia. It is recommended in patients with incessant ventricular tachycardia and those who experience frequent appropriate ICD shocks despite maximal tolerable medical therapy [48].

Preventing SCD is the most important goal of treatment [42]. The only therapy that has been proven to be life-saving is ICD, but the benefit must be weighed against the significant morbidity due to inappropriate shocks and device-related complications [42]. Indications for ICD are based on risk stratification, where patients are divided into one of three categories based on their risk factors for major arrhythmic events. As a final option, when patients suffer from severe congestive heart failure unresponsive to other treatment, or recurrent ventricular tachycardia or -fibrillation despite ablation and/or ICD therapy, heart transplantation is recommended [48].

Patients should be followed-up clinically and with ECG, echocardiography, 24-h Holter monitoring, and exercise-testing at regular intervals throughout their lives [48].

7. Unclassified cardiomyopathy

In the 2008 position statement from the ESC regarding classification of the cardiomyopathies, left ventricular non-compaction (LVNC) and takotsubo cardiomyopathy are regarded as unclassified cardiomyopathies [3]. Since this chapter is structurally based on the position statement, these two conditions will be briefly described. The group of cardiomyopathies that are deemed unclassified, however, has varied over time. In 1980, the WHO included, among others, endocardial fibroelastosis and Fiedler's myocarditis [2]. 15 years later, when the updated classification by the WHO was published, non-compaction cardiomyopathy, systolic dysfunction with minimal dilatation and mitochondrial cardiomyopathies were added to the unclassified cardiomyopathies [11, 55]. The future most certainly holds exciting advances in this field, and it is not a stretch of the imagination to think that this category will continue to evolve in the years to come.

7.1 Takotsubo cardiomyopathy

7.1.1 Definition

Takotsubo cardiomyopathy was first described in 1990. The name refers to a Japanese octopus-trap that bears likeness to the end-systolic left ventriculogram seen in the condition [56]. Sometimes referred to as transient left ventricular apical ballooning syndrome, takotsubo cardiomyopathy leads to regional systolic dysfunction of the left ventricular apex and/or mid-ventricle. For diagnosis, coronary disease should be excluded by coronary angiography [3]. Since ST-segment elevation and positive troponin is seen in more than 80% of patients [57], the diagnosis is often not considered until after coronary angiography is performed. In their 2016 position statement, the ESC refers to takotsubo as a syndrome rather than a cardiomyopathy, with the motivation that the diagnosis is based on a set of clinical observations - which is what defines a clinical syndrome. Since the patients do not appear to have a primary heart muscle disorder, no common genetic etiology has been identified, and most recover fully - takotsubo is likely different from the primary cardiomyopathies [58].

7.1.2 Clinical features

The first symptom is usually chest pain, which affects most of the patients. The condition highly resembles an acute coronary syndrome. Dyspnea is another common presentation [57]. Although the disease is generally considered benign, more than half of patients experience some form of complication [58]. Between 4% and 20% of patients develop cardiogenic shock [58], and 1.5% go into ventricular fibrillation [57]. Most patients have clear left ventricular dysfunction when they are admitted, but in weeks the cardiac function improves drastically [57]. Left ventricular EF usually recovers within three months, while ECG and elevated BNP levels may persist for up to a year or, sometimes, become permanent [58]. However, one retrospective observational study has found that early and late mortality in takotsubo cardiomyopathy is similar to the numbers seen in acute myocardial infarction [59].

7.1.3 Epidemiology

It has been estimated that approximately 2% of ST-segment elevation myocardial infarctions are in fact takotsubo cardiomyopathy. Out of all patients, most are post-menopausal women, about 90% [57].

7.1.4 Etiology

The exact pathophysiology is unknown, although several theories have been presented. Multivessel coronary vasospasm, coronary microvascular dysfunction and elevated levels of catecholamines leading to cardiotoxicity are found among these [57]. Often, the debut is preceded by emotional or physical stress, but in a minority of patients no such stressor can be identified [57]. Because of this, the term broken heart syndrome is sometimes used for the condition [60]. However, in a small number of patients takotsubo is triggered by a positive emotional experience [61].

7.1.5 Treatment

No randomized clinical trials that can form a basis for treatment recommendations exist. The ESC Heart Failure Association has proposed a risk stratification system, including among others age, systolic blood pressure, and pulmonary congestion, to be used for choosing the appropriate approach. In patients without complications and a left ventricular EF of over 45%, early discharge from hospital may be considered. Heart failure medications, including beta-blockers, should be considered in patients with an EF between 35 and 45%, who are otherwise at low risk. According to some experts, vasoactive drugs such as ACE inhibitors, should not be given to patients with a normal cardiac output, as takotsubo may be associated with low peripheral vascular resistance [58].

Higher risk patients (risk factors include, but are not limited to, age 75 or above, EF below 35%, and systolic blood pressure less than 110 mmHg) with takotsubo cardiomyopathy should be monitored for at least 72 hours after presentation with continuous ECG. It is recommended to avoid sympathomimetic drugs. Beta-blockers may be considered in hemodynamically stable patients, and patients with tachyarrhythmias. Patients with a hemodynamically significant left ventricular outflow tract obstruction should be considered for treatment with a beta-blocker of selective alpha1-agonist. Cardiogenic shock in patients with takotsubo cardiomyopathy can be managed with temporary left ventricular assist devices and extracorporeal membrane oxygenation, or low-dose levosimendan infusion. Other inotropes are generally contraindicated, owing to the possible worsening of status and outcome due to their activation of catecholamine receptors [58].

Low risk patients should be followed-up for 3 to 6 months, with cardiac imaging and a review of the medication [58].

7.2 Left ventricular non-compaction

7.2.1 Definition

LVNC is characterized by deep intertrabecular recesses in the left ventricle [62], resulting in a "spongy" morphological appearance [6]. LNVC often leads to a thickened myocardial wall, due to thickening of the endocardial layer, but the epicardium is compacted and thin (**Figure 4**). Dilation of the left ventricle and systolic dysfunction occur in some patients [3]. In their 2008 classification, the ESC commented that it is unclear whether LVNC is a distinct cardiomyopathy or a morphology seen in several different cardiomyopathies. Echocardiographic diagnosis is based on the Jenni criteria consisting of four criteria: absence of other cardiac abnormalities, end-systolic ratio between non-compacted endocardial myocardium and compacted epicardial myocardium of >2, hyper-trabeculation localized to the apex/mid-inferior/mid-lateral areas, and color doppler with blood flow from the ventricle into deep intertrabecular recesses that do not communicate with coronary vessels [64].

7.2.2 Clinical features

The dominating clinical manifestations are heart failure, arrhythmias and embolism due to thrombi forming within the intertrabecular recesses, but the presentation varies and some patients are asymptomatic [65]. One study reports chronic atrial fibrillation in 26% of LVNC patients, and ventricular tachycardia in 41% [66]. In the same study, 50% of all deaths were SCD. Non-compaction of both ventricles has been reported [67], but since the right ventricular apex is often highly trabeculated, the distinction between normal and pathological patterns is difficult and the existence of right ventricular non-compaction is therefore disputed [65, 66].

7.2.3 Epidemiology

The prevalence is unknown, and the results of studies vary. One echocardiographic study estimated a prevalence in the general population of 0.05% [67], another prevalence estimation based on patients referred to an echocardiography laboratory was 0.014% [66].

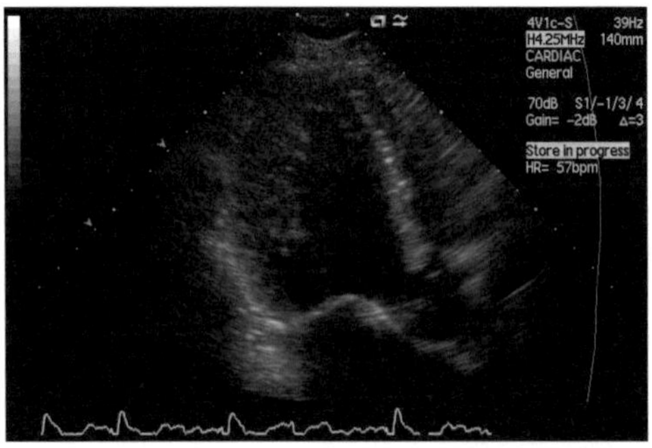

Figure 4.
A thick, non-compacted myocardium in the left ventricular wall. Transthoracic echocardiogram, during systole, apical long-axis view. Image from Mattsson et al. [63]. Published by BMC Cardiovascular Disorders under open access https://creativecommons.org/licenses/by/4.0/.

7.2.4 Etiology

LVNC is believed to occur when compaction of the myocardial fibers and meshwork is arrested during intrauterine development [62]. Normally, the intertrabecular recesses seen in LVNC are transformed to capillaries during 5 to 8 weeks of fetal development [68]. Serial echocardiographic studies where LVNC was not diagnosed in the first echocardiogram, however, suggest that it could be an acquired condition. The fact that LVNC is associated with mutations in sarcomere protein genes found in patients with both DCM and HCM, is another reason to ask the question whether LVNC could develop later in life [69].

There are descriptions of both familial and non-familial cases, and LVNC can be isolated or associated with other congenital heart anomalies [6]. The disease is classified as a primary genetic cardiomyopathy by the AHA [6]. Apart from mutations in sarcomeric proteins, LVNC can be linked to mutations in mitochondrial, Z-disc or cytoskeletal proteins [69]. The predominant mode of inheritance is autosomal dominant with incomplete penetrance, but autosomal recessive and X-linked patterns occur as well. Approximately one in four patients has a familial form [70].

7.2.5 Treatment

No specific treatment for LVNC exists [69]. Heart failure is treated with standard medical therapy. Yearly ambulatory ECGs for monitoring to assess rhythm disturbances, since these occur frequently in LVNC, should be performed [65]. In a long-term follow-up of 34 adult LVNC patients, thromboembolic complications were reported in 24%; thus the authors recommended that oral anticoagulation for all patients diagnosed with LVNC should be considered [66]. Another study found systemic embolization in 3 of their 8 patients [71]. In an article published in 2011, the authors recommend oral anticoagulation only in patients with an EF <40%, since they have never observed thromboembolic complications in a patient in sinus rhythm with a preserved EF [69]. There are no guidelines regarding anticoagulation in LVNC patients, and there is no general consensus in clinical practice [72].

8. Conclusions

The vast complexity that surrounds the diseases of the heart muscle can make the diagnosis and management of cardiomyopathy patients challenging. However, since the prevalence of heart failure and life-threatening arrhythmias is high among patients with cardiomyopathy it is crucial to correctly identify the patients and risk stratify. So far, as guidelines specific for heart muscle disease are not available for all its forms, treatment follows general guidelines for arrhythmias and heart failure. European or world-wide registries would offer most valuable insights and illuminate the future management of cardiomyopathies.

Conflict of interest

IK and ML report no conflicts of interest. GM has received speaker's fee from Alnylam, MSD, and Internetmedicin. Peter Magnusson has received speaker's fees or grants from Abbott, Alnylam, Amicus Therapeutics, AstraZeneca, Bayer, Boehringer-Ingelheim, Coala Life, Internetmedicin, Lilly, MSD, Novo Nordisk, Octopus Medical, Orion Pharma, Pfizer, Vifor Pharma, and Zoll.

Acronyms and abbreviations

ACM	arrhythmogenic cardiomyopathy
ACE	angiotensin-converting enzyme
AHA	American Heart Association
ARB	angiotensin receptor blocker
ARVC	arrhythmogenic right ventricle cardiomyopathy
DCM	dilated cardiomyopathy
EF	ejection fraction
ESC	European Society of Cardiology
HCM	hypertrophic cardiomyopathy
ICD	implantable cardioverter defibrillator
LVNC	left ventricular non-compaction
MRA	mineralocorticoid receptor antagonist
NYHA	New York Heart Association
RCM	restrictive cardiomyopathy
SCD	sudden cardiac death
WHO	World Health Organization

Author details

Ida Kåks[1]*, Marianna Leopoulou[2], Gustav Mattsson[1] and Peter Magnusson[1,3]

1 Centre for Research and Development, Uppsala University/Region Gävleborg, Gävle, Sweden

2 Cardiology Department, Athens General Hospital 'Elpis', Athens, Greece

3 Cardiology Research Unit, Department of Medicine, Solna, Karolinska Institutet, Stockholm, Sweden

*Address all correspondence to: ida.kaks@regiongavleborg.se

References

[1] Brigden W. Uncommon myocardial diseases: The non-coronary cardiomyopathies. Lancet. 1957;270(7008):1243-1249. DOI: 10.1016/S0140-6736(57)91537-4.

[2] Report of the WHO/ISFC task force on the definition and classification of cardiomyopathies. Br Heart J. 1980;44(6):672-3. DOI: 10.1136/hrt.44.6.672.

[3] Elliott P, Andersson B, Arbustini E, Bilinska Z, Cecchi F, Charron P, et al. Classification of the cardiomyopathies: a position statement from the european society of cardiology working group on myocardial and pericardial diseases. Eur Heart J. 2008;29(2):270-6. DOI: 10.1093/eurheartj/ehm342.

[4] Arbustini E, Narula N, Dec GW, Reddy KS, Greenberg B, Kushwaha S, et al. The MOGE(S) Classification for a Phenotype–Genotype Nomenclature of Cardiomyopathy: Endorsed by the World Heart Federation. J Am Coll Cardiol. 2013;62(22):2046-2072. DOI: 10.1016/j.jacc.2013.08.1644.

[5] Charron P, Arad M, Arbustini E, Basso C, Bilinska Z, Elliott P, et al. Genetic counselling and testing in cardiomyopathies: a position statement of the European Society of Cardiology Working Group on Myocardial and Pericardial Diseases. Eur Heart J. 2010;31(22):2715-2726. DOI: 10.1093/eurheartj/ehq271.

[6] Maron BJ, Towbin JA, Thiene G, Antzelevitch C, Corrado D, Arnett D, et al. Contemporary definitions and classification of the cardiomyopathies: an American Heart Association Scientific Statement from the Council on Clinical Cardiology, Heart Failure and Transplantation Committee; Quality of Care and Outcomes Research and Functional Genomics and Translational Biology Interdisciplinary Working Groups; and Council on Epidemiology and Prevention. Circulation. 2006;113(14):1807-1816. DOI: 10.1161/CIRCULATIONAHA.106.174287.

[7] Sharkey SW, Lesser JR, Maron MS, Maron BJ. Why Not Just Call It Tako-Tsubo Cardiomyopathy: a discussion of nomenclature. J Am Coll Cardiol. 2011;57(13):1496-1497. DOI:10.1016/j.jacc.2010.11.029.

[8] Maron BJ, Seidman CE, Ackerman MJ, Towbin JA, Maron MS, Ommen SR, et al. How should hypertrophic cardiomyopathy be classified?: What's in a name? Dilemmas in nomenclature characterizing hypertrophic cardiomyopathy and left ventricular hypertrophy. Circ. Cardiovasc. Genet. 2009;2(1):81-85. DOI:10.1161/CIRCGENETICS.108.788703.

[9] Goodwin JF, Gordon H, Hollman A, Bishop MB. Clinical aspects of cardiomyopathy. Br Med J. 1961;1(5219):69-79. DOI:10.1136/bmj.1.5219.69.

[10] Braunwald E. Cardiomyopathies: an overview. Circ Res. 2017;121(7):711-721. DOI:10.1161/CIRCRESAHA.117.311812.

[11] Richardson P, McKenna W, Bristow M, Maisch B, Mautner B, O'Connell J, et al. Report of the 1995 World Health Organization/International Society and Federation of Cardiology Task Force on the Definition and Classification of Cardiomyopathies. Circulation. 1996;93(5):841-2. DOI:10.1161/01.CIR.93.5.841.

[12] Mattsson G, Magnusson P. Familial Dilated Cardiomyopathy: Risk Stratification for Sudden Cardiac Death. In: Magnusson P, LeQuang JA, editors. Sudden Cardiac Death. IntechOpen. 2020. DOI: 10.5772/intechopen.94437.

[13] Pinto YM, Elliott PM, Arbustini E, Adler Y, Anastasakis A, Böhm M, et al. Proposal for a revised definition of dilated cardiomyopathy, hypokinetic non-dilated cardiomyopathy, and its implications for clinical practice: a position statement of the ESC working group on myocardial and pericardial diseases. Eur Heart J. 2016;37(23):1850-1858. DOI: 10.1093/eurheartj/ehv727.

[14] Jamil G, Abbas A, Shehab A, Qureshi A. Echocardiography Findings in Common Primary and Secondary Cardiomyopathies. In: Milei J, Ambrosio G, editors. Cardiomyopathies. IntechOpen. 2013. DOI: 10.5772/55036.

[15] Jefferies JL, Towbin JA. Dilated cardiomyopathy. The Lancet. 2010;375(9716):752-762. DOI:10.1016/S0140-6736(09)62023-7.

[16] Dec GW, Fuster V. Idiopathic Dilated Cardiomyopathy. N Engl J. Med. 1994;331(23):1564-1575. DOI: 10.1056/NEJM199412083312307.

[17] Weintraub RG, Semsarian C, Macdonald P. Dilated cardiomyopathy. The Lancet. 2017;390(10092):400-414. DOI:10.1016/S0140-6736(16)31713-5.

[18] Priori SG, Blomström-Lundqvist C, Mazzanti A, Blom N, Borggrefe M, Camm J, et al. 2015 ESC Guidelines for the management of patients with ventricular arrhythmias and the prevention of sudden cardiac death: The Task Force for the Management of Patients with Ventricular Arrhythmias and the Prevention of Sudden Cardiac Death of the European Society of Cardiology (ESC)Endorsed by: Association for European Paediatric and Congenital Cardiology (AEPC). Eur Heart J. 2015;36(41):2793-2867. DOI:10.1093/eurheartj/ehv316.

[19] Bern C. Chagas' Disease. N Engl J Med. 2015;373:456-466. DOI:10.1056/NEJMra1410150.

[20] World Health Organization. Working to overcome the global impact of neglected tropical diseases: first WHO report on neglected tropical diseases. 2010. Geneva. ISBN: 978 92 4 1564090

[21] McNally EM, Mestroni L. Dilated Cardiomyopathy. Circ Res. 2017;121(7):731-748. DOI: 10.1161/CIRCRESAHA.116.309396.

[22] Ponikowski P, Voors AA, Anker SD, Bueno H, Cleland JGF, Coats AJS, et al. 2016 ESC Guidelines for the diagnosis and treatment of acute and chronic heart failure: The Task Force for the diagnosis and treatment of acute and chronic heart failure of the European Society of Cardiology (ESC)Developed with the special contribution of the Heart Failure Association (HFA) of the ESC. Eur Heart J. 2016;37(27):2129-2200. DOI:10.1093/eurheartj/ehw128.

[23] Zinman B, Wanner C, Lachin JM, Fitchett D, Bluhmki E, Hantel S, et al. Empagliflozin, Cardiovascular Outcomes, and Mortality in Type 2 Diabetes. N Engl J Med. 2015;373(22):2117-2128. DOI: 10.1056/NEJMoa1504720.

[24] Huynh K. Dapagliflozin — a breakthrough in the search for drugs to treat HFrEF. Nat Rev Cardiol. 2019;16(12):700. DOI: 10.1038/s41569-019-0291-1.

[25] Elliott PM, Anastasakis A, Borger MA, Borggrefe M, Cecchi F, Charron P, et al. 2014 ESC Guidelines on diagnosis and management of hypertrophic cardiomyopathy: The Task Force for the Diagnosis and Management of Hypertrophic Cardiomyopathy of the European Society of Cardiology (ESC)," Eur Heart J. 2014;35(39):2733-79. DOI: 10.1093/eurheartj/ehu284.

[26] Gersh BJ, Maron BJ, Bonow RO, Dearani JA, Fifer MA, Link MS,

et al. 2011 ACCF/AHA Guideline for the Diagnosis and Treatment of Hypertrophic Cardiomyopathy. Circulation. 2011;124(24):e783-831. DOI: 10.1161/CIR.0b013e318223e2bd.

[27] Maron BJ, Maron MS. Hypertrophic cardiomyopathy. Lancet. 2013;381(9862): 242-255. DOI:10.1016/S0140-6736(12)60397-3.

[28] Wigle ED, Rakowski H, Kimball BP, Williams WG. Hypertrophic Cardiomyopathy: Clinical Spectrum and Treatment. Circulation. 1995;92(7):1680-1692. DOI:10.1161/01.CIR.92.7.1680.

[29] Finocchiaro G, Papadakis M, Robertus J-L, Dhutia H, Steriotis AK, Tome M, et al. Etiology of Sudden Death in Sports: Insights From a United Kingdom Regional Registry. J Am Coll Cardiol. 2016;67(18):2108-2115. DOI:10.1016/j.jacc.2016.02.062.

[30] Vassalini M, Verzeletti A, Restori M, De Ferrari F. An autopsy study of sudden cardiac death in persons aged 1-40 years in Brescia (Italy). J Cardiovasc Med (Hagerstown). 2016;17(6):446-453. DOI:10.2459/JCM.0000000000000234.

[31] Maron BJ, Gardin JM, Flack JM, Gidding SS, Kurosaki TT, Bild DE. Prevalence of Hypertrophic Cardiomyopathy in a General Population of Young Adults. Echocardiographic analysis of 4111 subjects in the CARDIA Study. Coronary Artery Risk Development in (Young) AdultsCirculation. 1995;92(4):785-789. DOI:10.1161/01.CIR.92.4.785.

[32] Adalsteinsdottir B, Teekakirikul P, Maron BJ, Burke MA, Gudbjartsson DF, Holm H, et al. Nationwide Study on Hypertrophic Cardiomyopathy in Iceland. Circulation. 2014;130(14):1158-1167. DOI:10.1161/CIRCULATIONAHA.114.011207.

[33] Semsarian C, Ingles J, Maron MS, Maron BJ, New Perspectives on the Prevalence of Hypertrophic Cardiomyopathy. J Am Coll Cardiol. 2015;65(12):1249-1254. DOI:10.1016/j.jacc.2015.01.019.

[34] Magnusson P, Palm A, Branden E, Mörner S. Misclassification of hypertrophic cardiomyopathy: validation of diagnostic codes. Clin Epidemiol. 2017;9:403-410. DOI:10.2147/CLEP.S139300.

[35] O'Mahony C, Jichi F, Ommen SR, Christiaans I, Arbustini E, Garcia-Pavia P, et al. International External Validation Study of the 2014 European Society of Cardiology Guidelines on Sudden Cardiac Death Prevention in Hypertrophic Cardiomyopathy (EVIDENCE-HCM). Circulation. 2018;137(10):1015-1023. DOI:10.1161/CIRCULATIONAHA.117.030437.

[36] Kushwaha SS, Fallon JT, Fuster VT. Restrictive Cardiomyopathy. N Engl J Med. 1997;336(4):267-276. DOI:10.1056/NEJM199701233360407.

[37] Nakata T, Shimamoto K, Yonekura S, Kobayashi N, Sugiyama T, Imai K, et al. Cardiac Sympathetic Denervation in Transthyretin-Related Familial Amyloidotic Polyneuropathy: Detection with Iodine-123-MIBG. J Nucl Med. 1995;36(6):1040-2. PMID:7769425.

[38] Muchtar E, Blauwet LA, Gertz MA. Restrictive Cardiomyopathy: Genetics, Pathogenesis, Clinical Manifestations, Diagnosis, and Therapy. Circ Res. 2017;121(7):819-837. DOI:10.1161/CIRCRESAHA.117.310982.

[39] Schoenfeld MH, Supple EW, Dec GW, Fallon JT, Palacios IF. Restrictive cardiomyopathy versus constrictive pericarditis: role of endomyocardial biopsy in avoiding unnecessary thoracotomy. Circulation. 1987;75(5):1012-1017. DOI: 10.1161/01.CIR.75.5.1012.

[40] Mocumbi AO, Yacoub S, Yacoub MH. Neglected tropical cardiomyopathies: II. Endomyocardial fibrosis. Heart. 2008;94(3):384-390. DOI: 10.1136/hrt.2007.136101.

[41] Rivenes SM, Kearney DL, Smith EO, Towbin JA, Denfield SW. Sudden Death and Cardiovascular Collapse in Children With Restrictive Cardiomyopathy. Circulation. 2000;102(8):876-882. DOI:10.1161/01.CIR.102.8.876.

[42] Corrado D, Basso C, Judge DP. Arrhythmogenic Cardiomyopathy. Circ Res. 2017;121(7):784-802. DOI:10.1161/CIRCRESAHA.117.309345.

[43] Towbin JA, McKenna WJ, Abrams DJ, Ackerman MJ, Calkins H, Darrieux FCC, et al. 2019 HRS expert consensus statement on evaluation, risk stratification, and management of arrhythmogenic cardiomyopathy. Heart Rhythm. 2019;16(11):e301–e372. DOI:10.1016/j.hrthm.2019.05.007.

[44] Marcus FI, McKenna WJ, Sherrill D, Basso C, Bauce B, Bluemke DA, et al. Diagnosis of arrhythmogenic right ventricular cardiomyopathy/dysplasia: proposed modification of the Task Force Criteria. Eur Heart J. 2010;31(7):806-814. DOI:10.1093/eurheartj/ehq025.

[45] Protonotarios N, Tsatsopoulou A, Patsourakos P, Alexopoulos D, Gezerlis P, Simitsis S, et al. Cardiac abnormalities in familial palmoplantar keratosis. Br Heart J. 1986;56(4):321-6. DOI:10.1136/hrt.56.4.321.

[46] Carvajal-Huerta L. Epidermolytic palmoplantar keratoderma with woolly hair and dilated cardiomyopathy. J Am Acad Dermatol. 1998;39(3):418-421. DOI:10.1016/S0190-9622(98)70317-2.

[47] Tabib A, Loire R, Chalabreysse L, Meyronnet D, Miras A, Malicier D, et al. Circumstances of Death and Gross and Microscopic Observations in a Series of 200 Cases of Sudden Death Associated With Arrhythmogenic Right Ventricular Cardiomyopathy and/or Dysplasia. Circulation. 2003;108(24):3000-3005. DOI:10.1161/01.CIR.0000108396.65446.21.

[48] Corrado D, Wichter T, Link MS, Hauer R, Marchlinski F, Anastasakis A, et al. Treatment of arrhythmogenic right ventricular cardiomyopathy/dysplasia: an international task force consensus statement. Eur Heart J. 2015;36(46):3227-37. DOI:10.1093/eurheartj/ehv162.

[49] Hulot JS , Jouven X, Empana JP, Frank R, Fontaine G. Natural History and Risk Stratification of Arrhythmogenic Right Ventricular Dysplasia/Cardiomyopathy. Circulation. 2004;110(14):1879-1884. DOI:10.1161/01.CIR.0000143375.93288.82.

[50] McKenna WJ, Maron BJ, Thiene G. Classification, Epidemiology, and Global Burden of Cardiomyopathies. Circ Res. 2017;121(7):722-730. DOI:10.1161/CIRCRESAHA.117.309711.

[51] Peters S, Trümmel S, Meyners W. Prevalence of right ventricular dysplasia-cardiomyopathy in a non-referral hospital. Int J Cardiol. 2004;97(3):499-501. DOI: 10.1016/j.ijcard.2003.10.037.

[52] McKoy G, Protonotarios N, Crosby A, Tsatsopoulou A, Anastasakis A, Coonar A, et al. Identification of a deletion in plakoglobin in arrhythmogenic right ventricular cardiomyopathy with palmoplantar keratoderma and woolly hair (Naxos disease). The Lancet. 2000;355(9221):2119-2124. DOI: 10.1016/S0140-6736(00)02379-5.

[53] Corrado D, Basso C, Rizzoli G, Schiavon M, Thiene G. Does sports activity enhance the risk of sudden death in adolescents and young adults?. J Am Coll Cardiol.

2003;42(11):1959-1963. DOI:10.1016/j.jacc.2003.03.002.

[54] James CA, Bhonsale A, Tichnell C, Murray B, Russell SD, Tandri H, et al. Exercise Increases Age-Related Penetrance and Arrhythmic Risk in Arrhythmogenic Right Ventricular Dysplasia/Cardiomyopathy–Associated Desmosomal Mutation Carriers. J Am Coll Cardiol. 2013;62(14):1290-1297. DOI:10.1016/j.jacc.2013.06.033.

[55] Thiene G, Corrado D, Basso C. Cardiomyopathies: is it time for a molecular classification? Eur Heart J. 2004;25(20):1772-1775. DOI:10.1016/j.ehj.2004.07.026.

[56] Kurisu S, Sato H, Kawagoe T, Ishihara M, Shimatani Y, Nishioka K, et al. Tako-tsubo-like left ventricular dysfunction with ST-segment elevation: A novel cardiac syndrome mimicking acute myocardial infarction. Am Heart J. 2002;143(3):448-455. DOI:10.1067/mhj.2002.120403.

[57] Gianni M, Dentali F, Grandi AM, Sumner G, Hiralal R, Lonn E. Apical ballooning syndrome or takotsubo cardiomyopathy: a systematic review. Eur Heart J. 2006;27(13):1523-1529. DOI:10.1093/eurheartj/ehl032.

[58] Lyon AR, Bossone E, Schneider B, Sechtem U, Citro R, Underwood SR, et al. Current state of knowledge on Takotsubo syndrome: a Position Statement from the Taskforce on Takotsubo Syndrome of the Heart Failure Association of the European Society of Cardiology. Eur J Heart Fail. 2016;18(1):8-27. DOI:10.1002/ejhf.424.

[59] Redfors B, Vedad R, Angerås O, Råmunddal T, Petursson P, Haraldsson I, et al. Mortality in takotsubo syndrome is similar to mortality in myocardial infarction — A report from the SWEDEHEART registry. Int J Cardiol. 2015;185:282-9. DOI:10.1016/j.ijcard.2015.03.162.

[60] Mukherjee A, Sünkel-Laing B, Dewhurst N. 'Broken Heart' syndrome in Scotland: a case of Takotsubo cardiomyopathy in a recently widowed lady. Scott Med J. 2013;58(1):e15–e19. DOI:10.1177/0036933012474605.

[61] Ghadri JR, Sarcon A, Diekmann J, Bataiosu DR, Cammann VL, Jurisic S, et al. Happy heart syndrome: role of positive emotional stress in takotsubo syndrome. Eur Heart J. 2016;37(37:)2823-2829. DOI:10.1093/eurheartj/ehv757.

[62] Jenni R, Oechslin EN, van der Loo B. Isolated ventricular non-compaction of the myocardium in adults. Heart. 2007;93(1):11-15. DOI:10.1136/hrt.2005.082271.

[63] Mattsson G, Baroudi A, Tawfiq H, Magnusson P. Left ventricular non-compaction cardiomyopathy with coronary artery anomaly complicated by ventricular tachycardia. BMC Cardiovasc Disord. 2017;17(1):263. DOI: 10.1186/s12872-017-0699-7.

[64] Jenni R, Oechslin E, Schneider J, Attenhofer Jost C, Kaufmann PA. Echocardiographic and pathoanatomical characteristics of isolated left ventricular non-compaction: a step towards classification as a distinct cardiomyopathy. Heart. 2001;86(6): 666-71. DOI:10.1136/heart.86.6.666.

[65] Weiford BC, Subbarao VD, Mulhern KM. Noncompaction of the Ventricular Myocardium. Circulation. 2004;109(24):2965-2971. DOI:10.1161/01.CIR.0000132478.60674.D0.

[66] Oechslin EN, Attenhofer Jost CH, Rojas JR, Kaufmann PA, Jenni R. Long-term follow-up of 34 adults with isolated left ventricular noncompaction: a distinct cardiomyopathy with poor prognosis. J Am Coll Cardiol. 2000;36(2):493-500. DOI:10.1016/S0735-1097(00)00755-5.

[67] Ritter M, Oechslin E, Sütsch G, Attenhofer C, Schneider J, Jenni R. Isolated Noncompaction of the Myocardium in Adults. Mayo Clin Proc. 1997;72(1):26-31. DOI:10.4065/72.1.26.

[68] Udeoji DU, Philip KJ, Morrissey RP, Phan A, Schwarz ER. Left ventricular noncompaction cardiomyopathy: updated review. Ther Adv Cardiovasc Dis. 2013;7(5):260-273. DOI:10.1177/1753944713504639.

[69] Oechslin E, Jenni R. Left ventricular non-compaction revisited: a distinct phenotype with genetic heterogeneity? Eur Heart J. 2011;32(12):1446-1456. DOI:10.1093/eurheartj/ehq508.

[70] Sen-Chowdhry S, McKenna WJ. Left ventricular noncompaction and cardiomyopathy: cause, contributor, or epiphenomenon? Curr Opin Cardiol. 2008;23(3):171-175. DOI:10.1097/HCO.0b013e3282fdc939.

[71] Chin TK, Perloff JK, Williams RG, Jue K, Mohrmann R. Isolated noncompaction of left ventricular myocardium. A study of eight cases. Circulation. 1990;82(2):507-513. DOI: 10.1161/01.cir.82.2.507.

[72] Kido K, Guglin M. Anticoagulation Therapy in Specific Cardiomyopathies: Isolated Left Ventricular Noncompaction and Peripartum Cardiomyopathy. J Cardiovasc Pharmacol Ther. 2018;24(1):31-36. DOI:10.1177/1074248418783745.

Chapter 2

Cardiomyopathy: Recent Findings

Yoshihiro Yamada, Keiki Sugi, Hiroyuki Nakajima and Takaaki Senbonmatsu

Abstract

In 1957, Wallace Brigden published an article on the Lancet, such as uncommon myocardial diseases: the non-coronary cardiomyopathy. In this article, he mentioned that "the term cardiomyopathy is used here to indicate isolated noncoronary myocardial disease." Then "cardiomyopathy" has become a commonly used term in the cardiovascular field, and has been defined and classified by many researchers and academic societies. The basic concept of cardiomyopathy is a group of diseases with mechanical and/or electrophysiological dysfunction of the ventricles, and cardiomyopathy is distinguished with normal ischemic heart disease, valvular disease, and hypertensive heart disease. It can often cause heart failure and cardiac death. In this chapter, we describe the classification, details, and treatment of cardiomyopathy, and iPS cell from pathological myocardium.

Keywords: cardiomyopathy, classification, dilated cardiomyopathy, differentiation of dilated cardiomyopathy, hypertrophic cardiomyopathy, treatment of cardiomyopathy, human- induced pluripotent stem cell

1. Introduction

Goodwin et al. stated that, "the term cardiomyopathy has come into use to describe disorders of the heart, not primarily due to rheumatic, hypertensive, coronary-artery, thyroid, or congenital disease" [1]. They mentioned that the definition of cardiomyopathy is not completely satisfactory, but cardiomyopathy is a subacute or chronic disorder of the myocardium of unknown or unclear etiology, often with associated endocardium and sometimes with pericardial involvement. However, atherosclerosis does not cause cardiomyopathy. They described that the classification of cardiomyopathy consists of congestive heart failure including dilated, constrictive, restrictive, obstructive, and hypertrophic cardiomyopathy. Inheriting the concept of cardiomyopathy proposed by Goodwin et al., in 1980, the World Health Organization (WHO)/International Society and Federation of Cardiology (ISFC) task force defined "cardiomyopathies are heart muscle diseases of unknown cause" and classified into dilated cardiomyopathy, hypertrophic cardiomyopathy, restrictive cardiomyopathy and unclassifiable cardiomyopathy [2]. In 1982, arrhythmogenic right ventricular dysplasia (formerly known as ARVC, currently known as arrhythmogenic cardiomyopathy), which is an inherited form of heart disease characterized pathologically by fibrofatty myocardial replacement and clinically by prominent ventricular arrhythmias and impairment of ventricular systolic function, was reported [3]. Since arrhythmogenic right ventricular dysplasia means a genetically determined heart muscle disorder, the term dysplasia was replaced by cardiomyopathy. In 1995, the WHO/ISFC task force newly defined cardiomyopathies as "diseases of the myocardium associated with cardiac dysfunction." classified into dilated cardiomyopathy, hypertrophic cardiomyopathy, restrictive cardiomyopathy and arrhythmogenic right ventricular cardiomyopathy, unclassified cardiomyopathy [4]. And then, they used the term specific cardiomyopathy for heart muscle disease that is clearly associated with specific cardiac or systemic disorders.

In 2006, the American Heart Association (AHA) proposed a definition and classification of cardiomyopathy as following: "Cardiomyopathies are a heterogeneous group of diseases of the myocardium associated with mechanical and/or electric dysfunction that usually (but not invariably) exhibit inappropriate ventricular hypertrophy or dilatation and are due to a variety of causes that frequently are genetic. Cardiomyopathies either are confined to the heart or are part of generalized systemic disorders" [5]. AHA cardiomyopathy classification roughly divided into primary cardiomyopathy which has main lesion in the heart, and secondary cardiomyopathy which is a systemic heart lesion. Primary cardiomyopathy is classified into three categories: hereditary, mixed (hereditary and acquired), and acquired (**Figure 1**). Genetic cardiomyopathy includes HCM, ARVC, LVNC, glucose accumulation disease, cardiac conduction disorders, mitochondrial cardiomyopathy, and ion channel disease such as LQTS, Brugada, SQTS, CPVT, IVF (**Table 1**). The ion channelopathy are primary electrical diseases without gross or histopathological abnormalities in which the functional and structural myocardial abnormalities responsible for arrhythmogenesis are at the molecular level in the cell membrane itself. Therefore, the basic pathological abnormality in these diseases is not identifiable by either conventional noninvasive imaging or myocardial biopsy during life or even by autopsy examination of tissue. This is a new concept of cardiomyopathy adopted in the AHA classification. Mixed cardiomyopathy includes DCM, restrictive (non-hypertrophied and non-dilated), and acquired cardiomyopathy includes myocarditis, stress-provoked (tako-tsubo), peripartum, tachycardia-induced,

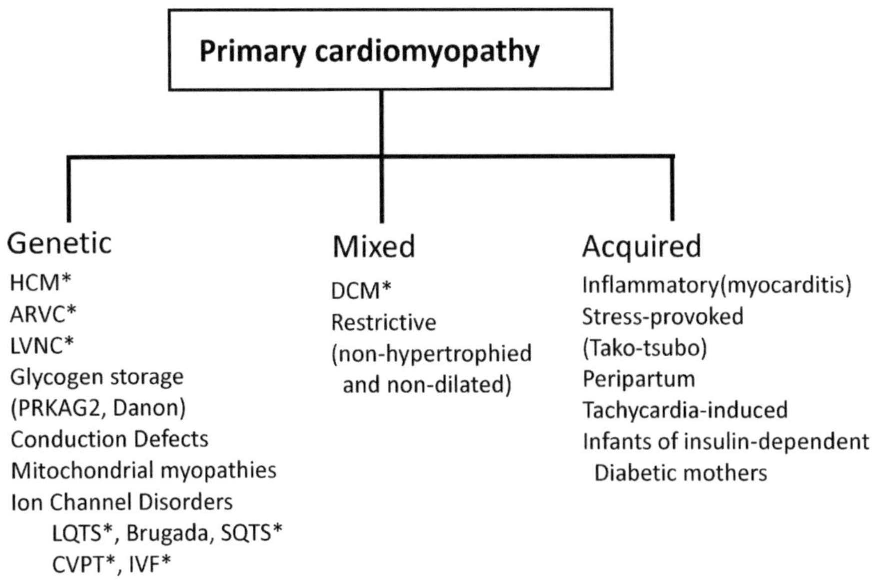

Figure 1.
Definition and classification of cardiomyopathy proposed by AHA in 2006. Modified citation from Ref. [5]. See* **Table 1**. *© 2006 American Heart Association, Inc.*

ARVC: Arrhythmogenic Right Ventricular Cardiomyopathy
CPVT: Catecholaminergic Polymorphic Ventricular Tachycardia
DCM: Dilated Cardiomyopathy
HCM: Hypertrophic Cardiomyopathy
IVF: Idiopathic Ventricular Fibrillation
LVNC: Left Ventricular Noncompaction Cardiomyopathy
LQTS: Long QT Syndrome
RCM: Restrictive Cardiomyopathy
SQTS: Short-QT Syndrome

Table 1.
List of abbreviations

infants of insulin-dependent diabetic mothers. **Tables 2** and **3** display secondary cardiomyopathy that is almost equivalent to the previous specific cardiomyopathy of the WHO/ISFC task force. This looks like a classification from a genetic, biomolecular point of view.

On the other hand, in 2008 European Society of Cardiology (ESC) defined a cardiomyopathy as, "a myocardial disorder in which the heart muscle is structurally and functionally abnormal, in the absence of coronary artery disease, hypertension, valvular disease and congenital heart disease sufficient to cause the observed myocardial abnormality" [6]. Cardiomyopathies are grouped into specific

Infiltrative (Accumulation of abnormal substances between myocytes (ie, extracellular))
Amyloidosis (primary, familial autosomal dominant†, senile, secondary forms)
Gaucher disease (Genetic (familial) origin)
Hurler's disease (Genetic (familial) origin)
Hunter's disease (Genetic (familial) origin)
Storage (Accumulation of abnormal substances within myocytes (ie, intracellular))
Hemochromatosis
Fabry's disease (Genetic (familial) origin)
Glycogen storage disease (type II, Pompe) (Genetic (familial) origin)
Niemann-Pick disease (Genetic (familial) origin)
Toxicity
Drugs, heavy metals, chemical agents
Endomyocardial
Endomyocardial fibrosis
Hypereosinophilic syndrome (Löeffler's endocarditis)
Inflammatory (granulomatous)
Sarcoidosis
Endocrine
Diabetes mellitus
Hyperthyroidism
Hypothyroidism

Hyperparathyroidism
Pheochromocytoma
Acromegaly
Modified citation from Reference [5]. ©2006 American Heart Association, Inc.

Table 2.
Secondary Cardiomyopathies.

Cardiofacial
Noonan syndrome (Genetic (familial) origin)
Lentiginosis (Genetic (familial) origin)
Neuromuscular/neurological
Friedreich's ataxia (Genetic (familial) origin)
Duchenne-Becker muscular dystrophy (Genetic (familial) origin)
Emery-Dreifuss muscular dystrophy (Genetic (familial) origin)
Myotonic dystrophy (Genetic (familial) origin)
Neurofibromatosis (Genetic (familial) origin)
Tuberous sclerosis (Genetic (familial) origin)
Nutritional deficiencies
Beriberi (thiamine), pallagra, scurvy, selenium, carnitine, kwashiorkor
Autoimmune/collagen
Systemic lupus erythematosis
Dermatomyositis
Rheumatoid arthritis
Scleroderma
Polyarteritis nodosa
Electrolyte imbalance
Consequence of cancer therapy
Anthracyclines: doxorubicin (adriamycin), daunorubicin
Cyclophosphamide
Radiation
Modified citation from Reference [5]. ©2006 American Heart Association, Inc.

Table 3.
Secondary Cardiomyopathies continued.

morphological and functional phenotypes. Each phenotype is then sub-classified into familial and non-familial forms (**Figure 2**). This classification is an extension of the WHO/ISFC classification, with genetic and non-genetic classifications based on morphological and functional abnormalities. In 2018, Japanese Circulation Society (JCS) has revised the cardiomyopathy clinical practice guidelines [7]. JCS defined a cardiomyopathy as so-called primary cardiomyopathy, is divided into four types: hypertrophic cardiomyopathy, dilated cardiomyopathy, arrhythmogenic right ventricular cardiomyopathy, and restrictive cardiomyopathy (**Figure 3**). Some of the

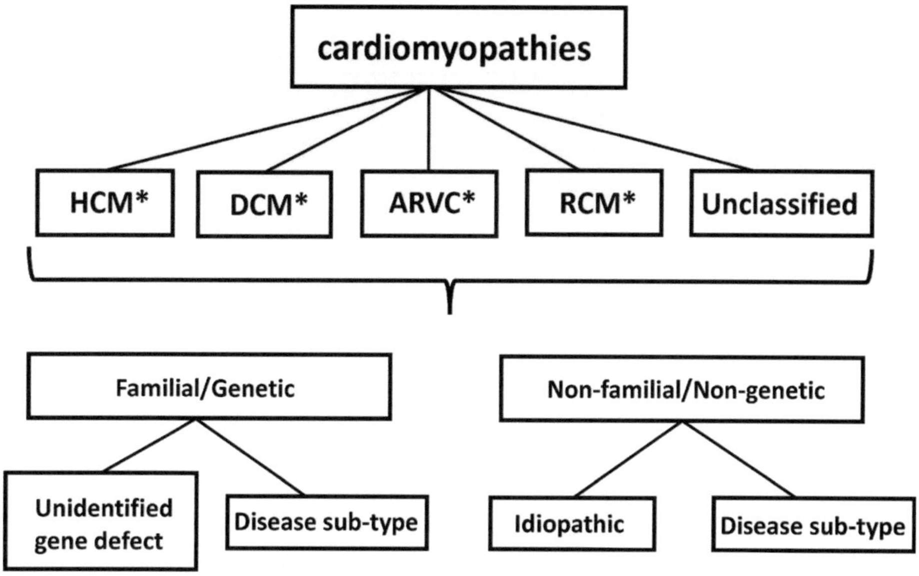

Figure 2.
*Definition and classification of cardiomyopathy proposed by ESCA in 2008. Modified citation from Ref. [6]. * See* ***Table 1****.*

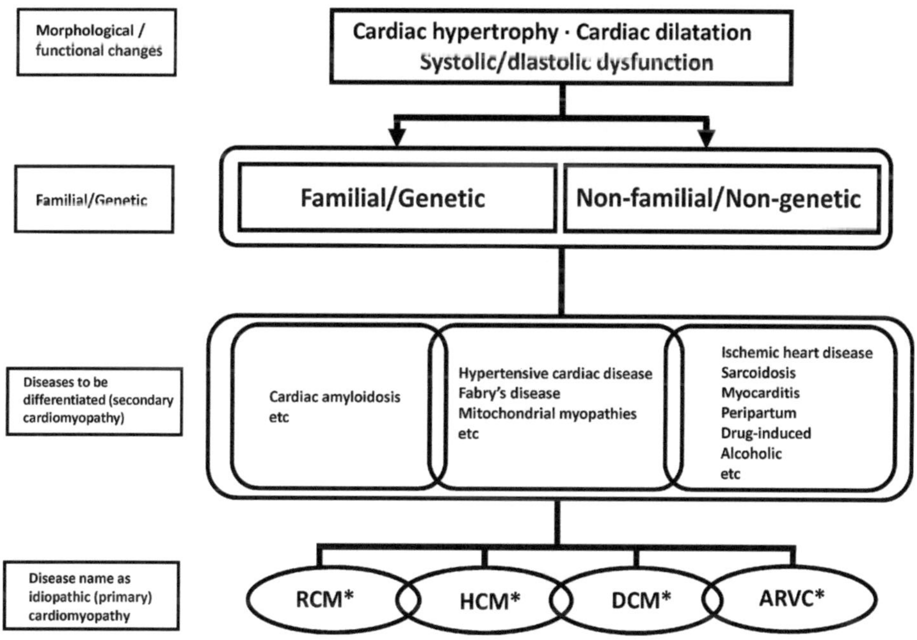

Figure 3.
*Revised definition and classification of cardiomyopathy proposed by JSC in 2018. Modified citation from Ref. [7]. * See* ***Table 1****.*

four basic pathologies of primary cardiomyopathy overlap and are often difficult to distinguish from each other. Diagnosis of these four primary cardiomyopathies should be confirmed after distinguishing secondary cardiomyopathy as much as possible. Cardiomyopathy that cannot be classified into four basic pathological conditions at present is called unclassifiable cardiomyopathy. The classification of JCS may be close to that of ESC.

M Morphofunctional Phenotype	O Organ/System Involvement	G Genetic	E Etiological Annotation	S Stage; ACC/AHA Stage, NYHA Functional Class
(D) Dilated (H) Hypertrophic (R) Restrictive (A) ARVC (NC) LVNC Overlapping (H+R), (D+A), (NC+H), (H+D), (D+NC) or more complex combinations such as (H+R+NC) (E) Early, with type in parentheses (NS) Nonspecific phenotype (NA) Information not available (0) Unaffected	(H) Heart (M) Muscle, skeletal (N) Nervous (C) Cutaneous (E) Eye (A) Auditory (K) Kidney (G) Gastrointestinal (S) Skeletal (0) Absence of organ/ system involvement, e.g., in family members who are healthy mutation carriers; the mutation is specified in E and inheritance in G	(N) Family history negative (U) Family history unknown (AD) Autosomal dominant (AR) Autosomal recessive (XLR) X-linked recessive (XLD) X-linked dominant (XL) X-linked (M) Matrilineal (DN) De novo (0) Family history not investigated	(G) Genetic etiology-add gene and mutation; (NC) Individual noncarrier plus the gene that tested negative (OC) Obligate carrier (ONC) Obligate noncarrier (DN) De novo (C) Complex genetics when >1 mutation (provide additional gene and mutation) (Neg) Genetic test negative for the known familial mutation (NA) Genetic test not yet available (N) Genetic defect not identified (0) No genetic test, any reason (no blood sample, no informed consent, etc.) Genetic amyloidosis (A-TTR) or hemochromatosis (HFE) Nongenetic etiologies: (M) Myocarditis (V) Viral infection (add the virus identified in affected heart) (AI) Autoimmune/immune-mediated; suspected (AI-S), proven (AI-P); (A) Amyloidosis (add type of amyloidosis: A-K; A-L, A-SAA) (I) Infectious, nonviral (add the infectious agent) (T) Toxicity (add toxic cause/drug) (Eo) Hypereosinophilic heart disease	ACC/AHA stage represented as letter (A, B, C, D) To be followed by NYHA Functional class represented in Roman numerals (I, II, III, IV) Modified citation from Reference 8
M_D, M_H, M_R, M_A, M_{NC}, M_0, M_{H+R}, M_{D+A}	O_H, O_M, O_K, O_C	G_N, G_U, G_{AD}, G_{AR}, G_{XLR}, G_{XLD}, G_{XD}, G_M, G_{DN}	$E_{G\text{-}MYH7[R403E]}$, $E_{G\text{-}HFE[Cys282Tyr+/+]}$, $E_{V\text{-}HCMV}$, $E_{G\text{-}A\text{-}TTR[V30M]}$, $E_{M\text{-}sarcoidosis}$	$S_{A\text{-}I}$, $S_{A\text{-}II}$

Figure 4.
The MOGE(S) nomenclature of cardiomyopathy. Modified citation from Ref. [8].

In 2013, Arbustini et al proposed the MOGE (S) classification of cardiomyopathy approved by the World Heart Federation [8] (**Figure 4**). This is a classification system similar to the TMM system, which is a system for staging cancers in oncology. This is a classification that integrates cardiomyopathy by morphology and function (M:Morpho-functional phenotype), affected organs (O:Organ/system involvement), gene mutation (G:Genetic inheritance pattern), cause and pathology E: Etiology), and severity (S: Stage) and obtains information necessary for treatment in an easy-to-understand manner. In this way, there are many cardiomyopathy classifications in the world, but it is difficult to say that they are sufficiently unified, including the usage of terms.

2. Dilated cardiomyopathy (DCM)

DCM is a group of diseases characterized by myocardial contractile dysfunction and dilatation of the left ventricular lumen and has a poor prognosis and progressive disease with symptoms of chronic heart failure and repeated acute deterioration. It also causes sudden death due to fatal arrhythmias. The initial report on the prevalence of DCM was published in 1989. This study was analyzed using data from Mayo Clinic and identified 45 new cases of DCM in Olmsted County, Minnesota between 1975 and 1984. The incidence of DCM doubled from 3.9 per 100,000 person-years to 7.9 per 100,000 person-years during the first 5 years. The prevalence of DCM in people younger than 55 years was 17.9 per 100,000, and more than one-third of them were in New York Heart Association functional III or IV at diagnosis [9].

The etiology of DCM has been unknown for a long time, but it has been divided into familial and non-familial categories. In particular, most cases of adult-onset DCM are considered to be caused by both familial and non-familial factors.

Advances in molecular genetic analysis have revealed causative mutations of DCM in more than 60 genes and truncating mutations in the titin (TTN) gene were shown to be present 25% of familial or severe transplant DCM cases [10]. In another report, truncation of the TTN gene was found in about 13% of non-familial DCM cases, but also 2% of the general population [11]. Recently, a polygenic risk score has been developed to predict the cumulative effect of multiple susceptibility genes identified by genome-wide association studies using mathematical models, and it has become clear that genetic variation can be affected by exogenous or environmental factors [12]. In addition, the clinical impact differed by genetic mutation, DCM patients with truncating mutations in TTN having a milder disease phenotype at baseline and a higher incidence of reverse remodeling compared with patients with a pathogenic lamin A/C (LMNA) mutation [13], which is one of the DCM with poor prognosis due to the risk of sudden death [14]. Recently, other mutations such as carriers of a specific phospholamban (PLN) mutation or truncating filamin C (FLNC) mutations have been reported as a risk of sudden death in DCM patients [15, 16]. The causes of non-familial DCM are still unknown. The etiology is considered to be inflammation and necrosis of cardiomyocytes caused by infectious factors such as viruses and bacteria and non-infectious factors such as autoimmunity, drugs and stress. In fact, it has been reported that viral genomes have been detected in the tissues of patients diagnosed with DCM [17].

3. Differentiation of DCM

As mentioned above, DCM is defined as a group of diseases characterized by diffuse contractility disorder and dilatation of the left ventricle. Therefore, it is necessary to exclude specific heart muscle diseases for definitive diagnosis. Specific heart muscle indicates ischemic cardiomyopathy, valvular heart disease, and hypertensive heart disease, inflammatory heart disease, metabolic heart disease, myocardial disease associated with neuromuscular disease or myocardial disease with clear association with systemic disease [4].

3.1 Ischemic cardiomyopathy

Ischemic cardiomyopathy is caused by ischemia due to coronary atherosclerosis and it is characterized by left ventricular dilatation and contractile dysfunction, similar to DCM. Ischemic cardiomyopathy is the most common cause of heart failure in clinical cases and should be excluded initially. In addition to a history of ischemic heart disease, coronary angiography or coronary computed tomography is necessary to be differentiated. If contrast medium is not available, scintigraphy can be used as a substitute. In rare cases, left ventricular dysfunction such as DCM may occur due to multiple vessel coronary artery spasm, even in the absence of coronary artery stenosis. If this is suspected on symptoms, an acetylcholine provocation test should be considered [18].

3.2 Hypertensive cardiomyopathy

Hypertensive cardiomyopathy is similar to DCM, which presents with systolic dysfunction as a result of histological abnormalities such as left ventricular hypertrophy and myocardial cell hypertrophy, interstitial proliferation and perivascular fibrosis due to persistent hypertensive conditions. It is a pathological condition and is characterized by efferent hypertrophy with left ventricular enlargement. In addition to the histological and functional disorders of the heart, other organ disorders due to sustained hypertension such as blood vessels and kidneys often contribute to the onset of heart failure.

3.3 Amyloidosis Cardiomyopathy

Amyloidosis indicates a general team of diseases characterized by the extracellular deposition of misfolded amyloid fibrils in organs. Clinically, it is roughly divided into systemic amyloidosis in which multiple organs and peripheral nerves are damaged, and focal amyloidosis in which amyloid deposits occur locally in an organ or organs. Cardiac amyloidosis is one of the common infiltrative or restrictive cardiomyopathies associated with an unfavorable prognosis. The pathophysiology of amyloidosis is the misfolding of abnormal protein that is amyloid fibrils resulting in its accumulation to extracellular on the affected tissues. Although there are multiple causes of the misfolding, one of them is a gene mutation that encodes a different amino-acid leading to the conformational change of protein [19].

Clinical outcome depends on the extent of tissue involvement and on the type of amyloid fibril deposits. The major subtypes of systemic amyloidosis classified based on the underlying etiologies are as follows: primary (AL) amyloidosis, Secondary (AA) amyloidosis (or reactive amyloidosis), familial transthyretin-associated amyloidosis (ATTR or hereditary amyloidosis), dialysis-related amyloidosis, and senile systemic amyloidosis. AL amyloidosis has an incidence of 1 case per 100,000 person-years in western countries. ATTR is a less common systemic type of amyloidosis with unknown incidence

Cardiac manifestations predominantly include symptoms of right heart failure. Infiltration of amyloid fibrils results in stiffening and thickening of ventricles causing decreased compliance and increased pressure altering the mechanics of ventricular function manifesting as diastolic dysfunction. Furthermore, cytotoxic effects of amyloid fibrils result in apoptotic and fibrotic changes of the heart. Finally, these changes lead to heart failure. Amyloid deposits to cardiac conduction system result in heart block or arrhythmias [20]. Syncope due to heart block or arrhythmia may be a marker of prognosis [20]. Atrial fibrillation (AF) is the most common arrhythmia described in approximately 10%-20% of patients who have cardiac amyloidosis [21].

It is possible that patients of cardiac amyloidosis are completely asymptomatic or may present with various signs and symptoms. Therefore, a diagnostic approach is important in cases of suspected cardiac amyloidosis. Pseudoinfarction, which is low voltage in limb leads and poor R wave progression in ECG, is one of the most common electrocardiographic characteristics in cardiac amyloidosis. This finding has been demonstrated in up to half of patients with AL [22]. Furthermore, amyloid deposits also result in various arrhythmias, such as various heart blocks, AF, and complex ventricular tachycardia [23].

The echocardiography is recommended in all patients with suspected amyloidosis, and findings include bilateral dilatation and thickening of ventricular wall and valves, decreased diastolic filling, and classic granular sparkling appearance. The wall thickness is attributed to infiltrative amyloid deposition instead of myocyte hypertrophy [24]. Decreased left ventricular ejection fraction is of grim prognostic significance [25]. Cardiovascular magnetic resonance imaging (CMR) is an important diagnostic and prognostic tool in the assessment of severity of cardiac amyloidosis. Injury to the myocardium secondary to deposition of amyloid fibrils in the interstitium denotes a reservoir for gadolinium accumulation leading to characteristic late gadolinium enhancement (LGE) [26]. This technique has a sensitivity of close to 80% and impressive specificity of 94% [27]. Strain analysis based on CMR can be accomplished with the recent advances, a technique known as Displacement Encoding with Stimulated Echoes with high sensitivity and specificity close to echo

[28]. It is a highly precise modality and hold promises in generation of strain time curves with "tissue tracking" techniques. Use of radiotracers has been used to diagnose amyloidosis. Most commonly, 99mTc-DPD (technetium-3,3-diphosphono-1,2-propanodicarboxylic acid) and 99mTc-PYP is used. As 99mTc-PYP preferentially binds to ATTR relative to AL fibrils, this technique also serves as an on invasive way to distinguish the aforementioned amyloidosis subtypes [29]. Biopsy with histopathology remains the gold standard showing deposition of amorphous deposits of amyloid fibrils.

Treatment can be divided into HF therapy, specific therapy for each amyloidosis. Chemotherapy is based on the concept of reducing the number of amyloid fibrils and retarding the disease process. In AL, chemotherapy and autologous hematopoietic stem cell transplant is the main stay of treatment. Chemotherapy in AL is aimed at reducing free light chains. Bortezomib is a proteasome inhibitor that induces rapid hematological response either alone or in combination with dexamethasone [30]. As mutant amyloid ATTR is produced in liver, orthotropic liver transplantation is the established treatment since 1990. Transthyretin (TTR) tetramer stabilizers (tafamidis and diflunisal) work by binding to TTR and by stabilizing its normal tetrameric structure preventing amyloid fibril formation [31]. Drugs such as tafamidis and diflunisal, could have role in the treatment of senile systemic amyloidosis (SSA) which is amyloidosis that mainly affects the heart of the elderly.

3.4 Sarcoidosis

Sarcoidosis is a systemic inflammatory disease characterized by the formation of granulomas in affected organs, especially the lungs. Diagnosis is challenging for clinicians because various organs can be affected. The exact prevalence of cardiac lesions in sarcoidosis is unknown due to ethnic differences, but the incidence of sarcoidosis has been reported to 11-24 cases per 100,000 per a year in Scandinavian countries and 1 case per 100,000 per a year [32, 33]. The incidence is higher in women (45-60%) and the average age of diagnosis is younger in men (30-50 years) compared to women (50-60 years) [34]. The etiology of sarcoidosis is unknown, however, it has been reported that not only genetic factors but also living environment and lifestyle are contributing factors [35]. The inflammatory response in sarcoidosis is thought to involve autoimmunity, possibly including autoantigens, although there are no specific diagnostic markers or biomarkers for activity.

Cardiac sarcoidosis is present 2-7% of patients with sarcoidosis, and cardiac sarcoidosis can occur without pulmonary or systemic involvement [36]. In the early stages of the disease, ventricular wall thickening coinciding with regions of granulomatous inflammation and interstitial edema is observed, and as inflammation gradually fades and fibrosis of the lesions progresses, the base of the ventricular septum often shows characteristic wall thinning. Regional hypokinesia of the left and right ventricles and ventricular aneurysm are observed and if the lesion is extensive, DCM-like pathology may be observed [37].

The detection rate of myocardial biopsies is low, and currently gadolinium-enhanced cardiac magnetic resonance imaging is the optimal test for determining the presence and extent of cardiac lesions. 18F-FDG-PET is useful for evaluating the degree of granulomatous inflammation and activity of cardiac lesions [38].

3.5 Drug-induced cardiomyopathy

Drug-induced cardiomyopathy is commonly seen in clinical situations as a serious side effect of anticancer drugs and antiretroviral therapy. In particular, patients with a history of cancer treatment need to be asked about what kind of anticancer drug treatment they have received and whether they have received radiation therapy.

The most commonly identified chemotherapeutic drugs with cardiotoxicity are anthracyclines and these drugs are still used in clinical practice [39]. It has been reported that cutoff value for anthracycline administration to affect cardiovascular risk is 250 mg/m^2 or higher, but even lower doses can cause cardiac dysfunction [40, 41]. With the improvement of chemotherapy outcomes, the number of long-term survivors of childhood cancer has increased and delayed drug-induced cardiomyopathy often develops in adulthood after anthracycline treatment in childhood [42].

Trastuzumab (Herceptin) is a humanized IgG kappa monoclonal antibody that targets the extracellular domain of human epidermal growth factor receptor 2 (HER2) [43]. The HER2 has been found to be amplified 2 to 20 times or more in 30% of breast cancer patients, and gene amplification has been reported to be a significant predictor of both survival and time to recurrence [44]. Trastuzumab-induced cardiomyopathy usually presents as an asymptomatic decrease in left ventricular ejection fraction and can lead to complications such as heart failure, but the cardiotoxicity is transient and reversible, in addition it isn't dose-dependent as with anthracyclines [45, 46].

To evaluate such drug-induced cardiomyopathy, American Society of Echocardiography has defined that cancer therapeutics-related cardiac dysfunction as decrease in left ventricular ejection fraction (LVEF) or greater to less than 53%. In addition, LVEF is reevaluated after 2 to 3 weeks and is considered reversible if the decline is within 5% of baseline, and irreversible if the improvement in EF is less than 10% and remains below 5% of baseline. In particular, it is recommended that the LVEF and global strain be evaluated in combination [47]. Even in facilities that do not have echocardiography, troponin I has been reported to be elevated indicating the possibility of cardiotoxicity and measurement of troponin I is also recommended [48].

3.6 Myocarditis

Myocarditis is an inflammatory disease in which inflammation spreads to cardiomyocytes. Most of them are viral infections, and adenovirus, enterovirus including the coxsackievirus B, parvovirus, cytomegalovirus and HIV are the most frequent as causative virus of myocarditis [49]. Bacteria that causes non-viral myocarditis include corynebacterium infection, streptococcal infection, tuberculosis, Whipple's disease, and Lyme carditis. The definitive diagnosis of myocarditis is based on myocardial biopsy and histological diagnosis. A typical finding of myocardial biopsy of myocarditis is infiltration of inflammatory cells such as neutrophils and mononuclear cells between myocardial fibers, and a necrotic lesion such as rupture/melting of adjacent cardiomyocytes. The interstitium becomes edematous and capillary angiogenesis occurs. The prevalence of cardiomyopathy during whole heart failure varies by age and region, but ranges from approximately 0.5% to 4.0% [50]. Although about half of myocarditis patients are cured, sudden death due to myocarditis is not uncommon.

3.7 Alcoholic cardiomyopathy

It is one of addictive cardiomyopathy caused by long-term and heavy drinking. In general, it is estimated that the onset occurs when 80 to 90 g/day of pure ethanol equivalent is ingested daily for 5 years or more. Initially, diastolic dysfunction and left ventricular hypertrophy occur, and then the left ventricle is dilated as it progresses of pathologic state. Treatment is complete abstinence first.

3.8 Left ventricular noncompaction cardiomyopathy

Left ventricular noncompaction cardiomyopathy (LVNC) is a structural abnormality of the left ventricular myocardium of unknown cause. Since LVNC is associated with genetic disease, particularly neuromuscular disorders (NMDs) and chromosomal defects in the majority of patients, in the AHA cardiomyopathy classification, LVNC is classified as one of the genetic primary cardiomyopathies [5]. Mortality of patients with LVNC ranges from 5% to 47% [51]. LVNC is characterized by a two-layered structure usually of the apical and lateral left ventricular myocardium, distal to the papillary muscles. The two-layered structure consists of an excessive spongy endocardial layer (noncompacted layer: NC) and a compacted epicardial layer (compacted layer: C), which is usually thinner than the endocardial layer and NC/C ratio is 2 or more by echocardiography. In LVNC, many genetic abnormalities have been reported such as TAZ, DTNA and LDB3 gene mutation, and many genetic abnormalities of sarcomere protein have also been reported [51]. LVNC is usually asymptomatic, but can be complicated by heart failure, thromboembolism, or ventricular arrhythmias, including sudden cardiac death. LVNC is diagnosed primarily by echocardiography, and is frequently associated with myocardial fibrosis, as shown by the presence of late gadolinium enhancement (LGE) on CMR [51, 52].

3.9 Beriberi heart

Vitamin B1 (thiamine) is a coenzyme essential for glucose metabolism. It is thought that thiamine supplementation is insufficient due to high-calorie infusion and unbalanced diet during the growth period, and then deficiency occurs [53]. If this deficiency lasts for more than 3 months, beriberi occurs.

3.10 Mitochondrial cardiomyopathy

Mitochondrial disease is a multi-organ disease characterized by oxidative phosphorylation disorders caused by mitochondrial dysfunction due to mutations in the nucleus and mitochondrial DNA. Therefore, mitochondrial cardiomyopathy is often recognized as a symptom of mitochondrial disease. The prevalence of inherited mitochondrial disease has been estimated to be greater than 1 in 5,000 births [54]. A common pathology of mitochondrial cardiomyopathy is a decrease in mitochondrial ATP production capacity per one cardiomyocyte [55]. Since the myocardium is an organ that continuously consumes energy through aerobic metabolism, ATP deficiency is directly linked to a decrease in myocardial contractility. Many nuclear and mitochondrial DNA mutations associated with mitochondrial cardiomyopathy have been reported. Typical mitochondrial diseases MELAS (mitochondrial myopathy, encephalopathy, lactic acidosis and stroke-like episodes), MERRF (myoclonus epilepsy associated with ragged-red fibers), CPEO (chronic progressive external ophthalmoplegia), and KSS (Kearns-Sayre syndrome) also develop mitochondrial cardiomyopathy. The typical cardiac manifestations of mitochondrial cardiomyopathy are diverse such as hypertrophic and dilated cardiomyopathy, arrhythmias, left ventricular myocardial noncompaction, and heart failure, and may worsen rapidly due to infection or sudden death due to lethal arrhythmia [55].

3.11 Anderson-Fabry disease

Anderson-Fabry disease (AFD) is an X-linked hereditary glycolipid metabolism disorders due to deficient activity of the enzyme alpha-galactosidase A (α-Gal A) located on the X-chromosome (Xq22.1) resulting in progressive lysosomal deposition of globotriaosylceramide (GL-3) in cells throughout the body [56]. AFD is one of sex-linked recessive inheritance diseases. This indicates that all hemizygous men are affected, whereas their daughters are obligate heterozygous carriers. However, AFD is a disease that is more likely to onset the disease in heterozygotes (female). In female, it is thought that one of the two X chromosomes is inactivated. In a female who is heterozygotes, when the rate of inactivation of the X chromosome with the mutant allele is high, it is close to normal. On the other hand, when the rate of inactivation of the X chromosome with normal allele is high, symptoms of AFD will appear. Females with AFD tend to develop and diagnose symptoms later than males. In classic of AFD, glycosphingolipid accumulates in organs throughout the body especially in the skin, kidneys, nerves, eyes, and heart, on the other hand, a cardiac variant phenotype or a renal variant phenotype lack systemic findings and present with organ-specific symptoms [56, 57]. Since the heart is involved in up to 70% of patients who have AFD, the diagnostic procurer of AFD include the cardiac diagnosis strategy such as baseline ECG, echocardiography and CMR with or without symptoms. The typical cardiac manifestations of AFD often mimic hypertrophic cardiomyopathy [58]. That is, it is recognized as a disease that causes cardiac hypertrophy and is classified as one of secondary cardiomyopathy. So clinically, the distinction between sarcometic HCM and AFD is extremely important. CMR is an excellent way to non-invasively diagnose cardiac involvement in AFD. Non-contrast T1 mapping of CMR significantly displays lower value in AFD, compared to healthy volunteers and patients with other confounding diseases [59].

3.12 Peripartum cardiomyopathy

Peripartum cardiomyopathy is a dilated cardiomyopathy-like state in women who have no history of heart disease during pregnancy or childbirth. In some cases, severe heart failure associated with postpartum cardiomyopathy is developed. Although the detailed mechanisms of postpartum cardiomyopathy are still unknown, the causes are thought to be hemodynamic changes due to pregnancy, preeclampsia, viral infections, allergies, nutritional disorders, etc. In Japan, the prevalence of peripartum cardiomyopathy has been estimated 1 in 10,000 to 20,000 births [60]. This is a lower rate than that of the United States [61]. However, the prevalence rate is increasing year by year due to the aging of pregnant women, improvement of reproductive technology, and improvement of cardiomyopathy diagnosis rate.

3.13 Cardiomyopathy in muscular dystrophy

Muscle dystrophy is heterogeneous group of disorders characterized by genetic and progressive degeneration of skeletal muscle and muscle weakness [62]. In Japan the overall incidence of this disease is estimated as 2 to 3 out of 100,000. Duchenne muscular dystrophy (DMD), Becker muscular dystrophy (BMD) are X-linked recessive (Xp21), Emery- Dreifuss Muscular Dystrophy (EDMD) is X-linked recessive (Xq28 in EDMD1, Xq26 in EDMD 6), Autosomal dominant (EDMD2; LMNA gene at 1q21), autosomal recessive (EDMD3, also involving the LMNA gene at 1q21), Limb Girdle Muscular Dystrophy (LGMD) is usually autosomal recessive (LGMD2C. 2D, 2E & 2F: sarcoglycanopathies; LGMD2I: mutation of fukutin-related protein gene; 19q), Rarely autosomal dominant (LGDM1; 1B due to mutation of the LMNA gene encoding lamin A/C), and Myotonic Dystrophy (DM) is autosomal dominant: type 1 (DM1, Steinert's disease): unstable expansion of CTG the myotonic dystrophy protein kinase gene (DMPK) on chromosome 19q13.3, type 2 (DM2): CCTG tetranucleotide repeat expansion in intron 1 of the zinc finger protein 9 gene (ZNF9) on chromosome 3q21.3 [63]. Almost all DMD patients develop cardiomyopathy early on, on the other hand, symptom progression in BMD patients is slow but may present with severe heart failure [64, 65]. Cardiomyopathy in EDMD patients develops in the same way as that of DMD patients [66]. LGMD patients develop sinus node dysfunction, atrioventricular node dysfunction, ventricular arrhythmias as cardiomyopathy manifestations [67]. Common cardiomyopathy manifestations in DM1 and DM2 patients are atrioventricular and intraventricular conduction defects. Infra-hisian block is likely an important cause of sudden death in these patients [68, 69].

4. Hypertrophic cardiomyopathy (HCM)

Hypertrophic cardiomyopathy (HCM) is the common primary cardiomyopathy, with a prevalence of 1:500 persons [64]. It is defined as left ventricular hypertrophy without chamber dilation and is caused by gene mutations that encode 8 sarcomere proteins: beta-myosin heavy chain (MYH7), cardiac myosin-binding protein C (MYPBC3), cardiac troponin T (TNNT2), cardiac troponin I (TNNI3), cardiac actin (ACTC), alpha-tropomyosin (TPM1), essential myosin light chain (MYL3) and regulatory myosin light chain (MYL2) [70]. Mutations in MYH7 and MYPBC3 often occur and account for approximately 50% of HCM cases, while mutations in TNNT2, TNNI3, ACTC, TPM1, MYL3 and MYL2 collectively account for less than 20% of HCM cases [71]. Septal thickening predominates and may cause left ventricular outflow tract obstruction or mitral valve dysfunction [65]. Phenotypic expression is variable. Many patients with HCM are asymptomatic and are diagnosed during family screening, by incidentally after an abnormal result on electrocardiography. Presenting signs and symptoms most characteristic of HCM include atypical chest pain and sudden cardiac death (SCD). Patients who are diagnosed with HCM may have a family history of unexplained sudden cardiac death. ECG often show left ventricular hypertrophy and Q waves, and echocardiography often show hypertrophy of the left ventricle coupled with reduction in ventricular chamber volume [66].

The natural history of HCM is quite variable. Signs and symptoms range from none, to atrial fibrillation, heart failure, embolic stroke and SCD. In heart failure in HCM, since decreased left ventricular diastolic function due to cardiac hypertrophy is the basic pathology of HCM, three categories of HCM patients emerged [67]: (1) patients with obstruction at all times, (2) patients without obstruction in the basal state in whom obstruction could be provoked, (3) patients without obstruction in whom obstruction could not be provoked. The severity of the outflow gradient is related to prognosis, and diastolic failure is a common dysfunction of HCM patients [68]. Ventricular fibrillation is one of cause of SCD in HCM. All patients with HCM should undergo risk stratification for SCD and be evaluated for placement of an implantable cardioverter-defibrillator [69]. Additionally, these devices are recommended for secondary prevention of SCD when there is any personal history of ventricular fibrillation or sustained ventricular tachycardia [64]. Although the main goals of therapy in HCM patients are to decrease exertional dyspnea and chest pain and prevent SCD, about 25% of HCM patients achieve normal longevity. Particular the MYPBC3 variant carries a good prognosis.

5. Arrthymogenic cardiomyopathy (ACM)

As mentioned in history of classification in cardiomyopathy, ARVC was one of cardiomyopathies characterized by right ventricular enlargement, decreased right ventricular wall contractility, and right ventricular tachycardia due to myocardial cell shedding and fibrofatty replacement in right ventricle. However, although the original article defines as disease phenotype characterized by predominant involvement of right ventricular dysfunction, recent reports show increased left dominant and biventricular forms. Therefore, the recent recognition of the term of ARVC has been replaced by arrthymogenic cardiomyopathy (ACM) [72].

ACM is an inherited heart disease characterized pathologically by fibrofatty myocardial replacement and clinically by prominent ventricular arrhythmias and impairment of ventricular function including both ventricles. The classical ARVC phenotype in ACM shows the right ventricle with fibrofatty infiltration, regional dilatation and aneurysm formation at the right ventricular inflow tract, outflow tract and the right ventricular apex which are called as triangle of dysplasia. Phenotype of left ventricular dominant type of ACM is characterized by the early left ventricular (LV) involvement with arrhythmias prior to gross structural alterations, on the other hand global RV function of this type is preserved. Biventricular ACM is characterized by early involvement of both ventricles with disease progression characterized by systolic impairment and biventricular dilation, with clinical features of global congestive heart failure, and ventricular arrhythmias originating from either ventricle at an early stage. Frequency of occurrence of ACM has been estimated at 1:1000 to 5,000, and it often occurs in the 30s, and the Sudden Cardiac Death in the Young |Ten Points to Remember disease declared by American College of Cardiology includes ACM as ARVC [73–75]. In ACM, there are gene abnormalities of the desmosome proteins which works in adhesion between cardiomyocytes, and gene abnormalities in the ryanodine receptor (RyR2) gene, which is a Ca^{2+} handling protein. The desmosomal complex is formed the trans-membrane proteins (cadherins), desmocollin-2 (DSC2), desmoglein-2 (DSG2), desmoplakin (DSP), the linker armadillo proteins plakoglobin (JUP) and plakophi-lin-2 (PKP2). JUP and PKP2 are mediators between the cadherins and DSP. Mutations in PKP2, DSP, and DSG2 are identified in up to 80% of confirmed pathogenic mutations. PKP2 accounts for 36–92% of mutations identified in desmosomal genes [72].

6. Restricted cardiomyopathy (RCM)

RCM is characterized by limited filling of one or both ventricles, reduced diastolic volume, and normal or near-normal contractility and wall thickness [76]. Ventricular wall thickness and contractility are almost normal, but diastolic volume decreases due to decreased myocardial compliance, resulting in heart failure. Endocardial fibrotic thickening and myocardial fibrosis may also be present.

7. Treatment of cardiomyopathy

7.1 Medical treatment of cardiomyopathy

Treatment of symptomatic heart failure associated with various cardiomyopathy should follow current guideline for the management of heart failure from American College of Cardiology/American Heart Association or guidelines for the diagnosis and treatment of acute and chronic heart failure from European Society of Cardiology [77, 78]. Beta blocker, angiotensin-converting enzyme inhibitor (ACEi), angiotensin receptor blocker (ARB), diuretics, angiotensin receptor-neprilysin inhibitor (ARNI), or sodium/glucose cotransporter 2 (SGLT2) blocker are used as pharmacologic therapy, when cardiomyopathy is associated with systolic dysfunction [79]. Patients with more severe heart failure symptoms should be evaluated for placement of an implantable cardioverter-defibrillator, and may require cardiac transplantation in refractory cases.

7.2 Mavacamten: new treatment for HCM

Mavacamten selectively inhibits cardiac myosin ATPase leading to reducing actin–myosin cross-bridge formation [80]. As a result, it is expected that mavacamten will improve pathophysiology of hypertrophic cardiomyopathy such as left ventricular outflow tract (LOVT) obstruction, decreased left ventricular filling. In preclinical and early clinical studies of mavacamten succeeded reduction of LVOT gradients and improved parameters of left ventricular filling [81, 82]. In the phase 2, PIONEER-HCM study revealed that mavacamten was well tolerated and significantly reduced post-exercise LVOT gradients in obstructive HCM [83]. On the basis of these results, the short-term results of the phase 3 EXPLORER-HCM trial have been published. EXPLORER-HCM was a phase 3, multicentre, randomised, double-blind, placebo-controlled trial [84]. Eligible patients were aged at least 18 years with a diagnosis of obstructive HCM; peak LVOT gradient at least 50 mm Hg at rest, after Valsalva manoeuvre or exercise; left ventricular ejection fraction (LVEF) at least 55%; and NYHA class II–III symptoms. The patients had to be able to safely perform upright cardiopulmonary exercise testing (CPET). Finally, 429 adults were assessed for eligibility, of whom 251 (59%) were enrolled. In the placebo group, post-exercise LVOT gradient had changed from 84mmHg to 73mmHg after 30weeks, meanwhile that of the mavacamten group improved from 86 mmHg to 38 mmHg (difference from the placebo group: -36 mmHg, 95% CI:-43.2 to -28.1 mmHg, $P < 0.0001$). The average increase in pVO2 was also significantly greater in the mavacamten group than in the placebo group (1.4 mL / kg / min, 95% CI: 0.6-2.1 mL/kg/min, $P = 0.0006$). The number of patients whose NYHA classification improved by 1 degree or more was 40 of 128 (31%) in the placebo group and 80 of 123 (65%) in the mavacamten group (difference between groups: 33.8%, 95% CI: 22.2-45.4%, $P < 0.0001$). Treatment with mavacamten improved exercise capacity, LVOT obstruction, NYHA functional class, and health status in patients with obstructive HCM. EXPLORER-HCM trial is ongoing to assess long-term (5 year) efficacy and safety.

7.3 Surgery for dilated and hypertrophic cardiomyopathy

Cardiomyopathy is categorized as a disease of the cardiomyocytes and is complicated with heart failure due to reduced ejection fraction or diastolic dysfunction.

Moreover, mitral valve regurgitation (MR) and ventricular arrhythmia are commonly associated with cardiomyopathy. Surgical treatment for cardiomyopathy is a combination of maneuvers on the ventricle, mitral annulus and leaflets. We herein summarize the current surgical management of dilated and hypertrophic obstructive cardiomyopathy (HOCM).

7.4 Hypertrophic cardiomyopathy

In patients with HOCM, heart failure is caused by left ventricular outflow tract (LVOT) obstruction, mitral valve dysfunction due to systolic anterior motion and diastolic dysfunction. Surgical treatment should relieve such dysfunctions, and the use of a mitral prosthetic valve should be avoided if possible.

7.4.1 Procedures on the left ventricle

Septal hypertrophy is a typical physiological feature of HOCM. Echocardiography during exercise is a reliable diagnostic modality and could provide significant prognostic information [85]. Peteiro and colleagues reported that, as only 13% of patients presented with LVOT obstruction at rest, 27% developed exercise-induced LVOT obstruction [85]. Cui and colleagues proved that septal hypertrophy with a significant LVOT pressure gradient truly generated obstruction of blood flow to the aorta [86]. Different from aortic valve stenosis, increased LVOT gradient caused decreased stroke volume [86]. In addition, the efficacy of septal myectomy was compared with valvular aortic stenosis. After myectomy with a normalized LVOT gradient, the aortic flow pattern returned to normal [86]. Therefore, septal myectomy is the principal surgical maneuver for HOCM. The improvement in stroke volume after myectomy explains the improvement in exercise capacity postoperatively [86]. Furthermore, Parbhudayal and colleagues compared myectomy for HOCM with aortic valve replacement for valvular stenosis and reported reverse remodeling after surgery [87]. They reported that recovery of systolic function was only observed after aortic valve replacement, while patients with HOCM demonstrated systolic functional deterioration, which was a negative impact of septal myectomy on cardiac function and was associated with ongoing pathophysiological conditions [87].

The spectrum of HOCM is of great variety in terms of location and severity of hypertrophy, positional relationship between the septum and anterior mitral leaflet and papillary muscles. For patients with mid-ventricular hypertrophy, broad myectomy concomitant with mitral valve replacement is necessary to relieve dilatation dysfunction.

7.4.2 Procedures on the mitral valve

Both ventricular hypertrophy and structural abnormalities of the mitral valve are frequently found in HOCM. An elongated anterior mitral leaflet is commonly associated with systolic anterior motion and MR. Regarding surgery for MR, analysis of the Society of Thoracic Surgeons database suggested that mitral etiology was not significantly associated with an incremental risk of early mortality [88].

Systolic anterior motion is associated with anomalously elongated anterior mitral leaflet. Balaram and colleagues recommended that the standard maneuver for the mitral leaflet was horizontal plication through the aortic valve when the anterior mitral leaflet was elongated by 30 mm, and the standard technique is plication of the leaflet, usually performed through the aortic valve [89, 90]. The plication can shorten the leaflet length by 2–5 mm [91]. Recently, the edge-to-edge technique was reported to be useful in HOCM and can be applied through either the aortic valve [92] or the left atrium [93]. Chordal cutting was also reported to be effective for relieving LVOT obstruction through geometric modification [94].

Septal myectomy is the primary maneuver for HOCM. In addition to myectomy, the maneuvers for the leaflet and sub-valvular apparatus are viable surgical options, especially when septal hypertrophy is not severe.

7.5 Idiopathic and ischemic dilated cardiomyopathies

For ischemic cardiomyopathy, MR was commonly found without any prolapse or deformity of the leaflets and chordal elongation or rupture. Such MR is usually functional and associated with apical displacement of the papillary muscles and dilatation of the mitral annulus. The presence of MR causes heart failure during follow-up and significantly worsens patient prognosis. Therefore, it has been widely accepted that surgical management of MR is crucial.

7.5.1 Procedures on the mitral valve

Ischemic or dilated cardiomyopathy causes functional MR. Patients have severe dilatation of the left ventricle, which causes mitral annular dilatation, leaflet tethering and the gap between the leaflets. Consequently, severe MR causes volume overload, fibrosis and adverse remodeling of the ventricle [95, 96].

During mitral valve repair, annuloplasty is frequently performed for ischemic cardiomyopathy. In the procedure, the artificial full and semi-rigid ring is implanted to reduce the annular diameter. Noack and colleagues reported that even for patients with poor ventricular ejection fraction of <30%, mitral valve repair could be safely performed [97]. Xu and colleagues reported that under-sizing annuloplasty was effective for eliminating MR [98]. Kainuma and colleagues reported favorable remodeling, decreased tethering distance and inter-papillary muscle distance during the follow-up period [99]. Conversely, choosing a downsized artificial ring might cause functional mitral stenosis and recurrence of MR compared with mitral valve replacement [100]. In some cases, ventricular or sub-valvular reconstruction procedures are necessary to achieve successful and durable mitral valve repair.

7.5.2 Procedures on the left ventricle

In ischemic cardiomyopathy, surgical coronary revascularization is beneficial to achieve favorable remodeling after surgery and avoid clinical outcomes [101]. Surgical ventricular reconstruction (SVR) such as the Dor procedure and its modifications contributed to improved long-term clinical outcomes with a reasonable perioperative risk [102]. Moreover, appropriate surgical maneuver of SVR had a significant impact on prognosis after surgery [102]. However, the clinical advantage of SVR concomitant with coronary artery bypass graft was not demonstrated in the STICH (Surgical Treatment for ischemic Heart Failure) trial, which was a randomized study of SVR in ischemic cardiomyopathy [103]. Patient selection for SVR may be an issue in the future.

7.5.3 Summary of surgery for dilated and hypertrophic cardiomyopathy

The clinical and morphological manifestations of cardiomyopathy vary greatly depending on etiology, severity and cardiac function. Especially procedures on the ventricle are not necessarily beneficial in the long-term follow-up. Surgical treatment for cardiomyopathy should be individualized for patients.

8. iPS cell development from DCM heart

Induced pluripotent stem (iPS) cell development is one of the most promising technologies in regenerative medicine [104]. iPS cell is evoked via the epigenetic silencing of somatic cells by the Yamanaka factors, i.e., the four transcription factors Oct4, Sox2, Klf4, and c-Myc. Advances in iPS cell reprogramming technology could allow aging or damaged cells to be replaced by the patient's own rejuvenated cells; therefore, the clinical application of iPS cell reprogramming technology may be a solution to the problem of age-related degenerative diseases. However, senescent or pathologic tissue has a relatively low reprogramming efficiency compared with juvenile or robust tissue, resulting in incomplete cell reprogramming. Our laboratory developed a new reprogramming method for generating iPS cells using pathologic somatic cells from a recipient heart that states the severe heart failure associated with DCM [105].

For gene transfection of iPS cell differentiation, in addition to the Yamanaka factors, GLIS1 and TET-1 were added. Gli-similar transcription factors (Glis) belong to the group of Krüppel-like zinc-finger transcription factors, and three GLIS genes (GLIS1–3) have been identified [106]. Yoshioka et al. reported that Yamanaka factor RNAs with Glis-1 RNA that were purified from an RNA-replicative vector yielded high-efficiency iPS cell reprogramming from older adult human cells [107]. Tet-1, which is one of DNA demethylase, contributes to the differentiation of the inner cell mass at the blastocyst stage and regulates the maintenance of ES cells by altering the DNA methylation status [108]. Olariu et al. found that TET1 could replace OCT4 in the iPS cell reprogramming Yamanaka

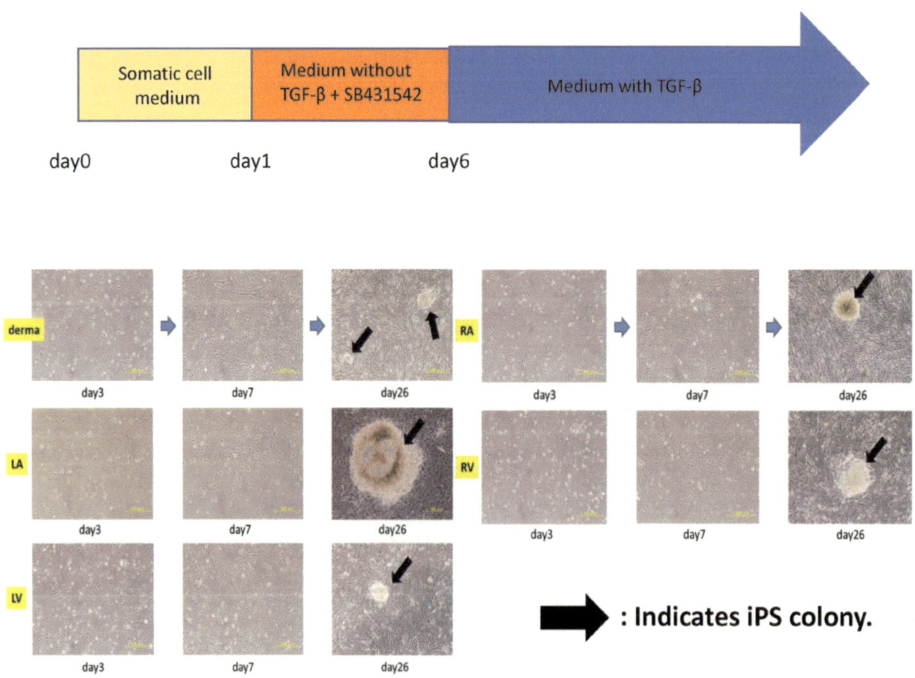

Figure 5.
Gene transfection.

cocktail and that DNA methylation is the key to regulating pluripotency genes [109]. Since Tet-1 may also evoke the induction of Dnmt3b expression upon transition to the epiblast stage, TET-1 was included in the final set of six genes to be transfected in our protocol.

Cardiac fibroblasts obtained from a recipient heart highly expressed α-smooth muscle actin (α-SMA) that is a representative marker of myofibroblast. Myofibroblasts occur at a converging spot of mesenchymal cells, resulting from acute or chronic inflammation caused by stimulation with TGF-β, Ang II, and cytokines [110]. Interestingly, the myofibroblasts from our patient's heart tissue did not differentiate into human iPS cells by previous methods [111]. Therefore, the cell culture medium for iPS cell induction was also prepared in detail. During the first 5 days post-transfection, TGF-β was removed from the cell culture medium for iPS cell induction, and selective TGF-β inhibitor SB431542 was added. Finally, by combining these methods, we developed a highly efficient method for inducing human iPS cells from pathologic somatic cells (**Figure 5**) [105].

9. Summary of cardiomyopathy recent findings

We outlined the recent findings of cardiomyopathy. In addition to the development of the cardiac devices and regenerative medicine, clinical trials of heart failure drugs such as ARNI, SGLT2 inhibitors and cardiac function improving drugs as mavacamten have shown effective results leading to desirable situation for cardiologists to expand their options. Our goal is to improve the QOL of cardiomyopathy patients.

Conflicts of interest

We confirm there are no conflicts of interest.

Author details

Yoshihiro Yamada[1], Keiki Sugi[1], Hiroyuki Nakajima[2] and Takaaki Senbonmatsu[1,3]*

1 Department of Cardiology, Saitama Medical University International Medical Center, Saitama, Japan

2 Department of Cardiovascular Surgery, Saitama Medical University International Medical Center, Saitama, Japan

3 Research Administration Center, Saitama Medical University, Saitama, Japan

*Address all correspondence to: senbont@saitama-med.ac.jp

References

[1] Goodwin JF, Gordon H, Hollman A, Bishop MB. Clinical aspects of cardiomyopathy. *Br Med J*. 1961; 1: 69–79.

[2] Report of the WHO/ISFC task force on the definition and classification of cardiomyopathies. *Br Heart J* 1980; 44: 672-673.

[3] Marcus FI, Fontaine GH, Guiraudon G, et al. Right ventricular dysplasia: a report of 24 adult cases. *Circulation*. 1982; 65: 384–398.

[4] Richardson P, McKenna W, Bristow M, et al. Report of the 1995 World Health Organization/ International Society and Federation of Cardiology Task Force on the Definition and Classification of cardiomyopathies. *Circulation* 1996; 93: 841-842.

[5] Maron BJ, Towbin JA, Thiene G, et al. Contemporary definitions and classification of the cardiomyopathies: an American Heart Association Scientific Statement from the Council on Clinical Cardiology, Heart Failure and Transplantation Committee; Quality of Care and Outcomes Research and Functional Genomics and Translational Biology Interdisciplinary Working Groups; and Council on Epidemiology and Prevention. *Circulation* 2006; 113: 1807-1816.

[6] Elliott P, Andersson B, Arbustini E, et al. Classification of the cardiomyopathies: a position statement from the European Society Of Cardiology Working Group on Myocardial and Pericardial Diseases. *Eur Heart J* 2008; 29: 270-276.

[7] *JCS 2018 Guideline on Diagnosis and Treatment of Cardiomyopathies*.

[8] Arbustini E, Narula N, Dec GW, et al. The MOGE(S) classification for a phenotype-genotype nomenclature of cardiomyopathy: endorsed by the World Heart Federation. *J Am Coll Cardiol*. 2013; 62:2046–2072.

[9] Codd MB, Sugrue DD, Gersh BJ, Melton LJ. Epidemiology of idiopathic dilated and hypertrophic cardiomyopathy: A population-based study in Olmsted County, Minnesota, 1975-1984. *Circulation*. 1989; 80(3): 564–572.

[10] Herman DS, Lam L, Taylor MRG, et al. Truncations of Titin Causing Dilated Cardiomyopathy. *N Engl J Med*. 2012; 366(7):619–628.

[11] Roberts AM, Ware JS, Herman DS, et al. Integrated allelic, transcriptional, and phenomic dissection of the cardiac effects of titin truncations in health and disease. *Sci Transl Med*. 2015; 7(270).

[12] Warren M. The approach to predictive medicine that is taking genomics research by storm. *Nature*. 2018; 562(7726):181–183.

[13] Jansweijer JA, Nieuwhof K, Russo F, et al. Truncating titin mutations are associated with a mild and treatable form of dilated cardiomyopathy. *Eur J Heart Fail*. 2017; 19(4):512–521.

[14] Van Rijsingen IAW, Arbustini E, Elliott PM, et al. Risk factors for malignant ventricular arrhythmias in Lamin A/C mutation carriers: A European cohort study. *J Am Coll Cardiol*. 2012; 59(5):493–500.

[15] Van Rijsingen IAW, Van Der Zwaag PA, Groeneweg JA, et al. Outcome in phospholamban R14del carriers results of a large multicentre cohort study. *Circ Cardiovasc Genet*. 2014; 7(4):455–465.

[16] Ortiz-Genga MF, Cuenca S, Dal Ferro M, et al. Truncating FLNC Mutations Are Associated With High-Risk Dilated and Arrhythmogenic

Cardiomyopathies. *J Am Coll Cardiol*. 2016; 68(22):2440–2451.

[17] Kühl U, Pauschinger M, Noutsias M, et al. High prevalence of viral genomes and multiple viral infections in the myocardium of adults with "idiopathic" left ventricular dysfunction. Circulation 2005;111(7):887–893.

[18] Inami T, Kataoka M, Shimura N, et al. Left ventricular dysfunction due to diffuse multiple vessel coronary artery spasm can be concealed in dilated cardiomyopathy. *Eur. J. Heart Fail*. 2012; 14(10):1130–1138.

[19] Eisenberg D, Jucker M. The amyloid state of proteins in human diseases. *Cell*. 2012; 148:1188-1203.

[20] Falk RH. Diagnosis and management of the cardiac amyloidoses. *Circulation*. 2005; 112:2047-2060.

[21] Dharmarajan K, Maurer MS. Transthyretin cardiac amyloidosis in older North Americans. *J Am Geriatr Soc*. 2012; 60:765-774.

[22] Cheng ZW, Tian Z, Kang L, et al. Electrocardiographic and echocardiographic features of patients with primary cardiac amyloidosis. *Zhonghua Xin Xue Guan Bing Za Zhi*. 2010; 38(7):606-609.

[23] Sokolow M, LyonTP. The ventricular complex in left ventricular hypertrophyas obtained by unipolar precordial and limb leads. *Am Heart J*. 1949; 37:161-186.

[24] Rapezzi C, Lorenzini M, Longhi S, et al. Cardiac amyloidosis: the great pretender. *Heart Fail Rev*. 2015; 20: 117-24.

[25] Connors LH, Sam F, Skinner M, et al. Heart failure resulting from age-related cardiac amyloid disease associated with wild-type transthyretin: a prospective, observational cohort study. *Circulation*. 2016; 133:282-290.

[26] White JA, Fine NM. Recent advances in cardiovascular imaging relevanttothe management of patients with suspected cardiac amyloidosis. *Curr Cardiol Rep*. 2016; 18:1-11.

[27] Vogelsberg H, Mahrholdt H, Deluigi CC, et al. Cardiovascular magnetic resonance in clinically suspected cardiac amyloidosis: noninvasive imaging compared to endomyocardial biopsy. *J Am Coll Cardiol*. 2008; 51:1022-1030.

[28] Simpson RM, Keegan J, Firmin DN. MR assessment of regional myocardial mechanics. *J Magn Reson Imaging*. 2013; 37:576-599.

[29] Bokhari S, Castaño A, Pozniakoff T, et al. 99mTc-pyrophosphate scintigraphy for differentiating light-chain cardiac amyloidosis from the transthyretin-related familial and senile cardiac amyloidoses. *Circ Cardiovasc Imaging*. 2013; 6:195-201.

[30] Kastritis E, Wechalekar AD, Dimopoulos MA, et al. Bortezomib with or without dexamethasone in primary systemic(light chain)amyloidosis. *J Clin Oncol*. 2010; 28: 1031-1037.

[31] Johnson SM, Connelly S, Fearns C, Powers ET, Kelly JW. The transthyretin amyloidoses: from delineating the molecular mechanism of aggregation linked to pathology to a regulatory-agency-approved drug. *J Mol Biol*. 2012; 421:185-203.

[32] Byg KE, Milman N, Hansen S. Sarcoidosis in Denmark 1980-1994. A registry-based incidence study comprising 5536 patients. *Sarcoidosis Vasc Diffuse Lung Dis*. 2003; 20(1):46-52.

[33] Morimoto T, Azuma A, Abe S, et al. Epidemiology of sarcoidosis in Japan. *Eur Respir J*. 2008; 31(2):372–379.

[34] Arkema EV, Cozier YC. Epidemiology of sarcoidosis: current findings and future directions. *Ther Adv Chronic Dis*. 2018; 24;9(11):227-240.

[35] Grunewald J, Grutters JC, Arkema E V, et al. Publisher Correction: Sarcoidosis. *Nat Rev Dis Prim*. 2019;5(1).

[36] Schupp JC, Freitag-Wolf S, Bargagli E, et al. Phenotypes of organ involvement in sarcoidosis. *Eur Respir J*. 2018; 51(1):1–11.

[37] Kosuge H, Noda M, Kakuta T, et al. Left ventricular apical aneurysm in cardiac sarcoidosis. *Jpn Heart J*. 2001; 42 (2):265-269.

[38] Hulten E, Aslam S, Osborne M, et al. Cardiac sarcoidosis-state of the art review. *Cardiovasc Diagn Ther*. 2016; 6 (1):50–63.

[39] Bozkurt B, Colvin M, Cook J, et al. Current Diagnostic and Treatment Strategies for Specific Dilated Cardiomyopathies: A Scientific Statement From the American Heart Association. *Circulation*. 2016 6;134(23): e579-e646.

[40] Armenian SH, Lacchetti C, Barac A, et al. Prevention and Monitoring of Cardiac Dysfunction in Survivors of Adult Cancers: American Society of Clinical Oncology Clinical Practice Guideline. *J Clin Oncol*. 2017 10; 35(8): 893-911.

[41] Chang HM, Moudgil R, Scarabelli T, Okwuosa TM, Yeh ETH. Cardiovascular Complications of Cancer Therapy: Best Practices in Diagnosis, Prevention, and Management: Part 1. *J Am Coll Cardiol*. 2017 14; 70(20):2536-2551.

[42] Lipshultz SE, Alvarez JA, Scully RE. Anthracycline associated cardiotoxicity in survivors of childhood cancer. *Heart*, 2008; 94(4):525–533.

[43] Garnock-Jones KP, Keating GM, Scott LJ. Trastuzumab: A review of its use as adjuvant treatment in human epidermal growth factor receptor 2 (HER2)-positive early breast cancer. *Drugs*. 2010; 70(2):215-239.

[44] Slamon DJ, Clark GM, Wong SG, et al. Human breast cancer: correlation of relapse and survival with amplification of the HER-2/neu oncogene. *Science*. 1987; 235(4785):177-182.

[45] Russell SD, Blackwell KL, Lawrence J, et al. Independent adjudication of symptomatic heart failure with the use of doxorubicin and cyclophosphamide followed by trastuzumab adjuvant therapy: a combined review of cardiac data from the National Surgical Adjuvant breast and Bowel Project B-31 and the North Central Cancer Treatment Group N9831 clinical trials. *J Clin Oncol*. 2010; 28(21): 3416-3421.

[46] Suter TM, Procter M, Van Veldhuisen DJ, et al. Trastuzumab-associated cardiac adverse effects in the herceptin adjuvant trial. *J Clin Oncol*. 2007; 25(25):3859–3865.

[47] Plana JC, Galderisi M, Barac A, et al. Expert consensus for multimodality imaging evaluation of adult patients during and after cancer therapy: A report from the American Society of Echocardiography and the European Association of Cardiovascular Imaging. *Eur Heart J Cardiovasc Imaging*. 2014; 15 (10):1063–1093.

[48] Cardinale D, Sandri MT, Colombo A, et al. Prognostic value of troponin I in cardiac risk stratification of cancer patients undergoing high-dose chemotherapy. *Circulation*. 2004; 109 (22):2749–2754.

[49] Elamm C, Fairweather D, Cooper LT. Pathogenesis and diagnosis of myocarditis. *Heart*. 2012; 98(11): 835-840.

[50] Cooper LT Jr, Keren A, Sliwa K, Matsumori A, Mensah GA. The global

burden of myocarditis: part 1: a systematic literature review for the Global Burden of Diseases, Injuries, and Risk Factors 2010 study. *Glob Heart*. 2014 Mar;9(1):121-129.

[51] Finsterer J, Stöllberger C, Towbin JA. Left ventricular noncompaction cardiomyopathy: cardiac, neuromuscular, and genetic factors. *Nat Rev Cardiol*. 2017;14(4): 224-237.

[52] Stöllberger C, Finsterer J, Blazek G. Left ventricular hypertrabeculation/ noncompaction and association with additional cardiac abnormalities and neuromuscular disorders. *Am. J. Cardiol.* 2002; 90, 899–902.

[53] Betrosian AP, Thireos E, Toutouzas K, et al. Occidental beriberi and sudden death. *Am J Med Sci*. 2004; 327: 250-252.

[54] Meyers DE, Basha HI, Koenig MK. Mitochondrial cardiomyopathy: pathophysiology, diagnosis, and management. *Tex Heart Inst J*. 2013; 40 (4):385-394.

[55] Meyers DE, Basha HI, Koenig MK. Cardiac manifestations of mitochondrial disorders. *Tex Heart Inst J*. 2013;40(5): 635-636.

[56] Schiffmann R. Fabry disease. *Handb Clin Neurol*. 2015; 132:231-248.

[57] Arends M, Wanner C, Hughes D, et al. Characterization of Classical and Nonclassical Fabry Disease: A Multicenter Study. *J Am Soc Nephrol*. 2017; 28(5):1631-1641.

[58] O'Mahony C, Elliott P. Anderson-Fabry disease and the heart. *Prog Cardiovasc Dis*. 2010; 52(4): 326-335.

[59] Niemann M, Herrmann S, Hu K, et al. Differences in Fabry cardiomyopathy between female and male patients: consequences for diagnostic assessment. *JACC Cardiovasc Imaging*. 2011; 4(6): 592-601.

[60] Kamiya CA, Kitakaze M, Ishibashi-Ueda H, et al. Different characteristics of peripartum cardiomyopathy between patients complicated with and without hypertensive disorders. –Results from the Japanese Nationwide survey of peripartum cardiomyopathy. *Circ J*. 2011; 75: 1975-1981.

[61] Sliwa K, Fett, J, Elkayam U. Peripartum cardiomyopathy. *Lancet*. 2006; 368: 687-693

[62] Muntoni F. Cardiomyopathy in muscular dystrophies. *Curr Opin Neurol*. 2003; 16(5):577-583.

[63] Verhaert D, Richards K, Rafael-Fortney JA, Raman SV. Cardiac involvement in patients with muscular dystrophies: magnetic resonance imaging phenotype and genotypic considerations. *Circ Cardiovasc Imaging*. 2011; 4(1):67-76.

[64] Argulian E, Sherrid MV, Messerli FH. Misconceptions and facts about hypertrophic cardiomyopathy. *Am J Med*. 2016; 129(2): 148-152.

[65] Spirito P, Seidman CE, McKenna WJ, Maron BJ. The management of hypertrophic cardiomyopathy. *N Engl J Med*. 1997; 336(11): 775-785.

[66] Gersh BJ, Maron BJ, Bonow RO, et al. American College of Cardiology Foundation/American Heart Association Task Force on Practice Guidelines; American Association for Thoracic Surgery; American Society of Echocardiography; American Society of Nuclear Cardiology; Heart Failure Society of America; Heart Rhythm Society; Society for Cardiovascular Angiography and Interventions; Society of Thoracic Surgeons. 2011 ACCF/AHA guideline for the diagnosis and treatment of hypertrophic cardiomyopathy: a report of the

American College of Cardiology Foundation/American Heart Association Task Force on Practice Guidelines. *Circulation*. 2011; 124(24): e783-e831.

[67] Effect of metoprolol CR/XL in chronic heart failure: Metoprolol CR/XL Randomised Intervention Trial in Congestive Heart Failure (MERIT-HF). *Lancet*. 1999; 353(9169): 2001-2007.

[68] Ryan TD, Madueme PC, Jefferies JL, et al. Utility of echocardiography in the assessment of left ventricular diastolic function and restrictive physiology in children and young adults with restrictive cardiomyopathy: a comparative echocardiography-catheterization study. *Pediatr Cardiol*. 2017; 38(2): 381-389.

[69] Dekker RL, Morton CH, Singleton P, Lyndon A. Women's experiences being diagnosed with peripartum cardiomyopathy: a qualitative study. *J Midwifery Womens Health*. 2016; 61(4): 467-473.

[70] Konno T, Chang S, Seidman JG, Seidman CE. Genetics of Hypertrophic Cardiomyopathy. *Curr Opin Cardiol*. 2010; 25(3): 10.

[71] Bos JM, Towbin JA, Ackerman MJ. Diagnostic, prognostic, and therapeutic implications of genetic testing for hypertrophic cardiomyopathy. J Am Coll Cardiol. 2009; 54(3): 201-211.

[72] Bennett RG, Haqqani HM, Berruezo A, et al. Arrhythmogenic Cardiomyopathy in 2018-2019: ARVC/ALVC or Both? *Heart Lung Circ*. 2019; 28(1):164-177.

[73] Corrado D, Basso C, Judge DP. Arrythmogenic cardiomyopathy. *Circ Res*. 2017;121(7):784-802.

[74] Romero J, Mejia-Lopez E, Manrique C, Lucariello R. Arrhythmogenic Right Ventricular Cardiomyopathy (ARVC/D): A Systematic Literature Review. *Clin Med Insights Cardiol*. 2013; 7: 97–114.

[75] Ackerman M, Atkins DL, Triedman JK. Sudden cardiac death in the young. *Circulation*. 2016; 133(10): 1006–1026.

[76] Muchtar E, Blauwet LA, Gertz MA. Restrictive cardiomyopathy Genetics, Pathogenesis, Clinical Manifestations, Diagnosis, and Therapy. *Circ Res*. 2017; 121:819–837

[77] Yancy CW, Jessup M, Bozkurt B, et al. 2017 ACC/AHA/HFSA Focused Update of the 2013 ACCF/AHA Guideline for the Management of Heart Failure: A Report of the American College of Cardiology/American Heart Association Task Force on Clinical Practice Guidelines and the Heart Failure Society of America. *Circulation*. 2017; 136(6): e137-e161.

[78] Ponikowski P, Voors AA, Anker SD, et al. ESC Scientific Document Group. 2016 ESC Guidelines for the diagnosis and treatment of acute and chronic heart failure: The Task Force for the diagnosis and treatment of acute and chronic heart failure of the European Society of Cardiology (ESC) Developed with the special contribution of the Heart Failure Association (HFA) of the ESC. *Eur Heart J*. 2016; 37(27): 2129-2200.

[79] Tomasoni D, Adamo M, Lombardi CM, Metra M. Highlight in heart failure. *ESC Heart Fail*. 2019; 6(6): 1105-1127.

[80] Kawas RF, Anderson RL, Ingle SRB, et al. A small-molecule modulator of cardiac myosin acts on multiple stages of the myosin chemomechanical cycle. *J Biol Chem* 2017; **292:** 16571–16577.

[81] Anderson RL, Trivedi DV, Sarkar SS, et al. Deciphering the super relaxed state of human β-cardiac myosin and the mode of action of mavacamten

from myosin molecules to muscle fibers. *Proc Natl Acad Sci U S A*. 2018; 115(35): E8143-E8152.

[82] Green EM, Wakimoto H, Anderson RL, et al. A small-molecule inhibitor of sarcomere contractility suppresses hypertrophic cardiomyopathy in mice. *Science*. 2016; 351(6273):617-621.

[83] Heitner SB, Jacoby D, Lester SJ, et al. Mavacamten treatment for obstructive hypertrophic cardiomyopathy: a clinical trial. *Ann Intern Med* 2019; 170: 741–748.

[84] Olivotto I, Oreziak A, Barriales-Villa R, et al. EXPLORER-HCM study investigators. Mavacamten for treatment of symptomatic obstructive hypertrophic cardiomyopathy (EXPLORER-HCM): a randomised, double-blind, placebo-controlled, phase 3 trial. *Lancet*. 2020; 396(10253): 759-769.

[85] Peteiro J, Barriales-Villa R, Larranaga-Moreira JM, et al. Value of a comprehensive exercise echocardiography assessment for patients with hypertrophic cardiomyopathy. *J Cardiol*. 2020; S0914-5087(20)30396-30398.

[86] Cui H, Schaff HV, Abel MD, et al. Left ventricular ejection hemodynamics before and after relief of outflow tract obstruction in patients with hypertrophic obstructive cardiomyopathy and valvular aortic stenosis. *J Thorac Cardiovasc Surg*. 2020; 159:844-852 e1.

[87] Biesbroek PB, Croisille P, Clarysse P, et al. Myocardial adaptation after surgical therapy differs for aortic valve stenosis and hypertrophic obstructive cardiomyopathy. *Int J Cardiovasc Imaging*. 2019; 35:1089-1100.

[88] Rankin JS, Grau-Sepulveda M, Shahian DM, et al. The Impact of Mitral Disease Etiology on Operative Mortality After Mitral Valve Operations. Ann Thorac Surg. 2018; 106:1406-1413.

[89] Balaram SK, Ross RE, Sherrid MV, et al. Role of mitral valve plication in the surgical management of hypertrophic cardiomyopathy. *Ann Thorac Surg*. 2012; 94:1990-1997; discussion 1997-8.

[90] Halpern DG, Swistel DG, Po JR, et al. Echocardiography before and after resect-plicate-release surgical myectomy for obstructive hypertrophic cardiomyopathy. *J Am Soc Echocardiogr*. 2015; 28:1318-1328.

[91] Balaram SK, Tyrie L, Sherrid MV, et al. Resection-plication-release for hypertrophic cardiomyopathy: clinical and echocardiographic follow-up. *Ann Thorac Surg*. 2008; 86:1539-1544; discussion 1544-5.

[92] Obadia JF, Basillais N, Armoiry X, et al. Hypertrophic cardiomyopathy: the edge-to-edge secures the correction of the systolic anterior motion. *Eur J Cardiothorac Surg*. 2017; 51:638-643.

[93] Nakajima H, Tokunaga C, Hayashi J, et al. Trapezoidal resection of an elongated anterior mitral leaflet and Alfieri stitch in hypertrophic cardiomyopathy. *J Cardiothorac Surg*. 2020; 15:311.

[94] Ferrazzi P, Spirito P, Iacovoni A, et al. Transaortic Chordal Cutting: Mitral Valve Repair for Obstructive Hypertrophic Cardiomyopathy With Mild Septal Hypertrophy. *J Am Coll Cardiol*. 2015; 66:1687-1696.

[95] Nishimura RA, Otto CM, Bonow RO, et al. 2017 AHA/ACC Focused Update of the 2014 AHA/ACC Guideline for the Management of Patients With Valvular Heart Disease: A Report of the American College of Cardiology/American Heart Association Task Force on Clinical Practice

Guidelines. *J Am Coll Cardiol.* 2017; 70: 252-289.

[96] Asgar AW, Mack MJ, Stone GW. Secondary mitral regurgitation in heart failure: pathophysiology, prognosis, and therapeutic considerations. J Am Coll Cardiol 2015; 65:1231-1248.

[97] Noack T, Marin Cuartas M, Kiefer P, et al. Isolated Mitral Valve Repair in Patients with Reduced Left Ventricular Ejection Fraction. *Ann Thorac Cardiovasc Surg*. 2019; 25:326-335.

[98] Xu D, McBride E, Kalra K, et al. Undersizing mitral annuloplasty alters left ventricular mechanics in a swine model of ischemic mitral regurgitation. *J Thorac Cardiovasc Surg*. 2020; S0022-5223(20)33010-33015.

[99] Kainuma S, Funatsu T, Kondoh H, et al. Beneficial effects of restrictive annuloplasty on subvalvular geometry in patients with functional mitral regurgitation and advanced cardiomyopathy. *J Thorac Cardiovasc Surg*. 2018; 156:630-638 e1.

[100] Theron A, Morera P, Resseguier N, et al. Long-term results of surgical treatment of secondary severe mitral regurgitation in patients with end-stage heart failure: Advantage of prosthesis insertion. *Arch Cardiovasc Dis*. 2019; 112: 95-103.

[101] Howlett JG, Stebbins A, Petrie MC, et al. STICH Trial Investigators. CABG Improves Outcomes in Patients With Ischemic Cardiomyopathy: 10-Year Follow-Up of the STICH Trial. *JACC Heart Fail*. 2019; 7:878-887.

[102] Stefanelli G, Bellisario A, Meli M, et al. Outcomes after surgical ventricular restoration for ischemic cardiomyopathy. *J Thorac Cardiovasc Surg*. 2020; S0022-5223(20)31236-31238.

[103] Jones RH, Velazquez EJ, Michler RE, et al. STICH Hypothesis 2 Investigators. Coronary bypass surgery with or without surgical ventricular reconstruction. *N Engl J Med*. 2009; 360: 1705-1717.

[104] Takahashi K, Tanab, K, Ohnuki M, et al. Induction of pluripotent stem cells from adult human fibroblasts by defined factors. *Cell*. 2007; 131, 861–872.

[105] Tanaka N, Kato H, Tsuda H, et al. Development of a High-Efficacy Reprogramming Method for Generating Human Induced Pluripotent Stem (iPS) Cells from Pathologic and Senescent Somatic Cells. *Int J Mol Sci*. 2020; 21 (18):6764.

[106] Jetten AM. GLIS1–3 transcription factors: Critical roles in the regulation of multiple physiological processes and diseases. *Cell Mol. Life Sci*. 2018; 75, 3473–3494.

[107] Yoshioka N, Dowdy SF. Enhanced generation of iPSCs from older adult human cells by a synthetic five-factor self-replicative RNA. *PLoS ONE*. 2017; 12, e182018.

[108] Ito S, D'Alessio AC, Taranova OV, et al. Role of Tet proteins in 5mC to 5hmC conversion, ES-cell self-renewal and inner cell mass specification. *Nature*. 2010; 466, 1129–1133.

[109] Olariu V, Lövkvist C, Sneppen K. Nanog, Oct4 and Tet1 interplay in establishing pluripotency. *Sci. Rep*. 2016; 6, 25438.

[110] Hinz B. Myofibroblasts. *Exp. Eye Res*. 2016; 142, 56–70.

[111] Khoo TS, Jamal R, Abdul Ghani NA, et al. Retention of somatic memory associated with cell identity, age and metabolism in induced pluripotent stem (iPS) cells reprogramming. *Stem Cell Rev. Rep*. 2020; 16, 251–261.

Chapter 3

Cardiomyopathy Etiologies, Symptoms and Management

Waleed Kian, Melanie Zemel, Emily H. Kestenbaum, Wafeek Alguayn, Boris Shvarts, Adam A. Sharb, Dina Levitas, Yousef Kian, Nir Peled and Alexander Yakobson

Abstract

Cardiomyopathy can be defined as a structural and functional myocardial disorder that is commonly genetic rather than due to coronary artery, valvular or congenital heart disease. It can be subcategorized into dilated, hypertrophic, restrictive, unclassified, and arrhythmogenic right ventricular cardiomyopathy/dysplasia. They can be further subdivided into primary and secondary cardiomyopathy. Primary includes genetics (HOCM, ARVC/D), mixed (DCM, RCM) or acquired (stress-induced, myocarditis) causes; while secondary cardiomyopathy is derived from the involvement of other organ systems. Cardiomyopathies can be identified by echocardiogram to display the anatomic and functional changes related to each subtype including systolic or diastolic dysfunction. In certain instances, cardiac-MRI or CT are used to further elucidate its specific characteristics such as fatty infiltration and focal hypertrophy. Treatment is very diverse and catered to each individual case. This will all be further elaborated on in the following chapter.

Keywords: cardiomyopathy, heart diseases, systolic dysfunction, diastolic dysfunction

1. Introduction

Cardiomyopathies are a heterogeneous group of diseases of the myocardium that are associated with mechanical and/or electrical dysfunction. They generally exhibit inappropriate ventricular hypertrophy or dilation and have multiple etiologies, which are often genetic [1]. They can be further subdivided into primary and secondary cardiomyopathy. Primary includes genetics, acquired or mixed causes; while secondary cardiomyopathy is derived from the involvement of other organ systems. Cardiomyopathies can be identified by echocardiogram to display the anatomic and functional changes related to each subtype including systolic or diastolic dysfunction. In certain instances, cardiac-Magnetic resonance imaging or Computer tomography scans are used to further elucidate its specific characteristics such as fatty infiltration and focal hypertrophy. Treatment is very diverse and catered to each individual case. This will all be further elaborated on in the following chapter.

IntechOpen

2. Primary and secondary cardiomyopathy

Cardiomyopathies can be characterized into two different groups, primary and secondary. Primary cardiomyopathies are defined by primary involvement of the heart while secondary cardiomyopathies are consequences of other medical disease states such as endocrine diseases or drug induced. Primary cardiomyopathies can be further divided by their causes. These include cardiomyopathies of genetic, acquired, or mixed origin [1].

Genetic sources of primary cardiomyopathy include hypertrophic cardiomyopathy (HCM), arrhythmogenic right ventricular cardiomyopathy/dysplasia (ARVC/D), mitochondrial myopathies and ion channel disorders. Mixed causes of primary cardiomyopathy can include dilated cardiomyopathy (DCM) and restrictive cardiomyopathy (RCM). Finally, the acquired causes of primary cardiomyopathy include a wide variety of diseases, such as myocarditis, peripartum cardiomyopathy, stress-induced cardiomyopathy (Takotsubo) and tachycardia-induced cardiomyopathy. These are all summarized in **Table 1**.

Primary Cardiomyopathy
Genetic Causes: Hypertrophic Cardiomyopathy, arrhythmogenic right ventricular cardiomyopathy/dysplasia, mitochondrial myopathies and ion channel disorders
Acquired Causes: Myocarditis, Peripartum cardiomyopathy, stress-induced cardiomyopathy and tachycardia-induced cardiomyopathy
Mixed Causes: Dilated cardiomyopathy and Restrictive cardiomyopathy
Secondary Cardiomyopathy
Toxin induced, medication induced, Endocrine disorders, autoimmune/collagen diseases, nutritional deficiencies.

Table 1.
Primary and secondary causes of cardiomyopathy.

3. Systolic and diastolic dysfunction

Systolic dysfunction is defined as a decrease in the contractility of the heart [2]. Contractility can be reduced throughout the left ventricle (LV), as seen in DCM, or only in a portion of the LV, as seen in stress-induced cardiomyopathy. Systolic dysfunction is also classically seen following myocardial ischemia. Initially, cardiac output is maintained through compensatory mechanisms which include an increased preload in order to improve contractility (Frank-Starling relationship) and enlargement of the LV to increase the stroke volume. However, these mechanisms ultimately fail and lead to the clinical manifestations of heart failure. Systolic dysfunction can be evaluated through echocardiogram (echo) and is characterized by a decreased left ventricular ejection fraction (LVEF) and increased end diastolic volume (EDV).

Diastolic dysfunction is characterized by abnormal myocardial filling and relaxation with concurrent elevated filling pressures. It can occur in combination with systolic dysfunction or it can be an isolated phenomenon. Its main features are due to impairment of active relaxation and/or passive compliance during LV diastole. This takes place during both isovolumetric relaxation and early rapid filling. Diastolic dysfunction is a common characteristic of both HCM and RCM and can sometimes be seen in patients with DCM. It is also found secondary to myocardial hypertrophy presenting with decreased compliance. An echo study is done to identify diastolic dysfunction where a normal LVEF and EDV are seen, however occasionally systolic function may be impaired. These two markers are one way to differentiate diastolic from systolic dysfunction, both of which lead to a common clinical endpoint of heart failure symptoms.

3.1 Dilated cardiomyopathy

Dilated cardiomyopathy (DCM) manifests as global dilation of one or both ventricles leading to systolic dysfunction. Left ventricular ejection fraction is ≤40% and affected patients can develop symptomatic heart failure (HF). DCM causes around 10,000 deaths and 46,000 hospitalizations in the United States each year. Idiopathic DCM is the leading indication for heart transplantation [3]. Affected patients are generally between 20 and 60 years of age [4]. Symptoms vary, but most patients present with HF symptoms of progressive dyspnea with exertion, peripheral edema, orthopnea, and/or paroxysmal nocturnal dyspnea. Conduction disturbances, cardiomegaly, thromboembolic disease, and sudden death can also be observed [5, 6].

There are many causes of DCM including idiopathic, stress-induced, myocarditis, infiltrative disease (amyloidosis, sarcoidosis, hemochromatosis), peripartum cardiomyopathy, tachycardia-mediated, infections, drugs (alcohol, cocaine, anthracyclines) [7], as well as others illustrated in the **Table 2**.

DCM is frequently idiopathic, indicated after exclusion of both primary and secondary causes of cardiac disease except genetic causes. Familial disease is seen in about 50% of patients with idiopathic DCM. The disease is generally inherited in autosomal dominant fashion but also other forms of inheritance (autosomal recessive, X-linked, and mitochondrial). Mutations in more than 30 genes were identified in the past 20 years. Sarcomere genes are responsible for about 30% of familial DCM cases. These include mutations in genes for beta myosin heavy chain (MYH7), cardiac troponin T (TNNT2), titin (TTN), alpha-tropomyosin (TPM1), and cardiac troponin C (TNNC1) [8].

Infectious diseases: adenovirus, HIV, influenza virus, coxsackie virus, streptococci-rheumatic fever, diphtheria, typhoid fever
Deposition diseases: amyloidosis, hemochromatosis
Medications: antiretroviral drugs (didanosine, zidovudine, zalcitabine), chemotherapeutic agents (cyclophosphamide, anthracyclines, trastuzumab), chloroquine, hydroxychloroquine, phenothiazines, clozapine
Toxins: ethanol, amphetamines, cocaine, lead, mercury, lithium, carbon monoxide
Nutritional deficiencies: niacin, selenium, thiamine, carnitine
Electrolyte and renal abnormalities: hypophosphatemia, uremia, hypocalcemia
Autoimmune/inflammatory: rheumatoid arthritis, systemic lupus erythematosis, scleroderma, dermatomyositis, sarcoidosis, giant cell arteritis, kawasaki disease
Endocrinologic disorders: growth hormone and thyroid hormone excess/deficiency, diabetes mellitus, pheochromocytoma, cushing's syndrome
Genetic: duchenne's muscular dystrophy, familial and sporadic genetic cardiomyopathies, friedreich's ataxia, myotonic dystrophy, arrhythmogenic right ventricular cardiomyopathy
Other: tachycardia, peripartum cardiomyopathy, hypothermia, heat stroke, sleep apnea

Table 2.
Etiologies of dilated cardiomyopathy.

3.2 Hypertrophic cardiomyopathy

Hypertrophic cardiomyopathy (HCM) is a disease of the heart muscle that is mainly due to genetic mutations in sarcomere genes, the contractile component of the heart. The prevalence of HCM is about 0.5% in adults and typically has an autosomal dominant transmission pattern [9]. HCM is defined by left ventricular hypertrophy (LVH), which manifests with a multitude of different clinical features. The location and amount of hypertrophy will determine the clinical presentation which can include left ventricular outflow tract (LVOT) obstruction, myocardial ischemia, diastolic dysfunction and mitral regurgitation.

HCM presents with a huge spectrum of signs and symptoms; patients can be asymptomatic or present with symptoms of chest pain, arrhythmias, or those related to HF [10]. Many patients are diagnosed with HCM incidentally during a routine doctor visit by identification of an abnormal ECG or murmur and through family screening protocols. Otherwise, patients can present with many different symptoms including dyspnea on exertion, fatigue, chest pain, palpitations, and presyncope or syncope commonly after exertion.

The most common presenting symptom is HF seen clinically as dyspnea on exertion. This is found in approximately 90% of symptomatic patients and can result from diastolic dysfunction caused by hypertrophy, impaired LV emptying from the LVOT obstruction, and mitral regurgitation. Concurrent systolic dysfunction is also seen in very extensive disease due to adverse LV remodeling [11].

Another common symptom is angina, both typical (following exertion) and atypical, which is frequently worsened after heavy meals. The pathophysiology behind this chest pain in HCM can be broken down into two categories: increased myocardial oxygen demand and decreased myocardial blood flow. HCM increases oxygen demand in several ways including increased muscle mass, myocardial hypertrophy and disarray, and increased diastolic pressures due to LVOT obstruction. Causes of decreased myocardial blood flow in HCM is due to decreased ability of coronary arterioles to vasodilate and myocardial fibrosis.

Arrhythmias are also a major complication of HCM as they can lead to sudden cardiac death (SCD) [12]. Both supraventricular and ventricular arrhythmias are found which can lead to palpitations, dyspnea, presyncope, syncope, and SCD. Of the supraventricular arrhythmias, atrial fibrillation (AF) is the most common [12].

Syncope occurs in around 15–25% of patients with HCM and is caused by a variety of mechanisms which ultimately lead to decreased cardiac output. Some of these include AF, LVOT obstruction and conduction abnormalities such as atrioventricular nodal block. Syncope not due to vasovagal or cardiogenic causes is an increased risk for SCD, especially when occurring in young patients. Predictors of SCD includes experiencing at least one syncopal episode include a family history of SCD from HCM, massive LVH, unexplained syncope, LV apical aneurysm, HCM with LV systolic dysfunction [13, 14].

Paradoxical Split of S2
Brisk and Bifid Carotid Pulse
Prominent a wave seen in neck veins
Diffuse, forceful LV apical impulse
Systolic thrill
Parasternal lift

Table 3.
Physical exam findings in hypertrophic cardiomyopathy.

Just as there are a variety of clinical symptoms, the physical exam of a patient with HCM can range from normal to several nonspecific findings. These findings include a systolic crescendo-decrescendo murmur that is similar to the murmur seen with aortic stenosis, a fourth heart sound. Physical exam findings are mainly caused by LVOT obstruction thus if there is minimal or no obstruction, the physical exam will commonly be normal. Other physical exam findings are not specific to HCM and can be seen with other heart diseases. They are listed in the following **Table 3**.

The histology of HCM is unique, showing myocyte hypertrophy and myofibrillar disarray with interstitial fibrosis. Coronary arterioles with decreased luminal cross-sectional area can also be seen. These arterioles have reduced ability to vasodilate leading to decreased myocardial blood flow during periods of stress [15].

3.3 Restrictive cardiomyopathy

Restrictive cardiomyopathy (RCM) presents as non-dilated ventricles and diastolic dysfunction. It causes a ventricular filling defect, leading to elevated pressure and biatrial enlargement. Systolic function is generally normal unless RCM becomes more severe.

RCM is significantly less common universally than both DCM and HCM. However, mortality from RCM is high in Africa, South and Central America, and Asia. This is due to a higher incidence of endomyocardial fibrosis, which is one of the major causes of RCM.

There are several causes of RCM including infiltrative, familial non-infiltrative, storage diseases, other disorders (scleroderma, endomyocardial fibrosis, diabetic cardiomyopathy), secondary causes, and idiopathic RCM [16]. The various etiologies are demonstrated in **Table 4**.

RCM presents as pulmonary and systemic congestion with peripheral edema, dyspnea, palpitations, weakness, and inadequate cardiac output with exercise. Severe RCM can have elevated central venous pressure, ascites, and hepatosplenomegaly [17]. In addition, autonomic dysfunction leading to arrhythmias can occur. During auscultation, a third heart sound can be heard. Jugular venous pressure (JVP) is often elevated with a prominent y descent. Kussmaul's sign with an increase in JVP with inspiration may be observed. These two JVP signs are seen in constrictive pericarditis as well.

3.4 Arrhythmogenic right ventricular cardiomyopathy

Arrhythmogenic right ventricular cardiomyopathy (ARVC) is defined by right ventricular (RV) origin arrhythmias and structural abnormalities. The myocardium

Infiltrative disorders: amyloidosis, Gaucher disease, sarcoidosis, fatty infiltration, and Hurler syndrome
Familial: familial cardiomyopathy with unknown gene, sarcomeric protein mutations (troponin I, essential light chain of myosin), familial amyloidosis, pseudoxanthoma elasticum, and desminopathy, hemochromatosis, Fabry disease, glycogen storage disease
Storage diseases: Fabry disease, hemochromatosis, and glycogen storage disease.
Other disorders: scleroderma, diabetic cardiomyopathy, endomyocardial fibrosis (caused by hypereosinophilic syndrome, drugs, or idiopathic), chemotherapy, radiation, metastatic cancers, and carcinoid heart disease.
Secondary causes: hypertension, dilated cardiomyopathy, or ischemic heart disease
Idiopathic RCM

Table 4.
Etiologies of restrictive cardiomyopathy.

is scarred and replaced with fibrous or fibro-fatty tissue. Scarring can occur first regionally and then become global leading to RV dilation, RV dysfunction, and wall motion abnormalities. Demonstration of biventricular myocardial injury is illustrated through the use of autopsy investigations, genotype and phenotype correlation studies and cardiac MRI. However, these diagnostic tools show an equal or increased extent of left ventricular severity when compared to the right ventricular involvement. This development has led to a new understanding of arrhythmogenic cardiomyopathy(ACM) [18]. ACM/ARVC is generally inherited in an autosomal dominant fashion. However, autosomal recessive inheritance has also been noted as in the cardiocutaneous syndrome, Naxos disease [19]. Patients can present with palpitations, dizziness, syncope, atypical chest pain, and dyspnea, but many are asymptomatic. The most common arrhythmia of ARVC is monomorphic ventricular tachycardia with a left bundle branch block. SCD can be the initial presentation of ARVC [20].

3.5 Stress-induced cardiomyopathy

Stress-induced cardiomyopathy, also known as takotsubo cardiomyopathy or broken heart syndrome, is characterized as brief systolic dysfunction in the absence of coronary artery disease that is usually brought on by stress. The systolic dysfunction is focal and mainly limited to the cardiac apex which is in contrast to DCM where we see global systolic dysfunction.

Patient presentation is similar to that of a patient with ST-elevation myocardial infarction (STEMI). It is more common in elderly women. About 1–2 percent of patients that are troponin positive with a suspected STEMI are diagnosed with stress-induced cardiomyopathy [21]. As in a STEMI, the most common presenting symptom is substernal chest pain with or without dyspnea. The pathophysiology of this disease is not very well understood but it is thought to be in part due to catecholamine excess thus cocaine-related ACS should be ruled out.

3.6 Cirrhotic cardiomyopathy

Cirrhosis which leads to systolic and/or diastolic myocardial dysfunction independent of alcohol consumption has been termed cirrhotic cardiomyopathy. The pathophysiology of this disease is not well established. Patients may have normal or increased cardiac output at rest but the myocardium inadequately responds when placed under stress. ECG findings can include QT interval prolongation and mechanical and electrical desynchrony. Structurally, the LV is normal, but the left atrium is generally dilated. Treatment is mostly supportive but the orthotropic liver transplantation has been shown to improve patient's condition [22].

4. Diagnosis

Diagnosis of the various cardiomyopathies are done by clinical presentation (chest pain, fatigue, dyspnea, syncope, etc.), physical exam, diagnostic tools (12-lead ECG, chest radiograph, echocardiography, cardiac MRI, doppler ultrasound), genetic testing, endomyocardial biopsy, and/or plasma BNP. Systolic dysfunction is observed in DCM and stress-induced cardiomyopathy as decreased LVEF and increased EDV on echo. Diastolic dysfunction is observed in HCM and RCM and can sometimes occur in DCM. An echo of diastolic dysfunction demonstrates normal LVEF and EDV.

Dilated cardiomyopathy demonstrates systolic dysfunction, ventricular dilation, myocyte hypertrophy and fibrosis, and possible conduction system involvement.

Familial DCM is diagnosed when idiopathic DCM is seen in two or more close relatives. A three to four generation family history and clinical screening (history, exam, electrocardiogram, echocardiogram) of first-degree relatives is done when a new diagnosis is made to identify asymptomatic/undetected disease. Genetic testing is also done for known familial DCM and nonfamilial without an obvious alternative cause. Screening for specific mutations does not necessarily determine therapy, but certain genes are related to clinical characteristics. This may affect family counseling, screening, and influence of primary prevention or pre-symptomatic therapy [23].

Hypertrophic cardiomyopathy should be suspected if there is a positive family history of the disease, clinical symptoms, an abnormal 12-lead ECG, or if a systolic ejection murmur is heard. In addition, increased LV wall thickness (≥15 mm) seen anywhere in the LV wall without any identifiable cause such as valvular disease or hypertension is suggestive of the HCM [24]. Other findings are not required to make a diagnosis of HCM but may include a hyperdynamic LV or systolic anterior motion of the mitral valve seen on echo.

Restrictive cardiomyopathy is diagnosed as non-dilated, non-hypertrophied ventricles with biatrial enlargement seen on echo. Abnormal ventricular filling is visualized with Doppler imaging. Although RCM is generally characterized as non-hypertrophied, the LV may have increased wall thickness if due to infiltrative or storage disease. Echo, cardiac MRI, and endomyocardial biopsy can all be used to differentiate various types of RCM. Chest radiograph can demonstrate cardiomegaly with atrial enlargement, pulmonary venous congestion, and pleural effusions.

RCM appears similar to constrictive pericarditis with impaired ventricular filling but is distinguished by echo, MRI, CT, and endomyocardial biopsy. A patient history can also differentiate the two since possible causes of constrictive pericarditis include different causes such as tuberculosis, malignancy, connective tissue disease. Plasma BNP indicates LV wall stretching and helps separate RCM from constrictive pericarditis. Levels of ≥400 pg./mL indicate RCM due to the limited wall stretch in constrictive pericarditis from very stiff and thickened endocardium [25].

Arrhythmogenic right ventricular cardiomyopathy echo shows dilation of the RV and its outflow tract, aneurysm, akinesis, and dyskinesis. Genetic testing is recommended (DSC2, DSP, DSG2, JUP, TMEM43, and PKP2).

In order to identify stress-induced cardiomyopathy, it is very important to take a thorough history as a physical stress or emotional trigger may sometimes be identified and can help lead to the diagnosis. Stress induced cardiomyopathy should be considered when a patient presents with signs and symptoms of acute coronary syndrome along with an abnormal ECG that are out of proportion to elevations in cardiac biomarkers [26]. The diagnostic criteria consist of four required findings: transient LV systolic dysfunction that is typically regional and contains more than one epicardial coronary distribution, no obstructive coronary disease in the area of the wall motion abnormality, new ECG abnormalities including ST-elevation and/or T wave inversion or moderately elevated cardiac troponin and lastly no pheochromocytoma or myocarditis present [27]. Apical ballooning is also commonly seen as a result of wall akinesia. Therefore, in order to diagnose stress induced cardiomyopathy, the patient must undergo an ECG, coronary angiography and an echo in order to assess LV systolic function.

5. Management

Management of the cardiomyopathies are generally directed towards relieving symptoms, slowing progression of the disease, and preventing SCD. The specific therapy depends on whether the patient is suffering from systolic dysfunction, diastolic dysfunction, fluid overload and/or arrhythmias.

Patients with HF with reduced ejection fraction, like DCM, are managed with beta blockers(BBs), nondihydropyridine calcium channel blocker (ndCCB), angiotensin converting enzyme inhibitors (ACEi), angiotensin II receptor blockers (ARBs), pacemakers, and implantable cardioverter-defibrillators (ICD) for arrhythmias [28].

HCM and RCM present mainly with diastolic dysfunction. Therefore, treatment is aimed at lowering heart rate to increase diastolic filling time and decreasing venous pressure [28]. Loop diuretics are used to relieve congestion, but careful monitoring is needed to prevent hypoperfusion. In HCM they are generally avoided since it can worsen the LVOT obstruction. In both HCM and RCM, BBs and CCBs can improve the patient's diastolic dysfunction by decreasing heart rate and increasing filling time. For HCM, they are generally only given when a patient is symptomatic.

For patients with HCM, if symptoms continue despite adequate medical management, dual therapy with another negative inotrope is recommended. This can include beta blocker + disopyramide, nondihydropyridine calcium channel blocker + disopyramide, or beta blocker + nondihydropyridine calcium channel blocker. If patients still have refractory symptoms and have a LVOT gradient of ≥50 mmHg then septal reduction therapy can be considered [29].

In addition, patients with RCM can benefit from ACEi/ARBs, which might reduce myocardial stiffness. Dual chamber pacemaker is used with advanced AV block, anticoagulants are used for patients with atrial fibrillation, and cardiac transplantation is indicated for patients with intractable heart failure [28].

Patients suffering from ARVC should minimize their strenuous physical activity since there is a significant association between exercise and ARVC. Beta blockers are recommended for patients with clinical symptoms but not asymptomatic patients with a positive genotype. ICDs are indicated for patients who were previously resuscitated from SCD and those with sustained ventricular arrhythmias. If beta blockers and ICDs are not helpful, antiarrhythmic drugs or radiofrequency ablation can serve as adjunct therapy. Management of patients with RV dysfunction is similar to other patients with HF with reduced ejection fraction (ACEi, ARBs, mineralocorticoid receptor antagonist, diuretics, and BBs).

Stress-induced cardiomyopathy is a transient disorder that will likely resolve within a couple of weeks and thus its mainstay in management is supportive. However, the mortality rate is about 3–4 percent. During the acute onset and following stabilization, heart failure management is started following current guidelines. Anticoagulation is also provided similarly to patients that are post-myocardial infarction [30].

Author contributions

Conception and design: All authors. Manuscript writing: All authors. Final approval of manuscript: All authors.

Funding

None.

Conflicts of interest

All the authors have no conflicts of interest to declare.

DOI: http://dx.doi.org/10.5772/intechopen.95566

Ethical statement

The authors are accountable for all aspects of the work in ensuring that questions related to the accuracy or integrity of any part of the work are appropriately investigated and resolved.

Author details

Waleed Kian[1†], Melanie Zemel[2†], Emily H. Kestenbaum[2†], Wafeek Alguayn[3], Boris Shvarts[4], Adam A. Sharb[2], Dina Levitas[1], Yousef Kian[5], Nir Peled[1*] and Alexander Yakobson[1]

1 The Legacy Heritage Oncology Center and Dr. Larry Norton Institute, Soroka Medical Center and Ben-Gurion University, Beer-Sheva, Israel

2 Faculty of Health Sciences, Ben-Gurion University of the Negev, Beer-Sheva, Israel

3 Department of Cardiac Surgery, Soroka Medical Center, Beer-Sheva, Israel

4 Internal Medicine Ward, Soroka Medical Center and Ben-Gurion University, Beer-Sheva, Israel

5 Internal Medicine Ward, Barzilai Medical Center, Ashkelon, Israel

*Address all correspondence to: peled.nir@gmail.com

† These three authors equally contributed to this work.

References

[1] B.J. Maron, J.A. Towbin, G. Thiene, C. Antzelevitch, D. Corrado, D. Arnett, A.J. Moss, C.E. Seidman, J.B. Young, Contemporary definitions and classification of the cardiomyopathies: An American Heart Association Scientific Statement from the Council on Clinical Cardiology, Heart Failure and Transplantation Committee; Quality of Care and Outcomes Research and Functional Genomics and Translational Biology Interdisciplinary Working Groups; and Council on Epidemiology and Prevention, Circulation. 113 (2006) 1807-1816. https://doi.org/10.1161/CIRCULATIONAHA.106.174287.

[2] A. Albakri, Systolic heart failure: A review of clinical status and meta-analysis of diagnosis and clinical management methods, Trends Res. 1 (2018). https://doi.org/10.15761/tr.1000124.

[3] T.A. Manolio, K.L. Baughman, R. Rodeheffer, T.A. Pearson, J.D. Bristow, V. V. Michels, W.H. Abelmann, W.R. Harlan, Prevalence and etiology of idiopathic dilated cardiomyopathy (summary of a National Heart, Lung, and Blood Institute Workshop), Am. J. Cardiol. 69 (1992) 1458-1466. https://doi.org/10.1016/0002-9149(92)90901-A.

[4] G.W. Dec, V. Fuster, Idiopathic Dilated Cardiomyopathy, N. Engl. J. Med. 331 (1994) 1564-1575. https://doi.org/10.1056/nejm199412083312307.

[5] W.H. Abelmann, B.H. Lorell, The challenge of cardiomyopathy, in: J. Am. Coll. Cardiol., J Am Coll Cardiol, 1989: pp. 1219-1239. https://doi.org/10.1016/0735-1097(89)90293-3.

[6] S.F. Nagueh, O.A. Smiseth, C.P. Appleton, B.F. Byrd, H. Dokainish, T. Edvardsen, F.A. Flachskampf, T.C. Gillebert, A.L. Klein, P. Lancellotti, P. Marino, J.K. Oh, B.A. Popescu, A.D. Waggoner, Recommendations for the Evaluation of Left Ventricular Diastolic Function by Echocardiography: An Update from the American Society of Echocardiography and the European Association of Cardiovascular Imaging, J. Am. Soc. Echocardiogr. 29 (2016) 277-314. https://doi.org/10.1016/j.echo.2016.01.011.

[7] G.M. Felker, R.E. Thompson, J.M. Hare, R.H. Hruban, D.E. Clemetson, D.L. Howard, K.L. Baughman, E.K. Kasper, Underlying Causes and Long-Term Survival in Patients with Initially Unexplained Cardiomyopathy, N. Engl. J. Med. 342 (2000) 1077-1084. https://doi.org/10.1056/nejm200004133421502.

[8] J. Haas, K.S. Frese, B. Peil, W. Kloos, A. Keller, R. Nietsch, Z. Feng, S. Müller, E. Kayvanpour, B. Vogel, F. Sedaghat-Hamedani, W.K. Lim, X. Zhao, D. Fradkin, D. Köhler, S. Fischer, J. Franke, S. Marquart, I. Barb, D.T. Li, A. Amr, P. Ehlermann, D. Mereles, T. Weis, S. Hassel, A. Kremer, V. King, E. Wirsz, R. Isnard, M. Komajda, A. Serio, M. Grasso, P. Syrris, E. Wicks, V. Plagnol, L. Lopes, T. Gadgaard, H. Eiskjær, M. Jørgensen, D. Garcia-Giustiniani, M. Ortiz-Genga, M.G. Crespo-Leiro, R.H.L.D. Deprez, I. Christiaans, I.A. Van Rijsingen, A.A. Wilde, A. Waldenstrom, M. Bolognesi, R. Bellazzi, S. Mörner, J.L. Bermejo, L. Monserrat, E. Villard, J. Mogensen, Y.M. Pinto, P. Charron, P. Elliott, E. Arbustini, H.A. Katus, B. Meder, Atlas of the clinical genetics of human dilated cardiomyopathy, Eur. Heart J. 36 (2015) 1123-1135. https://doi.org/10.1093/eurheartj/ehu301.

[9] C. Semsarian, J. Ingles, M.S. Maron, B.J. Maron, New perspectives on the prevalence of hypertrophic cardiomyopathy, J. Am. Coll. Cardiol. 65 (2015) 1249-1254. https://doi.org/10.1016/j.jacc.2015.01.019.

[10] B.J. Maron, S.A. Casey, L.C. Poliac, T.E. Gohman, A.K. Almquist, D.M. Aeppli, Clinical course of hypertrophic cardiomyopathy in a regional United States cohort, J. Am. Med. Assoc. 281 (1999) 650-655. https://doi.org/10.1001/jama.281.7.650.

[11] E.D. Wigle, H. Rakowski, B.P. Kimball, W.G. Williams, Hypertrophic cardiomyopathy: Clinical spectrum and treatment, Circulation. 92 (1995) 1680-1692. https://doi.org/10.1161/01.CIR.92.7.1680.

[12] E.J. Rowin, A. Orfanos, N.A.M. Estes, W. Wang, M.S. Link, M.S. Maron, B.J. Maron, Occurrence and Natural History of Clinically Silent Episodes of Atrial Fibrillation in Hypertrophic Cardiomyopathy, Am. J. Cardiol. 119 (2017) 1862-1865. https://doi.org/10.1016/j.amjcard.2017.02.040.

[13] M.S. Maron, E.J. Rowin, B.S. Wessler, P.J. Mooney, A. Fatima, P. Patel, B.C. Koethe, M. Romashko, M.S. Link, B.J. Maron, Enhanced American College of Cardiology/American Heart Association Strategy for Prevention of Sudden Cardiac Death in High-Risk Patients with Hypertrophic Cardiomyopathy, JAMA Cardiol. 4 (2019) 644-657. https://doi.org/10.1001/jamacardio.2019.1391.

[14] S.R. Ommen, S. Mital, M.A. Burke, S.M. Day, A. Deswal, P. Elliott, L.L. Evanovich, J. Hung, J.A. Joglar, P. Kantor, C. Kimmelstiel, M. Kittleson, M.S. Link, M.S. Maron, M.W. Martinez, C.Y. Miyake, H. V. Schaff, C. Semsarian, S. Paul, 2020 AHA/ACC Guideline for the Diagnosis and Treatment of Patients With Hypertrophic Cardiomyopathy: Executive Summary, Circulation. (2020). https://doi.org/10.1161/cir.0000000000000938.

[15] J. Shirani, R. Pick, W.C. Roberts, B.J. Maron, Morphology and significance of the left ventricular collagen network in young patients with hypertrophic cardiomyopathy and sudden cardiac death, J. Am. Coll. Cardiol. 35 (2000) 36-44. https://doi.org/10.1016/S0735-1097(99)00492-1.

[16] S.S. Kushwaha, J.T. Fallon, V. Fuster, Restrictive Cardiomyopathy, N. Engl. J. Med. 336 (1997) 267-276. https://doi.org/10.1056/NEJM199701233360407.

[17] K.N. Brown, V.S. Pendela, R.R. Diaz, Restrictive (Infiltrative) Cardiomyopathy, StatPearls Publishing, 2020. http://www.ncbi.nlm.nih.gov/pubmed/30725919 (accessed December 12, 2020).

[18] D. Corrado, M. Perazzolo Marra, A. Zorzi, G. Beffagna, A. Cipriani, M. De Lazzari, F. Migliore, K. Pilichou, A. Rampazzo, I. Rigato, S. Rizzo, G. Thiene, A. Anastasakis, A. Asimaki, C. Bucciarelli-Ducci, K.H. Haugaa, F.E. Marchlinski, A. Mazzanti, W.J. McKenna, A. Pantazis, A. Pelliccia, C. Schmied, S. Sharma, T. Wichter, B. Bauce, C. Basso, Diagnosis of arrhythmogenic cardiomyopathy: The Padua criteria, Int. J. Cardiol. 319 (2020) 106-114. https://doi.org/10.1016/j.ijcard.2020.06.005.

[19] M. Leopoulou, G. Mattsson, J.A. LeQuang, J. V. Pergolizzi, G. Varrassi, M. Wallhagen, P. Magnusson, Naxos disease–a narrative review, Expert Rev. Cardiovasc. Ther. (2020). https://doi.org/10.1080/14779072.2020.1828064.

[20] D. Corrado, P.J. Van Tintelen, W.J. McKenna, R.N.W. Hauer, A. Anastastakis, A. Asimaki, C. Basso, B. Bauce, C. Brunckhorst, C. Bucciarelli-Ducci, F. Duru, P. Elliott, R.M. Hamilton, K.H. Haugaa, C.A. James, D. Judge, M.S. Link, F.E. Marchlinski, A. Mazzanti, L. Mestroni, A. Pantazis, A. Pelliccia, M.P. Marra, K. Pilichou, P.G.A. Platonov, A. Protonotarios, A. Rampazzo, J.E. Saffitz, A.M. Saguner, C. Schmied, S. Sharma, H. Tandri, A.S.J.M. Te Riele, G. Thiene, A. Tsatsopoulou, W. Zareba, A. Zorzi,

T. Wichter, F.I. Marcus, H. Calkins, OUP accepted manuscript, Eur. Heart J. 41 (2019) 1414-1427b. https://doi.org/10.1093/eurheartj/ehz669.

[21] V. Kurowski, A. Kaiser, K. Von Hof, D.P. Killermann, B. Mayer, F. Hartmann, H. Schunkert, P.W. Radke, Apical and midventricular transient left ventricular dysfunction syndrome (Tako-Tsubo cardiomyopathy): Frequency, mechanisms, and prognosis, Chest. 132 (2007) 809-816. https://doi.org/10.1378/chest.07-0608.

[22] E.M. Zardi, A. Abbate, D.M. Zardi, A. Dobrina, D. Margiotta, B.W. Van Tassel, A. Afeltra, A.J. Sanyal, Cirrhotic cardiomyopathy, J. Am. Coll. Cardiol. 56 (2010) 539-549. https://doi.org/10.1016/j.jacc.2009.12.075.

[23] Familial Dilated Cardiomyopathy - The Cardiology Advisor, (n.d.). https://www.thecardiologyadvisor.com/home/decision-support-in-medicine/cardiology/familial-dilated-cardiomyopathy/ (accessed December 12, 2020).

[24] B.J. Maron, Clinical Course and Management of Hypertrophic Cardiomyopathy, N. Engl. J. Med. 379 (2018) 655-668. https://doi.org/10.1056/nejmra1710575.

[25] P.P. Sengupta, V.K. Krishnamoorthy, W.P. Abhayaratna, J. Korinek, M. Belohlavek, T.M. Sundt, K. Chandrasekaran, J.B. Seward, A.J. Tajik, B.K. Khandheria, Comparison of Usefulness of Tissue Doppler Imaging Versus Brain Natriuretic Peptide for Differentiation of Constrictive Pericardial Disease from Restrictive Cardiomyopathy, Am. J. Cardiol. 102 (2008) 357-362. https://doi.org/10.1016/j.amjcard.2008.03.068.

[26] G.W. Dec, Recognition of the apical ballooning syndrome in the United States, Circulation. 111 (2005) 388-390. https://doi.org/10.1161/01.CIR.0000155234.69439.E4.

[27] A. Prasad, A. Lerman, C.S. Rihal, Apical ballooning syndrome (Tako-Tsubo or stress cardiomyopathy): A mimic of acute myocardial infarction, Am. Heart J. 155 (2008) 408-417. https://doi.org/10.1016/j.ahj.2007.11.008.

[28] P. Ponikowski, A.A. Voors, S.D. Anker, H. Bueno, J.G.F. Cleland, A.J.S. Coats, V. Falk, J.R. González-Juanatey, V.P. Harjola, E.A. Jankowska, M. Jessup, C. Linde, P. Nihoyannopoulos, J.T. Parissis, B. Pieske, J.P. Riley, G.M.C. Rosano, L.M. Ruilope, F. Ruschitzka, F.H. Rutten, P. Van Der Meer, H.S. Sisakian, E. Isayev, A. Kurlianskaya, W. Mullens, M. Tokmakova, P. Agathangelou, V. Melenovsky, H. Wiggers, M. Hassanein, T. Uuetoa, J. Lommi, E.S. Kostovska, Y. Juilliere, A. Aladashvili, A. Luchner, C. Chrysohoou, N. Nyolczas, G. Thorgeirsson, J.M. Weinstein, A. Di Lenarda, N. Aidargaliyeva, G. Bajraktari, M. Beishenkulov, G. Kamzola, T. Abdel-Massih, J. Celutkiene, S. Noppe, A. Cassar, E. Vataman, S. AbirKhalil, P. van Pol, R. Mo, E. Straburzynska-Migaj, C. Fonseca, O. Chioncel, E. Shlyakhto, M. Zavatta, P. Otasevic, E. Goncalvesova, M. Lainscak, B.D. Molina, M. Schaufelberger, T. Suter, M.B. Yılmaz, L. Voronkov, C. Davies, 2016 ESC Guidelines for the diagnosis and treatment of acute and chronic heart failure, Eur. Heart J. 37 (2016) 2129-2200m. https://doi.org/10.1093/eurheartj/ehw128.

[29] D.M. Anderson, G.L. Raff, T.A. Ports, B.H. Brundage, W.W. Parmley, K. Chatterjee, Hypertrophic obstructive cardiomyopathy. Effects of acute and chronic verapamil treatment on left ventricular systolic and diastolic function, Heart. 51 (1984) 523-529. https://doi.org/10.1136/hrt.51.5.523.

[30] C. Templin, J.R. Ghadri, J. Diekmann, L.C. Napp, D.R. Bataiosu, M. Jaguszewski, V.L. Cammann, A. Sarcon, V. Geyer, C.A. Neumann, B. Seifert, J. Hellermann, M. Schwyzer, K. Eisenhardt, J. Jenewein, J. Franke, H.A. Katus, C. Burgdorf, H. Schunkert, C. Moeller, H. Thiele, J. Bauersachs, C. Tschöpe, H.-P. Schultheiss, C.A. Laney, L. Rajan, G. Michels, R. Pfister, C. Ukena, M. Böhm, R. Erbel, A. Cuneo, K.-H. Kuck, C. Jacobshagen, G. Hasenfuss, M. Karakas, W. Koenig, W. Rottbauer, S.M. Said, R.C. Braun-Dullaeus, F. Cuculi, A. Banning, T.A. Fischer, T. Vasankari, K.E.J. Airaksinen, M. Fijalkowski, A. Rynkiewicz, M. Pawlak, G. Opolski, R. Dworakowski, P. MacCarthy, C. Kaiser, S. Osswald, L. Galiuto, F. Crea, W. Dichtl, W.M. Franz, K. Empen, S.B. Felix, C. Delmas, O. Lairez, P. Erne, J.J. Bax, I. Ford, F. Ruschitzka, A. Prasad, T.F. Lüscher, Clinical Features and Outcomes of Takotsubo (Stress) Cardiomyopathy, N. Engl. J. Med. 373 (2015) 929-938, https://doi.org/10.1056/nejmoa1406761.

Chapter 4

The Role of Neurohormonal Systems, Inflammatory Mediators and Oxydative Stress in Cardiomyopathy

Ronald Zolty

Abstract

Cardiomyopathy and more specifically the dilated cardiomyopathy, regardless of severity, is associated with activation of neuro-hormonal, cytokine and oxidative stress signaling pathways that alter the structure and function of cardiac myocytes and non-myocyte cells. These cellular alterations culminate in the morphological changes in cardiac structure termed as cardiac remodeling, a maladaptive process that contributes to further left ventricular dysfunction and heart failure development. This pathological progression is mainly driven by circulating mediators, in particular angiotensin II and norepinephrine. Natriuretic peptides, endothelin-1, vasopressin play also an important role in the progression of the cardiomyopathy. Cardiac inflammation, mediated by cytokines such as tumor necrosis factor-α (TNF-α), interleukins 1 (IL-1) and 6 (IL-6), as well as the oxidative stress were also shown to worsen the cardiac function. Although these pathways have been described separately, they are critically inter-dependent in the response to the development and progression of the dilated cardiomyopathy. This chapter reviews the cellular basis for cardiac remodeling and the mechanisms that contribute to these cellular abnormalities and, more broadly, to the pathophysiology of dilated cardiomyopathy, its progression and its potential treatments.

Keywords: Angiotensin II, Adrenergic signaling, Natriuretic peptides, Vasopressin, Prostaglandin, Endothelin, Nitric Oxide, Cytokines, ROS, Oxidative stress

1. Introduction

Cardiomyopathy is a group of diseases that affect the heart muscle [1]. As the disease worsens, symptoms of heart failure will occur including shortness of breath, fatigue, and fluid retention with pulmonary congestion and peripheral edema.

The majority of patients with heart failure have an underlying cardiomyopathy as the causative etiology. In the US, the most common cause of heart failure (HF) is a primary or secondary dilated cardiomyopathy [1, 2] encompassing approximately 60% of the HF cases.

Whether the etiology of the cardiomyopathy is idiopathic, inflammatory, viral, or ischemic, the pathological processes leading to the clinical syndrome of heart failure begin with myocardial injury. The hemodynamic consequences of the initial

IntechOpen

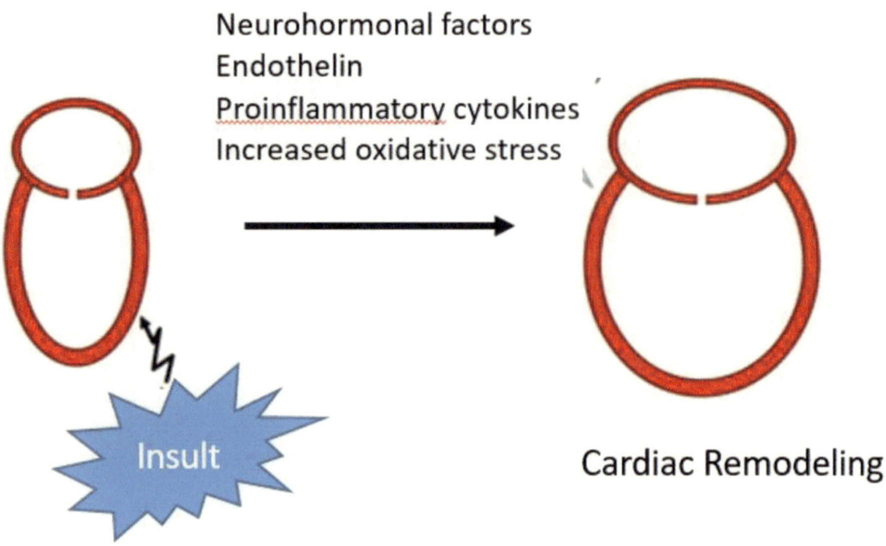

Figure 1.
Schematic representation of cardiac remodeling in dilated cardiomyopathy and HF.

injury will lead to a decline in myocardial contractility. The reduction of cardiac output will elicit a complex humoral and inflammatory response. The humoral response comprises two major components, the renin-angiotensin-aldosterone (RAA) pathway [3] and the sympathetic nervous (SN) system and is referred as neuro-hormonal activation [4]. Additional circulating mediators, such as natriuretic peptides, nitric oxide, endothelin and vasopressin also play a role in the circulatory adaptation to the heart failure state. Furthermore, the initial myocardial injury leading to the development of cardiomyopathy stimulates the production of cytokines, such as tumor necrosis factor-α (TNF-α) and interleukin-6 (IL-6) [5]. Finally, oxidative stress, defined as an excess production of reactive oxygen species (ROS) relative to antioxidant defense, is enhanced in HF [6–9].

For neuro-hormonal and cytokine activation, these pathways are initially compensatory in response to acute injury but have ultimately maladaptive consequences on the long term, leading to cardiac remodeling and worsening heart failure.

Cardiac remodeling refers to changes in the size, shape, structure and function of the heart. Ventricular remodeling involves hypertrophy and apoptosis of myocytes, regression to a fetal phenotype, as well as modification of the extracellular matrix (**Figure 1**).

2. Neuro-hormonal activation in cardiomyopathy and heart failure

Heart failure associated with cardiomyopathy is a highly complex syndrome in which the insufficient cardiac output leads to neuro-hormonal activation and subsequent ventricular remodeling [10]. The characteristic hemodynamic abnormalities in patients with HF are a reduction in stroke volume with concomitant increase in systemic vascular resistance. In the early phase of heart failure, neuro-hormonal activation, with the stimulation of the SN and RAA systems, helps maintaining adequate cardiac output and peripheral perfusion. Sustained neuro-hormonal activation, however, will result in increased cardiac wall stress, ventricular dilatation and adverse remodeling effects [11, 12]. A variety of endogenously produced mediators, including norepinephrine, angiotensin II, aldosterone, endothelin and vasopressin have been implicated as biologically active molecules which will contribute to disease progression of the failing heart.

Stimulation of these neuro-hormones and their receptors influences myocardial contractility, heart rate and conduction, cardiac metabolism, and cellular growth. Therefore, these cardiac neuro-mediator and neuro-receptors play a key role in cardiac physiology and myocyte function in healthy and diseased heart. For example, cardiac hypertrophy is produced by a combination of increased myocyte stretch, neurotransmitter release, and several types of autocrine, paracrine, and hormonal stimulation that mediate myocyte growth. In this context, the α-1 receptor pathway, the angiotensin II AT1 receptor pathway, the endothelin 1 receptor pathway, and the β-adrenergic receptor pathway have all been implicated in the pathogenesis of myocyte hypertrophy.

Activation of the adrenergic nervous system and the renin-angiotensin systems appears to be of primary importance in producing major adaptive cardiac receptor-signal transduction changes in the failing heart.

The most important modulated function mechanisms responsible for the stimulation of cardiac function appears to be the adrenergic signaling pathway. In addition to the adrenergic stimulation, an increase in plasma volume will take place, resulting in an increased ventricular preload as well as an increase in cardiac myocyte hypertrophy, which results in more contractile elements, increased wall thickness with a subsequent decrease in wall tension. The plasma volume increase is associated with stimulation of the RAA system and production of angiotensin II and aldosterone which will enhance sodium and water reabsorption in both the proximal and distal renal tubules [13].

2.1 Activation of the renin-angiotensin system with LV dysfunction

When the heart fails, the RAA system is activated as demonstrated with increased of the renin activity with production of angiotensin II and aldosterone [14–18].

The RAA system consists of a cascade of enzymatic reactions involving three components, angiotensinogen, renin and angiotensin-converting enzyme (ACE), which generate angiotensin (Ang) II as the biologically active product. Ang II binds to two types of specific receptors, angiotensin type-1 (AT1R) and type-2 (AT2R). Both receptor belong to the family of seven transmembrane domain heterotrimeric G protein-coupled receptors (GPCR). The majority of the deleterious mitogenic and hypertrophic actions of Ang II have been attributed to interaction with the AT1 receptor, which is the predominant receptor, while AT2 generally produces beneficial effects.

The deleterious effects of the activation of the RAA system are mediated primarily through increased circulating and tissue levels of the neuro-hormonal angiotensin II (**Figure 2**). Ang II is an extremely potent vasoconstrictor, acting directly on vascular smooth muscles and indirectly by increasing sympathetic tone [19, 20]. In addition, it produces sodium retention (through aldosterone and renal vasoconstriction), as well as fluid retention through anti-diuretic hormone [21, 22]. At the cellular level, Ang II promotes migration, proliferation, and hypertrophy, thus producing numerous adverse effects, including remodeling of the left ventricle, and development of endothelial dysfunction [23, 24].

Ang II promotes cardiac remodeling in several ways. By increasing arterial smooth muscle tone and causing salt and water retention, it increases cardiac preload and afterload. Also, increased wall stress is a potent stimulus for remodeling. In addition, Ang II has direct effects on the myocardium; it causes hypertrophy of cardiac myocytes and hyperplasia of cardiac fibroblasts as well as an increase

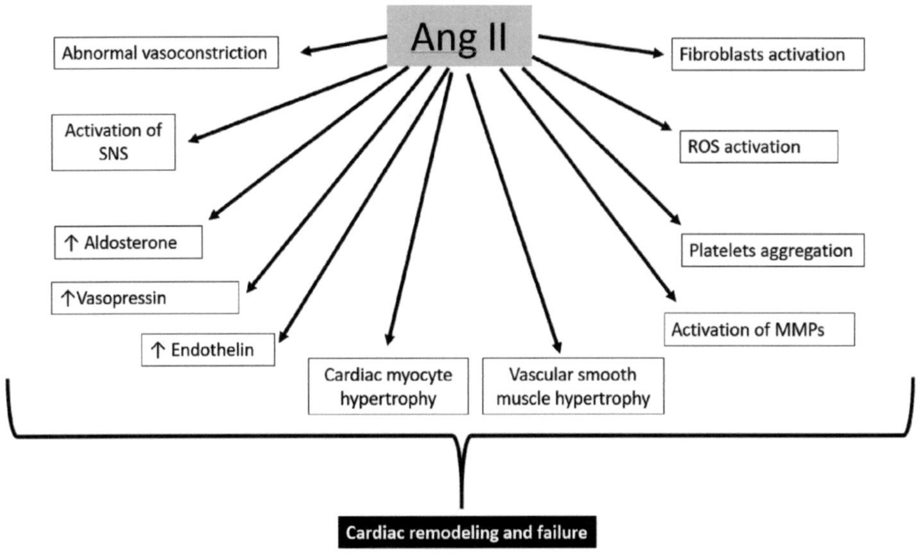

Figure 2.
Deleterious pathophysiologic effects of angiotensin II in dilated cardiomyopathy and heart failure. MMP: Matrix metalloproteinases, ROS: Reactive oxygen species.

in extracellular matrix deposition, [25] and stimulates the release of other growth factors, including norepinephrine and endothelin, which in turn stimulate cardiac remodeling [26]. These actions of Ang II are largely mediated through the angiotensin type 1 (AT1) receptor. Thus RAA system inhibition by ACE inhibitors or by angiotensin receptor blockers, attenuates many of the key hemodynamic, mechanical and functional disturbances crucial to the pathophysiology of cardiac dysfunction. ACE inhibitors are therefore a mainstay of therapy in patients with symptomatic and asymptomatic LV systolic dysfunction.

2.2 Sympathetic nervous system activation with LV dysfunction

Similarly to the RAA system, when the cardiac function fails, the adrenergic nervous system is activated. Numerous studies have documented elevated circulating norepinephrine levels with LV myocardial dysfunction [14–17, 27]. Even in asymptomatic patients with left ventricular dysfunction, an 35% increase in plasma norepinephrine was demonstrated [18]. In the failing heart, the increase of adrenergic activity seems to occur as a consequence of increased central sympathetic release at the pre-synaptic level [28].

Pre-synaptic facilitation of norepinephrine release by angiotensin II may also play an important role in adrenergic activation, [29] thus demonstrating a positive feedback of angiotensin II on cardiac adrenergic activity. Conversely, the adrenergic nervous system provides a major stimulus for activation of the RAA system, as activation of renal nerves by the SN system results in renal renin release [30, 31]. Thus activation of the adrenergic and renin-angiotensin systems appears to be co-regulated with cardiac dysfunction. Activation of one system stimulates the other and maneuvers that decrease the activity of one system may inhibit the other [32]. For example, administration of an ACE inhibitor to patients with heart failure with reduced ejection fraction (HFrEF) results not only in a decrease in plasma angiotensin II levels but also in a fall in circulating norepinephrine [33, 34].

Activation of cardiac β-adrenergic receptor (AR) represents the body's most powerful principle to increase cardiac contractility and heart rate [35] (**Figure 3**).

Adrenergic receptors are a family of G-protein-coupled receptors with nine members, three α1, three α2, and three β: β1, β2 and β3. When the first subdivision of adrenergic receptors was defined on the basis of pharmacological experiments, [36] the α-subtype was defined as the one that causes smooth muscle contraction, whereas the β-subtype mediates smooth muscle relaxation. Twenty years later, the β-receptors were subdivided again, into the β1-subtype, which stimulates cardiac muscle, and the β2-subtype, which relaxes smooth muscle [37].

The mammalian heart expresses all three β-adrenergic receptor subtypes [38–40]. In the healthy heart, the majority (i.e. 60–80%) of receptors are the β1-subtype in most species, while the β2-subtype accounts for a minor fraction of total βARs. A third β-adrenergic receptor subtype, the β3-subtype, was initially thought to be limited to adipose tissue, [40] but was later also detected in the heart [39]. This subtype is generally perceived as less important due to its very low expression level and relatively minor functional effects. There is evidence that the β1-subtype is preferentially located on cardiac myocytes, whereas the β2-subtype is expressed to a significant extent on non-cardiomyocyte cells, including vascular smooth muscle cells and synaptic nerve endings.

β1- and β2-adrenergic receptors are potent stimulators of cardiac contraction and relaxation in the human heart [35, 41]. As direct effectors of the sympathetic nervous system, they serve to rapidly adapt cardiac performance to an increased hemodynamic demand. Both β1 and β2 receptors couple to the stimulatory G protein Gs, thereby activating adenylyl cyclase. The formation of the second messenger cAMP then leads to activation of PKA (cAMP protein kinase A), which phosphorylates several key regulators of the cardiac excitation-contraction machinery. This includes phospholamban, [42] the L-type Ca-channel, [42, 43] the

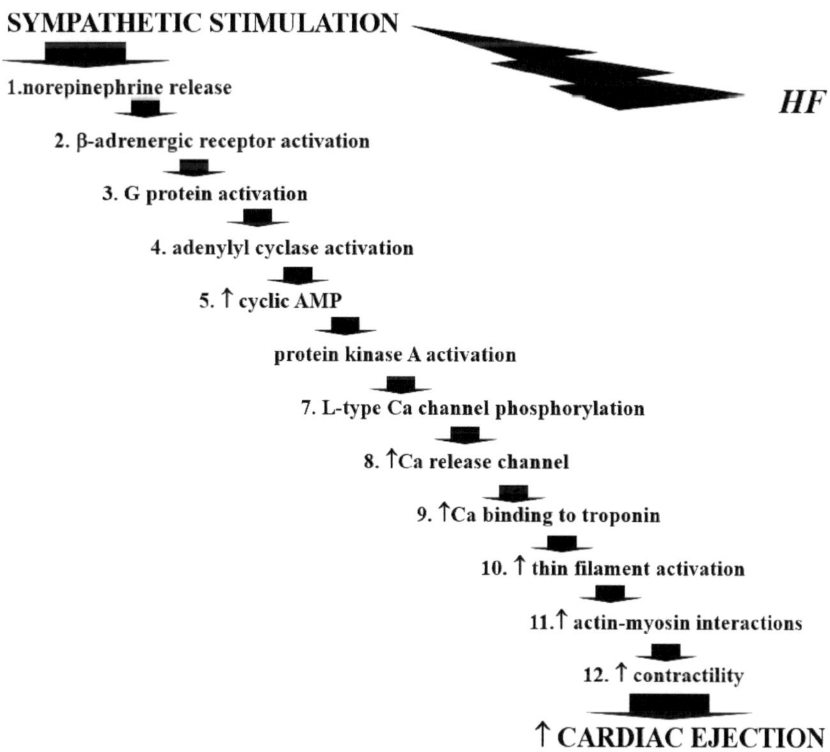

Figure 3.
Shematic representation of the cascade of reactions to increase cardiomyocyte contractility by the sympathetic nervous activation.

ryanodine receptor, [44] troponin T and I, [45] myosin binding protein C [46] and the small protein phosphatase inhibitor-1 [47]. These events lead to rapid changes of the cardiomyocyte calcium transient and enhanced myofilament sensitivity for calcium, resulting in a potent inotropic effect.

Data indicate that sustained stimulation of the β1-receptor system, which is ideally suited to provide short-term increases in cardiac function, causes marked structural and functional damage to the heart on the long term. Thus the chronic activation by the adrenergic system in heart failure represents a maladaptive response.

Also, the β-adrenergic signaling in dilated cardiomyopathy is characterized by the fact that it is desensitized in failing human hearts. In HF, there is a reduction of the density of β1ARs in in failing human myocardium, [48] a decrease of norepinephrine-re-uptake [49] and ultimately an increase in Ginhibitory (Gi) protein expression [50] and in GRK2 (βARK)-activity [51], a receptor kinase that phosphorylates and thereby inactivates βARs. The observed desensitization of βAR receptors represents an adaptation process to the highly increased levels of catecholamines in heart failure. This phenomenon is considered a beneficial readjustment of the signaling cascade to minimize the detrimental effects of chronic stimulation of the myocardium by catecholamines.

β-adrenergic receptor blockade is now regarded as one of the most effective therapeutic principle in dilated cardiomyopathy and heart failure [52].

Several large clinical trials with carvedilol, metoprolol succinate and bisoprolol have demonstrated a significant benefit in large placebo-controlled trial [53–55]. On the contrary, two β-blockers (xamoterol and bucindolol) have failed to significantly reduce mortality or even increased mortality [56, 57]. The most likely explanation for the failure of xamoterol is the pronounced partial agonism exerted by this agent [58]. Bucindolol led to a non-significant reduction of mortality in the BEST trial. Two main reasons might account for this finding. First, the study population differed markedly from the other large heart failure trials. It included a high percentage of African-Americans and of women, and both of these groups are underrepresented in other trials [56]. In the other trials, the beneficial effects of β-blockade were less pronounced compared with the effects in Caucasians [56]. Second bucindolol might display some degree of partial agonism.

2.3 Aldosterone

The pivotal role played by aldosterone in the pathogenesis of dilated cardiomyopathy and HF is well-recognized. Activation of the RAA system leads to marked elevations in plasma aldosterone levels, which have been shown to correlate with increased mortality [59]. Elevated aldosterone levels lead to excessive sodium retention, with expansion of the extracellular volume, worsening hemodynamic conditions, and a fall in cardiac output. Decreased renal blood flow further stimulates the RAA system, causing secondary hyperaldosteronism and further sodium retention. In addition, by contributing to hypokalemia and hypomagnesemia, aldosterone increases the sensitivity of cardiac tissue to arrhythmias, with a resultant increase in sudden death [60, 61].

A growing body of evidence suggests that aldosterone may contribute to endothelial dysfunction, possibly through reduced nitric oxide bioavailability [62]. Since the endothelium plays a critical role in the regulation of vascular tone, platelet aggregation and thrombosis, endothelial dysfunction predicts subsequent cardiovascular events [63]. Furthermore, aldosterone contributes to the development of HF by promoting myocardial fibrosis. In vitro studies have demonstrated that administration of aldosterone to cardiac fibroblasts significantly enhances collagen synthesis, [64] a finding that has been confirmed in rat models [65]. Another potentially harmful effect of aldosterone is its ability to blunt baroreflex response. Administration of aldosterone to dogs [66] and to healthy human volunteers [67] resulted in an elevation in the threshold for baroreflex activation and a reduction in peak discharge rate. Finally aldosterone has been shown to promote the activation and aggregation of platelets and to enhance arteriolar constriction [68].

The clinical trial Randomized Aldosterone Evaluation Study (RALES) demonstrated the benefits of aldosterone receptor blockade in HF. 1633 patients with NYHA Class III-IV chronic HF, already receiving ACEIs, were randomized to spironolactone versus placebo [69]. The relative risk of death was reduced by 30% over two years (RR 0.7, 95% CI 0.60–0.82; $p < 0.001$) with a 35% reduction in HF hospitalizations and an improvement in functional class.

2.4 Endothelin

Endothelin is a potent vasoconstrictor peptide and its synthesis is stimulated by hypoxia, ischemia, neurohormones (norepinephrine, angiotensin II, arginine vasopressin), and inflammatory cytokines [70–72].

Tissue and plasma levels of endothelin-1 and its precursor (big endothelin-1) are elevated in patients with cardiomyopathy and HF [73–78]. These increases are due to increased endothelin synthesis primarily in the pulmonary vascular bed [79] and the myocardium [80]. The vascular distension seen in HF (especially in the pulmonary vascular bed) appears to a stimulus for increased endothelin-1 production [81]. Another potential contributor to the increased endothelin-1 concentration in HF, is the downregulation of endothelin-B receptors, which has been observed in the lung tissue of experimental animals with HF [82, 83]. Endothelin B receptors appear to play a role in the clearance of endothelin-1. Pulmonary vascular tone in HF are largely mediated by endothelin-A receptor [84, 85]. Increased levels of endothelin-1 are associated with increased angiotensin II levels, more advanced HF symptoms, worse hemodynamics, and decreased survival [70, 75, 78, 81, 85–94].

Endothelin-A receptor antagonists prevent remodeling, improve LV function, and prolong survival in rats [95–97].

The Value of Endothelin Receptor Inhibition with Tezosentan in Acute Heart Failure Study (VERITAS), the largest clinical trial of an endothelin receptor antagonist for ADHF, enrolled 1435 patients. Patients treated with tezosentan experienced significant reduction in pulmonary arterial pressures and pulmonary capillary wedge pressures as well as an increase in cardiac index. Despite these significant improvements in hemodynamics, use of tozosentan did not improve the composite primary end point of dyspnea at 24 hours, worsening HF or death at 7 days [98].

The Resource utilization Among Congestive Heart Failure Study (REACH) was another clinical trial investigating the effects of bosentan in 370 patients with advanced HF and an LVEF <35%. The trial was stopped prematurely due to elevations in liver transaminases. At the time of the study termination, there was no significant differences in outcomes between the bosentan compared to the placebo group. Nevertheless, a post-hoc analysis of 174 patients who completed the 6-month follow up demonstrated significant clinical improvement ($p = 0.045$) [99].

Finally, the Enrasentan Cooperative Randomized Evaluation (ENCOR) trial studied enrasentan, a dual A/B endothelin receptor antagonist in 419 patients with stable NYHA Class II and II with LVEF ≤35%. There was no significant improvement in the primary endpoint of clinical HF score with the active drug [100].

2.5 Vasopressin

Arginine vasopressin (AVP) is a peptide hormone that is elevated in heart failure, and associated with a poor prognosis [18, 101]. AVP contributes to fluid retention and hyponatremia [102, 103]. AVP exerts its cardiao-vascular effects trough two receptors subtypes V1a and V2. V1a is found on vascular smooth muscle cells and cardiac myocytes. Whereas, vasopressin V1A receptors mediate vasoconstriction, positive inotropic and mitogenic effects, the V2 receptors inhibit free water clearance [104–106]. Stimulation of the V1a-receptor, initially leads to increased myocardial protein synthesis resulting in myocardial hypertrophy [107, 108]. V2-receptors are found in the distal tubule of the kidney, and their activation results in water retention via upregulation of aquaporin channels [104, 109].

The control of Vasopressin secretion is complex and involves both osmotic and nonosmotic stimuli [110]. Factors causing vasopressin release include plasma osmolality, intra-cardiac and arterial pressures, as well as Angiotensin II levels [111]. Under most circumstances, Vasopressin is coupled to osmolality levels, making osmo-receptor the major determinant of Vasopressin release.

When the pressure within the heart or arterial vessels decreases, tonic inhibitory restraint of vasopressin is diminished and plasma vasopressin levels rise. Inversely, elevated blood pressure leads to decrease plasma vasopressin level [112–114].

Despite their hypo-osmolar hyponatremia state, patients with HF have inappropriately elevated plasma vasopressin levels [101, 115, 116].

Agents that antagonize V1A receptor reduce vascular tone and the mitogenic myocardial effects of AVP. Because V2 antagonists increase aquaresis, the addition of an AVP V2 antagonist improves free water clearance, and reduces hyponatremia.

Conivaptan is a dual V1a/V2 receptor antagonist that has been investigated in the treatment of HF. One hundred and forty-two patients with NYHA class III or IV HF were randomized to either a single IV dose of conivaptan or placebo and evaluated over 12 hours for changes in hemodynamics. Both capillary wedge pressure and right atrial pressure were significantly reduced in the treatment group compared to placebo. However, cardiac index did not improve [117].

The EVEREST study investigated whether short term and long term blockade of the V2 receptor with Tolvaptan is beneficial in patients with HF. The results confirmed that Tolvapatan when added to standard therapy improved symptoms and signs of HF, however no benefit was observed on all-cause mortality or the combined endpoint of cardiovascular mortality or hospitalization for worsening HF The drug had no significant effect on long term LV remodeling in patient with LVEF <30% [118].

2.6 Natriuretic peptides

While the activation of the RAA and SN system is detrimental in HF, other counter-regulatory pathways are activated in HF, including the natriuretic peptide (NP) system. The NP system consists of atrial (ANP) [119]. B-type (BNP) [120] and C-type (CNP) NPs. These hormones regulate blood pressure and fluid homeostasis [121–123]. ANP is synthesized and secreted in atria. BNP is secreted from the ventricles in response to mechanical stretch and increased intra-cardiac volume and pressure, while CNP mostly originates from endothelial and renal cells and is secreted in response to endothelium-dependent agonists and pro-inflammatory cytokines [121, 122, 124].

NPs activate three transmembrane receptors: natriuretic peptide receptor (NPR)-A, NPR-B and NPR-C.27 The binding of NPs to type A (NPR-A) and type B

(NPR-B) receptors activates guanylate cyclase, increasing levels of the second messenger cyclic guanosine monophosphate (cGMP) and its effector molecule protein kinase G. This induces natriuresis, diuresis, vasodilation and inhibition of the RAA and the SN systems, as well as antifibrotic, antiproliferative and antithrombotic effects [121, 122, 124].

Blockade of NP breakdown by neprilysin inhibitors has, therefore, been investigated [125]. Oral neprilysin inhibitors, such as candoxatril, produced clinical benefit in patients with chronic HF [126, 127]. However, candoxatril has no effect on, or increases, systolic BP (SBP) in normotensives, an effect prevented by enalapril, and does not reduce BP in hypertensive subjects, probably because its vasodilatory effect may be offset by an increased activity of the RAAS and sympathetic nervous system and/or by downregulation of NP receptors [128, 129]. In addition, since neprilysin acts on numerous physiological targets, the effect of candoxatril was broader than anticipated [128].

Neprilysin inhibition results in activation of the RAAS, therefore, in order to be clinically beneficial, neprilysin inhibition requires concomitant inhibition of the RAAS [130]. Vasopeptidase inhibitors are dual inhibitors of ACE and neprilysin and, therefore, emerged as a new therapeutic option in HF and hypertension, but their pharmacological profile is complex [131]. Omapatrilat was more effective than either lisinopril or amlodipine in reducing BP, [131] but in patients with chronic HF it was not more effective than enalapril in reducing the combined risk of death or hospitalization for HF requiring intravenous treatment [132]. However, omapatrilat was discontinued due to the risk of angioedema, possibly due to excessive inhibition of bradykinin degradation (presumably via neprilysin, ACE and aminopeptidase P) [133, 134].

Sacubutril/Valsartan is an oral combination medication consisting of the neprilysin inhibitor sacubitril and the angiotensin receptor blocker valsartan. The combination is called angiotensin receptor-neprilysin inhibitor (ARNi). The PARADIGM-HF trial compared sacubitril/valsartan to enalapril [37] in heart failure patients with reduced LVEF. The trial was stopped early after a prespecified interim analysis revealed a significant reduction in the primary endpoint of cardiovascular death or heart failure in the sacubitril/valsartan group compared to enalapril [135].

3. Inflammation

Ample evidence exists that dilated cardiomyopathy and HF are associated with the activation of the immune system resulting in elevated levels of pro-inflammatory cytokines. In patients with cardiomyopathy and HF, elevated levels of tumor necrosis factor-α (TNF-α), interleukin-1 (IL-1), and interleukin-6 (IL-6) are found [136–138]. The best characterized inflammatory molecule in DCM and HF is TNF-α.

The importance in understanding the role of inflammation in the pathogenesis of dilated cardiomyopathy arises from the observation that many aspects of the development of dilated cardiomyopathy can be explained by the biological effects of pro-inflammatory cytokines. Cytokines, when expressed at sufficiently high concentrations, can mimic the development of the dilated cardiomyopathy phenotype features, which include left ventricular remodeling and dysfunction with myocyte hypertrophy, changes in fetal gene expression, alteration of the extracellular matrix, and cardiac myocyte apoptosis [139–143]. As it is the case with neuro-hormonal activation, overexpression of cytokines results in cardiac direct toxicity [144, 145].

Clinically, the progressive increase in inflammatory cytokine levels is in direct relation with NYHA functional class deterioration. Also, data from the VEST trial demonstrated a strong correlation between survival and TNF-α levels [146]. Similar findings were observed with levels of IL-6 [146].

One of the marks of pro-inflammatory cytokines is their ability to depress LV function. Preclinical studies in rodents showed that circulating levels of TNF-α that correspond with those observed in patients with HF were sufficient to produce negative inotropic effects [139]. Also, transgenic mice with TNF-α overexpression studies resulted in depressed LV function [140, 147].

The cytokine hypothesis proposes that cardiomyopathy progression is an inflammatory process and that amplification of pro-inflammatory cytokines worsens left ventricular dysfunction and facilitates the development of HF [10, 148].

There is significant cross-talk between the neuro-hormonal and the cytokine systems [144]. Data have shown that these cytokine signaling pathways augment local neuro-hormonal activation, which in turn promotes the enhanced expression of these same cytokines [144]. For instance adrenergic stimulation as seen in HF, induces myocardial TNF-α expression, [149] which in turn attenuates beta-adrenergic responsiveness. Also, Angiotensin II is known to activate nuclear factor-kappa B (NF-kB), a redox-sensitive transcription factor that is important in stimulating the myocardial inflammatory response, [150] including activation of inflammatory cytokines, NO, chemokines and cell adhesion molecules [150, 151].

Clinical studies that have examined the effect of ACE-inhibitors have shown that while ACE inhibitors have mixed results in terms of inhibiting pro-inflammatory cytokines, Angiotensin Receptor Blockers (ARBs) have consistently led to significant decrease in circulating levels of inflammatory mediators such as TNF-α in patients with cardiomyopathy and HF [152, 153]. Similar findings have been reported with the use of beta-blockers in experimental animal models and clinical heart failure studies. Beta-adrenergic blockade with a beta-1-selective adrenergic antagonist has demonstrated partial inhibition of the expression of pro-inflammatory mediators in an experimental model of post-infarct LV heart failure remodeling model [55]. In sub-group analysis of the MERIT-HF, treatment with metoprolol did not lead to a decrease in the level of pro-inflammatory mediators, whereas in a different trial, the use of carvedilol, a non-selective beta-1 and beta-2 adrenergic antagonist with anti-oxidant properties resulted in a significant reduction in the production of TNF-α [154–156]. These data suggest that here are interactions between the renin-angiotensin and adrenergic systems with pro-inflammatory cytokines.

3.1 Tumor necrosis factor-α (TNF-α)

TNF-α is recognized as a cytokine with pleiotropic biologic capacities [157, 158]. TNF affects growth, differentiation and function of every cell type, including cardiomyocytes.

TNF-α binds to a lower affinity the type 1 receptor called TNFR1 and a higher affinity type 2 receptor called TNFR2. Intracellular signaling occurs as a result of TNF-induced cross-linking (oligomerization) of the receptors. Previous studies have identified the presence of both types of TNF receptors in the non-failing and failing heart [159, 160]. Normal myocardium does not contain TNF-α. In the failing heart, with the increased expression of TNF-α, the receptors for TNF-α, TNFR1 and TNFR2, are downregulated, [159] similar to the β1 adrenergic receptor downregulation and the SN system in heart failure.

The majority of the deleterious effects of TNF-α are coupled to activation of TNFR1, whereas activation of TNFR2 appears to exert protective effects. Activation of TNFR1 is responsible for mediating negative inotropic effects, and cardiac myocyte apopotosis [142, 159, 161]. In contrast activation of the type 2 TNF receptor appears to protect the cardiomyocyte against hypoxic stress and ischemic injury [159, 162]. Previous studies have shown that both TNFR1 and TNFR2 exist in the circulation as circulating soluble receptors and are referred as sTNFR1 and sTNFR2. Elevated levels of sTNFR1 and sTNFR2 have been shown to be strong independent predictors of adverse outcomes in hospitalized HF patients [146, 163, 164].

Early in the disease process, much of circulating TNF-α is derived from immune cell line such as activated macrophages. However, late in disease progression much of the TNF-α is produced by the cardiac myocytes themselves [165]. Transgenic mice overexpressing TNF will develop an early inflammatory myocarditis that later progresses to myocyte hypertrophy, left ventricular dilatation, and progressive left ventricular dysfunction [140]. In this model, TNF also activate expression of matrix metalloproteinases, [166] which contribute to LV remodeling and dilatation. Administration of TNF in experimental animal models at concentrations comparable to those observed in clinical heart failure, produces significant declines in myocardial contractility with worsening left ventricular function [139]. In another rat model, the infusion of TNF, caused progressive left ventricular enlargement with significant degradation of the extra-cellular matrix [167].

The negative inotropic effects of TNF-α on cardiac myocytes are mediated through increased expression of iNOS with production of nitric oxide [168, 169] and activation of norepinephrine and angiotensinogen II. TNF-α was shown to increase the expression of the AT1 receptor in cardiac fibroblasts by a mechanism dependent on NF-ĶB, thereby augmenting Ang II effects on cells via an increase in AT1 receptor density [170]. Increase of Ang II stimulates the synthesis of cardiac fibroblasts and the inhibition of MMP2 activity. Ang II activates NF-ĶB, via the AT1 receptor and thus increases the production of pro-inflammatory cytokines [171]. Transgenic mice with TNF-α overexpression demonstrate increased levels of both ACE and Ang II [172]. These different studies support the presence of cross-talk between the RAA and cytokine signaling pathways. TNF-α also augments sympathetic activation. Isoproterenol administration in rodents increases the expression of TNF-α, IL-1β, and IL-6 [163, 173]. These studies support that the sympathetic nervous system regulates positively the cytokine gene expression, while cytokines potentiate the effects of catecholamines on the myocardium.

3.2 Interleukin-1 (IL-1)

There are three members of the interleukin-1 (IL-1) family: IL-1α, IL-β, and IL-1 receptor antagonist (IL-1Ra) [158]. IL-1α and IL-β are agonist and IL-1 Ra is a specific receptor antagonist. Similar to TNF-α, IL-1β appears to be activated in response to stressful environmental stimuli [136, 174].

IL-1β expression is elevated in the myocardium of failing hearts and is present at high circulating concentrations in patients with dilated cardiomyopathy. The primary sources of IL-1β within the myocardium are macrophages and cardiac fibroblasts [175, 176]. Similar to TNF-α and IL-6, IL-1β inhibits fibroblast-mediated production of collagen and suppresses proliferation of fibroblasts [177, 178]. IL-1β also increases the expression and activity of MMP's which cause destruction of the fibrillary collagen network. Moreover, IL-1β induces the expression of nitric oxide synthase. Furthermore, IL-1β causes cardiac myocytes hypertrophy and inhibits the expression of the fetal genes, β-MHC and skeletal α-actin. In summary, IL-1β alters the phenotype and genotype of cardiac myocytes, [177, 178] while also disrupting the composition of the extracellular matrix.

3.3 Interleukin IL-6

Similar to TNF-α and IL-1β, levels of IL-6 are elevated in patients with dilated cardiomyopathy and HF. The degree of IL-6 elevation correlates to heart failure severity and prognosis [179]. IL-6 signals through its receptor, IL-6R, associates with the gp130 cytokine receptor, and forms a membrane complex that activates downstream signaling pathways. The source of IL-6 production are cardiac myocytes, fibroblasts and mononuclear inflammatory cells [175]. IL-6 stimulation of fibroblasts decreases collagen synthesis and increases MMP activity, contributing to disintegration of extracellular matrix [175]. Transgenic mice expressing both IL-6 and IL-6R develop LV hypertrophy, resulting from activation of the gp130 receptor. Other cytokines within the IL-6 family, including cardiotropin 1 and leukemia inhibitor factor, induce cardiomyocyte hypertrophy [180–182]. Thus IL-6 participates to the alterations of the extracellular matrix and cardiomyocyte hypertrophy.

3.4 Nitric oxide synthases

While the contributions of neuro-hormonal and cytokine signaling pathways to ventricular remodeling are well-established, cytokine-mediated increase in inducible nitric oxide synthase may be an important downstream pathway that contributes significantly to the cardiac remodeling [183, 184]. There are three known members of the nitric oxide synthase (NOS) family, [183] neuronal NOS (nNOS or NOS 1), inducible NOS (iNOS or NOS II) and endothelial NOS (eNOS or NOS III). Cardiac myocytes in the normal heart express mainly eNOS [185]. However, studies have shown that iNOS is expressed at high levels in the myocardium of failing hearts [186–188].

Evidence from in vivo studies supports a detrimental effect of iNOS in the failing heart. Cardiac specific over-expression of iNOS in transgenic mice leads to cardiac fibrosis, dilatation and premature death, [189] although Heger et all reported no demonstrable phenotype accompanying iNOS overexpression in the mouse heart [190]. Sam et al. demonstrated that 6 months after an MI, the extent of LV dysfunction and myo-cardiac apoptosis was significantly diminished in iNOS knockout mice, supporting a detrimental role of iNOS in this ischemic cardiomyopathy model [191]. These data suggest that iNOS may play an important role in ventricular remodeling and cardiac myocyte apoptosis. Supporting this concept, iNOS expression in end-stage failing heart normalized after placement of ventricular assist device [188].

3.5 Anti-inflammation treatment in cardiomyopathy and heart failure

Despite an abundance of evidence implicating the inflammatory pathway in HF and cardiomyopathy, and numerous examples of anti-inflammatory therapies improving HF in experimental animal models, these agents have been largely unsuccessful in treating human cardiomyopathy and HF.

3.5.1 Prednisone

Prednisone was shown to suppress TN-Fα biosynthesis at the translational and transcriptional levels. Parrillo et al. randomized 102 patients to prednisone versus placebo to 102 patient with dilated cardiomyopathy. Following three months of therapy, an increase in LVEF of >5% was observed in 53% of patients receiving prednisone. All patients were categorized prospectively in two separately randomized subgroups. "Reactive" patients (n = 60) were those who had fibroblastic (n = 36) or lymphocytic (n = 2) infiltration or immunoglobulin deposition (n = 16) on endomyocardial biopsy, a positive gallium scan (n = 7), or an elevated erythrocyte sedimentation rate (n = 18). Nonreactive patients (n = 42) had none of these features. At three months, 67 percent of the reactive patients who received prednisone had LVEF improvement, as compared with 28 percent of the reactive controls (P = 0.004) [192]. The data of this study suggested that patients with idiopathic dilated cardiomyopathy may have some improvement when given a high dose of prednisone. However, the increase in the ejection fraction was overall small with limited duration, and the side effects were important. In conclusion, prednisone was judged to have only a marginal clinical benefit, and should not be administered as standard therapy for dilated cardiomyopathy.

3.5.2 Etarnecept

TNF-α inhibitors are immunomodulators that are used in a wide variety of rheumatological/autoimmune diseases including RA, [193, 194], inflammatory bowel disease, [195] and psoriasis/psoriatic arthritis [196].

Etanercept is a human recombinant TNF-α receptor that binds and inactivates circulating TNF-α molecules.

Preclinical experimental studies have demonstrated that etanercept reversed the deleterious negative inotropic effect of TNF-α [139, 197].

A series of phase I clinical studies in patients with moderate to advanced HF showed improvements in 6 –minute walk distance, quality of life and LV cardiac function following treatment with etanercept for up to 3 months [198, 199]. Subsequently, two large multicenter quality of life clinical trials RENAISSANCE (Randomized Etanercept North American Strategy to Study Antogonism of Cytokines) and RECOVER (Research into Etanercept Cytokine Antagonism in Ventricular Dysfunction) were conducted in HF patients with NYHA class II-IV and demonstrated no clinical benefit [200]. The RENEWAL (Randomized Etanercept World-wide EvALuation) clinical trial with all cause mortality and hospitalization for HF as primary end-point, did not reveal any benefit either with etarnecept [201].

3.5.3 Infliximab

Infliximab is a chimeric monoclonal antibody that binds and inactivates circulating TNF-α that has been shown to be effective in the treatment of Crohn disease and rheumatoid arthritis. The ATTACH clinical trial (Anti-TNF-α Therapy Against CHF), a phase II study enrolled 150 patients with NYHA class III-IV HF. The results of this trial revealed no beneficial effects on clinical status with infliximab. There was even a dose related increase in mortality and HF hospitalizations with infliximab when compared to placebo at 14 and 28 weeks, resulting in early termination of the trial [202].

3.5.4 Intravenous immunoglobulin

Although the exact mechanism of intravenous immunoglobulin (IVIg) therapy is not known, IVig therapy is being used in a wide range of immune-mediated disorders, such as dermatomyosis, Kawasaki and multiple sclerosis [203, 204]. Based on an initial report that IVIg was beneficial in acute cardiomyopathy, [205] Gullestad et al. conducted a double-blind clinical trial with IVIg for 26 weeks in 47 patients with Class II-III HF, who were receiving standard HF therapy including ACE inhibitors and β-blockers. In this study, IVIg induced a marked rise in plasma levels of the anti-inflammatory mediators (IL-10, IL-1 receptor antagonist and soluble TNF receptors) and was associated with a significant increase in LVEF [206]. Thus in this small study, therapy with IVIg was potentially effective in patients with cardiomyopathy and HF, but these results should be confirmed in a larger subset of patients and also needs to examine the effect on morbidity and mortality of this therapy.

4. Oxydative Stress

Oxidative stress, defined as an excess production of reactive oxygen species (ROS) relative to antioxidant defense (**Figure 4**), has been shown to play an important role in the pathophysiology of cardiac remodeling in HF, [6–9, 207]. Specifically, ROS activate a broad variety of hypertrophy signaling kinases and transcription factors and mediate apoptosis. They also stimulate cardiac fibroblast proliferation and activate the matrix metalloproteinases (MMPs), leading to the extracellular matrix remodeling. Moreover, ROS can directly impair the cardiac contractile function by modifying proteins involved in excitation-contraction coupling. These cellular events are involved in the development and progression of maladaptive myocardial remodeling and failure.

Oxidation products of several organic molecules including lipids, proteins, and nucleic acids have been implicated in the pathogenesis of dilated cardiomyopathy and their levels are found to be increased in heart failure. The severity of heart failure and levels of oxidative stress increase concurrently, which suggests that oxidative stress could be utilized as a biomarker for dilated cardiomyopathy progression.

Oxidative stress is associated with increased production of ROS and reactive nitrogen species (RNS), diminished nitric oxide (NO) bioavaibility and reduced superoxide dismutase (SOD), glutathione peroxidase and catalase activity. ROS are formed as products of oxidation–reduction reactions and include free radical molecules such as superoxide (O2−), hydroxyl radical (OH−), lipid peroxyl and non-free radical species like hydrogen peroxide (H2O2). RNS like (ONOO−) are

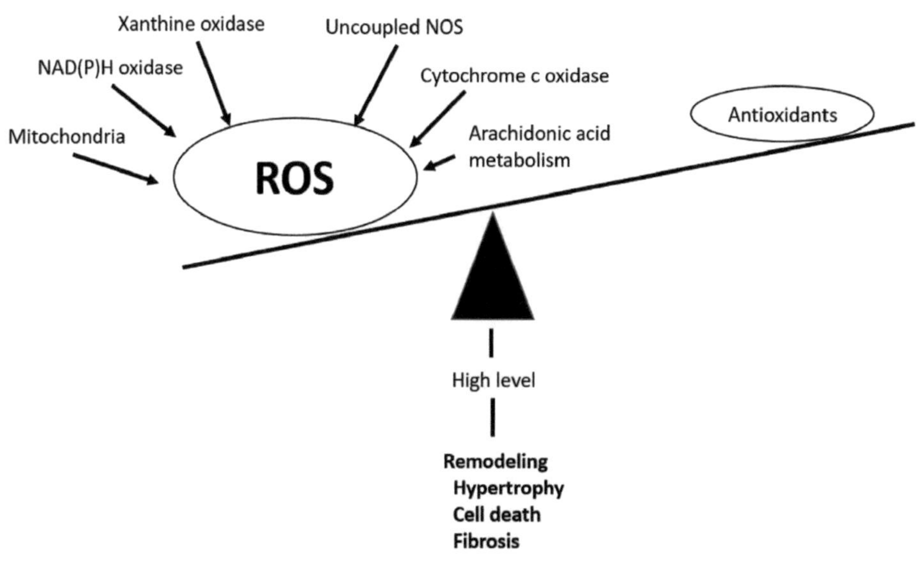

Figure 4.
Source of reactive oxygen species (ROS) and their pathophysiological role in heart failure. NOS: Nitric oxide synthase.

formed by the reaction between nitric oxide (NO) and O2− [208]. Cellular ROS are generated predominantly as by-products of mitochondrial respiration, NADPH oxidase, endothelial nitric oxide synthase (eNOS) [209] and xanthine oxidase activity [210].

Clinically, oxydative stress markers have prognostic values as they correlate with worsening NYHA functional class and cardiac dysfunction [211, 212]. Several studies have demonstrated that the lipid peroxidation products such as malondialdehyde [MDA] [211] and 4-hydroxynonenal [213] are increased in patients with dilated cardiomyopathies compared to normal controls. Myeloperoxidase, a peroxidase enzyme present in granulocytes is increased in the serum of patients with dilated cardiomyopathy. Increased myeloperidase levels correlate with HF severity. Finally, plasma myeloperidase appears also to be an independent predictor of mortality and HF hospitalization [212]. Uric acid, produced by the ubiquitous ROS-generating xanthine oxidase, is considered as a marker for oxidative stress in the cardiovascular system. It is released from the failing human heart, with an inverse correlation between the level of uric acid and left ventricular ejection fraction [214]. Increased serum uric acid levels are associated with increased filling pressures, reduced cardiac index and plasma NT-proBNP [215]. Uric acid is also a strong independent predictor of mortality in patients with dilated cardiomyopathy [216].

One consequence of myocardial oxidative stress is myocardial remodeling, including myocyte hypertrophy, myocyte apoptosis and alteration of the extracellular matrix.

Oxidative stress has direct effects on cellular structure and function and activates integral signaling molecules leading to myocardial remodeling and failure (**Figure 5**). Oxidative stress stimulates myocardial growth, matrix remodeling, and cellular dysfunction, which involve the activation of several downstream signaling pathways. First, ROS activate a broad variety of hypertrophy signaling kinases and

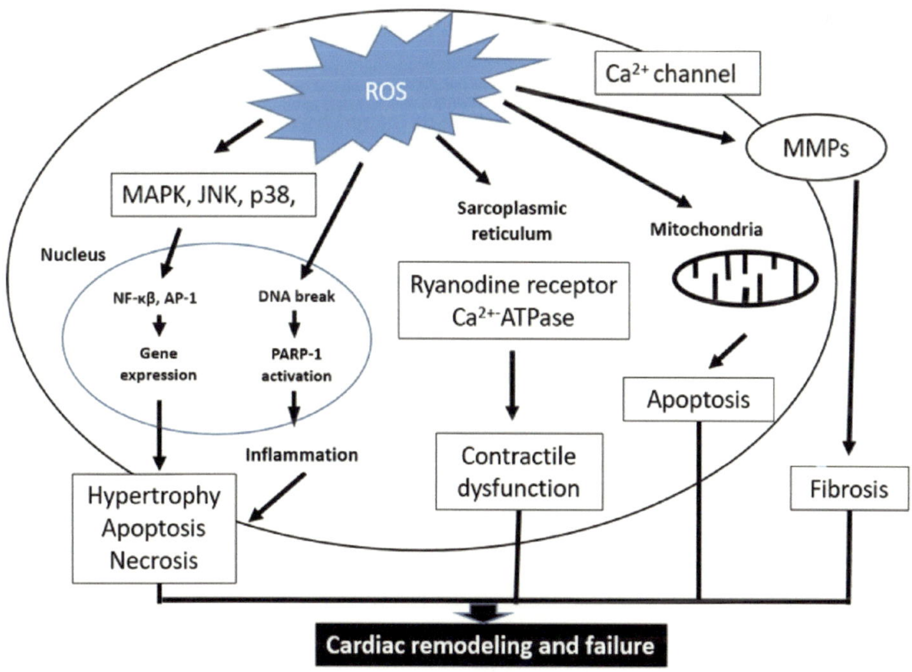

Figure 5.
Oxidative stress and heart failure. MAPK: Mitogen-activated protein kinases; JNK: Jun-nuclear kinase; PARP-1: Poly(ADP-ribose) polymerase-1; MMP: Matrix metalloproteinases; AP-1: Activator protein-1.

transcription factors [217]. Oxidative stress stimulates the tyrosine kinase Src, GTP-binding protein Ras, protein kinase C, mitogen-activated protein kinases (MAPK), Jun-nuclear kinase (JNK) and p38. Second, Oxidative stress induces apoptosis, another important contributor to remodeling and dysfunction, which is induced by ROS-mediated DNA and mitochondrial damage and activation of pro-apoptotic signaling kinases [218]. Third, Oxidative stress causes DNA strand breaks, activating the nuclear enzyme poly(ADP-ribose) polymerase-1 (PARP-1). PARP-1 regulates the expression of a variety of inflammatory mediators, which facilitate the progression of cardiac remodeling [219]. Fourth, oxidative stress can activate matrix metalloproteinases (MMPs), a family of proteolytic enzymes [220]. MMPs play a pivotal role in normal tissue remodeling processes, such as cell migration, invasion, proliferation, and apoptosis. MMP activity has been shown to be increased in the failing hearts [220, 221]. MMPs are generally produced in an inactive form and are activated by reactive oxygen species (ROS). Because MMP can be activated by ROS, one mechanism of LV remodeling is the activation of MMPs secondary to increased ROS [222]. Sustained MMP activation will lead to extracellular matrix remodeling. Fifth, ROS mediate growth responses in ventricular myocytes by stimulating the activity of several growth factors including transforming growth factor-β1 (TGF-β1), [223, 224] VEGF, [225] fibroblast growth factor-2 (FGF-2), [226], and PDGF [227]. Sixth, oxidative stress promotes vasoconstriction by increasing the production of endothelin-1 [228] and angiotensin II by increased production of 02- via the NADPH oxidase [229]. Seventh, oxidative stress upregulates the transcription of the factors HIF-1α and HIF-2α expression, [230] factors that are also implicated in the development of cardiomyopathy and HF. Eighth, increased oxidative stress leads to inflammation and cell injuries due to oxidation of proteins, lipids and DNA [209]. Finally, ROS directly influence myocyte contractile function by modifying proteins involved in excitation-contraction coupling. Zima and Blatter [231] including the ryanodine receptor, the L-type calcium channel, and the Ca2 + ATPase.

4.1 Oxidative stress and mitochondrial DNA damage

In addition to the role of mitochondria as a source of reactive oxygene species (ROS), the mitochondria themselves can be damaged by ROS. Increased generation of ROS in the failing hearts was associated with mitochondrial damage and dysfunction, characterized by an increased lipid peroxidation in the mitochondria, a reduction in the number of the mitochondrial DNA copy, a decrease in the number of mitochondrial RNA transcripts and a reduced oxidative capacity due to low complex enzyme activities [232]. They thus can lead to a catastrophic cycle of mitochondrial functional decline, further ROS generation, and cellular injury.

4.2 Therapies targeting oxidative stress

To date, there are no positive large-scale clinical trials of antioxidant therapy in cardiomyopathy and heart failure.

4.2.1 Coenzyme Q

Coenzyme Q (CoQ) is an antioxidant via the redox cycle. CoQ inhibits both the initiation and the propagation of lipid and protein oxidation.

Preclinical data has provided information across a variety of models supporting the pathophysiological role of CoQ10 depletion in HF and the concept of improved outcomes with CoQ10 supplementation [233].

There have been a large number of trials examining the effect of CoQ10 in HF. Two meta-analyses have examined the potential benefit of CoQ10. Fotino et al. [234] analysis from 13 trials and 395 patients demonstrated an improvement in LVEF of 3.67% (95% CI, 1.6%–5.74%) in those receiving CoQ10 versus placebo. The majority of benefit of LVEF improvement was in trials published before 1993. The other meta-analysis by Madmani et al. [235] looked at 7 studies data with 914 patients and did not show any significant improvement in LVEF or exercise capacity. Given the significant heterogeneity of the data, it was not possible to make any significant conclusion.

The most recent clinical trial with CoQ10l, Q-SYMBIO (Coenzyme Q10 as Adjunctive Treatment of Chronic Heart Failure: A Randomized, Double-blind, Multicenter Trial With Focus on Symptoms, Biomarker Status) enrolled 420 patients and demonstrated that compared with placebo, CoQ10 reduced the primary 2-year end point of cardiovascular death, hospital stays for HF, or mechanical support or cardiac transplant ($P = 0.005$; hazard ratio, 0.5; 95% CI, 0.32–0.80) [236]. Although having limitations, this study has renewed interest in evaluating CoQ10 supplementation in patients with HF. The results of the trial warrants future adequately powered randomized controlled trials of CoQ10 supplementation in patients with HF.

4.2.2 Allopurinol

Under normal conditions, the enzyme xanthine oxidase (XO) exists primarily in its dehydrogenase form, serving as the rate-limiting step in purine degradation to uric acid. Xanthine oxidase catalyzes the transformation of hypoxanthine to xanthine and then to uric acid with the associated production of four superoxide anions [237]. Xanthine oxidase is therefore a potential major regulator of cellular oxidative stress [238].

A large body of experimental and clinical data suggests that oxidative stress contributes to ventricular and vascular remodeling and disease progression in HF. XO is a potent source of oxidative stress, and therefore an obvious target for therapy.

Significant hyperuricemia is present in ≈25% of patients with HF with reduced ejection fraction, [215, 216] and it is associated with worsening symptoms, exercise intolerance, and reduced survival [239–241].

Under conditions of tissue hypoxia similar to HF in an experimental model, [242] the breakdown of ATP to AMP to hypoxanthine provides substrate to XO. Subsequently, XO uses oxygen rather than NAD as an oxidant. As a result, XO produces superoxide and hydrogen peroxide (H2O2) rather than NADH [243, 244]. Increased vascular O2• – production has been attributed in major part to XO, which has been found to adversely impact endothelial function by impairing nitric oxide (NO) signaling [245] and to directly contribute to experimental cardiac remodeling.

The Xanthine Oxidase Inhibition for Hyperuricemic Heart Failure Patients (EXACT-HF) Study, a randomized trial with 243 HF patients with reduced ejection fraction and elevated uric acid levels, xanthine oxidase inhibition with allopurinol compared to placebo failed to improve clinical status, exercise capacity, quality of life, or left ventricular ejection fraction after 24 weeks.of treatment [246].

In summary, oxidative stress appears to play an important role in the pathophysiology of cardiac remodeling and cardiomyopathy. Thus therapeutic strategies to modulate this maladaptive oxidative stress response as seen in cardiomyopathy and HF should become a target for future extensive investigation.

5. Conclusions

Cardiac remodeling represents the culmination of complex interactions between neuro-hormonal, stress activated cytokine and oxidative stress signaling pathways. These different signaling pathways feedback positively on one another and act in concert to initiate and propagate the cellular changes taking place within the remodeling ventricle. These pathways stimulate myocyte hypertrophy, increase the rate at which myocytes undergo hypertrophy, apoptotic cell death as well as proliferation of fibroblasts, some of which may differentiate into contractile myofibroblasts.

This constellation of cellular changes ultimately leads to gross morphological features of cardiac dilatation, progressive cardiac dysfunction and worsening heart failure. In this manner, these complex series of signaling events that lead to cardiac remodeling may very well represent the central pathophysiological mechanisms underlying cardiomyopathy progression.

Author details

Ronald Zolty
University of Nebraska Medical Center (UNMC), Omaha, NE, USA

*Address all correspondence to: ronald.zolty@unmc.edu

References

[1] Richardson P, McKenna W, Bristow M, Maisch B, Mautner B, O'Connell J, et al .Report of the 1995 World Health Organization/ International Society and Federation of Cardiology Task Force on the Definition and Classification of cardiomyopathies. Circulation. 1996 Mar 1;93(5):841-842. doi: 10.1161/01.cir.93.5.841.

[2] Bristow MR, Mestroni L, Bohlmeyer T, Gilbert EM. Chapter 66. Dilated Cardiomyopathies. Hurst's the Heart, 10th Edition, McGraw-Hill NY, 2001: 1947-1966.

[3] Dzau VJ Tissue renin-angiotensin system in myocardial hypertrophy and failure. Arch Intern Med. 1993 Apr 26;153(8):937-42.PMID: 8386920

[4] Packer M. The neurohormonal hypothesis: a theory to explain the mechanism of disease progression in heart failure. J Am Coll Cardiol. 1992 Jul;20(1):248-54. doi: 10.1016/0735-1097(92)90167-l. PMID: 1351488 DOI: 10.1016/0735-1097(92)90167-l.

[5] Mann DL. Inflammatory mediators and the failing heart: past, present, and the foreseeable future. Circ Res. 2002 Nov 29;91(11):988-98. doi: 10.1161/01.res.0000043825.01705.1b.PMID: 12456484

[6] Belch JJ, Bridges AB, Scott N, Chopra M.Oxygen free radicals and congestive heart failure.Br Heart J. 1991; 65: 245-248.

[7] Hill MF, Singal PK. Antioxidant and oxidative stress changes during heart failure subsequent to myocardial infarction in rats. Am J Pathol 1996; 148: 291-300.

[8] Hill MF, Singal PK. Right and left myocardial antioxidant responses during heart failure subsequent to myocardial infarction. Circulation 1997; 96:2414-2420.

[9] Mallat Z, Philip I, Lebret M, Chatel D, Maclouf J, Tedgui A. Elevated levels of 8-iso-prostaglandin F2alpha in pericardial fluid of patients with heart failure: a potential role for in vivo oxidant stress in ventricular dilatation and progression to heart failure. Circulation 1998; 97: 1536-1539.

[10] Klein L, O'Connor CM, Gattis WA, Zampino M, de Luca L, Vitarelli A, et al. M.Pharmacologic therapy for patients with chronic heart failure and reduced systolic function: review of trials and practical considerations. Am J Cardiol. 2003 May 8;91(9A):18F–40F. doi: 10.1016/s0002-9149(02)03336-2. PMID: 12729848

[11] Sutton MG, Sharpe. Left ventricular remodeling after myocardial infarction: pathophysiology and therapy. Circulation. 2000 Jun 27;101(25):2981-2988. doi: 10.1161/01.cir.101.25.2981.

[12] Weber KT. Extracellular matrix remodeling in heart failure: a role for de novo angiotensin II generation. Circulation. 1997 Dec 2;96(11):4065-4082. doi: 10.1161/01.cir.96.11.4065.

[13] Shchekochikhin D, Schrier RW, Lindenfeld J. Cardiorenal syndrome: pathophysiology and treatment. Curr Cardiol Rep. 2013 Jul;15(7):380. doi: 10.1007/s11886-013-0380-4. PMID: 23700289

[14] Levine TB , Francis GS, Goldsmith SR, Simon AB, Cohn JN. Activity of the sympathetic nervous system and renin-angiotensin system assessed by plasma hormone levels and their relation to hemodynamic abnormalities in congestive heart failure. Am J Cardiol. 1982 May;49(7):1659-1666. doi: 10.1016/0002-9149(82)90243-0.

[15] Hasking GJ, Esler MD, Jennings GL, Burton D, Johns JA, Korner PI. Norepinephrine spillover to plasma in patients with congestive heart failure: evidence of increased overall and cardiorenal sympathetic nervous activity. Circulation. 1986 Apr;73(4):615-621. doi: 10.1161/01.cir.73.4.615.

[16] Davis D, Baily R, Zelis R. Abnormalities in systemic norepinephrine kinetics in human congestive heart failure.Am J Physiol. 1988 Jun;254(6 Pt 1):E760–E766. doi: 10.1152/ajpendo.1988.254.6.E760. PMID: 3377075

[17] Abraham WT, Hensen J, Schrier RW. Elevated plasma noradrenaline concentrations in patients with low-output cardiac failure: dependence on increased noradrenaline secretion rates Clin Sci (Lond). 1990 Nov;79(5):429-435. doi: 10.1042/cs0790429.

[18] Francis GS , Benedict C, Johnstone DE, Kirlin PC, Nicklas J, Liang CS, et al. Comparison of neuroendocrine activation in patients with left ventricular dysfunction with and without congestive heart failure. A substudy of the Studies of Left Ventricular Dysfunction (SOLVD). Circulation. 1990 Nov;82(5):1724-1729. doi: 10.1161/01.cir.82.5.1724.

[19] Folkow B, Johansson B, Mellander S. The comparative effects of angiotensin and noradrenaline on consecutive vascular sections. Acta Physiol Scand. 1961; 53:99-104 PMID: 13893844

[20] Zimmerman BG, Sybertz EJ, Wong PC. Interaction between sympathetic and renin-angiotensin system. J Hypertens. 1984 Dec;2(6): 581-587. doi: 10.1097/00004872-198412000-00002.

[21] Weber KT. Aldosterone in congestive heart failure. N Engl J Med. 2001 Dec 6;345(23):1689-1697. doi: 10.1056/NEJMra000050.

[22] Brown JJ, Fraser R, Leckie B, Lever AF, Morton JJ, Padfield PL, Semple PF, Robertson JI. Significance of renin and angiotensin in hypertension. Cardiovasc Clin. 1978;9(1):55-89. PMID: 352522.

[23] Williams B. Angiotensin II and the pathophysiology of cardiovascular remodeling. Am J Cardiol. 2001 Apr 19;87(8A):10C-17C. doi: 10.1016/s0002-9149(01)01507-7.PMID: 11334763.

[24] Brown NJ, Vaughan DE. Angiotensin-converting enzyme inhibitors. Circulation. 1998 Apr 14;97(14):1411-1420. doi: 10.1161/01.cir.97.14.1411. PMID: 9577953.

[25] Sadoshima J, Izumo S. Molecular characterization of angiotensin II--induced hypertrophy of cardiac myocytes and hyperplasia of cardiac fibroblasts. Critical role of the AT1 receptor subtype. Circ Res. 1993 Sep;73(3):413-423. doi: 10.1161/01.res.73.3.413.

[26] Greenberg BH. Effects of angiotensin converting enzyme inhibitors on remodeling in clinical trials.J Card Fail. 2002 Dec;8(6 Suppl):S486-90. doi: 10.1054/jcaf.2002.129251.PMID: 12555162

[27] Thomas JA, Marks BH. Plasma norepinephrine in congestive heart failure. Am J Cardiol. 1978 Feb;41(2):233-243. doi: 10.1016/0002-9149(78)90162-5. PMID: 203177

[28] Meredith IT, Eisenhofer G, Lambert GW, Dewar EM, Jennings GL, Esler MD. Cardiac sympathetic nervous activity in congestive heart failure. Evidence for increased neuronal norepinephrine release and preserved neuronal uptake. Circulation. 1993

Jul;88(1):136-145. doi: 10.1161/01.cir.88.1.136. PMID: 8391399

[29] Abraham WT, Lowes BD, Rose CP, Larrabee P, Bristow MR. Angiotensin II selectively increases cardiac adrenergic activity in patients with heart failure. J Am Coll Cardiol 1994; 23: 215A

[30] Berl T, Henrich WL, Erickson AL, Schrier RW. Prostaglandins in the beta-adrenergic and baroreceptor-mediated secretion of renin. Am J Physiol. 1979 May;236(5):F472–F477. doi: 10.1152/ajprenal.1979.236.5.F472. PMID: 220882

[31] Weber F, Brodde OE, Anlauf M, Bock KD. Subclassification of human beta-adrenergic receptors mediating renin release.Clin Exp Hypertens A. 1983;5(2):225-238. doi: 10.3109/10641968309048823. PMID: 6131758

[32] Bristow MR, Abraham WT. Anti-adrenergic effects of angiotensin converting enzyme inhibitors. Eur Heart J. 1995 Nov;16 Suppl K:37-41. doi: 10.1093/eurheartj/16.suppl_k.37. PMID: 8869134

[33] Cody RJ, Franklin KW, Kluger J, Laragh JH. Sympathetic responsiveness and plasma norepinephrine during therapy of chronic congestive heart failure with captopril. Am J Med. 1982 May;72(5):791-7. doi: 10.1016/0002-9343(82)90547-2.PMID: 7044120

[34] Gilbert EM, Sandoval A, Larrabee P, Renlund DG, O'Connell JB, Bristow MR. Lisinopril lowers cardiac adrenergic drive and increases beta-receptor density in the failing human heart. Circulation. 1993 Aug;88(2):472-480. doi: 10.1161/01.cir.88.2.472. PMID: 8393389

[35] Brodde OE, Michel MC. Adrenergic and muscarinic receptors in the human heart. Pharmacol Rev. 1999 Dec;51(4):651-90.PMID: 10581327

[36] Ahlquist RP A study of the adrenotropic receptors. Am J Physiol. 1948 Jun;153(3):586-600. doi: 10.1152/ajplegacy.1948.153.3.586. PMID: 18882199

[37] Lands AM, Arnold A, McAuliff JP, Luduena FP, Brown TG Jr.Differentiation of receptor systems activated by sympathomimetic amines. Nature. 1967 May 6;214(5088):597-598. doi: 10.1038/214597a0. PMID: 6036174

[38] Brodde OE. Beta-adrenoceptors in cardiac disease. Pharmacol Ther. 1993 Dec;60(3):405-430. doi: 10.1016/0163-7258(93)90030-h. PMID: 7915424

[39] Gauthier C, Langin D, Balligand JL. Beta3-adrenoceptors in the cardiovascular system.Trends Pharmacol Sci. 2000 Nov;21(11):426-31. doi: 10.1016/s0165-6147(00)01562-5. PMID: 11121573

[40] Arch JR, Ainsworth AT, Cawthorne MA, Piercy V, Sennitt MV, Thody VE, et al. Atypical beta-adrenoceptor on brown adipocytes as target for anti-obesity drugs. Nature. 1984 May 10-16;309(5964):163-5. doi: 10.1038/309163a0. PMID: 6325935

[41] Kaumann A, Bartel S, Molenaar P, Sanders L, Burrell K, Vetter D, et al. Activation of beta2-adrenergic receptors hastens relaxation and mediates phosphorylation of phospholamban, troponin I, and C-protein in ventricular myocardium from patients with terminal heart failure. Circulation. 1999 Jan 5-12;99(1):65-72. doi: 10.1161/01.cir.99.1.65. PMID: 9884381

[42] Zhao XL, Gutierrez LM, Chang CF, Hosey MM. The alpha 1-subunit of skeletal muscle L-type Ca channels is the key target for regulation by A-kinase and protein phosphatase-1C. Biochem Biophys Res Commun. 1994 Jan 14;198(1):166-173. doi: 10.1006/bbrc.1994.1024. PMID: 8292020

[43] Gerhardstein BL, Puri TS, Chien AJ, Hosey MM. Identification of the sites phosphorylated by cyclic AMP-dependent protein kinase on the beta 2 subunit of L-type voltage-dependent calcium channels. Biochemistry. 1999 Aug 10;38(32):10361-10370. doi: 10.1021/bi990896o. PMID: 10441130

[44] Marx SO, Reiken S, Hisamatsu Y, Jayaraman T, Burkhoff D, Rosemblit N, Marks AR. PKA phosphorylation dissociates FKBP12.6 from the calcium release channel (ryanodine receptor): defective regulation in failing hearts. Cell. 2000 May 12;101(4):365-376. doi: 10.1016/s0092-8674(00)80847-8.

[45] Sulakhe PV, Vo XT. Regulation of phospholamban and troponin-I phosphorylation in the intact rat cardiomyocytes by adrenergic and cholinergic stimuli: roles of cyclic nucleotides, calcium, protein kinases and phosphatases and depolarization. Mol Cell Biochem. 1995 Aug-Sep;149-150:103-26. doi: 10.1007/BF01076569. PMID: 8569720

[46] Kunst G, Kress KR, Gruen M, Uttenweiler D, Gautel M, Fink RH. Myosin binding protein C, a phosphorylation-dependent force regulator in muscle that controls the attachment of myosin heads by its interaction with myosin S2.Circ Res. 2000 Jan 7-21;86(1):51-8. doi: 10.1161/01.res.86.1.51. PMID: 10625305

[47] Zhang ZY, Zhou B, Xie L. Modulation of protein kinase signaling by protein phosphatases and inhibitors. Pharmacol Ther. 2002 Feb-Mar;93(2-3):307-317. doi: 10.1016/s0163-7258(02)00199-7. PMID: 12191622

[48] Bristow MR, Ginsburg R, Minobe W, Cubicciotti RS, Sageman WS, Lurie K, et al .Decreased catecholamine sensitivity and beta-adrenergic-receptor density in failing human hearts. N Engl J Med. 1982 Jul 22;307(4):205-211. doi: 10.1056/NEJM198207223070401. PMID: 6283349

[49] Böhm M, La Rosée K, Schwinger RH, Erdmann E . Evidence for reduction of norepinephrine uptake sites in the failing human heart. J Am Coll Cardiol. 1995 Jan;25(1):146-153. doi: 10.1016/0735-1097(94)00353-r. PMID: 7798493

[50] Bristow MR, Ginsburg R, Umans V, Fowler M, Minobe W, Rasmussen R, et al. Beta 1- and beta 2-adrenergic-receptor subpopulations in nonfailing and failing human ventricular myocardium: coupling of both receptor subtypes to muscle contraction and selective beta 1-receptor down-regulation in heart failure. Circ Res. 1986 Sep;59(3):297-309. doi: 10.1161/01.res.59.3.297. PMID: 2876788

[51] Ungerer M, Böhm M, Elce JS, Erdmann E, Lohse MJ. Altered expression of beta-adrenergic receptor kinase and beta 1-adrenergic receptors in the failing human heart. Circulation. 1993 Feb;87(2):454-463. doi: 10.1161/01.cir.87.2.454. PMID: 8381058

[52] Bristow MR. beta-adrenergic receptor blockade in chronic heart failure. Circulation. 2000 Feb 8;101(5):558-569. doi: 10.1161/01.cir.101.5.558. PMID: 10662755

[53] Packer M, Bristow MR, Cohn JN, Colucci WS, Fowler MB, Gilbert EM, Shusterman NH. The effect of carvedilol on morbidity and mortality in patients with chronic heart failure. U.S. Carvedilol Heart Failure Study Group. N Engl J Med. 1996 May 23;334(21):1349-55. doi: 10.1056/NEJM199605233342101. PMID: 8614419

[54] CIBIS II Investigators and Committees: The Cardiac Insufficiency Bisoprolol Study II (CIBIS-II): a randomised trial. Lancet. 1999 Jan 2;353(9146):9-13. PMID: 10023943

[55] MERIT-HF Study Group Effect of metoprolol CR/XL in chronic heart failureEffect of metoprolol CR/XL in chronic heart failure: Metoprolol CR/XL Randomised Intervention Trial in Congestive Heart Failure (MERIT-HF). Lancet. 1999 Jun 12;353(9169):2001-7. PMID: 10376614

[56] Beta-Blocker Evaluation of Survival Trial Investigators, Eichhorn EJ, Domanski MJ, Krause-Steinrauf H, Bristow MR, Lavori PW. A trial of the beta-blocker bucindolol in patients with advanced chronic heart failure.N Engl J Med. 2001 May 31;344(22):1659-67. doi:10.1056/NEJM200105313442202. PMID: 11386264

[57] Xamoterol in severe heart failure. The Xamoterol in Severe Heart Failure Study Group. Lancet. 1990 Jul 7;336(8706):1-6. PMID: 1694945

[58] Engelhardt S, Grimmer Y, Fan GH, Lohse MJ. Constitutive activity of the human beta(1)-adrenergic receptor in beta(1)-receptor transgenic mice. Engelhardt S, Grimmer Y, Fan GH, Lohse MJ. Mol Pharmacol. 2001 Oct;60(4):712-717. PMID: 11562432

[59] Swedberg K, Eneroth P, Kjekshus J, Wilhelmsen L. Hormones regulating cardiovascular function in patients with severe congestive heart failure and their relation to mortality. CONSENSUS Trial Study GroupCirculation. 1990 Nov;82(5):1730-1736. doi: 10.1161/01.cir.82.5.1730.

[60] Tsuji H, Venditti FJ Jr, Evans JC, Larson MG, Levy D. The associations of levels of serum potassium and magnesium with ventricular premature complexes (the Framingham Heart Study). Am J Cardiol. 1994 Aug 1;74(3):232-235. doi: 10.1016/0002-9149(94)90362-x. PMID: 7518645

[61] Gottlieb SS, Baruch L, Kukin ML, Bernstein JL, Fisher ML, Packer M. Prognostic importance of the serum magnesium concentration in patients with congestive heart failure.J Am Coll Cardiol. 1990 Oct;16(4):827-831. doi: 10.1016/s0735-1097(10)80329-8. PMID: 2212365

[62] Farquharson CA, Struthers AD. Spironolactone increases nitric oxide bioactivity, improves endothelial vasodilator dysfunction, and suppresses vascular angiotensin I/angiotensin II conversion in patients with chronic heart failure. Circulation. 2000 Feb 15;101(6):594-597. doi: 10.1161/01.cir.101.6.594. PMID: 10673249

[63] Heitzer T, Schlinzig T, Krohn K, Meinertz T, Münzel T. Endothelial dysfunction, oxidative stress, and risk of cardiovascular events in patients with coronary artery disease. Circulation. 2001 Nov 27;104(22):2673-2678. doi: 10.1161/hc4601.099485. PMID: 11723017

[64] Brilla CG, Zhou G, Matsubara L, Weber KT. Collagen metabolism in cultured adult rat cardiac fibroblasts: response to angiotensin II and aldosterone. J Mol Cell Cardiol. 1994 Jul;26(7):809-820. doi: 10.1006/jmcc.1994.1098. PMID: 7966349

[65] Brilla CG, Pick R, Tan LB, Janicki JS, Weber KT. Remodeling of the rat right and left ventricles in experimental hypertension. Circ Res. 1990 Dec;67(6):1355-1364. doi: 10.1161/01.res.67.6.1355. PMID: 1700933

[66] Wang W. Chronic administration of aldosterone depresses baroreceptor reflex function in the dog. Hypertension. 1994 Nov;24(5):571-575. doi: 10.1161/01.hyp.24.5.571. PMID: 7960015

[67] Yee KM, Struthers AD. Aldosterone blunts the baroreflex response in man. Clin Sci (Lond). 1998 Dec;95(6):687-692. doi: 10.1042/cs0950687. PMID: 9831693

[68] Vaughan DE, Lazos SA, Tong K. Angiotensin II regulates the expression of plasminogen activator inhibitor-1 in cultured endothelial cells. A potential link between the renin-angiotensin system and thrombosis. J Clin Invest. 1995 Mar;95(3):995-1001. doi: 10.1172/JCI117809. PMID: 7884001

[69] Pitt B, Zannad F, Remme WJ, Cody R, Castaigne A, Perez A, et al. The effect of spironolactone on morbidity and mortality in patients with severe heart failure. Randomized Aldactone Evaluation Study Investigators N Engl J Med. 1999 Sep 2;341(10):709-717. doi: 10.1056/NEJM199909023411001.

[70] Clavell AL, Mattingly MT, Stevens TL, Nir A, Wright S, Aarhus LL, et al. Angiotensin converting enzyme inhibition modulates endogenous endothelin in chronic canine thoracic inferior vena caval constriction. J Clin Invest. 1996 Mar 1;97(5):1286-1292. doi: 10.1172/JCI118544. PMID: 8636441

[71] Noll G, Wenzel RR, Lüscher TF. Endothelin and endothelin antagonists: potential role in cardiovascular and renal disease. Mol Cell Biochem. 1996 Apr 12-26;157(1-2):259-67. doi: 10.1007/BF00227908. PMID: 8739256

[72] Fukuroda T, Fujikawa T, Ozaki S, Ishikawa K, Yano M, Nishikibe M. Clearance of circulating endothelin-1 by ETB receptors in rats. Biochem Biophys Res Commun. 1994 Mar 30;199(3):1461-1465. doi: 10.1006/bbrc.1994.1395. PMID: 8147891

[73] Fukuchi M, Giaid A. Expression of endothelin-1 and endothelin-converting enzyme-1 mRNAs and proteins in failing human hearts. J Cardiovasc Pharmacol. 1998;31 Suppl 1:S421–S423. doi: 10.1097/00005344-199800001-00120. PMID: 9595501

[74] Genth-Zotz S, Zotz RJ, Cobaugh M, van Veldhuisen DJ, Netzer T, Meyer J, Darius H. Changes of neurohumoral parameters and endothelin-1 in response to exercise in patients with mild to moderate congestive heart failure. Int J Cardiol. 1998 Sep 30;66(2):137-142. doi: 10.1016/s0167-5273(98)00225-3. PMID: 9829325

[75] Kiowski W, Sütsch G, Hunziker P, Müller P, Kim J, Oechslin E et al. Evidence for endothelin-1-mediated vasoconstriction in severe chronic heart failure. Lancet. 1995 Sep 16;346(8977):732-736. doi: 10.1016/s0140-6736(95)91504-4. PMID: 7658874

[76] Good JM, Nihoyannopoulos P, Ghatei MA, Crossman D, Bloom SR, Clark P, et al. Elevated plasma endothelin concentrations in heart failure; an effect of angiotensin II? Eur Heart J. 1994 Dec;15(12):1634-1640. doi: 10.1093/oxfordjournals.eurheartj.a060446. PMID: 7698133

[77] Pacher R, Stanek B, Hülsmann M, Koller-Strametz J, Berger R, Schuller M, et al .Prognostic impact of big endothelin-1 plasma concentrations compared with invasive hemodynamic evaluation in severe heart failure. J Am Coll Cardiol. 1996 Mar 1;27(3):633-641. doi: 10.1016/0735-1097(95)00520-x. PMID: 8606275

[78] Tsutamoto T, Wada A, Maeda Y, Adachi T, Kinoshita M. Relation between endothelin-1 spillover in the lungs and pulmonary vascular resistance in patients with chronic heart failure. J Am Coll Cardiol. 1994 May;23(6):1427-1433. doi: 10.1016/0735-1097(94)90387-5. PMID: 8176102

[79] Sakai S, Miyauchi T, Sakurai T, Kasuya Y, Ihara M, Yamaguchi I, et al. Endogenous endothelin-1 participates in the maintenance of cardiac function in rats with congestive heart failure. Marked increase in endothelin-1 production in the failing heart. Circulation. 1996 Mar 15;93(6):1214-1222. doi: 10.1161/01.cir.93.6.1214. PMID: 8653844

[80] Cody RJ, Haas GJ, Binkley PF, Capers Q, Kelley R. Plasma endothelin correlates with the extent of pulmonary hypertension in patients with chronic congestive heart failure. Circulation. 1992 Feb;85(2):504-509. doi: 10.1161/01.cir.85.2.504. PMID: 1735147

[81] Takeda S, Takano T, Ogawa R. The effect of nasal continuous positive airway pressure on plasma endothelin-1 concentrations in patients with severe cardiogenic pulmonary edema. Anesth Analg. 1997 May;84(5):1091-1096. doi: 10.1097/00000539-199705000-00025. PMID: 9141937

[82] Kobayshi T, Miyauchi T, Sakai S, Maeda S, Yamaguchi I, Goto K, Sugishita Y Down-regulation of ET(B) receptor, but not ET(A) receptor, in congestive lung secondary to heart failure. Are marked increases in circulating endothelin-1 partly attributable to decreases in lung ET(B) receptor-mediated clearance of endothelin-1?Life Sci. 1998;62(2):185-93. doi: 10.1016/s0024-3205(97)01064-3. PMID: 9488116

[83] Ooi H, Colucci WS, Givertz MM. Endothelin mediates increased pulmonary vascular tone in patients with heart failure: demonstration by direct intrapulmonary infusion of sitaxsentan. Circulation. 2002 Sep 24;106(13):1618-1621. doi: 10.1161/01.cir.0000034444.31846.f4. PMID: 12270852

[84] Fleisch M, Sütsch G, Yan XW, Wenzel RR, Binggeli C, Bianchetti MG, et al Systemic, pulmonary, and renal hemodynamic effects of endothelin ET(A/B)-receptor blockade in patients with maintained left ventricular function J Cardiovasc Pharmacol. 2000 Sep;36(3):302-309. doi: 10.1097/00005344-200009000-00004. PMID: 10975586

[85] Rodeheffer RJ, Lerman A, Heublein DM, Burnett JC Jr. Increased plasma concentrations of endothelin in congestive heart failure in humans. Mayo Clin Proc. 1992 Aug;67(8):719-24. doi: 10.1016/s0025-6196(12)60795-2. PMID: 1434909

[86] Wei CM, Lerman A, Rodeheffer RJ, McGregor CG, Brandt RR, Wright S, et al. Endothelin in human congestive heart failure. Circulation. 1994 Apr;89(4):1580-1586. doi: 10.1161/01.cir.89.4.1580. PMID: 8149524

[87] Tsutamoto T, Hisanaga T, Fukai D, Wada A, Maeda Y, Maeda K, Kinoshita M. Prognostic value of plasma soluble intercellular adhesion molecule-1 and endothelin-1 concentration in patients with chronic congestive heart failure. Am J Cardiol. 1995 Oct 15;76(11):803-808. doi: 10.1016/s0002-9149(99)80231-8. PMID: 7572659

[88] Krum H, Goldsmith R, Wilshire-Clement M, Miller M, Packer M. Role of endothelin in the exercise intolerance of chronic heart failure. Am J Cardiol. 1995 Jun 15;75(17):1282-1283. doi: 10.1016/s0002-9149(99)80783-8. PMID: 7778560

[89] Omland T, Lie RT, Aakvaag A, Aarsland T, Dickstein K. Plasma endothelin determination as a prognostic indicator of 1-year mortality after acute myocardial infarction. Circulation. 1994 Apr;89(4):1573-1579. doi: 10.1161/01.cir.89.4.1573. PMID: 8149523

[90] Pousset F, Isnard R, Lechat P, Kalotka H, Carayon A, Maistre G, et al. Prognostic value of plasma endothelin-1 in patients with chronic heart failure. Eur Heart J. 1997 Feb;18(2):254-258. doi: 10.1093/oxfordjournals.eurheartj.a015228. PMID: 9043842

[91] Hülsmann M, Stanek B, Frey B, Sturm B, Putz D, Kos T, et al. Value of cardiopulmonary exercise testing and

big endothelin plasma levels to predict short-term prognosis of patients with chronic heart failure. J Am Coll Cardiol. 1998 Nov 15;32(6):1695-1700. doi: 10.1016/s0735-1097(98)00437-9. PMID: 9822098

[92] Frey B, Pacher R, Locker G, Bojic A, Hartter E, Woloszczuk W, Stanek B. Prognostic value of hemodynamic vs big endothelin measurements during long-term IV therapy in advanced heart failure patients. Chest. 2000 Jun;117(6):1713-1719. doi: 10.1378/chest.117.6.1713. PMID: 10858407

[93] Stanek B, Frey B, Hülsmann M, Koller-Strametz J, Hartter E, Schuller M, et al .Validation of big endothelin plasma levels compared with established neurohumoral markers in patients with severe chronic heart failure. Transplant Proc. 1997 Feb-Mar;29(1-2):595-6. doi: 10.1016/s0041 1345(96)00097-8. PMID: 9123146

[94] Sakai S, Miyauchi T, Kobayashi M, Yamaguchi I, Goto K, Sugishita Y. Inhibition of myocardial endothelin pathway improves long-term survival in heart failure. Nature. 1996 Nov 28;384(6607):353-355. doi: 10.1038/384353a0. PMID: 8934519

[95] Spinale FG, Walker JD, Mukherjee R, Iannini JP, Keever AT, Gallagher KP. Concomitant endothelin receptor subtype-A blockade during the progression of pacing-induced congestive heart failure in rabbits. Beneficial effects on left ventricular and myocyte function. Circulation. 1997 Apr 1;95(7):1918-1929. doi: 10.1161/01.cir.95.7.1918. PMID: 9107181

[96] Borgeson DD, Grantham JA, Williamson EE, Luchner A, Redfield MM, Opgenorth TJ, Burnett JC Jr. Chronic oral endothelin type A receptor antagonism in experimental heart failure. Hypertension. 1998 Mar;31(3):766-770. doi: 10.1161/01.hyp.31.3.766. PMID: 9495259

[97] Moe GW, Albernaz A, Naik GO, Kirchengast M, Stewart DJ. Beneficial effects of long-term selective endothelin type A receptor blockade in canine experimental heart failure. Cardiovasc Res. 1998 Sep;39(3):571-579. doi: 10.1016/s0008-6363(98)00169-2. PMID: 9861299

[98] Kalra PR, Moon JC, Coats AJ. Do results of the ENABLE (Endothelin Antagonist Bosentan for Lowering Cardiac Events in Heart Failure) study spell the end for non-selective endothelin antagonism in heart failure? Int J Cardiol. 2002 Oct;85(2-3):195-197. doi: 10.1016/s0167-5273(02)00182-1. PMID: 12208583

[99] Cosenzi A. Enrasentan, an antagonist of endothelin receptors. Cardiovasc Drug Rev. 2003 Spring;21(1):1-16. doi: 10.1111/j.1527-3466.2003.tb00102.x. PMID: 12595914

[100] Anand I, McMurray J, Cohn JN, Konstam MA, Notter T, Quitzau K, et al; EARTH investigators.Long-term effects of darusentan on left-ventricular remodelling and clinical outcomes in the EndothelinA Receptor Antagonist Trial in Heart Failure (EARTH): randomised, double-blind, placebo-controlled trial. Lancet. 2004 Jul 24-30;364(9431):347-54. doi: 10.1016/S0140-6736(04)16723-8. PMID: 15276394

[101] Goldsmith SR, Francis GS, Cowley AW Jr, Levine TB, Cohn JN. Increased plasma arginine vasopressin levels in patients with congestive heart failure. J Am Coll Cardiol. 1983 Jun;1(6):1385-1390. doi: 10.1016/s0735-1097(83)80040-0. PMID: 6343460

[102] Anand IS, Ferrari R, Kalra GS, Wahi PL, Poole-Wilson PA, Harris PC. Edema of cardiac origin. Studies of body water and sodium, renal function, hemodynamic indexes, and plasma hormones in untreated congestive cardiac failure. Circulation. 1989

Aug;80(2):299-305. doi: 10.1161/01.cir.80.2.299. PMID: 2752558

[103] Goldsmith SR, Gheorghiade M. Vasopressin antagonism in heart failure J Am Coll Cardiol. 2005 Nov 15;46(10):1785-1791. doi: 10.1016/j.jacc.2005.02.095. Epub 2005 Oct 21.

[104] Walker BR, Childs ME, Adams EM. Direct cardiac effects of vasopressin: role of V1- and V2-vasopressinergic receptors. Am J Physiol. 1988 Aug;255(2 Pt 2):H261–H265. doi: 10.1152/ajpheart.1988.255.2.H261. PMID: 2970231

[105] Kaygisiz Z, Kabadere TE, Dernek S, Erden SH.The effects of vasopressin in isolated rat hearts. Indian J Physiol Pharmacol. 2001 Jan;45(1):54-62. PMID: 11211571

[106] Briner VA, Tsai P, Choong HL, Schrier RW. Comparative effects of arginine vasopressin and oxytocin in cell culture systems. Am J Physiol. 1992 Aug;263(2 Pt 2):F222–F227. doi: 10.1152/ajprenal.1992.263.2.F222. PMID: 1510120

[107] Nakamura Y, Haneda T, Osaki J, Miyata S, Kikuchi K. Hypertrophic growth of cultured neonatal rat heart cells mediated by vasopressin V(1A) receptor Eur J Pharmacol. 2000 Mar 10;391(1-2):39-48. doi: 10.1016/s0014-2999(99)00775-x. PMID: 10720633

[108] Fukuzawa J, Haneda T, Kikuchi K. Arginine vasopressin increases the rate of protein synthesis in isolated perfused adult rat heart via the V1 receptor. Mol Cell Biochem. 1999 May;195(1-2):93-98. doi: 10.1023/a:1006980517557. PMID: 10395073

[109] Xu DL, Martin PY, Ohara M, St John J, Pattison T, Meng X, et al. Upregulation of aquaporin-2 water channel expression in chronic heart failure rat. J Clin Invest. 1997 Apr 1;99(7):1500-1505. doi: 10.1172/JCI119312. PMID: 9119993

[110] Schrier RW, Berl T, Anderson RJ. Osmotic and nonosmotic control of vasopressin release. Am J Physiol. 1979 Apr;236(4):F321–F332. doi: 10.1152/ajprenal.1979.236.4.F321. PMID: 373467

[111] Share L. Role of vasopressin in cardiovascular regulation. Physiol Rev. 1988 Oct;68(4):1248-1284. doi: 10.1152/physrev.1988.68.4.1248. PMID: 3054948

[112] Goldsmith SR. Baroreflex loading maneuvers do not suppress increased plasma arginine vasopressin in patients with congestive heart failure. J Am Coll Cardiol. 1992 May;19(6):1180-1184. doi: 10.1016/0735-1097(92)90321-d. PMID: 1532971

[113] Goldsmith SR, Francis GS, Cowley AW, Cohn N. Response of vasopressin and norepinephrine to lower body negative pressure in humans. Am J Physiol 1982; 243: H970

[114] Goldsmith SR, Cowley AW, Francis GS, Cohn N. Effects of increased intracardiac and arterial pressure on plasma vasopressin in humans. Am J Physiol 1984; 246: H647

[115] Szatalowicz VL, Arnold PE, Chaimovitz C, Bichet D, Berl T, Schrier RW. Radioimmunoassay of plasma arginine vasopressin in hyponatremic patients with congestive heart failure. N Engl J Med. 1981 Jul 30;305(5):263-266. doi: 10.1056/NEJM198107303050506. PMID: 7242616

[116] Riegger GA, Liebau G, Kochsiek K. Antidiuretic hormone in congestive heart failure. Am J Med. 1982 Jan;72(1):49-52. doi: 10.1016/0002-9343(82)90576-9. PMID: 7058822

[117] Udelson JE, Smith WB, Hendrix GH, Painchaud CA, Ghazzi M, Thomas I, et al . Acute hemodynamic effects of conivaptan, a dual V(1A) and

V(2) vasopressin receptor antagonist, in patients with advanced heart failure. Circulation. 2001 Nov 13;104(20):2417-2423. doi: 10.1161/hc4501.099313. PMID: 11705818

[118] Konstam MA, Gheorghiade M, Burnett JC Jr, Grinfeld L, Maggioni AP, Swedberg K, et al; Efficacy of Vasopressin Antagonism in Heart Failure Outcome Study With Tolvaptan (EVEREST) Investigators. Effects of oral tolvaptan in patients hospitalized for worsening heart failure: the EVEREST Outcome Trial. JAMA. 2007 Mar 28;297(12):1319-1331. doi: 10.1001/jama.297.12.1319. Epub 2007 Mar 25. PMID: 17384437

[119] de Bold AJ, Borenstein HB, Veress AT, et al. A rapid and potent natriuretic response to intravenous injection of atrial myocardial extract in rats. Life Sci. 1981;28:89-94.

[120] Sudoh T, Kangawa K, Minamino N, et al. A new natriuretic peptide in porcine brain. Nature. 1988;332:78-81.

[121] Potter LR, Abbey-Hosch S, Dickey DM. Natriuretic peptides, their receptors, and cyclic guanosine monophosphate-dependent signaling functions. Endocr Rev. 2006;27:47-72.

[122] Boerrigter G, Burnett JC., Jr Recent advances in natriuretic peptides in congestive heart failure. Expert Opin Investig Drugs. 2004;13:643-652.

[123] Zois NE, Bartels ED, Hunter I, et al. Natriuretic peptides in cardiometabolic regulation and disease. Nat Rev Cardiol. 2014;11:403-412. DOI: 10.1038/nrcardio.2014.64.

[124] Mangiafico S, Costello-Boerrigter LC, Andersen IA, et al. Neutral endopeptidase inhibition and the natriuretic peptide system: an evolving strategy in cardiovascular therapeutics. Eur Heart J. 2013;34:886-93c. DOI: 10.1093/eurheartj/ehs262.

[125] Chen HH, Burnett JC., Jr Therapeutic potential for existing and novel forms of natriuretic peptides. Heart Fail Clin. 2006;2:365-373.

[126] Northridge DB, Newby DE, Rooney E, et al. Comparison of the short-term effects of candoxatril, an orally active neutral endopeptidase inhibitor, and frusemide in the treatment of patients with chronic heart failure. Am Heart J. 1999;138:1149-1157.

[127] Westheim AS, Bostrøm P, Christensen CC, et al. Hemodynamic and neuroendocrine effects for candoxatril and frusemide in mild stable chronic heart failure. J Am Coll Cardiol. 1999;34:1794-1801.

[128] Ando S, Rahman MA, Butler GC, et al. Comparison of candoxatril and atrial natriuretic factor in healthy men. Effects on hemodynamics, sympathetic activity, heart rate variability, and endothelin. Hypertension. 1995;26:1160-1166. DOI: 10.1161/01.HYP.26.6.1160.

[129] Corti R, Burnett JC, Jr, Rouleau JL, et al. Vasopeptidase inhibitors: a new therapeutic concept in cardiovascular disease? Circulation. 2001;104:1856-1862. DOI: 10.1161/hc4001.097191.

[130] Margulies KB, Perrella MA, McKinley LJ, et al. Angiotensin inhibition potentiates the renal responses to neutral endopeptidase inhibition in dogs with congestive heart failure. J Clin Invest. 1991;88:1636-1642.

[131] Nathisuwan S, Talbert RL. A review of vasopeptidase inhibitors: a new modality in the treatment of hypertension and chronic heart failure. Pharmacotherapy. 2002;22:27-42.

[132] Packer M, Califf RM, Konstam MA, et al. Comparison of omapatrilat and enalapril in patients with chronic heart failure: the Omapatrilat Versus Enalapril

Randomized Trial of Utility in Reducing Events (OVERTURE). Circulation. 2002;106:920-926.

[133] Byrd JB, Touzin K, Sile S, et al. Dipeptidyl peptidase IV in angiotensin-converting enzyme inhibitor associated angioedema, Hypertension. 2008;51:141-147.

[134] Messerli FH, Nussberger J. Vasopeptidase inhibition and angio–oedema. Lancet. 2000;356:608-609.

[135] McMurray JJ, Packer M, Desai AS, Gong J, Lefkowitz MP, Rizkala AR, Rouleau JL, et al; PARADIGM-HF Investigators and Committees. Angiotensin-neprilysin inhibition versus enalapril in heart failure. N Engl J Med. 2014 Sep 11;371(11):993-1004. doi: 10.1056/NEJMoa1409077. Epub 2014 Aug 30. PMID: 25176015

[136] Francis SE, Holden H, Holt CM, Duff GW. Interleukin-1 in myocardium and coronary arteries of patients with dilated cardiomyopathy. J Mol Cell Cardiol. 1998 Feb;30(2):215-223. doi: 10.1006/jmcc.1997.0592. PMID: 9514998

[137] Munger MA, Johnson B, Amber IJ, Callahan KS, Gilbert EM. Circulating concentrations of proinflammatory cytokines in mild or moderate heart failure secondary to ischemic or idiopathic dilated cardiomyopathy. Am J Cardiol. 1996 Apr 1;77(9):723-727. doi: 10.1016/s0002-9149(97)89206-5. PMID: 8651123

[138] Levine B, Kalman J, Mayer L, Fillit HM, Packer M. Elevated circulating levels of tumor necrosis factor in severe chronic heart failure N Engl J Med. 1990 Jul 26;323(4):236-241. doi: 10.1056/NEJM199007263230405. PMID: 2195340

[139] Bozkurt B, Kribbs SB, Clubb FJ Jr, Michael LH, Didenko VV, Hornsby PJ, et al Pathophysiologically relevant concentrations of tumor necrosis factor-alpha promote progressive left ventricular dysfunction and remodeling in rats Circulation. 1998 Apr 14;97(14):1382-1391. doi: 10.1161/01.cir.97.14.1382. PMID: 9577950

[140] Kubota T, McTiernan CF, Frye CS, Slawson SE, Lemster BH, Koretsky AP, et al Dilated cardiomyopathy in transgenic mice with cardiac-specific overexpression of tumor necrosis factor-alpha Circ Res. 1997 Oct;81(4):627-635. doi: 10.1161/01.res.81.4.627. PMID: 9314845

[141] Yokoyama T, Nakano M, Bednarczyk JL, McIntyre BW, Entman M, Mann DL Tumor necrosis factor-alpha provokes a hypertrophic growth response in adult cardiac myocytes Circulation. 1997 Mar 4;95(5):1247-1252. doi: 10.1161/01.cir.95.5.1247. PMID: 9054856

[142] Krown KA, Page MT, Nguyen C, Zechner D, Gutierrez V, Comstock KL, et al. Tumor necrosis factor alpha-induced apoptosis in cardiac myocytes. Involvement of the sphingolipid signaling cascade in cardiac cell death J Clin Invest. 1996 Dec 15;98(12):2854-2865. doi: 10.1172/JCI119114. PMID: 8981934

[143] Thaik CM, Calderone A, Takahashi N, Colucci WS.Interleukin-1 beta modulates the growth and phenotype of neonatal rat cardiac myocytes. J Clin Invest. 1995 Aug;96(2):1093-1099. doi: 10.1172/JCI118095. PMID: 7635944

[144] Sekiguchi K, Li X, Coker M, Flesch M, Barger PM, Sivasubramanian N, Mann DL Cross-regulation between the renin-angiotensin system and inflammatory mediators in cardiac hypertrophy and failure Cardiovasc Res. 2004 Aug 15;63(3):433-442. doi: 10.1016/j.cardiores.2004.02.005. PMID: 15276468

[145] Bryant D, Becker L, Richardson J, Shelton J, Franco F, Peshock R, et al Cardiac failure in transgenic mice with myocardial expression of tumor necrosis factor-alphaCirculation. 1998 Apr 14;97(14):1375-1381. doi: 10.1161/01.cir.97.14.1375. PMID: 9577949

[146] Deswal A, Petersen NJ, Feldman AM, Young JB, White BG, Mann DL. Cytokines and cytokine receptors in advanced heart failure: an analysis of the cytokine database from the Vesnarinone trial (VEST). Circulation. 2001 Apr 24;103(16):2055-2059. doi: 10.1161/01.cir.103.16.2055. PMID: 11319194

[147] Franco F, Thomas GD, Giroir B, Bryant D, Bullock MC, Chwialkowski MC, et al. Magnetic resonance imaging and invasive evaluation of development of heart failure in transgenic mice with myocardial expression of tumor necrosis factor-alpha. Circulation. 1999 Jan 26;99(3):448-454. doi: 10.1161/01.cir.99.3.448. PMID: 9918534

[148] Seta Y, Shan K, Bozkurt B, Oral H, Mann DL. Basic mechanisms in heart failure: the cytokine hypothesis. J Card Fail. 1996 Sep;2(3):243-249. doi: 10.1016/s1071-9164(96)80047-9. PMID: 8891862

[149] Murray DR, Prabhu SD, Chandrasekar B. Chronic beta-adrenergic stimulation induces myocardial proinflammatory cytokine expression. Circulation. 2000 May 23;101(20):2338-2341. doi: 10.1161/01.cir.101.20.2338. PMID: 10821806

[150] Hernández-Presa M, Bustos C, Ortego M, Tuñon J, Renedo G, Ruiz-Ortega M, Egido J. Angiotensin-converting enzyme inhibition prevents arterial nuclear factor-kappa B activation, monocyte chemoattractant protein-1 expression, and macrophage infiltration in a rabbit model of early accelerated atherosclerosis Circulation. 1997 Mar 18;95(6):1532-41. doi: 10.1161/01.cir.95.6.1532. PMID: 9118522

[151] Brasier AR, Jamaluddin M, Han Y, Patterson C, Runge MS. Angiotensin II induces gene transcription through cell-type-dependent effects on the nuclear factor-kappaB (NF-kappaB) transcription factor. Mol Cell Biochem. 2000 Sep;212(1-2):155-169. PMID: 11108147

[152] Gullestad L, Aukrust P, Ueland T, Espevik T, Yee G, Vagelos R, et al Effect of high- versus low-dose angiotensin converting enzyme inhibition on cytokine levels in chronic heart failure. J Am Coll Cardiol. 1999 Dec;34(7):2061-2067. doi: 10.1016/s0735-1097(99)00495-7. PMID: 10588224

[153] Gurlek A, Kilickap M, Dincer I, Dandachi R, Tutkak H, Oral D. Effect of losartan on circulating TNFalpha levels and left ventricular systolic performance in patients with heart failure. J Cardiovasc Risk. 2001 Oct;8(5):279-282. doi: 10.1177/174182670100800506. PMID: 11702033

[154] Prabhu SD, Chandrasekar B, Murray DR, Freeman GL. beta-adrenergic blockade in developing heart failure: effects on myocardial inflammatory cytokines, nitric oxide, and remodeling. Circulation. 2000 May 2;101(17):2103-9. doi: 10.1161/01.cir.101.17.2103.PMID: 10790354

[155] Gullestad L, Ueland T, Brunsvig A, Kjekshus J, Simonsen S, Frøland SS, Aukrust P. Effect of metoprolol on cytokine levels in chronic heart failure--a substudy in the Metoprolol Controlled-Release Randomised Intervention Trial in Heart Failure (MERIT-HF). Am Heart J. 2001 Mar;141(3):418-421. doi: 10.1067/mhj.2001.112785. PMID: 11231439

[156] Tsutamoto T, Wada A, Matsumoto T, Maeda K, Mabuchi N, Hayashi M, et al. Relationship between

tumor necrosis factor-alpha production and oxidative stress in the failing hearts of patients with dilated cardiomyo pathy.J Am Coll Cardiol. 2001 Jun 15;37(8):2086-92. doi: 10.1016/s0735-1097(01)01299-2. PMID: 11419892

[157] Carswell EA, Old LJ, Kassel RL, Green S, Fiore N, Williamson B. An endotoxin-induced serum factor that causes necrosis of tumors. Proc Natl Acad Sci U S A. 1975 Sep;72(9):3666-3670. doi: 10.1073/pnas.72.9.3666. PMID: 1103152

[158] Old LJ. Tumor necrosis factor (TNF).Science. 1985 Nov 8;230(4726):630-632. doi: 10.1126/science.2413547. PMID: 2413547

[159] Torre-Amione G, Kapadia S, Lee J, Bies RD, Lebovitz R, Mann DL. Expression and functional significance of tumor necrosis factor receptors in human myocardium. Circulation. 1995 Sep 15;92(6):1487-1493. doi: 10.1161/01.cir.92.6.1487. PMID: 7664431

[160] Torre-Amione G, Kapadia S, Lee J, Durand JB, Bies RD, Young JB, Mann DL. Tumor necrosis factor-alpha and tumor necrosis factor receptors in the failing human heart. Circulation. 1996 Feb 15;93(4):704-711. doi: 10.1161/01.cir.93.4.704. PMID: 8640999

[161] Oral H, Dorn GW 2nd, Mann DL. Sphingosine mediates the immediate negative inotropic effects of tumor necrosis factor-alpha in the adult mammalian cardiac myocyte.J Biol Chem. 1997 Feb 21;272(8):4836-4842. doi: 10.1074/jbc.272.8.4836. PMID: 9030540

[162] Nakano M, Knowlton AA, Dibbs Z, Mann DL. Tumor necrosis factor-alpha confers resistance to hypoxic injury in the adult mammalian cardiac myocyte. Circulation. 1998 Apr 14;97(14):1392-1400. doi: 10.1161/01.cir.97.14.1392. PMID: 9577951

[163] Ferrari R, Bachetti T, Confortini R, Opasich C, Febo O, Corti A, et al. Tumor necrosis factor soluble receptors in patients with various degrees of congestive heart failure. Circulation. 1995 Sep 15;92(6):1479-1486. doi: 10.1161/01.cir.92.6.1479. PMID: 7664430

[164] Rauchhaus M, Doehner W, Francis DP, Davos C, Kemp M, Liebenthal C, et al. Plasma cytokine parameters and mortality in patients with chronic heart failure. Circulation. 2000 Dec 19;102(25):3060-3067. doi: 10.1161/01.cir.102.25.3060. PMID: 11120695

[165] Kubota T, Miyagishima M, Alvarez RJ, Kormos R, Rosenblum WD, Demetris AJ, et al. Expression of proinflammatory cytokines in the failing human heart: comparison of recent-onset and end-stage congestive heart failure Heart Lung Transplant. 2000 Sep;19(9):819-824. doi: 10.1016/s1053-2498(00)00173-x. PMID: 11008069

[166] Sivasubramanian N, Coker ML, Kurrelmeyer KM, MacLellan WR, DeMayo FJ, Spinale FG, Mann DL.Left ventricular remodeling in transgenic mice with cardiac restricted overexpression of tumor necrosis factor. Circulation. 2001 Aug 14;104(7):826-831. doi: 10.1161/hc3401.093154. PMID: 11502710

[167] Bradham WS, Bozkurt B, Gunasinghe H, Mann D, Spinale FG. Tumor necrosis factor-alpha and myocardial remodeling in progression of heart failure: a current perspective. Cardiovasc Res. 2002 Mar;53(4):822-830. doi: 10.1016/s0008-6363(01)00503-x. PMID: 11922892

[168] Funakoshi H, Kubota T, Machida Y, Kawamura N, Feldman AM, Tsutsui H, et al. Involvement of inducible nitric oxide synthase in cardiac dysfunction with tumor necrosis factor-alpha. Am J Physiol Heart Circ Physiol. 2002

Jun;282(6):H2159–H2166. doi: 10.1152/ajpheart.00872.2001. PMID: 12003824

[169] Ferdinandy P, Danial H, Ambrus I, Rothery RA, Schulz R. Peroxynitrite is a major contributor to cytokine-induced myocardial contractile failure. Circ Res. 2000 Aug 4;87(3):241-247. doi: 10.1161/01.res.87.3.241. PMID: 10926876

[170] Gurantz D, Cowling RT, Villarreal FJ, Greenberg BH. Tumor necrosis factor-alpha upregulates angiotensin II type 1 receptors on cardiac fibroblasts. Circ Res. 1999 Aug 6;85(3):272-279. doi: 10.1161/01.res.85.3.272. PMID: 10436170

[171] Cowling RT, Gurantz D, Peng J, Dillmann WH, Greenberg BH. Transcription factor NF-kappa B is necessary for up-regulation of type 1 angiotensin II receptor mRNA in rat cardiac fibroblasts treated with tumor necrosis factor-alpha or interleukin-1 beta. J Biol Chem. 2002 Feb 22;277(8):5719-5724. doi: 10.1074/jbc.M107515200. Epub 2001 Oct 12. PMID: 11600498

[172] Flesch M, Höper A, Dell'Italia L, Evans K, Bond R, Peshock R,et al. Activation and functional significance of the renin-angiotensin system in mice with cardiac restricted overexpression of tumor necrosis factor. Circulation. 2003 Aug 5;108(5):598-604. doi: 10.1161/01.CIR.0000081768.13378.BF. Epub 2003 Jul 21. PMID: 12874189

[173] Jaffré F, Callebert J, Sarre A, Etienne N, Nebigil CG, Launay JM, et al. Involvement of the serotonin 5-HT2B receptor in cardiac hypertrophy linked to sympathetic stimulation: control of interleukin-6, interleukin-1beta, and tumor necrosis factor-alpha cytokine production by ventricular fibroblasts. Circulation. 2004 Aug 24;110(8):969-974. doi: 10.1161/01.CIR.0000139856.20505.57. Epub 2004 Aug 9. PMID: 15302781

[174] Herskowitz A, Choi S, Ansari AA, Wesselingh S Cytokine mRNA expression in postischemic/reperfused myocardium Am J Pathol. 1995 Feb;146(2):419-28.PMID: 7856752

[175] Siwik DA, Colucci WS. Regulation of matrix metalloproteinases by cytokines and reactive oxygen/nitrogen species in the myocardium. Heart Fail Rev. 2004 Jan;9(1):43-51. doi: 10.1023/B:HREV.0000011393.40674.13. PMID: 14739767

[176] Long CS. The role of interleukin-1 in the failing heart. Heart Fail Rev. 2001 Mar;6(2):81-94. doi: 10.1023/a:1011428824771. PMID: 11309527

[177] Patten M, Hartogensis WE, Long CS. Interleukin-1beta is a negative transcriptional regulator of alpha1-adrenergic induced gene expression in cultured cardiac myocytes. J Biol Chem. 1996 Aug 30;271(35):21134-21141. doi: 10.1074/jbc.271.35.21134. PMID: 8702883

[178] Palmer JN, Hartogensis WE, Patten M, Fortuin FD, Long CS Interleukin-1 beta induces cardiac myocyte growth but inhibits cardiac fibroblast proliferation in culture J Clin Invest. 1995 Jun;95(6):2555-2564. doi: 10.1172/JCI117956. PMID: 7769098

[179] Tsutamoto T, Hisanaga T, Wada A, Maeda K, Ohnishi M, Fukai D, et al. Interleukin-6 spillover in the peripheral circulation increases with the severity of heart failure, and the high plasma level of interleukin-6 is an important prognostic predictor in patients with congestive heart failure. J Am Coll Cardiol. 1998 Feb;31(2):391-398. doi: 10.1016/s0735-1097(97)00494-4. PMID: 9462584

[180] Nicol RL, Frey N, Pearson G, Cobb M, Richardson J, Olson EN. Activated MEK5 induces serial assembly of sarcomeres and eccentric cardiac

hypertrophy. EMBO J. 2001 Jun 1;20(11):2757-2767. doi: 10.1093/emboj/20.11.2757. PMID: 11387209

[181] Kato T, Sano M, Miyoshi S, Sato T, Hakuno D, Ishida H, et al Calmodulin kinases II and IV and calcineurin are involved in leukemia inhibitory factor-induced cardiac hypertrophy in rats Circ Res. 2000 Nov 10;87(10):937-945. doi: 10.1161/01.res.87.10.937. PMID: 11073891

[182] Wollert KC, Taga T, Saito M, Narazaki M, Kishimoto T, Glembotski CC, et al Cardiotrophin-1 activates a distinct form of cardiac muscle cell hypertrophy. Assembly of sarcomeric units in series VIA gp130/leukemia inhibitory factor receptor-dependent pathways J Biol Chem. 1996 Apr 19;271(16):9535-9545. doi: 10.1074/jbc.271.16.9535. PMID: 8621626

[183] Balligand JL, Cannon PJ. Nitric oxide synthases and cardiac muscle. Autocrine and paracrine influences Arterioscler Thromb Vasc Biol. 1997 Oct;17(10):1846-58. doi: 10.1161/01.atv.17.10.1846 PMID: 9351345

[184] Sawyer DB, Colucci WS. Nitric oxide in the failing myocardium. Cardiol Clin. 1998 Nov;16(4):657-664, viii. doi: 10.1016/s0733-8651(05)70042-4. PMID: 9891595

[185] Feron O, Belhassen L, Kobzik L, Smith TW, Kelly RA, Michel T. Endothelial nitric oxide synthase targeting to caveolae. Specific interactions with caveolin isoforms in cardiac myocytes and endothelial cells. J Biol Chem. 1996 Sep 13;271(37):22810-22814. doi: 10.1074/jbc.271.37.22810. PMID: 8798458

[186] Fukuchi M, Hussain SN, Giaid A. Heterogeneous expression and activity of endothelial and inducible nitric oxide synthases in end-stage human heart failure: their relation to lesion site and beta-adrenergic receptor therapy Circulation. 1998 Jul 14;98(2):132-9. doi: 10.1161/01.cir.98.2.132.PMID: 9679719

[187] Haywood GA, Tsao PS, von der Leyen HE, Mann MJ, Keeling PJ, Trindade PT, et al. Expression of inducible nitric oxide synthase in human heart failure. Circulation. 1996 Mar 15;93(6):1087-1094. doi: 10.1161/01.cir.93.6.1087. PMID: 8653828

[188] Patten RD, Denofrio D, El-Zaru M, Kakkar R, Saunders J, Celestin F, et al. Ventricular assist device therapy normalizes inducible nitric oxide synthase expression and reduces cardiomyocyte apoptosis in the failing human heart. J Am Coll Cardiol. 2005 May 3;45(9):1419-1424. doi: 10.1016/j.jacc.2004.05.090. PMID: 15862412

[189] Mungrue IN, Gros R, You X, Pirani A, Azad A, Csont T, et al. Cardiomyocyte overexpression of iNOS in mice results in peroxynitrite generation, heart block, and sudden death. J Clin Invest. 2002 Mar;109(6):735-743. doi: 10.1172/JCI13265. PMID: 11901182

[190] Heger J, Gödecke A, Flögel U, Merx MW, Molojavyi A, Kühn-Velten WN, Schrader J. Cardiac-specific overexpression of inducible nitric oxide synthase does not result in severe cardiac dysfunction. Circ Res. 2002 Jan 11;90(1):93-99. doi: 10.1161/hh0102.102757. PMID: 11786524

[191] Sam F, Sawyer DB, Xie Z, Chang DL, Ngoy S, Brenner DA,et ak. Mice lacking inducible nitric oxide synthase have improved left ventricular contractile function and reduced apoptotic cell death late after myocardial infarction. Circ Res. 2001 Aug 17;89(4):351-356. doi: 10.1161/hh1601.094993. PMID: 11509452

[192] Parrillo JE, Cunnion RE, Epstein SE, Parker MM, Suffredini AF, Brenner M, et al. A prospective, randomized, controlled trial of

prednisone for dilated cardiomyopathy. N Engl J Med. 1989 Oct 19;321(16):1061-1068. doi: 10.1056/NEJM198910193211601. PMID: 2677721

[193] Weinblatt ME, Kremer JM, Bankhurst AD, et al. A trial of etanercept, a recombinant tumor necrosis factor receptor: Fc fusion protein, in patients with rheumatoid arthritis receiving methotrexate. N Engl J Med. 1999;340:253-259.

[194] Moreland LW, Schiff MH, Baumgartner SW, et al. Etanercept therapy in rheumatoid arthritis. A randomized, controlled trial. Ann Intern Med. 1999;130:478-486.

[195] Ford AC, Sandborn WJ, Khan KJ, et al. Efficacy of biological therapies in inflammatory bowel disease: systematic review and meta-analysis. Am J Gastroenterol. 2011;106:644-659.

[196] Mease PJ. Tumor necrosis factor (TNF) in psoriatic arthritis: pathophysiology and treatment with TNF inhibitors. Ann Rheum Dis. 2002;61:298-304.

[197] Kapadia S, Torre-Amione G, Yokoyama T, Mann DL. Soluble TNF binding proteins modulate the negative inotropic properties of TNF-alpha in vitro. Am J Physiol. 1995 Feb;268 (2 Pt 2):H517–H525. doi: 10.1152/ajpheart.1995.268.2.H517. PMID: 7864177

[198] Deswal A, Bozkurt B, Seta Y, Parilti-Eiswirth S, Hayes FA, Blosch C, Mann DL Safety and efficacy of a soluble P75 tumor necrosis factor receptor (Enbrel, etanercept) in patients with advanced heart failure Circulation. 1999 Jun 29;99(25):3224-6. doi: 10.1161/01.cir.99.25.3224.PMID: 10385494

[199] Bozkurt B, Torre-Amione G, Warren MS, Whitmore J, Soran OZ, Feldman AM, Mann DL Results of targeted anti-tumor necrosis factor therapy with etanercept (ENBREL) in patients with advanced heart failure Circulation . 2001 Feb 27;103(8):1044-1047. doi: 10.1161/01.cir.103.8.1044. PMID: 11222463

[200] Packer M. Proposal for a new clinical end point to evaluate the efficacy of drugs and devices in the treatment of chronic heart failure.J Card Fail. 2001 Jun;7(2):176-182. doi: 10.1054/jcaf.2001.25652. PMID: 11420770

[201] Mann DL, McMurray JJ, Packer M, Swedberg K, Borer JS, Colucci WS, et al Targeted anticytokine therapy in patients with chronic heart failure: results of the Randomized Etanercept Worldwide Evaluation (RENEWAL). Circulation. 2004 Apr 6;109(13):1594-1602. doi: 10.1161/01.CIR.0000124490.27666.B2. Epub 2004 Mar 15. PMID: 15023878

[202] Chung ES, Packer M, Lo KH, Fasanmade AA, Willerson JT; Anti-TNF Therapy Against Congestive Heart Failure Investigators. Randomized, double-blind, placebo-controlled, pilot trial of infliximab, a chimeric monoclonal antibody to tumor necrosis factor-alpha, in patients with moderate-to-severe heart failure: results of the anti-TNF Therapy Against Congestive Heart Failure (ATTACH) trial. Circulation. 2003 Jul 1;107(25):3133-40. doi: 10.1161/01.CIR.0000077913.60364.D2. Epub 2003 Jun 9. PMID: 12796126

[203] Dwyer JM. Manipulating the immune system with immune globulin.N Engl J Med. 1992;326:107-116.

[204] Mobini N, Sarela A, Ahmed AR. Intravenous immunoglobulins in thetherapy of autoimmune and systemic inflammatory disorders.Ann AllergyAsthma Immunol. 1995;74:119-128

[205] McNamara DM, Holubkov R, Starling RC, Dec GW, Loh E, Torre-Amione G, et al .Controlled trial of intravenous immune globulin in recent-onset dilated cardiomyopathy. Circulation. 2001 May 8;103(18):2254-2259. doi: 10.1161/01.cir.103.18.2254. PMID: 11342473

[206] Gullestad L, Aass H, Fjeld JG, Wikeby L, Andreassen AK, Ihlen H, et al. Immunomodulating therapy with intravenous immunoglobulin in patients with chronic heart failure. Circulation. 2001 Jan 16;103(2):220-225. doi: 10.1161/01.cir.103.2.220. PMID: 11208680

[207] Takimoto E, Kass DA.Role of oxidative stress in cardiac hypertrophyand remodeling. Hypertension 49: 241-248, 2007.

[208] Beckman JS, Beckman TW, J. Chen J, et al. Apparent hydroxyl radical production by peroxynitrite: implications for endothelial injury from nitric oxide and superoxide. Proc Natl Acad Sci U S A. 1990 Feb;87(4):1620-1624. doi: 10.1073/pnas.87.4.1620.

[209] Chen CA, Wang TY, Varadharaj S, et al. S-glutathionylation uncouples eNOS and regulates its cellular and vascular function. Nature. 2010 Dec 23;468(7327):1115-1118.doi: 10.1038/nature09599.

[210] Elahi MM, Kong YX, Matata BM. Oxidative stress as a mediator of cardiovascular disease. Oxid Med Cell Longev. Nov-Dec 2009;2(5):259-269. doi: 10.4161/oxim.2.5.9441.

[211] Díaz-Vélez CR, García-Castiñeiras S, Mendoza-Ramos E, Hernández-López E. Increased malondialdehyde in peripheral blood of patients with congestive heart failure. Am Heart J. 1996 Jan;131(1):146-152. doi: 10.1016/s0002-8703(96)90063-0.

[212] Tang WH, Brennan ML, Philip K, Tong W, Mann S, Van Lente F, et al. Plasma myeloperoxidase levels in patients with chronic heart failure. Am J Cardiol. 2006 Sep 15;98(6):796-799. doi: 10.1016/j.amjcard.2006.04.018. Epub 2006 Jul 28.

[213] Mak S, Lehotay DC, Yazdanpanah M, Azevedo ER, Liu PP, Newton GE.Unsaturated aldehydes including 4-OH-nonenal are elevated in patients with congestive heart failure. J Card Fail. 2000 Jun;6(2):108-14.PMID: 10908084

[214] Sakai H, Tsutamoto T, Tsutsui T, Tanaka T, Ishikawa C, Horie M. Serum level of uric acid, partly secreted from the failing heart, is a prognostic marker in patients with congestive heart failure. Circ J. 2006 Aug;70(8):1006-1011. doi: 10.1253/circj.70.1006. PMID: 16864933

[215] Kittleson MM, St John ME, Bead V, Champion HC, Kasper EK, Russell SD, et al. Increased levels of uric acid predict haemodynamic compromise in patients with heart failure independently of B-type natriuretic peptide levels. Heart. 2007 Mar;93(3):365-367. doi: 10.1136/hrt.2006.090845. PMID: 17322514

[216] Anker SD, Doehner W, Rauchhaus M, Sharma R, Francis D, Knosalla C, et al. Uric acid and survival in chronic heart failure: validation and application in metabolic, functional, and hemodynamic staging. Circulation. 2003 Apr 22;107(15):1991-1997. doi: 10.1161/01.CIR.0000065637.10517.A0. Epub 2003 Apr 21. PMID: 12707250

[217] Sabri A, Hughie HH, Lucchesi PA.Regulation of hypertrophic andapoptotic signaling pathways by reactive oxygen species in cardiacmyocytes.Antioxid Redox Signal 5: 731-740, 2003.

[218] Cesselli D, Jakoniuk I, Barlucchi L, Beltrami AP, Hintze TH, Nadal-Ginard B, Kajstura J, Leri A,

Anversa P.Oxidative stress-mediatedcardiac cell death is a major determinant of ventricular dysfunction andfailure in dog dilated cardiomyopathy. Circ Res. 2001; 89: 279-286.

[219] Xiao CY, Chen M, Zsengellér Z, Li H, Kiss L, Kollai M, Szabó C. Poly(ADP-Ribose) polymerase promotes cardiac remodeling, contractile failure, and translocation of apoptosis-inducing factor in a murine experimental model of aortic banding and heart failure. J Pharmacol Exp Ther. 2005 Mar;312(3):891-898. doi: 10.1124/jpet.104.077164. Epub 2004 Nov 2. PMID: 15523000

[220] Spinale FG, Coker ML, Thomas CV, Walker JD, Mukherjee R,Hebbar L.Time-dependent changes in matrix metalloproteinase activityand expression during the progression of congestive heart failure: relationto ventricular and myocyte function.Circ Res. 1998; 82: 482-495.

[221] Creemers EE, Cleutjens JP, Smits JF, Daemen MJ.Matrix metalloproteinase inhibition after myocardial infarction: a new approach toprevent heart failure? Circ Res. 2001; 89: 201-210.

[222] Rajagopalan S, Meng XP, Ramasamy S, Harrison DG, Galis ZS.Reactive oxygen species produced by macrophage-derived foam cellsregulate the activity of vascular matrix metalloproteinases in vitro. Implications for atherosclerotic plaque stability.J Clin Invest. 1996; 98: 2572-2579.

[223] Lim H, Zhu YZ. Role of transforming growth factor-beta in the progression of heart failure. Cell Mol Life Sci. 2006 Nov;63(22):2584-96. doi: 10.1007/s00018-006-6085-8.PMID: 17013566

[224] Purnomo Y, Piccart Y, Coenen T, Prihadi JS, Lijnen PJ. Oxidative stress and transforming growth factor-beta1-induced cardiac fibrosis.Cardiovasc Hematol Disord Drug Targets. 2013 Aug;13(2):165-72. doi: 10.2174/1871529x11313020010.PMID: 23988004

[225] Luo G, Wang R, Zhou H, Liu X. ALDOA protects cardiomyocytes against H/R-induced apoptosis and oxidative stress by regulating the VEGF/Notch 1/Jagged 1 pathway. Mol Cell Biochem. 2020 Oct 21. doi: 10.1007/s11010-020-03943-z. Online ahead of print. PMID: 33089381

[226] Moore JB 4th, Zhao J, Fischer AG, Keith MCL, Hagan D, Wysoczynski M, Bolli R. Histone Deacetylase 1 Depletion Activates Human Cardiac Mesenchymal Stromal Cell Proangiogenic Paracrine Signaling Through a Mechanism Requiring Enhanced Basic Fibroblast Growth Factor Synthesis and Secretion. J Am Heart Assoc. 2017 Jul 5;6(7):e006183. doi: 10.1161/JAHA.117.006183.PMID: 28679560

[227] Belviso I, Angelini F, Di Meglio F, Picchio V, Sacco AM, Nocella C,et al .The Microenvironment of Decellularized Extracellular Matrix from Heart Failure Myocardium Alters the Balance between Angiogenic and Fibrotic Signals from Stromal Primitive Cells. Int J Mol Sci. 2020 Oct 24;21(21):7903. doi: 10.3390/ijms21217903.PMID: 33114386

[228] Cheng TH, Shih NL, Chen SY, et al. Reactive oxygen species mediate cyclic strain-induced endothelin-1 gene expression via Ras/Raf/extracellular signal-regulated kinase pathway in endothelial cells. J. Mol. Cell. Cardiol. 2001;33:1805-1814. doi: 10.1006/jmcc.2001.1444.

[229] Griendling KK, Sorescu D, Ushio-Fukai M. NAD(P)H oxidase: role in cardiovascular biology and disease. Circ Res. 2000 Mar 17;86(5):494-501. doi: 10.1161/01.res.86.5.494. PMID: 10720409

[230] Packer M. Mutual Antagonism of Hypoxia-Inducible Factor Isoforms in Cardiac, Vascular, and Renal Disorders. JACC Basic Transl Sci. 2020 Sep 28;5(9):961-968. doi: 10.1016/j.jacbts.2020.05.006. eCollection 2020 Sep.PMID: 33015417

[231] Zima AV, Blatter LA.Redox regulation of cardiac calcium channelsand transporters.Cardiovasc Res. 2006; 71: 310-321.

[232] Ide T, Tsutsui H, Hayashidani S, Kang D, Suematsu N, Nakamura K,Utsumi H, Hamasaki N, Takeshita A. Mitochondrial DNA damage and dysfunction associated with oxidative stress in failing hearts after myocardial infarction. Circ Res 88: 529-535, 2001.

[233] Schmelzer C, Döring F. Micronutrient special issue: coenzyme Q(10) requirements for DNA damage prevention. Mutat Res. 2012;733:61-68. doi: 10.1016/j.mrfmmm.2011.09.004.

[234] Fotino AD, Thompson-Paul AM, Bazzano LA. Effect of coenzyme Q10 supplementation on heart failure: a meta-analysis. Am J Clin Nutr. 2013;97:268-275. doi: 10.3945/ajcn.112.040741.

[235] Madmani ME, Yousuf SA, Tamr AK, Madmani Y, Shahrour Y, Essali A, Kadro W. Coenzyme Q10 for heart failure (Review). Cochrane Review. 2013:1-35

[236] Mortensen SA, Rosenfeldt F, Kumar A, Dolliner P, Filipiak KJ, Pella D, Alehagen U, Steurer G, Littarru GP; Q-SYMBIO Study Investigators. The effect of coenzyme Q10 on morbidity and mortality in chronic heart failure: results from Q-SYMBIO: a randomized double-blind trial. JACC Heart Fail. 2014;2:641-649. doi: 10.1016/j.jchf.2014.06.008

[237] Archer SL, Nelson DP, Weir EK. Detection of activated O2 species in vitro and in rat lungs by chemiluminescence. J Appl Physiol (1985). 1989;67:1912-1921. doi: 10.1152/jappl.1989.67.5.1912.

[238] Pacher P, Nivorozhkin A, Szabó C. Therapeutic effects of xanthine oxidase inhibitors: renaissance half a century after the discovery of allopurinol. Pharmacol Rev. 2006;58:87-114.

[239] Ogino K, Kato M, Furuse Y, Kinugasa Y, Ishida K, Osaki S, Kinugawa T, Igawa O, Hisatome I, Shigemasa C, Anker SD, Doehner W. Uric acid-lowering treatment with benzbromarone in patients with heart failure: a double-blind placebo-controlled crossover preliminary study. Circ Heart Fail. 2010;3:73-81. doi: 10.1161/CIRCHEARTFAILURE.109.868604.

[240] Leyva F, Anker S, Swan JW, Godsland IF, Wingrove CS, Chua TP, Stevenson JC, Coats AJ. Serum uric acid as an index of impaired oxidative metabolism in chronic heart failure. Eur Heart J. 1997;18:858-865.

[241] Levy WC, Mozaffarian D, Linker DT, Sutradhar SC, Anker SD, Cropp AB, Anand I, Maggioni A, Burton P, Sullivan MD, Pitt B, Poole-Wilson PA, Mann DL, Packer M. The Seattle Heart Failure Model: prediction of survival in heart failure. Circulation. 2006;113:1424-1433. doi: 10.1161/CIRCULATIONAHA.105.584102.

[242] Poss WB, Huecksteadt TP, Panus PC, et al. Regulation of xanthine dehydrogenase and xanthine oxidase activity by hypoxia. Am J Physiol Lung Cell Mol Physiol. 1996; 270: L941–L946.

[243] Engerson TD, McKelvey TG, Rhyne DB, et al. Conversion of xanthine dehydrogenase to oxidase in ischemic rat tissues. J Clin Invest. 1987; 79: 1564-1570.

[244] Pritsos CA. Cellular distribution, metabolism and regulation of the xanthine oxidoreductase enzyme system. Chem Biol Interact. 2000; 129: 195-208.

[245] Houston M, Estevez A, Chumley P, et al. Binding of xanthine oxidase to vascular endothelium. Kinetic characterization and oxidative impairment of nitric oxide-dependent signaling. J Biol Chem. 1999; 274: 4985-4994.

[246] Givertz MM, Anstrom KJ, Redfield MM et al Effects of Xanthine Oxidase Inhibition in Hyperuricemic Heart Failure PatientsThe Xanthine Oxidase Inhibition for Hyperuricemic Heart Failure Patients (EXACT-HF) Study. Circulation. 2015;131:1763-1771. DOI: 10.1161/CIRCULATIONAHA. 114.014536.

Section 2

Genetics

Chapter 5

Genetics of Cardiomyopathy

Evan M. Harvey, Murad Almasri and Hugo R. Martinez

Abstract

Cardiomyopathies (CMs) encompass a heterogeneous group of structural and functional (systolic and diastolic) abnormalities of the myocardium and are either confined to the cardiovascular system or are part of a systemic disorder. CMs represent a leading cause of morbidity and mortality and account for a significant percentage of death and cardiac transplantation. The 2006 American Heart Association (AHA) classification grouped CMs into primary (genetic, mixed, or acquired) or secondary (i.e., infiltrative or autoimmune). In 2008, the European Society of Cardiology classification proposed subgrouping CM into familial or genetic and nonfamilial or nongenetic forms. In 2013, the World Heart Federation recommended the MOGES nosology system, which incorporates a morpho-functional phenotype (M), organ(s) involved (O), the genetic inheritance pattern (G), an etiological annotation (E) including genetic defects or underlying disease/substrates, and the functional status (S) of a particular patient based on heart failure symptoms. Rapid advancements in the biology of cardio-genetics have revealed substantial genetic and phenotypic heterogeneity in myocardial disease. Given the variety of disciplines in the scientific and clinical fields, any desired classification may face challenges to obtaining consensus. Nonetheless, the heritable phenotype-based CM classification offers the possibility of a simple, clinically useful diagnostic scheme. In this chapter, we will describe the genetic basis of dilated cardiomyopathy (DCM), hypertrophic cardiomyopathy (HCM), arrhythmogenic cardiomyopathy (ACM), LV noncompaction cardiomyopathy (LVNC), and restrictive cardiomyopathy (RCM). Although the descriptive morphologies of these types of CM differ, an overlapping phenotype is frequently encountered within the CM types and arrhythmogenic pathology in clinical practice. CMs appear to originate secondary to disruption of "final common pathways." These disruptions may have purely genetic causes. For example, single gene mutations result in dysfunctional protein synthesis causing downstream dysfunctional protein interactions at the level of the sarcomere and a CM phenotype. The sarcomere is a complex with multiple protein interactions, including thick myofilament proteins, thin myofilament proteins, and myosin-binding proteins. In addition, other proteins are involved in the surrounding architecture of the sarcomere such as the Z-disk and muscle LIM proteins. One or multiple genes can exhibit tissue-specific function, development, and physiologically regulated patterns of expression for each protein. Alternatively, multiple mutations in the same gene (compound heterozygosity) or in different genes (digenic heterozygosity) may lead to a phenotype that may be classic, more severe, or even overlapping with other disease forms.

Keywords: Inherited cardiovascular disease, Syndromic cardiovascular disease, Gene variants, Gene disorders, Genetic syndrome, Pathogenic mutation, Heritable cardiomyopathy, Sarcomeric cardiomyopathy, Metabolic disorders, Neuromuscular disease

IntechOpen

1. Introduction

Cardiomyopathies (CMs) encompass a heterogeneous group of structural and functional (systolic and diastolic) abnormalities of the myocardium and are either confined to the cardiovascular system or are part of a systemic disorder. CMs represent a leading cause of morbidity and mortality and account for a significant percentage of death and cardiac transplantation [1]. The 2006 American Heart Association (AHA) classification grouped CMs into primary (genetic, mixed, or acquired) or secondary (i.e., infiltrative or autoimmune). In 2008, the European Society of Cardiology classification proposed subgrouping CM into familial or genetic and nonfamilial or nongenetic forms. In 2013, the World Heart Federation recommended the MOGES nosology system, which incorporates a morpho-functional phenotype (M), organ(s) involved (O), the genetic inheritance pattern (G), an etiological annotation (E) including genetic defects or underlying disease/substrates, and the functional status (S) of a particular patient based on heart failure symptoms [2–4]. Rapid advancements in the biology of cardio-genetics have revealed substantial genetic and phenotypic heterogeneity in myocardial disease. Given the variety of disciplines in the scientific and clinical fields, any desired classification may face challenges to obtaining consensus. Nonetheless, the heritable phenotype-based CM classification offers the possibility of a simple, clinically useful diagnostic scheme (for an example, see [5]). In this chapter, we will describe the genetic basis of dilated cardiomyopathy (DCM), hypertrophic cardiomyopathy (HCM), arrhythmogenic cardiomyopathy (ACM), LV noncompaction cardiomyopathy (LVNC), and restrictive cardiomyopathy (RCM). Although the descriptive morphologies of these types of CM differ, an overlapping phenotype is frequently encountered within the CM types and arrhythmogenic pathology in clinical practice. CMs appear to originate secondary to disruption of "final common pathways." These disruptions may have purely genetic causes. For example, single gene mutations result in dysfunctional protein synthesis causing downstream dysfunctional protein interactions at the level of the sarcomere and a CM phenotype. The sarcomere is a complex with multiple protein interactions, including thick myofilament proteins, thin myofilament proteins, and myosin-binding proteins. In addition, other proteins are involved in the surrounding architecture of the sarcomere such as the Z-disk and muscle LIM proteins (**Figure 1**). One or multiple genes can exhibit tissue-specific function, development, and physiologically regulated patterns of expression for each protein. Alternatively, multiple mutations in the same gene (compound heterozygosity) or in different genes (digenic heterozygosity) may lead to a phenotype that may be classic, more severe, or even overlapping with other disease forms.

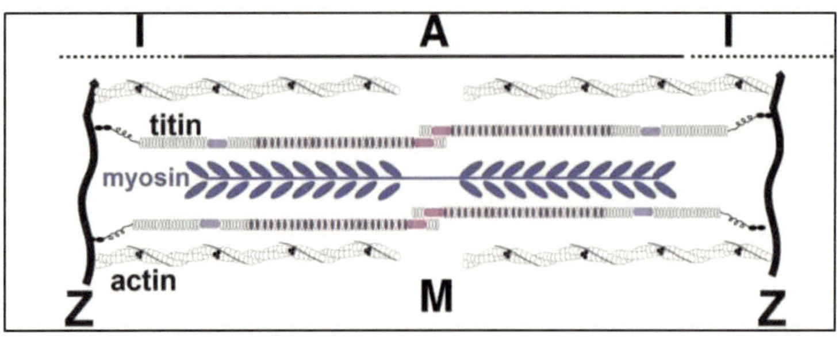

Figure 1.
Schematic image of the sarcomere featuring thick/thin filaments and surrounding protein architecture [13].

2. Heritable cardiomyopathies

2.1 Dilated cardiomyopathy

DCM is mainly characterized by left or biventricular dilatation, increased LV mass, and decreased systolic function (**Figure 2**) [6]. DCM can present with the clinical syndrome of systolic heart failure or with or without associated arrhythmias or thrombo-embolic disease. Additionally, DCM can be detected in asymptomatic individuals. Globally, DCM is the most common form of CM and the leading cause of heart transplantation in children and adults. The estimated incidence in the pediatric population is between 0.34 to 1.13 cases per 100,000 children per year with differences in demographic characteristics [7]. DCM has many known etiologies with many more to be discovered. Unfortunately, in many cases, no etiology can be found, and the CM is deemed idiopathic. Still, 25 to 50% of patients with idiopathic DCM have a positive family history, suggesting an underlying genetic predisposition [8]. The majority of genetically triggered cases of DCM are transmitted in an autosomal dominant pattern exhibiting variable penetrance. Other forms of inheritance include autosomal recessive, X-linked, and mitochondrial (maternally inherited), which are more frequent in the pediatric population [2]. Familial DCM occurs in 20 to 60% of cases, where approximately 40% of those cases may have a primary monogenic basis. However, this percentage is a variable approximation as a more critical evaluation of the genes linked to DCM continues to evolve and certain types of variations are

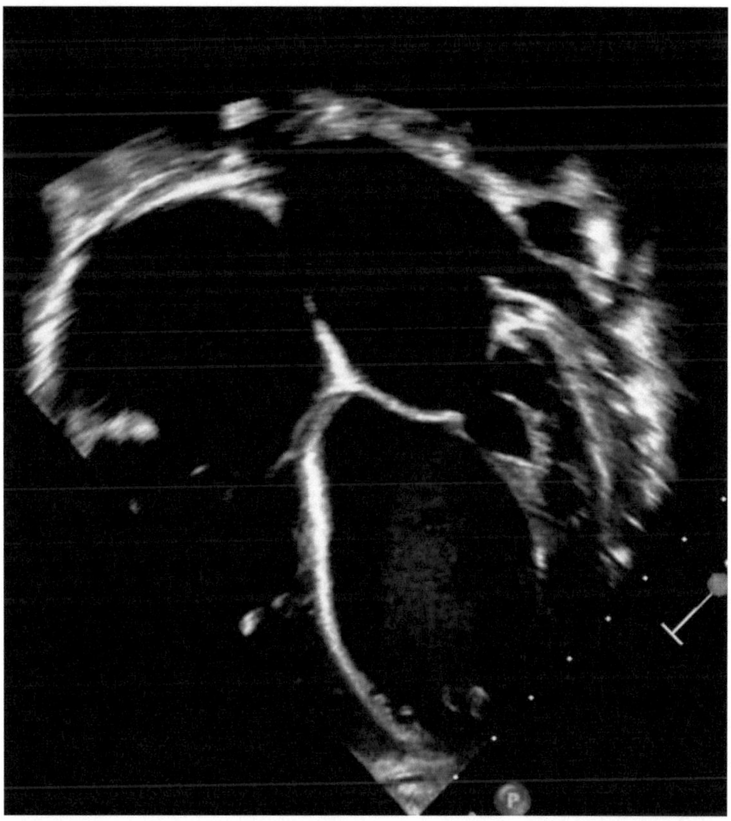

Figure 2.
Two-dimensional, apical 4-chamber echocardiographic image depicting an enlarged ventricle with spherical geometry and biatrial enlargement secondary to atrioventricular valve insufficiency in a patient with dilated cardiomyopathy.

excluded from being certified as pathogenic [8]. Another conventional classification of DCM is based on the presence or absence of systemic disease. Thus, dividing DCM into syndromic and non-syndromic forms is a practical approach to evaluating this highly heterogeneous disease. The diagnostic rate for gene testing in non-syndromic DCM is 46 to 73% [9], but this estimation may likely be confounded by insufficient control for population variation. Over the past decade, 47 new genes (for a total of 60 different genes) have been linked to DCM in the Human Gene Mutation Database (HGMD), see **Table 1**. From these genes, a large-scale analysis revealed truncating variants in the titin gene (*TNN*) were the most common pathogenic mutations in non-syndromic DCM [10, 11]. Other core-causative genes include *MYH7* (encoding beta myosin heavy chain), *TNNT2* (encoding troponin T2), *LMNA* (encoding a nuclear envelope protein, lamin A/C), and *TPM1* (encoding Tropomyosin 1). Other rare pathogenic variants (minor allele frequency) implicated in non-syndromic DCM include genes coding for the sarcomere and Z-disk (i.e., actin, myosin-binding protein C3, myopalladin, nebulette, ZASP), cytoskeleton (i.e., dystrophin, desmin), nuclear envelope (emerin), mitochondria (i.e., Tafazzin), sarcoplasmic reticulum, desmosomes, ion channels, and transcription factors [9, 12, 13].

Regardless of the mode of inheritance, pathogenic gene variants result in a cardiomyocyte milieu susceptible to stress, leading to downstream dysfunction of the contractile apparatus and heart failure, "the final common pathway" hypothesis [14]. The term "familial DCM" is frequently applied in the presence of DCM in two or more first-degree relatives. The incidence is likely underestimated due to the diversity of inheritance patterns, timing of presentation, variable penetrance, and lack of symptoms in subclinical disease [15, 16].

2.1.1 Autosomal dominant dilated cardiomyopathy

The most common form of familial DCM is inherited in an autosomal dominant pattern [6]. In this sub-type, arrhythmias associated with DCM (DCM-A) are frequently encountered [17]. Genetic heterogeneity exists with at least 30 unique genes identified in familial non-arrhythmogenic DCM and five genes for DCM-A [17, 18].

2.1.2 X-linked Cardiomyopathy (XLCM)

XLCM has been reported as an isolated disease of the heart or associated with skeletal myopathy such as with Duchenne muscular dystrophy (DMD) or Becker muscular dystrophy (BMD). All skeletal myopathies are frequently associated with the development of DCM and/or DCM-A. The causative gene codes for the protein dystrophin located at the short arm of the X chromosome at Xp21. Dystrophin is a cytoskeletal protein that provides structural support to the cardiomyocyte and plays a major role in linking the sarcomeric contractile apparatus to the sarcolemma and extracellular matrix (ECM) [19, 20]. DMD and BMD are severe muscular dystrophies of childhood, affecting ~1 in 3,500 males for DMD and 1 in 300,000 males for BMD. Typically, DMD and BMD are characterized by skeletal myopathy, elevated serum creatine kinase, and calf pseudo-hypertrophy. DMD is the more severe form due to the absence of functional dystrophin, leading to muscle weakness by 3 years of age and wheelchair dependence by 12 years of age [21]. Cardiac involvement varies with age but is nearly universal by 20 years in all DMD patients. The onset of clinical features starts later in life in BMD than in DMD. Histologic studies show cardiac muscle replacement with fibrosis. This fibrosis eventually leads to ventricular dysfunction/enlargement and is associated with conduction system abnormalities and ventricular arrhythmias. Molecular analysis of the *DMD* gene is indicated for diagnosis. If no mutation is detected, skeletal muscle biopsy should

DOI: http://dx.doi.org/10.5772/intechopen.97010

Gene	Protein	Pattern of Inheritance	Disease Association	OMIM#	Locus
ABCC9	ATP-Binding Cassette, Subfamily C, Member 9	AD	DCM	601439	14q12-q22
ACTC1	Actin, Alpha, Cardiac Muscle	AD	DCM, LVNC, ACM, HCM	102540	5q31.1
ACTN2	Actinin, Alpha-2	AD	DCM, HCM	102573	6q22.1
AKAP9	A-Kinase Anchor Protein 9	AD	DCM	604001	2q32.1-q32.3
ALMS1	Centrosome and Basal Body Associated Protein	AR	DCM	606844	10p14-p12
ALPK3	Alpha Kinase 3	AR	DCM, HCM	617608	1p36.32
ANKRD1	Ankyrin Repeat Domain-Containing Protein 1	AD	DCM, HCM	609599	7q36.1
BAG3	Bcl2-Associated Athanogene 3	AD	DCM, RCM, HCM	603883	14q24.3
CASQ2	Calsequestrin 2	AR, AD	DCM, LVNC	114251	6q22.31
CAV3	Caveolin 3	AD	DCM, HCM	601253	12q24.13
CHRM2	Cholinergic Receptor, Muscarinic, 2	AD	DCM	118493	10q25.2-q26.2
CRYAB	Crystallin, Alpha-B	AD	DCM	123590	11q23.1
CSRP3	Cysteine- And Glycine-Rich Protein 3	AD	DCM, HCM	600824	12p12.1
CTF1	Cardiotrophin 1	AR, AD	DCM	600435	1p13.1
DES	Desmin	AD, AR	DCM, ACM, RCM	125660	17q21
DMD	Dystrophin	XL	DCM	300377	3p25.3
DOLK	Dolichol Kinase	AR	DCM	610746	7q33
DSC2	Desmocollin 2	AD, AR	DCM, ACM	600271	Xq22
DSG2	Desmoglein 2	AD	DCM, ACM	125671	15q24.1
DSP	Desmoplakin	AD, AR	DCM, ACM	125485	11p15.5
DTNA	Dystrobrevin Alpha	AD	DCM, LVNC	601239	2q31
EMD	Emerin	XL	DCM	300384	11q23.1

Gene	Protein	Pattern of Inheritance	Disease Association	OMIM#	Locus
EYA4	Eyes Absent, Drosophila, Homolog Of, 4	AD	DCM	603550	11p15.1
FHL1	Four-And-A-Half LIM Domains 1	XL	DCM, HCM	300163	15q22.31
FHL2	Four-And-A-Half LIM Domains 2	Unknown	DCM	602633	16p11.2
FKRP	Fukutin-Related Protein	AR	DCM	606596	10q21.3
FKTN	Fukutin	AR	DCM	607440	2q35
FLNC	Filamin C	AD	DMC, RCM, HCM, ACM	102565	10q22.2
GATA4	Gata-Binding Protein 4	AD	DCM	600576	Xq21.2-p21.1
GATAD1	Gata Zinc Finger Domain-Containing Protein 1	AR	DCM	614518	9q34.11
GLA	Galactosidase, Alpha	XL	DCM, HCM	300644	18q11.2
ILK	Integrin-Linked Kinase	AD	DCM	602366	18q12.1
JUP	Junction Plakoglobin	AD, AR	DCM, ACM	173325	2p13.1
LAMA4	Laminin, Alpha-4	AD	DCM	600133	18q12.1
LAMP2	Lysosome-Associated Membrane Protein 2	XL	DCM, HCM	309060	3p25.2
LDB3	Lim Domain-Binding 3	AD	DCM, LVNC, ACM, HCM	605906	2p22.1
LMNA	Lamin A/C	AD, AR	DCM, LVNC, ACM, HCM	150330	1q22
LRRC10	Leucine-Rich Repeat-Containing Protein 10	AD, AR	DCM	610846	4q21.3
MURC/CAVIN4	Muscle-Related Coiled-Coil Protein/Caveolae-Associated Protein 4	AD	DCM	617714	18q12.1
MYBPC3	Myosin-Binding Protein C, Cardiac	AD	DCM, LVNC, RCM, HCM	600958	Xq28
MYH6	Myosin, Heavy Chain 6, Cardiac Muscle, Alpha	AD	DCM, HCM	160710	10q25.2

Gene	Protein	Pattern of Inheritance	Disease Association	OMIM#	Locus
MYH7	Myosin, Heavy Chain 7, Cardiac Muscle, Beta	AD	DCM, LVNC, RCM, HCM	160760	7p14.2
MYL2	Myosin, Light Chain 2, Regulatory, Cardiac, Slow	AD	DCM, HCM	160781	3p21.3-p21.2
MYL3	Myosin, Light Chain 3, Alkali, Ventricular, Skeletal, Slow	AD, AR	DCM, HCM, RCM	160790	1q32
MYLK2	Myosin Light Chain Kinase 2	AD	DCM, HCM	606566	20q13.31
MYOT	Myotilin	AD	DCM	604103	Xq28
MYOZ2	Myozenin 2	AD	DCM, RCM, HCM	605602	3p25.1
MYPN	Myopalladin	AD	DCM, RCM, HCM	608517	12q23.1
NEBL	Nebulette	AD	DCM	605491	6q23.2
NEXN	Nexilin (F Actin Binding Protein)	AD	DCM, HCM	613121	1q22
NKX2-5	Nk2 Homeobox 5	AD	DCM	600584	Xq26.3
PDLIM3	Pdz And Lim Domain Protein 3	AD	DCM, HCM	605899	1q43
PKP2	Plakophilin 2	AD	DCM, ACM	602861	11p15.4
PLN	Phospholamban	AD	DCM, ACM, HCM	172405	4q12
PRDM16	Pr Domain-Containing Protein 16	AD	DCM, LVNC	605557	6q21
PRKAG2	Protein Kinase, Amp-Activated, Noncatalytic, Gamma-2	AD	DCM, HCM	602743	4q26-q27
RBM20	RNA-Binding Motif Protein 20	AD	DCM	613171	2q12.2
RYR2	Ryanodine Receptor 2 (Cardiac)	AD	DCM, HCM, ACM	180902	12p11
SCN5A	Sodium Channel, Voltage-Gated, Type V, Alpha Subunit	AD	DCM, ACM	600163	20q13.12
SGCA	Sarcoglycan Alpha	AR	DCM	600119	1q25.2
SGCB	Sarcoglycan Beta	AR	DCM	600900	15q22.1
SGCD	Sarcoglycan, Delta (35kda Dystrophin-Associated Glycoprotein)	AD, AR	DCM	601411	19q13.32

Gene	Protein	Pattern of Inheritance	Disease Association	OMIM#	Locus
SLC25A4	Solute Carrier Family 25, Member 4 (Mitochondrial Carrier Adenine Nucleotide Translocator)	AD, AR	DCM	103220	7q21-q22
TAZ	Tafazzin	AR, XL	DCM, LVNC	300394	Xq24
TBX20	T-Box 20	AD	DCM, LVNC	606061	10q22.3-q23.2
TCAP	Titin-Cap (Telethonin)	AR	DCM, HCM	604488	3p21
TMEM43	Transmembrane Protein 43	AD	DCM, ACM	612048	10q23.3
TMPO	Thymopoietin	AD	DCM	188380	9q31.2
TNNC1	Troponin C Type 1 (Slow)	AD	DCM, HCM	191040	17q21.33
TNNI3	Troponin I Type 3 (Cardiac)	AD	DCM, RCM, HCM	191044	3p21.1
TNNT2	Troponin T Type 2 (Cardiac)	AD	DCM, LVNC, RCM, HCM	191045	17q12
TOR1AIP1	Torsin-1a-Interacting Protein 1	AR	DCM	614512	7q32.1
TPM1	Tropomyosin 1 (Alpha)	AD	DCM, RCM, HCM	191010	19q13.4
TRDN	Triadin	AR	DCM	603283	17q25.3
TTN	Titin	AD, AR	DCM, ACM, HCM	188840	5q33-q34
TTR	DCM	AD	DCM	176300	18q12.1
TXNRD2	Thioredoxin Reductase 2	AD, AR	DCM	606448	8p23.1
VCL	Vinculin	AD	DCM, LVNC, HCM	193065	10q25.2

AD – Autosomal dominant; AR – Autosomal Recessive; XL – X-linked; DCM – Dilated cardiomyopathy; HCM – Hypertrophic cardiomyopathy; LVNC – Left ventricular non-compaction cardiomyopathy; ACM – Arrhythmogenic cardiomyopathy; RCM – Restrictive cardiomyopathy.

Table 1.
List of common genes and patterns of inheritance in DCM, modified from Tayal et al. [9].

be considered for Western blot and immunohistochemistry studies, although this is rarely performed in current clinical practice [19, 20, 22–24]. Although less severe, female carriers with clinical DMD and BMD are also at risk to develop DCM but at a later age. Hence, a complete cardiac evaluation for carrier females every 3-5 years starting in adolescence or early adulthood is warranted with concomitant appropriate medical treatment if indicated [25].

2.1.3 Isolated X-Linked Dilated Cardiomyopathy

Isolated XLCM is characterized by consistent early expression and rapid progression of CM in males during childhood, later onset with slower progression in females, and no male-to-male transmission [26]. Linkage analysis of X-chromosome-specific DNA markers performed in suspected individuals demonstrated preferential involvement of cardiac muscle and normal dystrophin by Western blotting in skeletal muscle of the same affected individuals [27]. The phenotype and pathologic features described in this population do not differ from those in patients with DCM. Hence, the medical management should be provided according to the current heart failure guidelines.

2.1.4 Emery-Dreifuss Muscular Dystrophy

Emery-Dreifuss muscular dystrophy (EDMD), also known as humeroperoneal muscular dystrophy, is a heterogeneous disorder with X-linked recessive, autosomal dominant, and autosomal recessive forms of inheritance [28]. Several forms of this disease are considered nuclear envelopathies because they are associated with mutations in genes encoding nuclear membrane proteins, including the *EMD* gene encoding for emerin, the *LMNA* gene encoding for lamin A and lamin C, and the *SYNE1* and *SYNE2* genes encoding for nesprin 1 and nesprin 2, respectively [29]. The different forms of EDMD have identical symptoms that usually begin in the first or second decade of life. Extremity contractures are often the first manifestation. Muscle weakness and wasting has a humeroperoneal distribution and tends to be slowly progressive. DCM is seen in many patients with EDMD. This condition is typically associated with atrioventricular conduction abnormalities such as first-degree atrioventricular block, sinus bradycardia, or supraventricular tachycardia, which may be early signs of cardiac involvement and may be progressive. Symptoms of hypoperfusion (syncope or near syncope) often result from infranodal or atrioventricular conduction block with the development of slow junctional rhythms, which may require pacemaker placement [30]. The onset of cardiac abnormalities is usually in the third decade of life, but earlier onset during adolescence has been observed. Additionally, there is no correlation between the degree of neuromuscular involvement and the severity of cardiac abnormalities [31].

2.1.5 Barth Syndrome

Barth syndrome (BTS) is another X-linked cardioskeletal myopathy that encompasses abnormal mitochondrial function, short stature, cyclic neutropenia, cardiolipin deficiency, and variable degrees of 3-methylglutaconic aciduria. BTS is caused by mutations in the *TAZ* gene (previously called *G4.5*), which is located in the chromosome Xq28 region and encodes for the Tafazzin protein [32]. Pathologic gene variants may result in a wide variety of cardiac phenotypes including DCM, HCM, LVNC, and endocardial fibroelastosis. In many cases, affected infants succumb to heart failure, arrhythmias, or sepsis secondary to leukocyte dysfunction [33, 34].

2.2 Hypertrophic cardiomyopathy

HCM is the second most prevalent CM in children, representing 40% of cases, with an estimated incidence of 0.47 in 100,000 children [35]. HCM is more prevalent in boys than in girls and in African American children than in Caucasian or Hispanic children. In the pediatric population, the incidence of HCM is 10 times higher in patients under 1 year of age than in older children [36]. HCM is a primary myocardial disorder with mainly an autosomal dominant pattern of inheritance characterized by hypertrophy of the left ventricle (with or without hypertrophy of the right ventricle) and histologic features of myocyte hypertrophy, myofibrillar disarray, and interstitial fibrosis. While asymmetric septal hypertrophy is the most common pattern of hypertrophy, the degree and location of hypertrophy vary. Some patients exhibit concentric hypertrophy, harbored in other walls or confined to the left ventricular apex (**Figure 3**) [37].

The clinical presentation of HCM is highly variable, ranging from asymptomatic hypertrophy, to symptomatic arrhythmias, to refractory heart failure due to diastolic dysfunction, or "burned-out HCM" with the development of systolic dysfunction. Notably, diastolic dysfunction can even be detected in individuals with HCM who have normal LV wall thickness, suggesting that diastolic dysfunction is an early feature of HCM rather than a secondary consequence of hypertrophy [38]. Categorization of HCM includes non-syndromic HCM (without other systemic involvement) and the syndromic form of HCM (in association with inborn errors of metabolism, malformation syndromes, and neuromuscular disorders) [39].

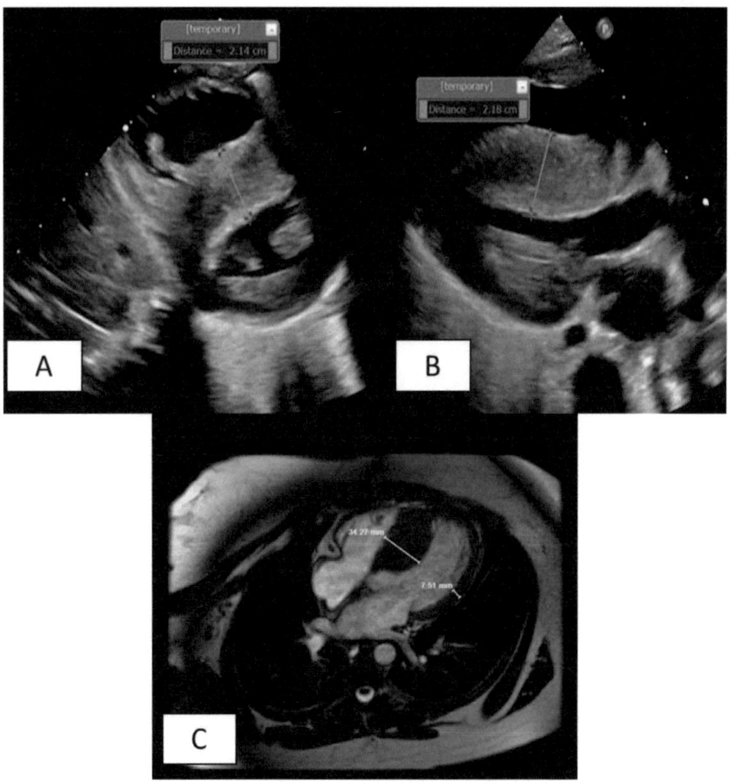

Figure 3.
Two dimensional images of HCM in the parasternal short axis (A) exhibiting concentric hypertrophy with significant involvement of the interventricular septum (IVS) and corroborated by the parasternal long axis view (B). Cardiac MRI also shows significant thickening of the IVS (C).

Approximately 20–30% of individuals with non-syndromic HCM and no family history of HCM harbor a pathogenic variant in a known gene encoding a component of the sarcomere. However, 50–60% of adults and children with a positive family history of HCM harbor a pathogenic gene variant. Furthermore, 3–5% of affected individuals have more than one sarcomere gene variant (either biallelic variants in 1 gene or heterozygous variants in >1 gene) [40, 41].

2.2.1 Non-syndromic Hypertrophic Cardiomyopathy

More than two decades ago, the first chromosome locus (14q11.2-q12) encoding components of the sarcomere (beta-myosin heavy chain) was elucidated as the pathogenic basis for familial HCM [42]. Since then, more than 1,400 mutations in 27 identified genes have been associated with HCM, see **Table 2** [43]. The vast majority have autosomal dominant transmission, but mitochondrial and autosomal recessive patterns have been also described [44–46]. Most of the disease-causing mutations implicated in HCM include mutations in the *MYH7* gene (encoding beta-myosin heavy chain) and in the *MYBPC3* gene (encoding cardiac myosin-binding protein C). These mutations account individually for 40%, and the remaining genes (*TNNT2, TPM1, ACTC1, TNNI3, TTN, MYL2,* and others) account collectively for 10% of cases [47]. Most of these mutations involve missense mutations (resulting in a direct amino acid change) and frameshift-type mutations (insertions or deletions of the number of nucleotides), which alter the properties of the protein involved. The prevalence of causal genes varies among different populations. Collective results of genetic epidemiologic studies suggest that up to 70% of the causal genes in familial cases and up to 40% in sporadic HCM cases have a genetic mutation identified [44–46]. In our experience in the past 10 years, approximately 70% of non-infantile individuals have an identifiable mutation in a sarcomere-encoding gene, whereas fewer mutations (approximately 20%) are identified in infants.

Mouse models of sarcomeric mutations have shown changes in cardiac chemistry and diastolic function well before myocardial hypertrophy is observed [48]. Moreover, the genetic defect in a gene encoding for a sarcomeric protein may disrupt normal contraction and relaxation with dysregulation of calcium in the sarcomere. Thus, reduced calcium reuptake and decreased stores in the sarcoplasmic reticulum will trigger a remodeling process by several transcription factors, resulting in the hypertrophy of the cardiomyocytes and increased energy demand, which eventually results in ischemia, fibrosis, and death [44]. There is no reliable correlation between the genotype and phenotype among the identified sarcomeric mutations, except for those patients harboring multiple mutations [49].

2.2.2 Syndromic hypertrophic cardiomyopathy

HCM has been associated with multiple phenotypically distinct disorders. Improvements in sequencing technologies and phenotypic characterization and the incorporation of epigenetics have expanded our understanding of syndromic CMs.

2.2.2.1 RAS/MAPK pathway syndromes

Since the discovery of the first gene (*PTPN11*) associated with Noonan syndrome in 2001, multiple genes (*RAF1, SOS1, KRAS, NRAS, BRAF, MAP2K1 [MEK1], MAP2K2 [MEK2], HRAS,* and *SHOC2*) have been identified in the RAS/mitogen-activated protein kinase (MAPK) pathway. This pathway is important for control of cell proliferation and differentiation. Thus, dysregulation results in

Gene	Protein	Pattern of Inheritance	Disease Association	OMIM#	Locus
ACTC1	Actin, Alpha, Cardiac Muscle	AD	HCM, DCM, LVNC, ACM	102540	5q31.1
ACTN2	Actinin, Alpha-2	AD	HCM, DCM	102573	6q22.1
ALPK3	Alpha Kinase 3	AR	HCM, DCM	617608	1p36.32
ANKRD1	Ankyrin Repeat Domain-Containing Protein 1	AD	HCM, DCM	609599	7q36.1
BAG3	Bcl2-Associated Athanogene 3	AD	HCM, DCM, RCM	603883	14q24.3
BRAF	V-Raf Murine Sarcoma Viral Oncogene Homolog B1	AD	HCM	164757	12q15
CAV3	Caveolin 3	AD	HCM, DCM	601253	12q24.13
CSRP3	Cysteine- And Glycine-Rich Protein 3	AD	HCM, DCM	600824	12p12.1
FHL1	Four-And-A-Half LIM Domains 1	XL	HCM	300163	15q22.31
FLNC	Filamin C	AD	HCM, ACM, DMC, RCM	102565	10q22.2
GAA	Glucosidase, Alpha, Acid	AR	HCM	606800	19p13.3
GLA	Galactosidase, Alpha	XL	HCM	300644	18q11.2
HRAS	V-Ha-Ras Harvey Rat Sarcoma Viral Oncogene Homolog	AD	HCM	190020	9q31.1
JPH2	Junctophilin 2	AD	HCM	605267	11p11.2
KRAS	V-Ki-Ras2	AD	HCM	190070	14q12
LAMP2	Lysosome-Associated Membrane Protein 2	XL	HCM, DCM	309060	3p25.2
LDB3	Lim Domain-Binding 3	AD	HCM, DCM, LVNC, ACM	605906	2p22.1
LMNA	Lamin A/C	AD, AR	HCM, DCM, LVNC, ACM	150330	1q22
MAP2K1	Mitogen-Activated Protein Kinase Kinase 1	AD	HCM	176872	14q12
MAP2K2	Mitogen-Activated Protein Kinase Kinase 2	AD	HCM	601263	12q24.11
MYBPC3	Myosin-Binding Protein C, Cardiac	AD	HCM, DCM, LVNC, RCM	600958	Xq28
MYH6	Myosin, Heavy Chain 6, Cardiac Muscle, Alpha	AD	HCM, DCM	160710	10q25.2

Gene	Protein	Pattern of Inheritance	Disease Association	OMIM#	Locus
MYH7	Myosin, Heavy Chain 7, Cardiac Muscle, Beta	AD	HCM, DCM, LVNC, RCM	160760	7p14.2
MYL2	Myosin, Light Chain 2, Regulatory, Cardiac, Slow	AD	HCM	160781	3p21.3-p21.2
MYL3	Myosin, Light Chain 3, Alkali, Ventricular, Skeletal, Slow	AD, AR	HCM, RCM	160790	1q32
MYLK2	Myosin Light Chain Kinase 2	AD	HCM	606566	20q13.31
MYOM1	Myomesin 1	AD	HCM	603508	18p11.31
MYOZ2	Myozenin 2	AD	HCM, DCM, RCM	605602	3p25.1
MYPN	Myopalladin	AD	HCM, DCM, RCM	608517	12q23.1
NEXN	Nexilin (F Actin Binding Protein)	AD	HCM, DCM	613121	1q22
NRAS	Neuroblastoma Ras Viral Oncogene Homolog	AD	HCM	164790	5q31.2
PDLIM3	Pdz And Lim Domain Protein 3	AD	HCM, DCM	605899	1q43
PLN	Phospholamban	AD	HCM, DCM, ACM	172405	4q12
PRKAG2	Protein Kinase, Amp-Activated, Noncatalytic, Gamma-2	AD	HCM	602743	4q26-q27
PTPN11	Protein-Tyrosine Phosphatase, Nonreceptor-Type, 11	AD	HCM	176876	10q21.3
RAF1	V-Raf-1 Murine Leukemia Viral Oncogene Homolog 1	AD	HCM	164760	10p12
RIT1	Ras-Like Without Caax 1	AD	HCM	609591	1p31.1
RYR2	Ryanodine Receptor 2 (Cardiac)	AD	HCM, ACM	180902	12p11
SHOC2	Soc-2 Homolog	AD	HCM	602775	5q35.1
SOS1	Son Of Sevenless, Drosophila, Homolog 1	AD	HCM	182530	1p13.2
TCAP	Titin-Cap (Telethonin)	AR	HCM, DCM	604488	3p21
TNNC1	Troponin C Type 1 (Slow)	AD	HCM, DCM	191040	17q21.33
TNNI3	Troponin I Type 3 (Cardiac)	AD	HCM, DCM, RCM	191044	3p21.1
TNNT2	Troponin T Type 2 (Cardiac)	AD	HCM, DCM, LVNC, RCM	191045	17q12
TPM1	Tropomyosin 1 (Alpha)	AD	HCM, DCM, RCM	191010	19q13.4

Gene	Protein	Pattern of Inheritance	Disease Association	OMIM#	Locus
TTN	Titin	AD, AR	HCM, DCM, ACM	188840	5q33-q34
TTR	Transthyretin	AD	HCM	176300	4q35.1
VCL	Vinculin	AD	HCM, DCM, LVNC	193065	10q25.2

AD – Autosomal dominant; AR – Autosomal Recessive; XL – X-linked; DCM – Dilated cardiomyopathy; HCM – Hypertrophic cardiomyopathy; LVNC – Left ventricular non-compaction cardiomyopathy; ACM – Arrhythmogenic cardiomyopathy; RCM – Restrictive cardiomyopathy.

Table 2.
List of common genes and patterns of inheritance in HCM.

a spectrum of disorders known as "RASopathies" including Noonan and Noonan-like syndromes such as LEOPARD, Costello, and cardiofaciocutaneous syndrome (CFC) [50].

The management of RASopathies should involve a multidisciplinary team with expertise in the assessment of cardiac structural defects, HCM, and arrhythmias. Surveillance with periodic echocardiography (HCM), electrocardiography (rhythm disturbances), neurologic and eye examination, evaluation for scoliosis, and assessment of growth and cognitive development is also recommended.

2.2.2.1.1 Noonan syndrome

Noonan syndrome is relatively common with a prevalence of ~1 in 3500 people. This disease is inherited in an autosomal dominant pattern, although new cases are common because the *de novo* mutation rate is high. Clinical manifestations of Noonan syndrome include short stature, as well as dysmorphic features including hypertelorism, down-slanting palpebral fissures, low-set posteriorly rotated ears, lymphatic anomalies, and webbing of the neck. The estimated frequency of cardiac disease is 50 to 80%, and the disease is mainly characterized by pulmonary valve stenosis, branch pulmonary artery stenosis and Tetralogy of Fallot, in addition to HCM. *PTPN11* gene mutations are more common in individuals with pulmonary stenosis, characteristic facial features, and short stature, while mutations in the *RAF1* gene are associated with HCM in up to 95% of individuals [51]. The myocardial involvement in these patients is typically diagnosed during infancy with findings of asymmetric septal hypertrophy associated with myocyte disarray [52, 53]. With progression of the disease, the combination of biventricular outflow track obstruction is poorly tolerated and associated with increased mortality. Presentation during infancy without congestive heart failure is associated with a 70% three-year survival rate; when associated with congestive heart failure, the 6-month survival rate decreases to 30% [54].

Surgical relief of right ventricular outflow tract obstruction (RVOTO) is recommended in patients with more than a mild degree of obstruction. Septal myectomy is also advised when left ventricular outflow tract obstruction (LVOTO) is associated with heart failure symptoms, although re-growth of the LVOTO is common when myectomy is performed in patients younger than one year of age. In some children, heart transplantation is necessary.

2.2.2.1.2 LEOPARD syndrome

LEOPARD syndrome, also called Noonan syndrome with multiple lentigines, is a rare autosomal dominant disorder caused by mutations in the protein tyrosine phosphatase gene, *PTPN11*. LEOPARD is an acronym for the major features of this disorder, including multiple lentigines, electrocardiogram conduction abnormalities, ocular hypertelorism, pulmonic stenosis, abnormal genitalia, retardation of growth, and sensorineural deafness [55]. Multiple lentigines, present in more than 90% of patients, are the most prominent manifestation of LEOPARD syndrome. Lentigines appear during infancy and early childhood and increase in number over time to involve a large portion of the skin, including the face, neck, and upper trunk. The diagnosis of LEOPARD is difficult, given the highly variable expressivity of the syndrome. In the first year of life, before the appearance of lentigines, the diagnosis can be clinically suspected in infants presenting with characteristic facial features, HCM, and café-au-lait macules. The diagnosis can be confirmed by molecular screening for *PTPN11* mutations [56].

2.2.2.1.3 Costello syndrome

Costello syndrome is a rare disorder with substantial clinical overlap with other RASopathy syndromes. This disorder is caused by mainly *de novo* heterozygous mutations in the *HRAS* gene, with more than 90% of the mutations clustered in codons 12 and 13 [57]. Costello syndrome is characterized by failure-to-thrive in infancy, short stature, characteristic facial features, curly/sparse hair, papillomata, osteoporosis, malignancies (such as embryonal rhabdomyosarcoma), cardiovascular malformations (such as pulmonary stenosis and HCM), rhythm disturbances (such as multifocal atrial tachycardia), and neurological abnormalities including intellectual disability [58].

2.2.2.1.4 Cardiofaciocutaneous (CFC) syndrome

Cardiofaciocutaneous (CFC) syndrome also has substantial clinical overlap with other RASopathy syndromes because of its common ectodermal involvement as well as findings of intellectual impairment and cardiac anomalies. Skin abnormalities can be extensive and include hyperkeratosis, eczema, palmoplantar hyperkeratosis, and keratosis pilaris. The hair is typically sparse and curly. CFC syndrome is characterized by cardiac abnormalities (pulmonary valve stenosis, other valve dysplasias, septal defects, HCM, and rhythm disturbances). HCM is identified in approximately 40% of cases and presents more commonly during infancy, but it can develop at any age [59]. Neoplasia, mostly acute lymphoblastic leukemia (ALL), has been reported in some individuals [50, 60]. Diagnosis is based on clinical findings and molecular genetic testing. Common genes associated with CFC syndrome include *BRAF* (~75%), *MAP2K1* and *MAP2K2* (~25%), and *MEK2* and *KRAS* (<2%) [61–63].

2.2.2.2 Metabolic disorders associated with cardiomyopathy

Congenital metabolic disorders result from absent or abnormal enzymes—or their cofactors—which can lead to accumulation or deficiency of a specific metabolite. Although these disorders exhibit different modes of inheritance, most are transmitted in an autosomal recessive or mitochondrial pattern. The possibility of an inborn error of metabolism should be considered in infants, children, and young adults who present with any of the cardiovascular phenotypes or laboratory features described below. Optimal outcomes for children with these disorders depend upon early recognition of the signs and symptoms of metabolic disease, prompt evaluation, and referral to a center with expertise in cardiovascular genetics. Delay in diagnosis may result in acute metabolic/hemodynamic decompensation, progressive neurologic injury, or death.

2.2.2.2.1 Pompe disease

Pompe disease, also known as glycogen storage disease type II, is an autosomal recessive metabolic disorder that affects muscle and nerve cells throughout the body. This condition occurs secondary to accumulation of glycogen in lysosomes due to a deficiency of the lysosomal acid alpha-glucosidase enzyme. The build-up of glycogen leads to progressive myopathy and weakness throughout the body affecting various tissues including the liver, nervous system, and—most notably—skeletal muscle and myocardium. The Pompe phenotype varies widely [64]. In the infantile form, muscles appear normal but are limp and weak, preventing normal development. Elevated creatine kinase, lactate dehydrogenase, and aspartate aminotransferase (AST) are common. ECG reveals a short PR interval with giant QRS complexes in all leads, suggesting biventricular hypertrophy. As the disease progresses, HCM may result in cardiorespiratory failure. Without treatment, death usually occurs due to heart failure and respiratory weakness within the first year of life [65]. The juvenile and adult forms present with a variable age of onset. The primary clinical finding is skeletal myopathy with a more protracted course, leading to respiratory failure. Affected children usually present with delayed gross-motor development and progressive weakness in a limb-girdle distribution. Early involvement of the diaphragm is a common feature leading to death in the second or third decade of life. In contrast to the infantile form, mild and non-specific cardiac abnormalities can be detected in patients with late-onset disease [66]. Enzyme replacement therapy usually results in decreased ventricular hypertrophy, reduced LV outflow tract obstruction, and normalization of the conduction system [67].

2.2.2.2.2 Danon disease

Danon disease, also known as glycogen storage disease type IIb, is an X-linked lysosomal and glycogen storage disorder associated with skeletal muscle weakness and intellectual disability. Danon disease involves a genetic defect in the *LAMP2* gene located at chromosome Xq24, which encodes the lysosome-associated membrane protein and alters the normal protein structure. While the function of the *LAMP2* gene is not well understood, LAMP2 protein is primarily located in lysosomes. HCM and electrophysiologic abnormalities are the major cardiovascular consequences of glycogen accumulation with resultant myocardial degeneration. Ventricular preexcitation is encountered at a much higher frequency in Danon disease than in sarcomere-related HCM [68, 69]. The cardiac degeneration is usually appreciated clinically by the presence of HCM during childhood or adolescence with subsequent transition to a DCM phenotype with progressive heart failure [70]. Female carriers have also been described in this disorder and are attributed to unfavorable lyonization [71]. They commonly develop symptoms in their 30s to 40s and can be afflicted with DCM.

2.2.2.2.3 Fabry disease

Fabry disease is considered the most prevalent lysosomal storage disorder. This disease is an X-linked inborn error of the glycosphingolipid metabolic pathway and involves deficiency of the lysosomal hydrolase alpha-galactosidase A (alpha-Gal A) mapped to the long arm of the X chromosome (Xq22.1) [72]. Several hundred mutations in the *GLA* gene have been identified. Most cases are familial and few originate from *de novo* mutations [73]. Patients with Fabry disease may present with a spectrum of clinical manifestations, ranging from the severe classic phenotype in males to asymptomatic disease in females. The enzyme deficiency results in accumulation of glycosphingolipids in the lysosomes in nearly all cell types and tissues, leading to multisystem disease including neurologic (paresthesia and pain crises), dermatologic (angiokeratomas and telangiectasias), ophthalmologic (corneal dystrophy), renal (proteinuria and renal insufficiency), and cardiac manifestations by the second to fifth decades of life [74]. Cardiac disease is relatively common in Fabry disease. Patients may develop HCM (similar to that seen in sarcomeric HCM), arrhythmias, and valvar abnormalities. Management of cardiovascular symptoms and the prevention of complications rely on conventional pharmacologic and device-based therapies, but data on the effect of enzyme replacement therapy suggest it has the potential to attenuate and possibly reverse some aspects of cardiac involvement [75, 76].

2.2.2.2.4 Friedreich's ataxia

Friedreich's ataxia is an autosomal recessive inherited disease with an estimated incidence of 1 in 50,000 in the general population. The genotype is characterized by trinucleotide repeat expansion of a normal codon affecting the protein frataxin, a mitochondrial inner membrane protein important for iron homeostasis. As the defect lies within an intron (which is removed from the mRNA transcript between transcription and translation), this mutation does not result in the production of abnormal frataxin. Instead, the mutation decreases the transcription of the gene through gene silencing. Low frataxin levels lead to insufficient biosynthesis of iron–sulfur clusters that are required for the mitochondrial electron transport chain to ultimately generate adenosine triphosphate (ATP). The major clinical manifestations of Friedreich's ataxia include progressive neurologic dysfunction (gait ataxia, optic atrophy, loss of position and vibration sense), diabetes mellitus, and myocardial involvement. The cardiac phenotype is manifested by arrhythmias and HCM. Heart failure remains the leading cause of death in this population [77, 78]. HCM is seen in approximately two-thirds of patients with Friedreich's ataxia, and one-third of those cases develop during childhood [79].

2.2.2.2.5 Mitochondrial cardiomyopathy

Mitochondria are the main energy source in cells due to the ability to perform oxidative phosphorylation via proteins in the mitochondrial respiratory chain. Several genes are involved in the role of cellular energy production. Mutations in these genes may result in severe involvement in organs that are heavily dependent on energy production, such as the brain, heart, and skeletal muscle. Mitochondrial DNA (mtDNA) is exclusively maternally inherited, whereas nuclear DNA follows Mendelian inheritance. The frequency of cardiac involvement in mitochondrial disease is 17–40%, and the estimated prevalence of inherited mitochondrial disease is at least 1 in 5,000 births [80]. More than 40 different types of mitochondrial disease have been associated with the development of HCM. Many forms of mitochondrial disease associated with HCM present during infancy. Because diagnosing mitochondrial disease can be challenging for clinicians, it is recommended that a multidisciplinary team (including a geneticist or mitochondrial specialist) be involved in the diagnosis and management [81]. Mitochondrial CM is characterized by abnormal heart-muscle structure, function, or both. These abnormalities result from genetic defects involving mitochondrial activity in the absence of concomitant coronary artery disease, hypertension, valvular disease, or CHD. The typical cardiac manifestations of mitochondrial disease include the presence of arrhythmias, hypertrophic HCM, LVNC and DCM. Worsening cardiovascular disease may occur during a metabolic crisis [80–82].

Barth syndrome, described earlier in this chapter, is an X-linked disorder caused by pathogenic variants in the *TAZ* gene on chromosome Xq28, resulting in an inborn error of lipid metabolism, cardiolipin deficiency, 3-methylglutaconic aciduria, and cyclic neutropenia. BTS patients may occasionally develop any form of CM, including HCM [32].

2.2.2.2.6 MELAS

MELAS (mitochondrial encephalopathy, lactic acidosis, and stroke-like episodes) is a multisystem clinical syndrome. Cardiac involvement is manifested by nonobstructive concentric hypertrophy (HCM), although DCM, Wolff-Parkinson-White (WPW) syndrome, and atrial tachycardia have also been reported [83–85]. Several genes have been postulated to cause MELAS, including the ones listed in **Table 3**.

2.3 Left ventricular noncompaction cardiomyopathy

LVNC is characterized by the presence of trabeculations, deep intertrabecular recesses, and a thin compacted myocardial layer in the left, right, or both ventricles. The incidence of LVNC is unknown, but some studies estimate 0.014% to 1.3% in the general population [4]. However, with improved echocardiographic and cardiac MRI quality and increasing awareness of LVNC in recent years, the incidence is likely underestimated [34]. Clinically, nine forms of LVNC have been described as follows: [1] the "benign" form of LVNC with normal systolic function, normal chamber sizes and thickness, and no history of arrhythmias; [2] the arrhythmogenic form of LVNC; [3] the DCM form of LVNC; [4] the HCM form of LVNC; [5] the mixed/undulating CM form of LVNC; [6] the RCM form of LVNC; [7] the biventricular noncompaction CM form; [8] the right ventricular noncompaction form (RVNC); and [9] LVNC associated with congenital heart disease [34, 81, 86, 87]. The various phenotypes are depicted in **Figure 4**. The clinical presentation may range from asymptomatic to a severe course accompanied by heart failure requiring heart transplant, arrhythmias, sudden cardiac death, and thromboembolic phenomena [88]. Familial cases are well-documented, and autosomal dominant transmission is the most common inheritance pattern (with variable penetrance and phenotypic heterogeneity). Other modes of inheritance include X-linked, autosomal recessive, and mitochondrial [43]. In pediatric and adult cohorts, the diagnostic rate of gene testing in patients with LVNC ranges from 17–41% depending on patient selection and the number of genes screened. An estimated 18 to 50% of probands have a family member with LVNC [89, 90]. One of the first genetic causes of isolated LVNC was described in 1997 in the gene *G4.5/TAZ* located at chromosome Xq28 [88]. Since then, multiple pathologic gene variants have been described as potential causes of LVNC. Genes encoding sarcomeric and cytoskeletal proteins (*TTN, ACTN2, RBM20, LMNA, DES,* DYS, *DTNA, LDB3, MYH7, MYBPC3, ACTC1)* as well as genes associated with

Gene/locus	Gene location
MTTL1	Mitochondrial
MTTQ	Mitochondrial
MTTH	Mitochondrial
MTTK	Mitochondrial
MTTC	Mitochondrial
MTTS1	Mitochondrial
MTND1	Mitochondrial
MTND5	Mitochondrial
MTND6	Mitochondrial
MTTS2	Mitochondrial

Table 3.
Genes associated with MELAS [83–85].

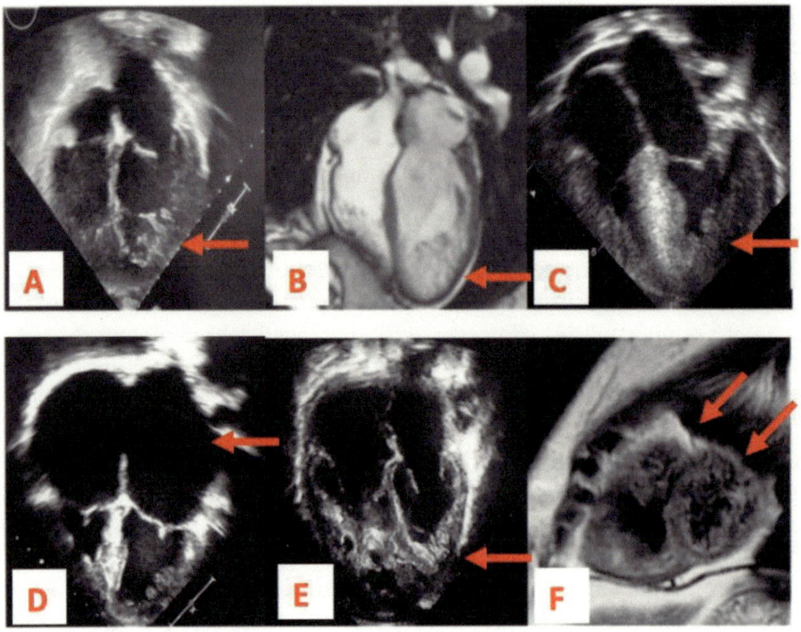

Figure 4.
LVNC phenotypes. (A) Echocardiographic 4-chamber view displays the benign type of LVNC characterized by the cardinal feature of left ventricular trabeculations (arrow) with normal anatomy and function; (B) cardiac magnetic resonance (cMRI) 4-chamber view displays the dilated type of LVNC, notice the enlargement of the LV and the presence of apical and lateral trabeculations (arrow); (C) echocardiographic 4-chamber view shows the hypertrophic type of LVNC represented by asymmetric hypertrophy of the interventricular septum and the presence of lateral LV trabeculations (arrow); (D) echocardiography displaying the restrictive type of LVNC, notice the significant bilateral atrial enlargement (arrows) and the left ventricular dysfunction showing spontaneous cavitary contrast; (E) echocardiography shows features suggestive of bilateral ventricular hypertrabeculations (arrows); (F) cMRI in a short axis view displays a mixed LVNC phenotype represented by dilated and dysfunctional ventricles in a patient with ventricular arrhythmias and biventricular trabeculations (arrows).

cardiac morphogenesis *(FKBP12, MIB1, Tbx20, Nkx2-5, Smad7, NF-ATc, Jarid2),* ion channels (*SCN5A*, *HCN4, RYR2),* and mitochondria (*NNT, TAZ)* have been implicated in the development of LVNC [90–93]. Along with sarcomere-encoding and cytoskeleton-encoding genes, pathogenic variants in a variety of genes, including *SCN5A*, *LMNA*, *RBM20*, *TTN*, and *DES*, have been associated with LVNC and rhythm disturbance [94–95]. In addition, homozygous deletions in desmoplakin (*DSP*) and plakophilin 2 (*PKP2*)—desmosomal protein-encoding genes that cause arrhythmogenic CM and DCM—have been identified in LVNC patients [96]. Moreover, mutations in the mitochondrial genome and chromosomal abnormalities have been associated with LVNC, including 1p36 deletion, 7p14.3p14.1 deletion, 18p subtelomeric deletion, 22q11.2 deletion, distal 22q11.2, trisomies 18 and 13, 8p23.1 deletion, and tetrasomy 5q35.2-5q35 (**Table 4**) [34, 47, 91, 97–99].

Additionally, LVNC has been associated with several genetic syndromes and inborn errors of metabolism such as Coffin-Lowry syndrome, Sotos syndrome, Charcot–Marie–Tooth disease, Noonan syndrome, and BTS [100–103]. A recent study also demonstrated a higher prevalence of LVNC among patients with heterotaxy than among the general population, suggesting possible common genetic mechanisms [104].

2.4 Arrhythmogenic Cardiomyopathy (ACM)

This CM is an arrhythmogenic myocardial disorder not explained by ischemia, hypertension, or valvular heart disease. ACM was previously referred to as

Gene	Protein	Pattern of Inheritance	Disease Association	OMIM#	Locus
ACTC1	Actin, Alpha, Cardiac Muscle	AD	LVNC, ACM, HCM, DCM	102540	5q31.1
CASQ2	Calsequestrin 2	AR, AD	LVNC	114251	6q22.31
DTNA	Dystrobrevin, Alpha	AD	LVNC	601239	2q31
HCN4	Hyperpolarization-Activated Cyclic Nucleotide-Gated Potassium Channel 4	AD	LVNC	605206	18q12.1
LDB3	Lim Domain-Binding 3	AD	LVNC, ACM, HCM, DCM	605906	2p22.1
LMNA	Lamin A/C	AD, AR	LVNC, ACM, HCM, DCM	150330	1q22
MIB1	E3 Ubiquitin Protein Ligase 1	AD	LVNC	608677	22q11.21
MYBPC3	Myosin-Binding Protein C, Cardiac	AD	LVNC, RCM, HCM, DCM	600958	Xq28
MYH7	Myosin, Heavy Chain 7, Cardiac Muscle, Beta	AD	LVNC, RCM, HCM, DCM	160760	7p14.2
PRDM16	Pr Domain-Containing Protein 16	AD	LVNC, DCM	605557	6q21
TAZ	Tafazzin	AR, XL	LVNC, DCM	300394	Xq24
TBX20	T-Box 20	AD	LVNC, DCM	606061	10q22.3-q23.2
TNNT2	Troponin T Type 2 (Cardiac)	AD	LVNC, RCM, HCM, DCM	191045	17q12
VCL	Vinculin	AD	LVNC, HCM, DCM	193065	10q25.2

AD – Autosomal dominant; AR – Autosomal Recessive; XL – X-linked; DCM – Dilated cardiomyopathy; HCM – Hypertrophic cardiomyopathy; LVNC – Left ventricular non-compaction cardiomyopathy; ACM – Arrhythmogenic cardiomyopathy; RCM – Restrictive cardiomyopathy.

Table 4.
List of common genes and patterns of inheritance in LVNC.

arrhythmogenic right ventricular dysplasia/cardiomyopathy (ARVD, ARVC). The reported prevalence of ACM is as common as 1 in 1,000-5,000 people [105]. The clinical diagnosis may be supported by evidence of conduction disease, supraventricular arrhythmias, and/or ventricular arrhythmias originating from any cardiac structure. ECG abnormalities include right bundle branch block pattern, an epsilon wave (defined as a low-amplitude deflection located between the end of the QRS and the onset of the T wave in leads V1–V3), and T wave inversion(s) recorded in leads V1–V4. Classically, the RV is dilated and contains fibro-fatty infiltration of the myocardium. The left ventricle is overtly affected with less frequent involvement. Notably, ACM clinically overlaps with other CM types, particularly DCM. However, ACM is distinct in that it is marked by arrhythmia at presentation with or without biventricular dilation and/or impaired systolic function [106]. This heritable disorder is usually transmitted in an autosomal dominant pattern (with variable penetrance), although autosomal recessive patterns reportedly affect junctional plakoglobin (JUP) and desmoplakin (DSP) in families with cardiocutaneous disease from Greece, Italy, India, Ecuador, Israel, and Turkey [107]. The most notable autosomal recessive diseases include Naxos disease (a homozygous pathogenic variant in the gene encoding the protein plakoglobin characterized by ACM, a non-epidermolytic palmoplantar keratoderma, and wooly hair) and Carvajal syndrome (caused by a homozygous pathogenic gene variant that truncates the DSP protein) [107, 108]. Analysis of first- and second-degree relatives of patients with ACM suggest that up to 50% of ACM cases are familial [109]. Pathogenic gene variants within the desmosomal proteins are the main cause of "classic" ACM [110]. Pathogenic gene variants in the three main classes of desmosomal proteins account for 60% of affected patients [111]. Overall, the three groups of desmosomal proteins include transmembrane desmosomal cadherins (including DSC2 and DSG2), DSP (a plakin family protein that attaches directly to the intermediate filament desmin in the myocardium), and linker proteins such as armadillo family proteins (including JUP and PKP2 that mediate interactions between the desmosomal cadherin tails and DSP) [112]. Pathogenic variants in the *PKP2, DSP* and *DSG2* genes are found in approximately 80% of classic ACM cases [112]. Overall, the most commonly mutated gene is plakophilin, which accounted for 46–61% of patients from two different registries [113]. In addition to desmosomal proteins, genes encoding proteins that interact with these desmosomal proteins have been found in ACM. These proteins include: transforming growth factor β3 (TGF-β3), which conveys cytokine-stimulating fibrosis and modulates cell adhesion and growth; transmembrane protein 43 (TMEM43), an adipogenic transcription factor; DES, which binds DSP; and TTN, which bridges the sarcomere along its longitudinal axis and forms a continuous filament along the myofibril [18]. To date, approximately 18 causative genes involved in ACM have been identified [106, 109], please see **Table 5**. Notably, compound and digenic heterozygosity is involved in ACM pathogenesis in up to 20% of cases and leads to more severe disease [114, 115]. Sarcoidosis and Brugada syndrome are commonly mistaken for ACM.

2.5 Restrictive cardiomyopathy (RCM)

RCM is rare, accounting for approximately 5% of all CMs. RCM is characterized by normal or decreased volume of both ventricles associated with atrial enlargement (left or bi-atrial), normal LV wall thickness, normal atrioventricular valve function/structure, impaired ventricular filling with restrictive physiology, and normal (or near normal) systolic function, please see **Figure 5** [4, 116].

The clinical course is defined by the inability to fill the ventricles due to poor ventricular relaxation, which limits the cardiac output. The disease may manifest

Gene	Protein	Pattern of Inheritance	Disease Association	OMIM#	Locus
ACTC1	Actin, Alpha, Cardiac Muscle	AD	ACM, HCM, DCM, LVNC	102540	5q31.1
ARVD3	Arrhythmogenic Right Ventricular Dysplasia, Familial, 3	AD	ACM	602086	12p12.1
ARVD4	Arrhythmogenic Right Ventricular Dysplasia, Familial, 4	AD	ACM	602087	15q14
ARVD6	Arrhythmogenic Right Ventricular Dysplasia, Familial, 6	AD	ACM	604401	1q42-q43
CTNNA3	Catenin Alpha 3	AD	ACM	607667	7q21.2
DES	Desmin	AD,AR	ACM, RCM, DCM	125660	17q21
DSC2	Desmocollin 2	AD, AR	ACM, DCM	600271	Xq22
DSG2	Desmoglein 2	AD	ACM, DCM	125671	15q24.1
DSP	Desmoplakin	AD, AR	ACM, DCM	125485	11p15.5
FLNC	Filamin C	AD	ACM, DMC, RCM, HCM	102565	10q22.2
JUP	Junction Plakoglobin	AD, AR	ACM	173325	2p13.1
LDB3	Lim Domain-Binding 3	AD	ACM, HCM, DCM, LVNC	605906	2p22.1
LMNA	Lamin A/C	AD, AR	ACM, HCM, DCM, LVNC	150330	1q22
PKP2	Plakophilin 2	AD	ACM, DCM	602861	11p15.4
PLN	Phospholamban	AD	ACM, HCM, DCM	172405	4q12
RYR2	Ryanodine Receptor 2 (Cardiac)	AD	ACM, HCM	180902	12p11
SCN5A	Sodium Channel, Voltage-Gated, Type V, Alpha Subunit	AD	ACM, DCM	600163	20q13.12
TGFB3	Transforming Growth Factor Beta 3	AD	ACM	190230	
TMEM43	Transmembrane Protein 43	AD	ACM	612048	10q23.3
TTN	Titin	AD, AR	ACM, HCM, DCM	188840	5q33-q34

AD – Autosomal dominant; AR – Autosomal Recessive; XL – X-linked; DCM – Dilated cardiomyopathy; HCM – Hypertrophic cardiomyopathy; LVNC – Left ventricular non-compaction cardiomyopathy; ACM – Arrhythmogenic cardiomyopathy; RCM – Restrictive cardiomyopathy.

Table 5.
List of common genes and patterns of inheritance in ACM.

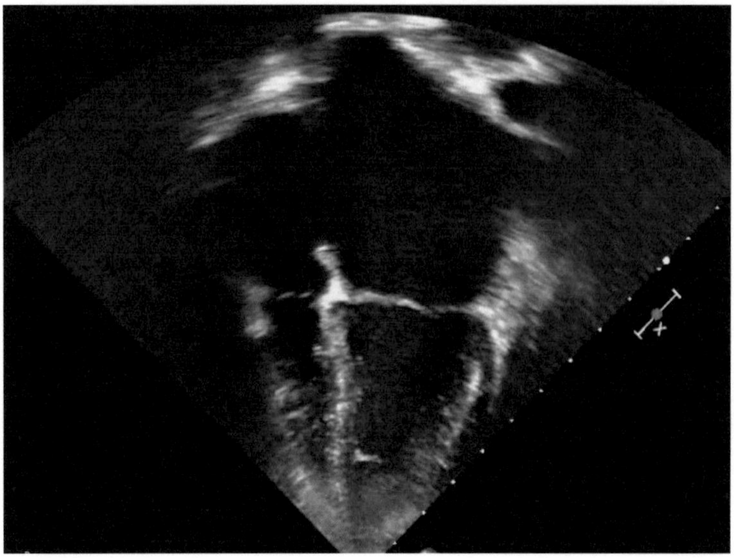

Figure 5.
Two-dimensional, apical 4-chamber echocardiographic image depicting small, restrictive ventricles and significant biatrial enlargement in a patient with restrictive cardiomyopathy.

with exercise intolerance, dyspnea, edema, atrial fibrillation, syncope, or sudden cardiac death. The hallmark of non-invasive imaging is atrial or bi-atrial enlargement. Normal or mild concentric hypertrophy with normal or reduced ventricular cavity can also be seen. Familial disease has been reported in 30% of cases and usually exhibits autosomal dominant inheritance. However, autosomal recessive, X-linked, and mitochondrial-transmitted disease have also been reported [117]. Most patients with RCM harbor gene mutations in sarcomere-encoding genes, such as *TNNI3* (most common), *TNNT2, MYH7, ACTC1, TPM1, MYL3,* and *MYL2*, see **Table 6** [18, 118]. Gene variants in the desmin gene have been reported in association with atrioventricular block and skeletal myopathy [119, 120].

RCM can be classified based on the underlying process: non-infiltrative; infiltrative; associated with storage diseases; idiopathic; or combined with DCM, HCM, and LVNC [116]. As with DCM, many previous cases deemed idiopathic are later found to harbor causative pathogenic variants in sarcomeric genes. Non-infiltrative causes of RCM include scleroderma and systemic sclerosis with well-described polymorphisms in genes coding for ECM proteins [121]. Pseudoxanthoma elasticum is an inherited disorder associated with accumulation of mineralized elastic fibers that may lead to blindness, coronary arterial occlusive disease, and RCM. The *ABCC6* gene on chromosome 16p13.1 is responsible for the calcification of elastic fibers [122]. Infiltrative causes of RCM include amyloidosis, a group of diseases characterized by extracellular deposition of insoluble fibrillar proteins with concomitant destruction of normal tissue structure and function. Approximately 20 different proteins cause cardiac amyloidosis. In the hereditary disease type, more than 100 gene mutations are known at present [123, 124]. The *Val122Ile* variant of transthyretin (*TTR*) is the most common [125]. Sarcoidosis can also cause systolic dysfunction and arrhythmias. The strongest genetic associations are found within the human leucocyte antigen (*HLA*) gene and functional polymorphisms within the butyrophilin-like 2 (*BTNL2*) gene [126].

Lysosomal storage disorders are characterized by abnormal lysosomal metabolism leading to accumulation of various glycosaminoglycans, glycoproteins, or glycolipids within lysosomes of various tissues, including the myocardium. Gaucher

Gene	Protein	Pattern of Inheritance	Disease Association	OMIM#	Locus
BAG3	Bcl2-Associated Athanogene 3	AD	LVNC, HCM, DCM	603883	14q24.3
DES	Desmin	AD, AR	RCM, DCM, ACM	125660	17q21
FLNC	Filamin C	AD	RCM, HCM, ACM, LVNC	102565	10q22.2
MYBPC3	Myosin-Binding Protein C, Cardiac	AD	RCM, HCM, DCM, LVNC	600958	Xq28
MYH7	Myosin, Heavy Chain 7, Cardiac Muscle, Beta	AD	RCM, HCM, DCM, LVNC	160760	7p14.2
MYL3	Myosin, Light Chain 3, Alkali, Ventricular, Skeletal, Slow	AD, AR	RCM, HCM	160790	1q32
MYOZ2	Myozenin 2	AD	RCM, HCM, DCM	605602	3p25.1
MYPN	Myopalladin	AD	RCM, HCM, DCM	608517	12q23.1
TNNI3	Troponin I Type 3 (Cardiac)	AD	RCM, HCM, DCM	191044	3p21.1
TNNT2	Troponin T Type 2 (Cardiac)	AD	RCM, HCM, DCM, LVNC	191045	17q12
TPM1	Tropomyosin 1 (Alpha)	AD	RCM, HCM, DCM	191010	19q13.4

AD – Autosomal dominant; AR – Autosomal Recessive; XL – X-linked; DCM – Dilated cardiomyopathy; HCM – Hypertrophic cardiomyopathy; LVNC – Left ventricular non-compaction cardiomyopathy; ACM – Arrhythmogenic cardiomyopathy; RCM – Restrictive cardiomyopathy.

Table 6.
List of common genes and patterns of inheritance in RCM.

disease and Fabry disease (two of the most common lysosomal disorders) may manifest as CM (HCM or RCM), valvular disease, coronary artery disease, and/or aortic enlargement [127].

Mucopolysaccharidoses (Hurler and Hunter diseases) are characterized by the deficiency of enzymes required for the breakdown of glycosaminoglycans. Thus, these diseases are considered lysosomal storage disorders. Cardiac manifestations start from childhood and include RCM, endocardial fibroelastosis, and valvular disease including thickening of the leaflets with resultant stenosis and/or insufficiency. Storage diseases such as hemochromatosis (mutation in the *HFE* gene) cause a mixture of systolic and diastolic dysfunction often accompanied by arrhythmias [128].

In summary, CM is a widely variable disease process with a similarly variable pattern of genetic inheritance. Our understanding of the interplay between genetic mutation and disease phenotype is ever-evolving and merits much deeper investigation.

Author details

Evan M. Harvey[1], Murad Almasri[2] and Hugo R. Martinez[1*]

1 Pediatric Cardiology, Le Bonheur Children's Hospital, University of Tennessee Health Science Center, Memphis, TN, United States

2 Department of Pediatrics, University of Texas Medical Branch, Galveston, TX, United States

*Address all correspondence to: hmartinez@uthsc.edu

References

[1] Wilkinson JD, Landy DC, Colan SD, Towbin JA, Sleeper LA, Orav EJ, et al. The pediatric cardiomyopathy registry and heart failure: key results from the first 15 years. Heart Fail Clin. 2010;6(4):401-13, vii.

[2] Arbustini E, Narula N, Dec GW, Reddy KS, Greenberg B, Kushwaha S, et al. The MOGE(S) Classification for a Phenotype-Genotype Nomenclature of Cardiomyopathy: Endorsed by the World Heart Federation. Glob Heart. 2013;8(4):355-82.

[3] Elliott P, Andersson B, Arbustini E, Bilinska Z, Cecchi F, Charron P, et al. Classification of the cardiomyopathies: a position statement from the European Society Of Cardiology Working Group on Myocardial and Pericardial Diseases. Eur Heart J. 2008;29(2): 270-6.

[4] Maron BJ, Towbin JA, Thiene G, Antzelevitch C, Corrado D, Arnett D, et al. Contemporary definitions and classification of the cardiomyopathies: an American Heart Association Scientific Statement from the Council on Clinical Cardiology, Heart Failure and Transplantation Committee; Quality of Care and Outcomes Research and Functional Genomics and Translational Biology Interdisciplinary Working Groups; and Council on Epidemiology and Prevention. Circulation. 2006;113(14):1807-16.

[5] Lipshultz SE, Law YM, Asante-Korang A, Austin ED, Dipchand AI, Everitt MD, et al. Cardiomyopathy in Children: Classification and Diagnosis: A Scientific Statement From the American Heart Association. Circulation. 2019;140(1):e9-e68.

[6] Jefferies JL, Towbin JA. Dilated cardiomyopathy. Lancet. 2010;375(9716):752-62.

[7] Towbin JA, Lowe AM, Colan SD, Sleeper LA, Orav EJ, Clunie S, et al. Incidence, causes, and outcomes of dilated cardiomyopathy in children. JAMA. 2006;296(15):1867-76.

[8] Petretta M, Pirozzi F, Sasso L, Paglia A, Bonaduce D. Review and metaanalysis of the frequency of familial dilated cardiomyopathy. Am J Cardiol. 2011;108(8):1171-6.

[9] Tayal U, Prasad S, Cook SA. Genetics and genomics of dilated cardiomyopathy and systolic heart failure. Genome Med. 2017;9(1):20.

[10] McNally EM, Golbus JR, Puckelwartz MJ. Genetic mutations and mechanisms in dilated cardiomyopathy. J Clin Invest. 2013;123(1):19-26.

[11] Nouhravesh N, Ahlberg G, Ghouse J, Andreasen C, Svendsen JH, Haunso S, et al. Analyses of more than 60,000 exomes questions the role of numerous genes previously associated with dilated cardiomyopathy. Mol Genet Genomic Med. 2016;4(6):617-23.

[12] Hershberger RE, Givertz MM, Ho CY, Judge DP, Kantor PF, McBride KL, et al. Genetic Evaluation of Cardiomyopathy-A Heart Failure Society of America Practice Guideline. J Card Fail. 2018;24(5):281-302.

[13] McNally EM, Mestroni L. Dilated Cardiomyopathy: Genetic Determinants and Mechanisms. Circ Res. 2017;121(7):731-48.

[14] Bowles NE, Bowles KR, Towbin JA. The "final common pathway" hypothesis and inherited cardiovascular disease. The role of cytoskeletal proteins in dilated cardiomyopathy. Herz. 2000;25(3):168-75.

[15] Fatkin D, Otway R, Richmond Z. Genetics of dilated cardiomyopathy. Heart Fail Clin. 2010;6(2):129-40.

[16] Ware SM. Evaluation of genetic causes of cardiomyopathy in childhood. Cardiol Young. 2015;25 Suppl 2:43-50.

[17] Towbin JA. Genetic arrhythmias complicating patients with dilated cardiomyopathy: How it happens. Heart Rhythm. 2020;17(2):313-4.

[18] Towbin JA. Inherited cardiomyopathies. Circ J. 2014;78(10):2347-56.

[19] Towbin JA, Ortiz-Lopez R. X-linked dilated cardiomyopathy. N Engl J Med. 1994;330(5):369-70.

[20] Davies KE, Nowak KJ. Molecular mechanisms of muscular dystrophies: old and new players. Nat Rev Mol Cell Biol. 2006;7(10):762-73.

[21] Wong BL, Rybalsky I, Shellenbarger KC, Tian C, McMahon MA, Rutter MM, et al. Long-Term Outcome of Interdisciplinary Management of Patients with Duchenne Muscular Dystrophy Receiving Daily Glucocorticoid Treatment. J Pediatr. 2017;182:296-303 e1.

[22] Feng J, Yan J, Buzin CH, Towbin JA, Sommer SS. Mutations in the dystrophin gene are associated with sporadic dilated cardiomyopathy. Mol Genet Metab. 2002;77(1-2):119-26.

[23] Hershberger RE, Givertz M, Ho CY, Judge DP, Kantor P, McBride KL, et al. Genetic Evaluation of Cardiomyopathy - a Heart Failure Society of America Practice Guideline. J Card Fail. 2018.

[24] American Academy of Pediatrics Section on C, Cardiac S. Cardiovascular health supervision for individuals affected by Duchenne or Becker muscular dystrophy. Pediatrics. 2005;116(6):1569-73.

[25] Martinez HR, Pignatelli R, Belmont JW, Craigen WJ, Jefferies JL. Childhood onset of left ventricular dysfunction in a female manifesting carrier of muscular dystrophy. Am J Med Genet A. 2011;155A(12):3025-9.

[26] Berko BA, Swift M. X-linked dilated cardiomyopathy. N Engl J Med. 1987;316(19):1186-91.

[27] Towbin JA, Hejtmancik JF, Brink P, Gelb B, Zhu XM, Chamberlain JS, et al. X-linked dilated cardiomyopathy. Molecular genetic evidence of linkage to the Duchenne muscular dystrophy (dystrophin) gene at the Xp21 locus. Circulation. 1993;87(6):1854-65.

[28] Puckelwartz M, McNally EM. Emery-Dreifuss muscular dystrophy. Handb Clin Neurol. 2011;101:155-66.

[29] Worman HJ, Ostlund C, Wang Y. Diseases of the nuclear envelope. Cold Spring Harb Perspect Biol. 2010;2(2):a000760.

[30] Rakovec P, Zidar J, Sinkovec M, Zupan I, Brecelj A. Cardiac involvement in Emery-Dreifuss muscular dystrophy: role of a diagnostic pacemaker. Pacing Clin Electrophysiol. 1995;18(9 Pt 1): 1721-4.

[31] Becane HM, Bonne G, Varnous S, Muchir A, Ortega V, Hammouda EH, et al. High incidence of sudden death with conduction system and myocardial disease due to lamins A and C gene mutation. Pacing Clin Electrophysiol. 2000;23(11 Pt 1):1661-6.

[32] Jefferies JL. Barth syndrome. Am J Med Genet C Semin Med Genet. 2013;163C(3):198-205.

[33] Barth PG, Scholte HR, Berden JA, Van der Klei-Van Moorsel JM, Luyt-Houwen IE, Van 't Veer-Korthof ET, et al. An X-linked mitochondrial disease affecting cardiac muscle, skeletal muscle and neutrophil leucocytes. J Neurol Sci. 1983;62(1-3):327-55.

[34] Towbin JA. Left ventricular noncompaction: a new form of heart

failure. Heart Fail Clin. 2010;6(4):453-69, viii.

[35] Lipshultz SE, Orav EJ, Wilkinson JD, Towbin JA, Messere JE, Lowe AM, et al. Risk stratification at diagnosis for children with hypertrophic cardiomyopathy: an analysis of data from the Pediatric Cardiomyopathy Registry. Lancet. 2013;382(9908):1889-97.

[36] Colan SD, Lipshultz SE, Lowe AM, Sleeper LA, Messere J, Cox GF, et al. Epidemiology and cause-specific outcome of hypertrophic cardiomyopathy in children: findings from the Pediatric Cardiomyopathy Registry. Circulation. 2007;115(6):773-81.

[37] Chun EJ, Choi SI, Jin KN, Kwag HJ, Kim YJ, Choi BW, et al. Hypertrophic cardiomyopathy: assessment with MR imaging and multidetector CT. Radiographics. 2010;30(5):1309-28.

[38] Rakowski H, Carasso S. Diastolic dysfunction and histopathology in hypertrophic cardiomyopathy: is relaxation in disarray? J Am Soc Echocardiogr. 2009;22(12):1335-7.

[39] Colan SD. Hypertrophic cardiomyopathy in childhood. Heart Fail Clin. 2010;6(4):433-44, vii-iii.

[40] Alfares AA, Kelly MA, McDermott G, Funke BH, Lebo MS, Baxter SB, et al. Results of clinical genetic testing of 2,912 probands with hypertrophic cardiomyopathy: expanded panels offer limited additional sensitivity. Genet Med. 2015;17(11):880-8.

[41] Burns C, Bagnall RD, Lam L, Semsarian C, Ingles J. Multiple Gene Variants in Hypertrophic Cardiomyopathy in the Era of Next-Generation Sequencing. Circ Cardiovasc Genet. 2017;10(4).

[42] Maass A, Konhilas JP, Stauffer BL, Leinwand LA. From sarcomeric mutations to heart disease: understanding familial hypertrophic cardiomyopathy. Cold Spring Harb Symp Quant Biol. 2002;67:409-15.

[43] Roma-Rodrigues C, Fernandes AR. Genetics of hypertrophic cardiomyopathy: advances and pitfalls in molecular diagnosis and therapy. Appl Clin Genet. 2014;7:195-208.

[44] Gersh BJ, Maron BJ, Bonow RO, Dearani JA, Fifer MA, Link MS, et al. 2011 ACCF/AHA guideline for the diagnosis and treatment of hypertrophic cardiomyopathy: a report of the American College of Cardiology Foundation/American Heart Association Task Force on Practice Guidelines. Circulation. 2011;124(24):e783-831.

[45] Konno T, Chang S, Seidman JG, Seidman CE. Genetics of hypertrophic cardiomyopathy. Curr Opin Cardiol. 2010;25(3):205-9.

[46] Jarcho JA, McKenna W, Pare JA, Solomon SD, Holcombe RF, Dickie S, et al. Mapping a gene for familial hypertrophic cardiomyopathy to chromosome 14q1. N Engl J Med. 1989;321(20):1372-8.

[47] Tariq M, Ware SM. Importance of genetic evaluation and testing in pediatric cardiomyopathy. World J Cardiol. 2014;6(11):1156-65.

[48] Ho CY. New Paradigms in Hypertrophic Cardiomyopathy: Insights from Genetics. Prog Pediatr Cardiol. 2011;31(2):93-8.

[49] Richard P, Charron P, Carrier L, Ledeuil C, Cheav T, Pichereau C, et al. Hypertrophic cardiomyopathy: distribution of disease genes, spectrum of mutations, and implications for a molecular diagnosis strategy. Circulation. 2003;107(17):2227-32.

[50] Rauen KA, Schoyer L, McCormick F, Lin AE, Allanson JE,

Stevenson DA, et al. Proceedings from the 2009 genetic syndromes of the Ras/MAPK pathway: From bedside to bench and back. Am J Med Genet A. 2010;152A(1):4-24.

[51] Thompson D, Patrick-Esteve J, Surcouf JW, Rivera D, Castellanos B, Desai P, et al. RAF1 variants causing biventricular hypertrophic cardiomyopathy in two preterm infants: further phenotypic delineation and review of literature. Clin Dysmorphol. 2017;26(4):195-9.

[52] Zenker M, Buheitel G, Rauch R, Koenig R, Bosse K, Kress W, et al. Genotype-phenotype correlations in Noonan syndrome. J Pediatr. 2004;144(3):368-74.

[53] Tafazoli A, Eshraghi P, Pantaleoni F, Vakili R, Moghaddassian M, Ghahraman M, et al. Novel mutations and their genotype-phenotype correlations in patients with Noonan syndrome, using next-generation sequencing. Adv Med Sci. 2017;63(1):87-93.

[54] Lee PA, Ross JL, Pedersen BT, Kotnik P, Germak JA, Christesen HT. Noonan syndrome and Turner syndrome patients respond similarly to 4 years' growth-hormone therapy: longitudinal analysis of growth-hormone-naive patients enrolled in the NordiNet(R) International Outcome Study and the ANSWER Program. Int J Pediatr Endocrinol. 2015;2015(1):17.

[55] Sarkozy A, Digilio MC, Dallapiccola B. Leopard syndrome. Orphanet J Rare Dis. 2008;3:13.

[56] Digilio MC, Sarkozy A, de Zorzi A, Pacileo G, Limongelli G, Mingarelli R, et al. LEOPARD syndrome: clinical diagnosis in the first year of life. Am J Med Genet A. 2006;140(7):740-6.

[57] Giannoulatou E, McVean G, Taylor IB, McGowan SJ, Maher GJ, Iqbal Z, et al. Contributions of intrinsic mutation rate and selfish selection to levels of de novo HRAS mutations in the paternal germline. Proc Natl Acad Sci U S A. 2013;110(50):20152-7.

[58] Bertola D, Buscarilli M, Stabley DL, Baker L, Doyle D, Bartholomew DW, et al. Phenotypic spectrum of Costello syndrome individuals harboring the rare HRAS mutation p.Gly13Asp. Am J Med Genet A. 2017;173(5):1309-18.

[59] Gelb BD, Roberts AE, Tartaglia M. Cardiomyopathies in Noonan syndrome and the other RASopathies. Prog Pediatr Cardiol. 2015;39(1):13-9.

[60] Rauen KA, Tidyman WE, Estep AL, Sampath S, Peltier HM, Bale SJ, et al. Molecular and functional analysis of a novel MEK2 mutation in cardio-facio-cutaneous syndrome: transmission through four generations. Am J Med Genet A. 2010;152A(4):807-14.

[61] Karaer K, Lissewski C, Zenker M. Familial cardiofaciocutaneous syndrome in a father and a son with a novel MEK2 mutation. Am J Med Genet A. 2015;167A(2):385-8.

[62] Pavithra S, Mallya H, Pai GS. Cardiofaciocutaneous syndrome: a rare entity. Indian J Dermatol. 2012;57(4):299-301.

[63] Terry J, Rauen KA, Nowaczyk MJ. Fetal autopsy findings of cardiofaciocutaneous syndrome with a unique BRAF mutation. Pediatr Dev Pathol. 2014;17(1):59-63.

[64] Hirschhorn R, Huie ML. Frequency of mutations for glycogen storage disease type II in different populations: the delta525T and deltaexon 18 mutations are not generally "common" in white populations. J Med Genet. 1999;36(1):85-6.

[65] Lim JA, Li L, Raben N. Pompe disease: from pathophysiology to

therapy and back again. Front Aging Neurosci. 2014;6:177.

[66] Boentert M, Florian A, Drager B, Young P, Yilmaz A. Pattern and prognostic value of cardiac involvement in patients with late-onset pompe disease: a comprehensive cardiovascular magnetic resonance approach. J Cardiovasc Magn Reson. 2016;18(1):91.

[67] Levine JC, Kishnani PS, Chen YT, Herlong JR, Li JS. Cardiac remodeling after enzyme replacement therapy with acid alpha-glucosidase for infants with Pompe disease. Pediatr Cardiol. 2008;29(6):1033-42.

[68] Arad M, Maron BJ, Gorham JM, Johnson WH, Jr., Saul JP, Perez-Atayde AR, et al. Glycogen storage diseases presenting as hypertrophic cardiomyopathy. N Engl J Med. 2005;352(4):362-72.

[69] Rowland TJ, Sweet ME, Mestroni L, Taylor MR. Danon disease - dysregulation of autophagy in a multisystem disorder with cardiomyopathy. J Cell Sci. 2016;129(11):2135-43.

[70] Maron BJ, Roberts WC, Arad M, Haas TS, Spirito P, Wright GB, et al. Clinical outcome and phenotypic expression in LAMP2 cardiomyopathy. JAMA. 2009;301(12):1253-9.

[71] Toib A, Grange DK, Kozel BA, Ewald GA, White FV, Canter CE. Distinct clinical and histopathological presentations of Danon cardiomyopathy in young women. J Am Coll Cardiol. 2010;55(4):408-10.

[72] Brady RO, Gal AE, Bradley RM, Martensson E, Warshaw AL, Laster L. Enzymatic defect in Fabry's disease. Ceramidetrihexosidase deficiency. N Engl J Med. 1967;276(21):1163-7.

[73] Garman SC, Garboczi DN. The molecular defect leading to Fabry disease: structure of human alpha-galactosidase. J Mol Biol. 2004;337(2):319-35.

[74] Mehta A, Ricci R, Widmer U, Dehout F, Garcia de Lorenzo A, Kampmann C, et al. Fabry disease defined: baseline clinical manifestations of 366 patients in the Fabry Outcome Survey. Eur J Clin Invest. 2004;34(3):236-42.

[75] Perrot A, Osterziel KJ, Beck M, Dietz R, Kampmann C. Fabry disease: focus on cardiac manifestations and molecular mechanisms. Herz. 2002;27(7):699-702.

[76] O'Mahony C, Elliott P. Anderson-Fabry disease and the heart. Prog Cardiovasc Dis. 2010;52(4):326-35.

[77] Weidemann F, Rummey C, Bijnens B, Stork S, Jasaityte R, Dhooge J, et al. The heart in Friedreich ataxia: definition of cardiomyopathy, disease severity, and correlation with neurological symptoms. Circulation. 2012;125(13):1626-34.

[78] Peverill RE. Letter by Peverill regarding article, "The heart in Friedreich ataxia: definition of cardiomyopathy, disease severity, and correlation with neurological symptoms". Circulation. 2012;126(17):e272.

[79] Kipps A, Alexander M, Colan SD, Gauvreau K, Smoot L, Crawford L, et al. The longitudinal course of cardiomyopathy in Friedreich's ataxia during childhood. Pediatr Cardiol. 2009;30(3):306-10.

[80] Brunel-Guitton C, Levtova A, Sasarman F. Mitochondrial Diseases and Cardiomyopathies. Can J Cardiol. 2015;31(11):1360-76.

[81] Towbin JA, Jefferies JL. Cardiomyopathies Due to Left Ventricular Noncompaction, Mitochondrial and

Storage Diseases, and Inborn Errors of Metabolism. Circ Res. 2017;121(7):838-54.

[82] Meyers DE, Basha HI, Koenig MK. Mitochondrial cardiomyopathy: pathophysiology, diagnosis, and management. Tex Heart Inst J. 2013;40(4):385-94.

[83] Sproule DM, Kaufmann P, Engelstad K, Starc TJ, Hordof AJ, De Vivo DC. Wolff-Parkinson-White syndrome in Patients With MELAS. Arch Neurol. 2007;64(11):1625-7.

[84] Okajima Y, Tanabe Y, Takayanagi M, Aotsuka H. A follow up study of myocardial involvement in patients with mitochondrial encephalomyopathy, lactic acidosis, and stroke-like episodes (MELAS). Heart. 1998;80(3):292-5.

[85] Thomas T, Craigen WJ, Moore R, Czosek R, Jefferies JL. Arrhythmia as a cardiac manifestation in MELAS syndrome. Mol Genet Metab Rep. 2015;4:9-10.

[86] Towbin JA. Ion channel dysfunction associated with arrhythmia, ventricular noncompaction, and mitral valve prolapse: a new overlapping phenotype. J Am Coll Cardiol. 2014;64(8):768-71.

[87] Towbin JA, Lorts A, Jefferies JL. Left ventricular non-compaction cardiomyopathy. Lancet. 2015;386(9995):813-25.

[88] Lee TM, Hsu DT, Kantor P, Towbin JA, Ware SM, Colan SD, et al. Pediatric Cardiomyopathies. Circ Res. 2017;121(7):855-73.

[89] Sedaghat-Hamedani F, Haas J, Zhu F, Geier C, Kayvanpour E, Liss M, et al. Clinical genetics and outcome of left ventricular non-compaction cardiomyopathy. Eur Heart J. 2017;38(46):3449-60.

[90] van Waning JI, Caliskan K, Michels M, Schinkel AFL, Hirsch A, Dalinghaus M, et al. Cardiac Phenotypes, Genetics, and Risks in Familial Noncompaction Cardiomyopathy. J Am Coll Cardiol. 2019;73(13):1601-11.

[91] van Waning JI, Caliskan K, Hoedemaekers YM, van Spaendonck-Zwarts KY, Baas AF, Boekholdt SM, et al. Genetics, Clinical Features, and Long-Term Outcome of Noncompaction Cardiomyopathy. J Am Coll Cardiol. 2018;71(7):711-22.

[92] Bagnall RD, Molloy LK, Kalman JM, Semsarian C. Exome sequencing identifies a mutation in the ACTN2 gene in a family with idiopathic ventricular fibrillation, left ventricular noncompaction, and sudden death. BMC Med Genet. 2014;15:99.

[93] Hastings R, de Villiers CP, Hooper C, Ormondroyd L, Pagnamenta A, Lise S, et al. Combination of Whole Genome Sequencing, Linkage, and Functional Studies Implicates a Missense Mutation in Titin as a Cause of Autosomal Dominant Cardiomyopathy With Features of Left Ventricular Noncompaction. Circ Cardiovasc Genet. 2016;9(5):426-35.

[94] Shan L, Makita N, Xing Y, Watanabe S, Futatani T, Ye F, et al. SCN5A variants in Japanese patients with left ventricular noncompaction and arrhythmia. Mol Genet Metab. 2008;93(4):468-74.

[95] Finsterer J, Stollberger C. Primary myopathies and the heart. Scand Cardiovasc J. 2008;42(1):9-24.

[96] Ramond F, Janin A, Di Filippo S, Chanavat V, Chalabreysse L, Roux-Buisson N, et al. Homozygous PKP2 deletion associated with neonatal left ventricle noncompaction. Clin Genet. 2017;91(1):126-30.

[97] Miller EM, Hinton RB, Czosek R, Lorts A, Parrott A, Shikany AR, et al.

Genetic Testing in Pediatric Left Ventricular Noncompaction. Circ Cardiovasc Genet. 2017;10(6).

[98] Dong X, Fan P, Tian T, Yang Y, Xiao Y, Yang K, et al. Recent advancements in the molecular genetics of left ventricular noncompaction cardiomyopathy. Clin Chim Acta. 2017;465:40-4.

[99] Miszalski-Jamka K, Jefferies JL, Mazur W, Glowacki J, Hu J, Lazar M, et al. Novel Genetic Triggers and Genotype-Phenotype Correlations in Patients With Left Ventricular Noncompaction. Circ Cardiovasc Genet. 2017;10(4).

[100] Oechslin E, Jenni R. Left ventricular non-compaction revisited: a distinct phenotype with genetic heterogeneity? Eur Heart J. 2011;32(12):1446-56.

[101] Blinder JJ, Martinez HR, Craigen WJ, Belmont J, Pignatelli RH, Jefferies JL. Noncompaction of the left ventricular myocardium in a boy with a novel chromosome 8p23.1 deletion. Am J Med Genet A. 2011;155A(9):2215-20.

[102] Martinez HR, Belmont JW, Craigen WJ, Taylor MD, Jefferies JL. Left ventricular noncompaction in Sotos syndrome. Am J Med Genet A. 2011;155A(5):1115-8.

[103] Martinez HR, Niu MC, Sutton VR, Pignatelli R, Vatta M, Jefferies JL. Coffin-Lowry syndrome and left ventricular noncompaction cardiomyopathy with a restrictive pattern. Am J Med Genet A. 2011;155A(12):3030-4.

[104] Martinez HR, Ware SM, Schamberger MS, Parent JJ. Noncompaction cardiomyopathy and heterotaxy syndrome. Prog Pediatr Cardiol. 2017;46:23-7.

[105] Peters S, Trummel M, Meyners W. Prevalence of right ventricular dysplasia-cardiomyopathy in a non-referral hospital. Int J Cardiol. 2004;97(3):499-501.

[106] Towbin JA, McKenna WJ, Abrams DJ, Ackerman MJ, Calkins H, Darrieux FCC, et al. 2019 HRS expert consensus statement on evaluation, risk stratification, and management of arrhythmogenic cardiomyopathy: Executive summary. Heart Rhythm. 2019;16(11):e373-e407.

[107] Protonotarios N, Tsatsopoulou A. Naxos disease and Carvajal syndrome: cardiocutaneous disorders that highlight the pathogenesis and broaden the spectrum of arrhythmogenic right ventricular cardiomyopathy. Cardiovasc Pathol. 2004;13(4):185-94.

[108] Marcus FI, McKenna WJ, Sherrill D, Basso C, Bauce B, Bluemke DA, et al. Diagnosis of arrhythmogenic right ventricular cardiomyopathy/dysplasia: proposed modification of the Task Force Criteria. Eur Heart J. 2010;31(7):806-14.

[109] Hamid MS, Norman M, Quraishi A, Firoozi S, Thaman R, Gimeno JR, et al. Prospective evaluation of relatives for familial arrhythmogenic right ventricular cardiomyopathy/dysplasia reveals a need to broaden diagnostic criteria. J Am Coll Cardiol. 2002;40(8):1445-50.

[110] Bauce B, Nava A, Beffagna G, Basso C, Lorenzon A, Smaniotto G, et al. Multiple mutations in desmosomal proteins encoding genes in arrhythmogenic right ventricular cardiomyopathy/dysplasia. Heart Rhythm. 2010;7(1):22-9.

[111] den Haan AD, Tan BY, Zikusoka MN, Llado LI, Jain R, Daly A, et al. Comprehensive desmosome mutation analysis in north americans with arrhythmogenic right ventricular dysplasia/cardiomyopathy. Circ Cardiovasc Genet. 2009;2(5):428-35.

[112] Delmar M, McKenna WJ. The cardiac desmosome and arrhythmogenic cardiomyopathies: from gene to disease. Circ Res. 2010;107(6):700-14.

[113] Groeneweg JA, Bhonsale A, James CA, te Riele AS, Dooijes D, Tichnell C, et al. Clinical Presentation, Long-Term Follow-Up, and Outcomes of 1001 Arrhythmogenic Right Ventricular Dysplasia/Cardiomyopathy Patients and Family Members. Circ Cardiovasc Genet. 2015;8(3):437-46.

[114] Rigato I, Bauce B, Rampazzo A, Zorzi A, Pilichou K, Mazzotti E, et al. Compound and digenic heterozygosity predicts lifetime arrhythmic outcome and sudden cardiac death in desmosomal gene-related arrhythmogenic right ventricular cardiomyopathy. Circ Cardiovasc Genet. 2013;6(6):533-42.

[115] Xu T, Yang Z, Vatta M, Rampazzo A, Beffagna G, Pilichou K, et al. Compound and digenic heterozygosity contributes to arrhythmogenic right ventricular cardiomyopathy. J Am Coll Cardiol. 2010;55(6):587-97.

[116] Denfield SW, Webber SA. Restrictive cardiomyopathy in childhood. Heart Fail Clin. 2010;6(4):445-52, viii.

[117] Kaski JP, Syrris P, Burch M, Tome-Esteban MT, Fenton M, Christiansen M, et al. Idiopathic restrictive cardiomyopathy in children is caused by mutations in cardiac sarcomere protein genes. Heart. 2008;94(11):1478-84.

[118] Caleshu C, Sakhuja R, Nussbaum RL, Schiller NB, Ursell PC, Eng C, et al. Furthering the link between the sarcomere and primary cardiomyopathies: restrictive cardiomyopathy associated with multiple mutations in genes previously associated with hypertrophic or dilated cardiomyopathy. Am J Med Genet A. 2011;155A(9):2229-35.

[119] Sen-Chowdhry S, Morgan RD, Chambers JC, McKenna WJ. Arrhythmogenic cardiomyopathy: etiology, diagnosis, and treatment. Annu Rev Med. 2010;61:233-53.

[120] Goldfarb LG, Vicart P, Goebel HH, Dalakas MC. Desmin myopathy. Brain. 2004;127(Pt 4):723-34.

[121] Worthley MI, Farouque HM, McNeil JD, Worthley SG. Scleroderma cardiomyopathy presenting with thromboembolism. Intern Med J. 2001;31(1):64-5.

[122] Nguyen LD, Terbah M, Daudon P, Martin L. Left ventricular systolic and diastolic function by echocardiogram in pseudoxanthoma elasticum. Am J Cardiol. 2006;97(10):1535-7.

[123] Lahuerta C, Menao S, Gracia-Gutierrez A, Bueno-Juana E, Guillen N, Sorribas V, et al. Diagnosis of genetic amyloidosis through the analysis of transthyretin gene mutation using high-resolution melting. Int J Cardiol. 2020;301:220-5.

[124] Rameev VV, Kozlovskaia LV, Sarkisova IA, Simonian A. [Genetic aspects of periodic diseases and associated amyloidosis]. Ter Arkh. 2002;74(6):80-3.

[125] Rapezzi C, Merlini G, Quarta CC, Riva L, Longhi S, Leone O, et al. Systemic cardiac amyloidoses: disease profiles and clinical courses of the 3 main types. Circulation. 2009;120(13):1203-12.

[126] Spagnolo P, Sato H, Grutters JC, Renzoni EA, Marshall SE, Ruven HJ, et al. Analysis of BTNL2 genetic polymorphisms in British and Dutch patients with sarcoidosis. Tissue Antigens. 2007;70(3):219-27.

[127] Lindor NM, Karnes PS. Initial assessment of infants and children with suspected inborn errors of metabolism. Mayo Clin Proc. 1995;70(10):987-8.

[128] Pietrangelo A. Hereditary hemochromatosis: pathogenesis, diagnosis, and treatment. Gastroenterology. 2010;139(2): 393-408, e1-2.

Chapter 6

The Role of Genetics in Cardiomyopaties: A Review

Luis Vernengo and Haluk Topaloglu

Abstract

Cardiomyopathies are defined as disorders of the myocardium which are always associated with cardiac dysfunction and are aggravated by arrhythmias, heart failure and sudden death. There are different ways of classifying them. The American Heart Association has classified them in either primary or secondary cardiomyopathies depending on whether the heart is the only organ involved or whether they are due to a systemic disorder. On the other hand, the European Society of Cardiology has classified them according to the different morphological and functional phenotypes associated with their pathophysiology. In 2013 the MOGE(S) classification started to be published and clinicians have started to adopt it. The purpose of this review is to update it.

Keywords: cardiomyopathy, primary and secondary cardiomyopathies, sarcomeric genes

1. Introduction

Cardiomyopathies can be defined as disorders of the myocardium associated with cardiac dysfunction and which are aggravated by arrhythmias, heart failure and sudden death [1]. The aim of this chapter is focused on updating and reviewing cardiomyopathies.

In 1957, Bridgen coined the word "cardiomyopathy" for the first time and in 1958, the British pathologist Teare reported nine cases of septum hypertrophy [2]. Genetics has played a key role in the understanding of these disorders. In general, the overall prevalence of cardiomyopathies in the world population is 3%.

The genetic forms of cardiomyopathies are characterized by both locus and allelic heterogeneity. The mutations of the genes which encode for a variety of proteins of the sarcomere, cytoskeleton, nuclear envelope, sarcolemma, ion channels and intercellular junctions alter many pathways and cellular structures affecting in a negative form the mechanism of muscle contraction and its function, and the sensitivity of ion channels to electrolytes, calcium homeostasis and how mechanic force in the myocardium is generated and transmitted [3, 4].

Panels of genes are performed to diagnose the different mutations of the genes that can be the cause of the disorders although it is not certain that these disorders might be caused by these mutations. Increasing insight has shown the overlapping of the different types of cardiomyopathies [3].

There are different ways of classifying them. In 2006, the American Heart Association classified them in either primary or secondary cardiomyopathies depending on whether the heart was the only organ involved or the disorder was a found in a systemic disease. On the other hand, in 2008, the European Society of

Cardiology classified them according to the different morphological and functional phenotypes associated with their pathophysiology. In 2013, the MOGE(S) classification was described [1, 5–11].

2. Classification

The American Heart Association (AHA) classified cardiomyopathies as primary those in which the heart is the only organ affected and can be genetic, mixed or acquired and secondary, those in which the heart is affected as part of a systemic disease. On the other hand, the European Society of Cardiology (ESC) classified them according to morphological and functional phenotypes involving their pathophysiology (**Tables 1** and **2**) [1, 7–12].

In 2013, MOGE(S), the new cardiomyopathy classification system, was developed. The MOGE(S) system, which is based on the TNM classification scheme for tumors, will be a useful tool for the diagnosis, management, and treatment of cardiomyopathies as well as the TNM classification is to the management of cancer. The nomenclature of the MOGE(S) classification system used in cardiomyopathies is easier to describe and understand. This latter configuration system has a descriptive language or code and it allows physicians to comprehend what the different types of cardiomyopathy are and what mutation each patient has It is a descriptive genotype–phenotype system. The MOGE(S) classification is based on five attributes and describes how it can be used on patients who have one of the disorders. Therefore, MOGE(S) stands for: (M) morphofunctional characteristic; (O) organ involvement; (G) genetic or familial inheritance pattern; (E) specific etiological characteristics; (S) Stage of heart failure (functional classes). The MOGE(S)

Genetic	Hypertrophic cardiomyopathy Arrhythmogenic Right Ventricular Cardiomyopathy/Dysplasia Left Ventricular Noncompaction Conduction defects (Lenegre-Lev disease) Ion channels disorders: Long QT syndrome Brugada syndrome Short QT syndrome Catecholaminergic polymorphic ventricular tachycardia Mitochondrial defects.
Mixed	Dilated cardiomyopathy Restrictive cardiomyopathy
Acquired	Inflammatory (cardiac amyloidosis) Takotsubo Peripartum Tachicardia-induced Infants of insulin-dependent diabetic mothers

Table 1.
Primary Cardiomyopathies

CARDIOMYOPATHIES	HCM DCM ACM RCM Unclassified	Genetic	Disease subtypes Unidentified gene defect
		Non genetic	Disease subtypes Unidentified gene defect

Table 2.
European Society of Cardiology. Classification of the cardiomyopathies.

classification system will, undoubtedly, not only help in the diagnosis, but in the management of the different cardiomyopathies as well. It will definitely help to diagnose a cardiomyopathy in the early stages that is to say when the disorder is not yet present allowing to physicians to start treatment quickly (**Table 3**) [5, 6, 13–16].

Let us show a couple of examples regarding the several cases in which this classification can be applied.

Let us discuss a patient with Friedriech's ataxia. The patient was a Caucasian male who had normal milestones and at age 10 he started with progressive gait. On examination he had Babinski reflex, pes cavus. The disorder progressed very quickly. He had limb ataxia and pyramidal signs appear. He underwent surgery because of the scoliosis and had his spine braced. At age 15, he had dysarthria, distal

M **Morphofunctional phenotype**	**O** **Organ involvement**	**G** **Genetic pattern**	**E** **Etiology**	**S** **Stage**
Cardiomyopathy diagnosis 1)HCM (H) a) H (obs) obstructive b) H (noObs) non Obstructive3) 2)DCM (D) 3)RCM (R) 4 R EMF 5) Endomyocardial fibrosis 6)ARVC/D (A) 7)LVNC (NC) 8)Early (specifyiing the different subgroups) a)E(H) b)E(D) c)E (R) d)E (A) Channelopaties (are not included) 0 Unaffected NA not available NS Non specific phenotype	0: Absence of involvement H: Heart M Skeletal Muscle A: Auditory C: Cutaneous E: Eye, Ocular G: Gastrointestinal K: Kidney Li: Liver Lu: Lung N: Nervous S: Skeletal	Inheritance A- Familial: AD: autosomal dominant AR: autosomal recessive XLD: X-inked dominant XLR: X-inked recessive Mit: mitochondrial B.Non familial: Phenotipically sporadic 1. Families: a) Informative b) non Informative 2. Family history not known by patient Family screening 1. affected asymptomatic relatives who do not know they have the disorder. 2. Abnormal ECG and echocardiogram detected in relatives 3.Normal ECG and echocardiogram in relatives who have no symptoms.	Index cases should be tested 1. If Positive relatives should also be tested 2.If Negative novel genes should be tested and relatives regular check-ups G-OC: Obligate carrier G ONC: Non carrier G-G-A-Genetic amyloidosis G-HFE Hemochromatosis DN *De novo* mutation G-Neg Test Negative for an unknown mutation G-N mutation not yet Identified 0 No genetic test performed *Non-genetic etiologies* A: amyloidosis (each type has to be stated) A: autimmune Eo: hypereosinophilic heart disease I: infectious diseases M: myocarditis V: viral infection state the gene that causes the disorder (if the molecular was performed) and the mutation found	The stage depicted by the letters A,B,C or D of the American College of cardiology- American Heart Association (ACC-AHA) NA: not applicable NU: not used Followed by the class of the New York Heart association (NYHA) which is described by I, II, II, IV stands for the functional status (and functional class. (This is optional).

Table 3.
The MOGE(S) system for classifying cardiomyopathy patients.

wasting, spasticity. The wasting of his muscles could be observed in his limbs. His fingers resembled aranodactyly.He was wheelchair-bound. Very intelligent person. Chest X ray: cardiomegaly. He never developed diabetes mellitus. He had several bouts of pneumonia. Serial ECGs showed repolarization wave abnormalities. Echocardiograms showed concentric left ventricular hypertrophy and normal ejection fraction. Pulmonary functional tests showed that he had restrictive pulmonary syndrome of scoliotic origin. Cranial CT scan demonstrated he had cerebellar atrophy. At age 19, he suffered from depression and he developed urinary urgency. Molecular test confirmed the diagnosis showing a GAA triplet repeat size over 2000.

$M_{H(T}$ wave abnormalities) for hypertrophic cardiomyopathy and T wave abnormalities.

$O_{H+M+N+Lu+S}$ The organs affected were the heart, skeletal muscles, neurological, lung and skeletal problems,

$G_{AR:}$ the disorder is inherited in an autosomal recessive pattern.

$E_{G\text{-}FXN}$ intron 1 GAA repeats >2000.

$S_{C\text{-}II}$.

Therefore, the patient could be classified as $M_{H(T\ wave\ abnormalities)}$ $O_{H+M+N+Lu+S}G_{AR}E_{G\text{-}FXN\ (intron\ 1\ GAArepeats\ >\ 2000)}\ S_{C\text{-}II}$.

The other case is a 17-year-old Caucasian male who had a mitochondrial myopathy presenting the typical clinical features of KSS. The patient had intellectual disability, short stature and hypogrowth. Bilateral palpebral ptosis. External ophtalmoplegia. Dyspnea at rest. Pigmentary retinal degeneration Sensorineural loss. Muscle weakness. Cerebellar syndrome. Ataxia. He denied having a disease and did not want to have any more tests performed. Atrioventricular block appeared in the different ECGs. Echocardiograms showed dilated cardiomyopathy. Muscle biopsy showed ragged-red cells. Electron microscopy and no molecular test was performed. No other family member had the disease.

$M_{D(AVB)}$. for dilated cardiomyopathy with atrioventricular block.

$O_{H+M+N+Lu+S}$ The organs affected were the heart and the skeletal muscles and had neurological, lung and skeletal problems,

$G_{AR:}$ the disorder is a mitochondrial disorder.

$E_{G\text{-}0}$: no molecular testing was run.

$S_{C\text{-}II}$.

The patient could be classified as followed $M_{D(AVB)}$ $O_{H+M+N+E+Li}G_{Mit}E_{G\text{-}0}S_{C\text{-}II.}$

3. Hypertrophic cardiomyopathy

Hypertrophic cardiomyopathy (HCM) has commonly been described as an unexplained hypertrophy of the left ventricle which develops in the absence of systemic hypertension, valvular heart disease or amyloidosis. The left ventricular hypertrophy (LVH) is usually asymmetric and involves the septum leading to a decrease of the left ventricular chamber [1, 4, 10, 12, 17].

The 2020 AHA/ACC guideline has defined it as the common definition of primary cardiomyopathies in which the heart is the only organ involved [18] while Europeans do not take into account the loading conditions in adult patients, but the wall thickness of the left ventricle which has to be greater than 13 mm and two standard deviations from the predicted mean (z-score > 2) [19, 20].

HCM is a familial disease which has locus heterogeneity. It is inherited in an autosomal dominant pattern in fifty percent of the cases, but autosomal recessive and X-linked HCM have also been described [1, 12, 17, 21–26]. The clinical presentation is variable and the clinical severity can even lead to, heart failure and sudden death. Many patients can be asymptomatic, whereas others will need a heart transplant [18, 27, 28]. It is the most common cause of death in young athletes while practicing sports [12, 27, 29, 30].

The prevalence of HCM varies from 1:200 to 1: 500 [4, 12, 31–33]. The cardiac sarcomere is a complex structure and it is a long way to completely unraveled the pathophysiology of HCM. Most mutations in HCM are private of each family thus presenting allelic heterogeneity, incomplete penetrance as well as myocyte hypertrophy and variable interstitial fibrosis. Genetic and environmental modifiers also play an important part in the development of the HCM [1, 4, 12, 18, 34–36].

A decade ago, there were thirty-three genes in the world literature that have been reported to be involved and caused the disease. The genetically based HCM are due to mutations in the cardiac sarcomere or the associated proteins (See **Table 4**). This has changed now and the classification of HCM is based on the ClinGen framework for evaluating gene-disease clinical validity. The genes that are considered to cause most likely HCM are *MYH7, TNNT2, TPM1, MYBPC3, ACTC1, TNNI3, MYL2* and *MYL3*. The different gene variants are now classified as definitive, strong, moderate, limited and no reported evidence. Conflicting evidence reported is defined when there is contradictory evidence reported and there are cases that were first described as HCM but later on they could not be confirmed [18, 19, 37–45].

There seems to be no correlation between the phenotype of the patients and the location of the mutations. Most of the mutations are usually missense with exception of the mutations in the *MYBPC3* gene in which it is common to find insertions, deletions and truncation mutations due to some frameshift mutations [1, 12, 17, 36, 46, 47].

There are syndromic phenotypes associated with HCM. Among them cardiofacial syndromes are commonly referred as RASopathies (Noonan, Leopard, Costello syndromes), neurological diseases (Frederich's ataxia which is caused by the expansion of GAA sequence in intron 1 of the frataxin gene), mitochondrial diseases caused by deletion syndromes (KSS, MELAS, MERFF; LOHN), metabolic disorders of lysosomal storage diseases (Anderson-Fabry disease (GLA mutations), Hurler's syndrome (absence of alpha-L-iduronidase,) and glycogen storage diseases (Wolf-Parkinson-White syndrome caused by mutations in the PRKAG2 gene), Forbes´ disease (mutations in the AGL gene) and Pompe disease [mutations in the alpha-1,4-glucosidase (GAA)]; infiltrative diseases (Danon disease that has mutations in LAMP2 gene). Other disorders that have HCM are Noonan syndrome caused by the syndromic genes PTPN11, RAF1 and RIT and myofibrillar myopathies caused by mutations in BAG3, FLNC and ZASP [11, 26, 36, 40, 48, 49].

4. Dilated cardiomyopathy

Dilated cardiomyopathy (DCM) is characterized by an enlargement of the left ventricular chamber with impaired left ventricular systolic function, which is progressive and, in some cases, has secondary diastolic dysfunction. The prevalence of DCM is greater than 1 in 2500. DCM is the most common cause of congestive heart failure in young patients. The prevalence is ~36: 100,000 in the U.S The most common feature is congestive heart failure, though, conduction impairment, syncope and sudden death may also occur. Cardiac transplantation is sometimes the only solution to the disease [12, 50–55].

HCM gene	Symbol	Locus name	Chromosome locus	Protein	Mode of inheritance	ClinGen Gene Validity Classification
Beta-myosin heavy chain	MYH7	CMH1	14q11.2	Myosin heavy chain, cardiac muscle beta isoform	AD	Definitive
Troponin T	TNNT2	CMH2	1q32.1	TroponinT, cardiac muscle	AD	Definitive
alpha-tropomyosin	TPM1	CMH3	15q22.1	Tropomyosin1 alpha chain		Definitive
Myosin-binding protein C	MYBPC3	CMH4	11p11.2	Myosin-binding protein C, cardiac-type	AD AR	Definitive
Troponin I	TNNI3	CMH7	19q13.42	TroponinI, cardiac muscle	AD	Definitive
Actin	ACTC1	CMH11	15q14	Actin, alpha cardiac muscle 1	AD	Definitive
Regulatory myosin light chain	*MYL2*	CMH10	12q.24.11	Myosin regulatory light chain 2, ventricular/ cardiacmuscle isoform	AD	Definitive
Essential myosin light chain	*MYL3*	CMH8	3p.21.31	Myosin light polypeptide 3	AD AR	Definitive
HGNC	*PLN*	CMH18	6q22.31	Phospholamban	AD	Definitive
Alpha kinase3	*ALPK3*	CMH27	15q25.3	Alpha-protein kinase 3	AR	Strong
Cysteine-rich protein 3	*CSRP3*	CMH12	11p15.1	Cysteine- and glycine-rich protein 3	AD	Moderate
slow-twitch skeletal	*TNNC1*	CMH13	3p21.1	Cardiac troponin C	AD	Moderate
junctophilin	*JPH2*	CMH17	20q13.12	Junctophilin-2	AD	Moderate
alpha-actinin-2	*ACTN2*	CMH23	1q43	Actinin, α2	AD	Moderate
NEXN gene	NEXN	CMH20	1p31.1	Nexilin	AD	Limited
Ankyrin repeat domain-containing 1	ARKD1		10q,21	Ankyrin repeat domain 1	AD	Limited
CALR3 gene	CALR3		19p13.11	Calreticulin	AD	Limited
Telethonin	TCAP	CMH25	17q.12	Telethonin	AD	Limited
MYOZ2 gene	*MYOZ2*	CMH16	4q26	Myozenin 2 (calsarcin 1)	AD	Limited
Titin	*TTN*	CMH9	2q.31.2	Titin	AD	Limited
Tripartite motif containing 63	*TRIM63*		1p36.11	Muscle ring finger protein 1	AD	Limited

HCM gene	Symbol	Locus name	Chromosome locus	Protein	Mode of inheritance	ClinGen Gene Validity Classification
Kruppel-like factor 10	KLF10		8q22.3		AD	Limited
Myosin heavy chain α gene	MYH6	CMH14	14q11.2	Myosin heavy chain α	AD	Limited
Myomesin 1	*MYOM1*		18p11.31		AD	Limited
Myoalladim	*MYPN*	CMH22	10q.21.3		AD	Limited
Obscurin	*OBSCN*		1q42.13		AD	Limited
	PDLIM3		4q35.1	PDZ and LIM domain protein 3	AD	Limited
Ryanodine	*RYR2*		1q43	Cardiac Ryanodine 2	AD	Limited
Myosin light chain kinase 2 gene	MYLK2	CMH1 digenic	20q11.21	Myosin heavy chain α	ADDD	Limited

Table 4.
Genes that cause HCM.

It is known that hypertension, valve disease, viral infections, toxins, drugs, metabolic disorders among others can cause DCM, but in almost 40% of DCM patients the cause of the disorder is due to a genetic mutation [12, 26, 53, 56].

The familial cases of DCM present autosomal dominant, autosomal recessive or X-linked inheritance so it can be stated that there is. both locus and allelic heterogeneity (See **Table 2**). The autosomal dominant pattern is undoubtedly the most frequent mode of inheritance. It has been demonstrated that DCM has reduced penetrance and expressivity is always variable. The mutations of the genes involved in DCM are those which encode cytoskeletal, sarcomeric, mitochondrial, desmosomal, nuclear membrane, and RNA-binding proteins [53, 54, 57, 58]. Generally speaking, the onset of DCM is in adulthood although its appearance has great variability [59, 60]. When the mutation is in one of the sarcomeric genes the affected patients are usually young adults [12, 61]. The most common genes that cause DCM are *FLNC*, *TTN* and *LMNA*. The truncating mutations found in *FLNC* and in *TTN* account for 4% and in 15–25% of the DCM cases respectively. 10% of cases are due to mutations in *LMNA*. It has been observed that patients with mutations in both *LMNA* and *FLNC* have a poor prognosis and are more susceptible to having an arrhythmogenic phenotype [12, 56, 62, 63].

The MOGE(S) classification can also be applied to patients that have been diagnosed with DCM and it has been observed there is a worse prognosis with the presence of multiple attributes [13, 64] (**Table 5**).

5. Restrictive cardiomyopathy

Familial restrictive cardiomyopathy (RCM) is a rare disease, which is inherited in autosomal dominant pattern with incomplete penetrance [65]. The exact prevalence of RCM is unknown [7]. In childhood, RCM accounts for 2–5% of cardiomyopathies and has a poor prognosis [10, 12, 66, 67].

DCM gene	Symbol	Locus name	Chromosome locus	Protein	Mode of inheritance
Lamin A/C gene	*LMNA*	CMD1A	1q21	lamin A and lamin C	AD
LDB3 gene		CMD1C	10q22-q23	LIM domain-binding protein 3	AD
TNNT2 gene	TNNT2	CMD1D	1q32	Troponin T, cardiac muscle	AD
SCN5A		CMD1E	3p	Sodium channel protein type 5 subunit alpha	AD
TTN gene	TTN	CMD1G	2q31	Titin	AD
DES gene	DES	CMD1I	2q35	Desmin	AD
EYA4 gene	EYA4	CMD1J	6q23-q24	Eyes absent homolog 4	AD
SGCD gene	SGCD	CMD1L	5q33	Delta-sarcoglycan	AD
CSRP3 gene	CSRP3	CMD1M	11p15.1	Cysteine and glycine-rich protein 3	AD
TCAP gene	TCAP	CMD1N	17q12;	Telethonin	AD
ABCC9 gene		CMD1O,	on 12p12.1;	ATP-binding cassette, subfamily C, member 9	AD
PLN gene	PLN	CMD1P	on 6q22.1;,	Cardiac phospholamban	AD
ACTC1 gene	ACTC1	CMD1R	15q14	Actin, alpha cardiac muscle 1	AD
MYH7 gene	MYH7	CMD1S	14q12;	Myosin 7	AD
TMPO gene	TMPO	CMD1T	12q22	Hymopoietin	AD
PSEN1 gene	PSEN1	CMD1U	14q24.3	Presenilin-1	AD
PSEN2 gene	PSEN2	CMD1V	1q31-q42;	Presenilin-2	AD
VCL		CMD1W	10q22-q23	Vinculin	AD
FKTN	FKTN	CMD1X	9q31	Fukutin	AR
TPM1 gene	TPM1	CMD1Y	15q22.1	tropomyosin-1	AD
TNNC1 gene	TNNC1	CMD1Z	3p21.3-p14.3	slow troponin-C	AD
ACTN2 gene	ACTN2	CMD1AA	1q42-q43;	Alpha-actinin-2	AD
DSG2 gene	DSG2	CMD1BB	18q12.1-q12.2;	desmoglein-2	AD
NEXN gene	NEXN	CMD1CC	1p31.1	Nelin	AD
RBM20 gene	RBM20	CMD1DD	10q25.2;	RNA-Binding motif protein 20	AD
MYH6 gene	MYH6	CMD1EE	14q12	Myosin 7	AD
TNNI3 gene	TNNI3	CMD1FF	19q13.4;	Troponin I,	AD
SDHA gene	SDHA	CMD1GG	5p15;	Succinate dehydrogenase complex subunit A	AD
BAG3 gene	BAG3	CMD1HH	10q25.2-q26.2	BCL2-associated athanogene 3	AD
TNNI3 gene	TNNI3	CMD2A,	*19q13.42*	Troponin I, cardiac muscle	AR

DCM gene	Symbol	Locus name	Chromosome locus	Protein	Mode of inheritance
GATAD1 gene.	GATAD1	CMD2	*7q21.2*	GATA zinc finger domain containing protein 1	AR
Dystrophin gene	*DMD*	CMD3B	Xp21.2	dystrophin	X-linked
LAMP2 gene	*LAMP2*	Danon disease	Xq24	lysosome-associated membrane protein-2	X-linked
TAZ gene	*TAZ*		Xq28	dystrophin	X-linked

Table 5.
Genes that cause DCM.

RCM is characterized by abnormal diastolic function, which has a restrictive filling pattern, a reduced diastolic volume of one of the ventricles or both ventricles, enlargement of the atria, pulmonary hypertension, and heart failure. In the early stages of the disorder the systolic function may be normal, but as the disease progresses, the systolic function generally declines [12, 68–70].

The list of RCM-associated genes includes sarcomeric and cytoskeletal genes often similar to those genes observed in HCM and DCM, but in total the genotyping success rate is quite low, corresponding approximately to 30%. The familial RCM is linked to the cardiac troponin genes. RCM1 is caused by a mutation in the *TNNI3* gene on chromosome 19q13. This gene encodes the cardiac muscle isoform of troponin 1. RCM2 has been mapped to chromosome 10q23. RCM3 is caused by mutation in the *TNNT2* gene. Mutations in the sarcomere gene, alpha-cardiac actin gene (ACTC) have also been reported to cause RCM. Cardiomyopathy, familial restrictive 5 is caused by mutations in the *FLNC* gene on chromosome 7q32. In many cases RCM can be observed overlapping with either HCM or DCM [10, 26, 66–68, 70–76].

Fabry's disease, Hurler syndrome, Gaucher's disease, haemochromatosis and glycogen storage diseases are among the diseases in which RCM can be observed [10, 26].

6. Arrhythmogenic cardiomyopathy

Arrhythmogenic cardiomyopathy (ACM) is a rather new word used to describe what previously was known as Arrhythmogenic right ventricular cardiomyopathy/dysplasia (ARVC/ARVD). The prevalence has been estimated 1:5000 in the general population.

Later on, it was observed that in many cases the left ventricle was also affected (ALVC) thus this disorder started to be called ACM.

The age of onset is between 10 and 50 years old. The clinical features include ventricular tachyarrhythmias, electrocardiographic abnormalities, systolic heart failure, syncope and sudden death. It is a frequent cause of sudden death in young people and athletes ACM is characterized by fibro-fatty replacement of the myocardium, apoptosis and inflammation [8, 12, 77, 78].

It is transmitted most of the time in an autosomal dominant pattern; though autosomal recessive families have also been reported. The data has shown the inheritance could be even be oligogenic or multifactorial where environmental

ARCV gene	Symbol	Locus name	Chromosome locus	Protein
Transforming growth factor beta- 3	*TGFB3*	ARVD1	14q24.3	Transforming growth factor beta-3
Ryanodine receptor 2	RYR2	ARVD2	1q43	RYR2
Unknown	Unknown	ARVD3	14q12-q22	Unknown
Unknown	Unknown	ARVD4	2q32.1-q32.3	Unknown
transmembrane protein 43	*TMEM43*	ARVD5	3p25.1	Transmembrane protein 43
Unknown	Unknown	ARVD6	10p14-p12	Unknownn
Desmin	*DES*	ARVD7	2q35	Desmin
Desmoplakin	*DSP*	ARVD8	6p24.3	Desmoplakin
Plakophilin-2	*PKP2*	ARVD9	12p11.21	Plakophilin-2
Desmoglein-2	*DSG2*	ARVD10	18q12.1	Desmoglein-2
Desmocollin-2	*DSC2*	ARVD11	18q12.1	Desmocollin-2
Junction plakoglobin	*JUP*	ARVD12	17q21.2	Junction plakoglobin
Alpha-T-catenin	*CTNNA3*	ARVC13	10q21.3	Catenin
Cadherin2	*CDH2*	ARVC14	18q12.1	Cadherin

Table 6.
Genes that cause ARVC.

factors intertwine to cause the disease. Incomplete penetrance and great variability in the symptoms have been observed [7, 12, 77–84].

The two first disorders to be described were Naxos disease and Carvajal syndrome, which are inherited in an autosomal recessive pattern. The former is caused by mutations in the plakoglobin gene on chromosome 17q21,2 and the latter by mutations in the desmoplakin gene on chromosome 6p24 [12, 77, 78, 80, 85–88].

Desmosomes are intercellular junctions that link intermediate filaments to the plasma membrane and are essential to tissues that experience mechanical stress such as the myocardium. Mutations in the cardiac desmosome genes are to be held responsible for most of the cases that cause the disorder (See **Table 6**). The prognosis of those who have a mutation in these genes is much worse [12, 79, 89–91].

There are overlapping syndromes. Myofrillar myopathies genes such as filamin C can cause ARLV [77]. The mutations p.S13F, p.E114del and p.N116S in the desmin gene have the same ARVC cardiac phenotype. In transfection cells aggresome formation in the cytoplasm was observed [12, 82, 92, 93]. The members of the Swedish family who were diagnosed with ARVC7 linked to chromosome 10q23.2 had instead the p.Pro419Ser mutation in *DES* [94, 95]. In mutations in the SCN5A gene the mutations can cause ARVC with Brugada syndrome, long QT syndrome or DCM. In both Titin and lamin A/C ACM overlaps with DCM [12, 77].

7. Non-compaction cardiomyopathy

Non-compaction cardiomyopathy (NCCM) has been classified as a primary cardiomyopathy with a genetic etiology. The age of onset varies from neonatal to adult hood. There is variability in the clinical features which include heart failure, arrhythmias and thromboembolism, but patients can also be asymptomatic.

The most common congenital heart defects in NCCM are Ebstein's anomaly, septal defects and patent ductus arteriosus.

The patients have a thickened two-layered myocardium with a thin, compact, epicardial layer and a severely thickened endocardial layer with a 'spongy' appearance due to prominent trabeculations and intertrabecular recesses [96–102].

The majority of the patients have an autosomal dominant mode of inheritance. Mutations in several genes coding for sarcomeric proteins such as β-myosin heavy chain (MYH7), cardiac myosin-binding protein C (*MYBPC3*), α-cardiac actin (*ACTC1*), cardiac troponin T (*TNNT2*), α-tropomyosin (*TPM1*) and cardiac troponin I (*TNNI3*). have been described in NCCM.

While mutations in the tail domain of *MYH7* and *TTN* have been reported to be associated to NCCM with DCM and have a poor patient ouycome, mutations in *MYBPC3* are linked to NCCM with HCM. Mutations in *DES, DSP, FKTN, HCN4, KCNQ1, LAMP2, LMNA, MIB1, NOTCH1, PLN, RYR2, SCN5A,* and *TAZ* have also been described [12, 98, 102–107].

8. Takotsubo cardiomyopathy

Takotsubo cardiomyopathy is characterized by an acute but transitient LV systolic dysfunction without atherosclerotic coronary artery disease and it is triggered by psychological stress. It is more common to find it in women than in men. Although some genes are considered to be involved in developing the disorder there is controversy about this and many believe Takotsubo cardiomyopathy is not genetically determined [108–112].

9. Ion channel disorders

The cell membrane transit of sodium and potassium ions is ruled by the ion channel genes which encode proteins responsible for the right transit of these ions. Mutations in these proteins lead to a group of familial disorders [113]. These ion channel disorders include long QT syndromes (LQTS), of which the Romano Ward syndrome is the commonest, the short-QT syndrome (SQTS), Brugada syndrome, and the catecholaminergic polymorphic ventricular tachycardia (CPVT). 5–10% of the sudden deaths in children can be associated to ion channel disorders [78, 114–117]. Many of the mutations found in these genes overlap in the different traits.

9.1 Long QT syndromes (LQTS)

LQTS is an arrhythmia syndrome characterized by a prolonged QT interval ECG, torsades de pointes and a higher chance of sudden cardiac death. In most of the cases it is inherited in an autosomal dominant pattern. The prevalence is 1:2000. The most common syndromes are LQT1 (40–55%), LQT2 (30–45%) and LQT3 (5–10%). The autosomal dominant mutations are found in genes *KCNQ1, KCNH2* and *SCN5A* respectively whereas TRDN is an autosomal recessive gene (**Table** 7). While in LQT1 cardiovascular symptoms that can lead to sudden death occur during exercise, in LQT2 the symptoms appear with auditory stimuli and in LQT3 during rest or sleep [71, 114, 118].

The Jervell and Lange-Nielsen syndrome (JLNS) is inherited as an autosomal recessive trait. The affected children present symptoms before the age of three and they died before the age of 15 if they are not treated. The prevalence can vary considerably and it depends on the population studied. The patients have a more

Long QT syndromes	Gene	Protein
LQT1	*KCNQ1*	Kv7.1 potassium channel
LQT2	*KCNH2*	k_V11./hERG Kv11.1 potassium channel
LQT3	*LQT3*	NaV1.5 sodium channel
LQT4	*ANK2*	ankyrin B
LQT5	*KCNE1*	minK
LQT6	*KCNE2*	MiRP1
LQT7 (Andersen-Tawil syndrome)	*KCNJ2*	Kir2.1
LQT8 (Timothy syndrome)	*CACNA1C*	Ca_V1.2
LQT9	*CAV3*	Caveolin-3
LQT10	*SCN4B*	B4-subunit of the voltage-dependent Na + channel
LQT11	*AKAP9*	A-kinase anchor protein-9
LQT12	*SNTA1*	α1-syntrophin
LQT13	*KCNJ5*	Kir3.4
LQT14	*CALM1*	calmodulin
LQT15	*CALM2*	calmodulin
	CALM3	calmodulin
	TRDN	Triadin
	RYR2	ryanodine receptor 2
	TRPM4	Transient receptor potential melastatin 4

Table 7.
Genes that cause long QT syndromes.

severe QT prolongation (greater than 500 msec) which is associated which tachiarrhythmias including torsade de pointes, ventricular fibrillation, syncope and sudden death. Mutations in the *KCNQ1* gene on chromosome 11p15.5-p15.4 and *KCNE1* gene on chromosome 21q22.12, have been reported in the affected individuals [116, 119].

Timothy syndrome is a rare autosomal dominant disorder that is due to either a *de novo* mutation or parent germline mosaicism. Mutations in the gene *CACNA1C* cause the two forms of the disorder: the classic, type 1, and type 2. The reported cases of the patients suffering type 1 syndrome have shown complete penetrance [120]. This complex multisystem disorder has a long QT syndrome associated with various forms of congenital heart defects such as tetralogy of Fallot and hypertrophic cardiomyopathy Webbing of both fingers and toes have been observed. Type 2 patients did not have syndactily [121]. Children died at age of 2.5 years due to ventricular tachycardia and ventricular fibrillation, infection or malignant hypoglycemia.

The Andersen–Tawil syndrome (LQT7) presents with QT interval prolongation, hypokalemic periodic paralysis and facial dysmorphism. The type 1 disorder disease is caused by mutations in KCNJ2 while type 2 is due to mutations in KCNJ5-GIRK4 gene [119, 120, 122–129].

9.2 Short-QT syndrome

Short-QT syndrome is a familial disease that is characterized by a high incidence of sudden death. Patients with this disease have QT intervals that are <300 ms, and increased risk of atrial and ventricular arrhythmia.

It is an autosomal dominant inherited disorder that affects patients of 30 years of age, but the fibrillation can even be observed in newborns and young patients.

Missense mutations in the *KCNH2* gene on chromosome 7q36.1 and mutations in the *KCNQ1* gene on chromosome ***11p15.5-p15.*** and the *KCNJ2* gene on chromosome 17q24.3 have shown that this is a genetically heterogeneous disease There also different variants in mutations of the genes *CACNA2D1, KCNH2, KCNJ2, KCNQ1* and *SLC4A3* which have been described in SQTS, but most of them are VUS [130–132].

9.3 Brugada síndrome

The Brugada syndrome is associated with sudden death in young people as the patients have malignant ventricular tachyarrhythmias and sudden cardiac death. The heart is not affected by either a structural heart or systemic disease. The cardiac differential diagnosis must be made with Duchenne muscular dystrophy, Freidreich's ataxia and ARVC. The age of appearance ranges from a two- day- old patient to 85 years. It was believed to be inherited in an autosomal dominant pattern with incomplete penetrance. Up to eighty different mutations were identified in the SCN5A gene. A family with a pathogenic variant in *KCNE5* which is inherited in an X-linked recessive pattern. The genetic variants in SCN5A-SCN10A and HEY2 have also been described [120, 125–127, 133–141].

9.4 Catecholaminergic polymorphic ventricular tachycardia

Catecholaminergic polymorphic ventricular tachycardia (CPVT) is an inherited tachyarrhythmia that is caused by acute adrenergic activation during exercise or acute emotion in young adolescents. The age of onset varies from 7 to 9 years to the fourth decade of life. It presents locus heterogeneity and in only approximately 50% of the cases the mutations in the genes causing the disease have been identified.

The prevalence of CPVT in the population is not known, but it could be estimated in approximately 1:10,000. In *CPVT, CALM1* and *RYR2* are inherited in an autosomal dominant manner while *CASQ2* and *TRDN* are inherited in an autosomal recessive manner [142–146].

10. Cardiomyopathy in muscular dystrophies

Muscular dystrophies are a heterogeneous group of inherited disorders, characterized by progressive weakness and wasting of the skeletal muscles. They are generally associated with cardiomyopathy. In many cases, there is no correlation between the skeletal myopathy and the involvement of the heart. The mutations of the genes that cause muscular dystrophies affect the skeletal and/or cardiac muscles. These include proteins which are associated with the dystrophin–glycoprotein complex, the nuclear lamina or the sarcomere [12, 147, 148].

Cardiomyopathy occurs in myofibrillar myopathy, myotonic dystrophies, myotonic myopathies, dystrophinopathies, Emery-Dreifuss muscular dystrophy, and limb girdle muscular dystrophies [147–149]. They are inherited in autosomal dominant, autosomal recessive and X-linked mode. (See **Table 4**). In this respect Duchenne muscular dystrophy and its allelic form Becker muscular dystrophy is of significant importance. These two conditions are the most common disorders in muscular dystrophies and cardiomyopathy can be a cardinal finding during the follow-up, thus requiring yearly evaluations.

The different forms of muscular dystrophies vary in the age of onset with no male or female prevalence and have different clinical features and severity.

Disease Name	Gene	Symbol	Locus name	Chromosome locus	Protein	Mode of inheritance	CMP
Desminopathy	Desmin	DES	MFM1	2q35	Desmin	AD/AR	HCM HCR
Alpha-B crystallinopathy	CRYAB gene	CRYAB	MFM2	11q23.1	alpha-B-crystallin	AR/AD	HCM
Myotilinopathy	Myotilinn	MYOT (TTID)	MFM3	5q31.2	Myotilin (titinmmunoglobulin domain protein)	AD	
ZASPopathy	ZASP	LDB3	MFM4	10q23.2	LIM domain-binding protein 3	AD	HCD
Filaminopathy	FilaminC	FLNC	MFM5	7q32.1	Filamin C	AD	HCM HCR
BAG3-Related Myofibrillar Myopathy	BCL2-associated athanogen 3	BAG3	BAG3	10q26.11	BAG family molecular chaperone regulator 3	AD	HCM HCD
Myotonic dystrophy type 1	myotonin-protein kinase (Mt-PK).	DMPK	DMPK	19q13.3	dystrophia myotonica-protein kinase	AD	HCD
Myotonic dystrophy type 2	zinc finger protein-9 gene	CNBP	ZNF9	3q21.3	zinc finger protein-9	AD	HCD
Duchenne/Becker muscular dystrophy	dystrophin	DMD	DMD	Xp21.2	emerin	X-linked	HCM
Rigid spine syndrome	Selenoprotein 1	SEPN1		1p36.11	Selenon	AR	HCD
LGMD1B	Lamin A/C	Lamin A		1q.22		AD	HCM
LGMD1C	Caveolin-3	CAV3				AR	HCM
LGMD2B	Dysferlin	Dysf		2p13.2	Dysferlin	AR	HCD
LGMD2E	Beta-sarcoglycan	SGCB	SGCB	4q12	Beta-sarcoglycan	AR	HCD
LGMD2I	Fukutin-related protein	FKRP				AR	HCD
LGMD2J	Titin	TTN		2q.31.2		AD AR	HCM
LGMD2M	Fukutin	FKTN		9q.31.2		AR	HCD
Barth syndrome	Tafazzin	TAZ		Xq28	Tazffin	XLR	HCM LVHT

Table 8.
Genes that cause cardiomyopathy in muscular dystrophies and limb girdle muscular dystrophies.

Mutations in the genes that are involved in muscular dystrophies can cause hypertrophic, dilated or restrictive cardiomyopathy depending on the mutations of the genes involved, but most cardiomyopathies in patients with a muscular dystrophy are of the dilated type. The progression of the disorders and life expectancy vary widely, even among different members of the same family. Patients die of sudden death due to conduction defects, and heart failure.

In dystrophinopathies, sarcoglycanopathies, and the disorders that are linked to mutations in the fukutin-related protein, the feature that stands out is the cardiomyopathy the patients suffer. In muscular dystrophies, the patients usually have a dilated cardiomyopathy. Hypertrophic cardiomyopathy can be observed in Danon disease, α-B crystallinopathy, and on patients or carriers of DMD and BMD. It has been proved that in spite of the fact that mutations in codon 92 (R92L and R92W) of the cardiac troponin T gene are in the same found in the same codon the severity and phenotypes are completely different due to fact that the mutated protein has a completely different function [4, 12, 48, 147, 148, 150–169] (**Table 8**).

11. Mitochondrial disorders

Mitochondrial disorders are a heterogeneous group of disorders that have common clinical features and are caused by the different mutations found in either the nuclear or mitochondrial DNA (mtDNA) genes which regulate the mitochondrial respiratory chain, the essential final common pathway of aerobic metabolism, tissues and organs. mtDNA is maternally inherited and the disorders can appear at any age. All the mitochondria have multiple copies of their own mtDNA and the mutation rate is much higher than in nuclear DNA [170–173].

Many mitochondrial disorders involve multiple organ systems such as the brain, the heart, the liver, and the skeletal muscles which are, therefore, affected due to the fact they depend on the energy and they are especially susceptible to energy metabolism impairment [170–173].

Mitochondrial dysfunction and clinical symptoms appear when the heteroplasmic levels are above 80–90% [170–172].

The different mitochondrial cardiomyopathies are a result of the heart being commonly affected. Sometimes, the cardiomyopathy is diagnosed during the first year of life even before the mitochondrial disorder has been diagnosed. HCM, DCM, LVNC cardiomyopathies have been reported [171, 173, 174].

11.1 Kearns-Sayre syndrome

The Kearns-Sayre syndrome (KSS), a mitochondrial deletion syndrome, is characterized by the triad: onset of the disorder before the age of 20, progressive external ophthalmoplegia and pigmentary retinopathy. A cerebrospinal fluid protein concentration greater than 100 mg/d, and a commonly elevated lactate and pyruvate concentrations in blood and cerebrospinal fluid are found.

The KSS has cardiac involvement with conduction defects such as right bundle branch block, left anterior hemiblock or complete A-V block. These patients can develop a cardiomyopathy usually dilated [170, 173, 175–177].

11.2 MELAS

It is a multisystem disorder with onset in childhood with mitochondrial encephalomyopathy, lactic acidosis, and recurrent stroke-like episodes. The variability of symptoms and the severity of the syndrome make it difficult to confirm the diagnosis.

MELAS is transmitted by maternal inheritance.

The cardiac involvement is considered to be 18–100% [178–180]. The first symptom the affected children have is the cardiomyopathy. The most common feature is a hypertrophic cardiomyopathy, although dilation has also been reported [134, 181, 182].

Mutations in the nuclear genes that also encode mitochondrial proteins can cause cardiomyopathies. These disorders are sometimes not considered among the group of mitochondrial primary disorders. Two of the most well-known disorders are Friedreich's ataxia and Barth syndrome [12, 171, 173, 183].

Friedreich's ataxia is an autosomal recessive disorder. Frataxin, the protein encoded by *FXN,* is involved in the mitochondrial transport and is needed for the synthesis of the enzymes of the respiratory chain complexes I – III and aconitase. HCM is found in this disorder [173].

In Barth syndrome, abnormal mitochondria and DCM are described as well as neutropenia [173].

12. The impact of genetics in the understanding of cardiomyopathy

Genetics started to play a key role with the advent of molecular genetics therefore physicians should not only base themselves on the family history of a patient, but with molecular genetics they have a tool that they could use and help them to diagnose and understand the disorders. Every year, new pathogenic mutations in the different genes are described, but it has not yet been figured out what the specific function and the pathogenic mechanisms the mutated proteins are.

The fact a molecular analysis can be performed does not mean the different steps physicians follow to evaluate and diagnose a cardiomyopathy should be left out, if one takes into account the fact that cardiomyopathies are in many cases inherited disorders. Therefore, a three generation family history looking for cardiac symptoms is essential as well as a thorough examination. Blood tests, ECGs, echocardiograms, cardiovascular magnetic resonance imaging, electromyography, and muscle biopsy should be carried out in order to provide us with the information that can help us to diagnose a cardiomyopathy. The suspected cardiomyopathy will have to be confirmed by DNA analysis not only in the patients, but also in asymptomatic carriers [12, 18, 51, 53, 59].

Multigene panels for molecular testing have been developed which allow physicians to diagnose the different disorders. If these tests are negative, exome sequencing, looking for point mutations and insertions as well as exome arrays checking for deletions and duplications should be performed. When performing the genetic testing the genes that should be tested are those that are considered to be the most common ones and are held responsible for the disorder. Cascade genetic testing of first degree relatives at risk seeking for a mutation that has been previously found in a patient should be performed. In children and adolescents, screening by means of serial ECGs, echocardiograms and genetic testing should be done every year or every two years while in adults it should be performed every three years There should be a lifelong surveillance of family members [18, 19, 51, 53, 54].

It has been observed that mutations in the same gene and in the same family can give rise to HCM; DCM, RCM, the three major types of cardiomyopathy, which in many cases overlap. It can be said that the different mutations of the genes plus modifier genes are liable to trigger the different pathways that lead to the remodeling of the heart. The different mechanisms are 11. still not clear and have to be cleared up [1, 12, 184, 185].

HCM is an autosomal dominant disorder in which mutations in the *MYH7, TNNT2, TPM1, MYBPC3, ACTC1, TNNI3, MYL2* and *MYL3* have been classified as definitive according to the new classification and most of the patients suffering from it are heterozygous. Mutations in MYH7 and/or MYBPC3 genes account for 80% of the mutations [1, 12, 40]. In some cases, patients have two different mutations, usually in MYH7 and/or MYBPC3 genes. These mutations result in the patients being compound heterozygous. The double heterozygotes that have also been observed have mutations in the MyBP-C/β –MHC, MyBP-C/TNNT2, MyBP-C/TNNT3, MyBP-C/TPM, β-MHC/TNNT2 genes. Sometimes, the patients can be homozygous for a mutation in the genes MyBP-C, β -MHC, and TNNT2 [1, 12, 17, 51, 186–188]. The genotype–phenotype correlations have been linked to specific mutations [1]. The different mutations in the MYH7gene show great variability in symptomatology. Patients with the R403Q, R719W and R719Q mutations have complete penetrance, severe hypertrophy and short life expectancy, whereas those with the V606M mutation have a mild progression [1, 12, 39, 189–191]. All the patients that have mutations in the TNNT2 gene seem to have a more severe course. In most cases, the affected patients carrying the mutations R92W, R92Q, TNNT2-I79N are young, and even though they have a mild LVH, they died of sudden death. The F110I mutation does not seem to have so severe a development as the rest of the mutations in this gene Arian, 1998; [1, 12, 192–194].

It was believed that patients having double mutations in HCM have a greater severity of the disorder due to a double dose effect [186], but in a study carried out later on the data has demonstrated that this is apparently not so with the exception of double mutations in *MYBPC3* [195, 196].

Incomplete or reduced penetrance has been observed in many cases (20 to 30%) as there are parents that are carriers of the mutations, but they do not develop the disease. It is unknown whether carriers will develop the disorder at a certain age or will remain asymptomatic throughout their lives. Symptoms show a great variability among the patients that have the same mutation and suffer the disorder. These may be due to gene interaction, environmental factors and modifier genes. After 15-year follow-up it is likely carriers will develop the disorder though it is not certain [1, 19, 197–199]. False positive reports have led to the misdiagnosis of HCM [200, 201]. It is the most common cause of sudden death in young people [12, 27–30, 44, 202].

In many cases RCM can be observed overlapping with either HCM or DCM. *An* autosomal dominant cardiomyopathy has been described where the single sarcomere *TNNT2* gene mutation can cause idiopathic RCM in some patients, or HCM or DCM in others. All affected members of a RCM-associated family have *the* I79N mutation in the *TNNT2* gene, thus showing the variability of the disorders [12, 203, 204].

It is very difficult to assess the genotype-phenotype correlation in NCCM. It seems that when there are mutations in the alpha-dystrobrevin gene *(DTNA)* on chromosome 18q12.1 taffazin gene on chromosome Xq28 (Barth syndrome), lamin A/C gene, *ZASP* and *SCN5A* gene can develop the disorder [12, 205].

As soon as the patients are diagnosed with the myopathies mentioned above they should be cardiac check-up should be performed and treated immediately as the cardiac therapy improves the cardiac involvement and life expectancy.

In the ion channels disorders the molecular diagnosis of Timothy syndrome where the gene *CACNA1C* gene is mutated it should be performed in several tissues, including sperm.

It has been observed that mutations in the lamin A/C gene cause CMD1A, LGMD1B or EDMD2 in the same family [12, 206, 207].

The mitochondrial deletion syndromes are generally not inherited. The *de novo* deletions that take place in the mother's oocytes during germline development or in the embryo during embryogenesis are to be held responsible for these syndromes. 90% of the patients with KSS have deletions of mtDNA. The deletions are present in all tissues in individuals with KSS. There is no correlation between the size or the location of the mtDNA deletion and the phenotype and penetrance because there are related to the mutation load. An overlap between KKS and MERRF has been observed due to point mutation in the tRNA [tRNALeu(UUR)] [208].

It has been suggested that the mutations in the nuclear gene *RRM2B* gene cause KSS following a Mendelian mode of inheritance. The patient had multiple mtDNA deletions and a normal left ventricular function with an increased thickness of the interventricular septum and left posterior ventricular wall [209].

Approximately 80% of cases of MELAS are due to mutations in the mtDNA gene *MT-TL1* which encodes tRNA leucine. The mutations in *MT-ND5* gene which encodes the NADH–ubiquinone oxidoreductase subunit 5 have also been found in individuals with MELAS or with overlap syndromes [181, 210].

In spite of the fact that there has been considerable improvement in the molecular diagnosis of the different mutations that lead to cardiomyopathies, we still have to learn more about the pathophysiology of these disorders. Genetic testing for these inherited disorders has provided us with an insight into the prevalence of the underlying mutations of the different cardiomyopathies. Even though many genes which cause cardiomyopathies have been identified and have led to a better understanding of the pathogenesis of cardiomyopathies, mutation analyses affecting the patients have proven not to be the panacea for the different family members [211]. Different variants within a specific gene can be associated with many different phenotypes, even within the same family, preventing physicians from having a clear genotype–phenotype correlation. It seems it is a long way ahead to unravel completely the pathophysiology of the different cardiomyopathies [212, 213].

13. What should the genetic counseling be in cardiomyopathy?

Genetic counseling to patients with cardiomyopathy is very complex due to the fact that there is locus heterogeneity and clinical variability. The geneticist has to be clear and explain that there are all sorts of disorders that cause it.

It is very important that when a numerical value is provided the patient and/or his family clearly understand that the value given it is the probability of having a another a child affected with the disorder. It is imperative they understand that chance has no memory. The numerical value given to them will be the same for every new offspring of an affected parent. It would be embarrassing to face a family that comes with a second affected child because they have misinterpreted the information given to them.

The different opinions regarding what steps should be taken when the consultants are less than 18 years of age and have a genetic disorder. Should we tell them when they are asymptomatic and are at risk of having the disorder when they are adults? If a mutation is found, the children will no longer lead a normal life and it will also have a negative effect on family life. In ACM, it is advised that the genetic test be run when the consultant is over 10 years of age. The decision will have to be made on the fact on whether the treatment could help to lead a better life.

In HCM, the first step the geneticist should take is to order the molecular analyses of *MYH7* and *MYBPC3*, the two genes that carry most of the mutations.

Should the mutations not be in these two genes, the genetic analysis has to be focused on those genes that are considered definite.

Sometimes, if no mutations are found in any of the genes tested, the disorder cannot be ruled out because it is likely that a new gene not yet discovered can be the cause of the disorder.

In DCM, the mode of inheritance has to be defined in order to provide a correct counseling as there is locus and allelic heterogeneity.

In the autosomal dominant cardiomyopathies most individuals diagnosed have an affected parent. However, the index case may have the disorder as the result of a *de novo* mutation [214].

In HCM, it is not known the number of cases that are caused by these *de novo* gene mutations. While in Brugada syndrome and in RWS *de novo* mutations are low, and in CPVT is almost 40%.

Timothy syndrome is due to either de *novo* mutations or parental germline mosaicism. The affected patients do not have offspring because they do not reach adult life. The siblings are at risk of inheriting the disorder. When there is a *de novo* mutation, alternate paternity and maternity as well as whether the patient is adopted have to be ruled out.

The offspring of a patient suffering autosomal dominant familial cardiomyopathy has a 50% chance of inheriting the mutation. Families in which penetrance appears to be incomplete or reduced have been observed; therefore, the parent with a mutation that causes the disorder is not affected whereas the son or daughter is. The severity and age of onset cannot be predicted [215–217].

The siblings of the index case depend on the genetic condition of their parents. If a parent is affected or has the mutation that causes the disorder, the risk to inherit the mutated allele is 50%.

In the cases reported where more than one mutation in one the genes encoding a sarcomere protein has been identified in a patient with HCM, it is very difficult to assess the mode of inheritance and makes it arduous for the geneticist to give an accurate risk assessment to another family member.

It is essential to provide patients and relatives that are at risk, the potential risk their offspring might have in these disorders and the reproductive options they have.

In the autosomal recessive traits, the parents are obligate carriers. The offspring of a patient suffering an autosomal recessive familial cardiomyopathy will be obligate carriers. The siblings have a 25% chance of inheriting the mutation.

The deletions in mtDNA are usually due to *de novo* mutations, so there is only one family member affected. The offspring of a male patient are not at risk whereas all females′ offspring are at risk of inheriting the mutation. There is not risk that any other family member will inherit the disease.

When there are multiple mtDNA deletions the analysis of *RRM2B* should be performed because it conditions the genetic counseling.

A prenatal diagnosis can be performed in those patients there are at risk of having any cardiomyopathy, if the mutation carried by the parents or the proband has been previously identified.

Preimplantation genetic diagnosis (PGD) may be available for families in which the mutation that causes the disorder has already been identified.

14. Conclusion

Genetic testing has undoubtedly broadened our knowledge of the mechanisms of cardiomyopathy and has to a certain extent helped physicians to understand to a certain extent the genotype–phenotype correlation. By having a deeper understanding of this genotype–phenotype correlation, it will be easier to get a clinical management of the patients. It has also aided to diagnose symptomatic and asymptomatic patients, be able to treat them when it is possible and to perform genetic counseling of the affected patients, their offspring and first degree relatives.

When a genetic test is performed and a patient is diagnosed with a disorder genetic counseling is essential for the patient and relatives at risk since this will allow an early identification of relatives who are at risk.

Not all the mutations that have been described over the last twenty have proven to be pathogenic. The new classification allows us to understand what mutations are really pathogenic. A deeper understanding of the genotype–phenotype correlation is necessary, because this could imply what steps should be taken in order to deal with the correct management of the patients.

Author details

Luis Vernengo[1*] and Haluk Topaloglu[2]

1 CASMU, Department of Medicine and Ethics Committee, Montevideo, Uruguay

2 Department of Pediatrics, Yeditepe University, İstanbul, Turkey

*Address all correspondence to: luvervi@gmail.com

References

[1] Richard P, Villard E, Charron P, Isnard R. The genetic bases of cardiomyopathies. J Am Coll Cardiol. 2006;48:A79–A78.

[2] Teare D.Asymmetrical hypertrophy of the heart Br heart J 1958;20:1–8 Postgrad Med J 1992;68 Suppl 1:S3–6.

[3] Dal Ferro, Severini G, Gigli M et al. Genetics of dilated cardiomyopathy: current knowledge and future perpectives. In Sinagra G, Merlo M, Pinamonti B, editors. Dilated Cardiomyopathy: From Genetics to Clinical Management, Chapter 5: Springer 2019.

[4] Spudich J. Three perspectives on the molecular basis of hypercontractility caused by hypertrophic cardiomyopathy mutations. Pflügers Archiv - European Journal of Physiology 2019; 471:701–717.

[5] Arbustini E, Narula N,Dec G et al. The MOGE(S) Classification for a Phenotype–Genotype Nomenclature of Cardiomyopathy. Journal of the American College of Cardiology 2013; 62: 2046–2072.

[6] Arbustini E, Narula N, Tavazzi L et al. The MOGE(S) Classification of Cardiomyopathy for Clinicians. Journal of the American College of Cardiology 2014; 64: 304–318.

[7] Elliott P, Andersson, B, Arbustini E et al. Classification of the cardiomyopathies: a position statement from the European Society Of Cardiology Working Group on Myocardial and Pericardial Diseases. Euro Heart Journal 2008; 29:270–276.

[8] Maron B, Towbin J, Thiene et al. Contemporary Definitions and Classification of the Cardiomyopathies an American Heart Association Scientific Statement from the Council on Clinical Cardiology, Heart Failure and Transplantation Committee; Quality of Care and Outcomes Research and Functional Genomics and Translational Biology Interdisciplinary Working Groups; and Council on Epidemiology and Prevention. Circulation 2006; 113: 1807-1816.

[9] Maron, B.J. The 2006 American Heart Association classification of cardiomyopathies is the gold standard. Circulation Heart Failure 2008; 1: 72-75.

[10] McCartan C, Mason R, Jayasinghe SR & Griffiths L. Cardiomyopathy Classification: Ongoing Debate in the Genomics Era. Biochemistry Research International 2012; Article ID 796926: 1-10.

[11] Cecchi F, Tomberli B, Olivotto I. Clinical and molecular classification of cardiomyopathies, Global Cardiology Science and Practice 2012:4.

[12] Vernengo L, Lilienbaum A, Agabulut O & Rodriguez, MM.. The role of geneties in cardiomyopathy .In Jos¨& Guiseppe Ambrosi, editors.: Cardiomyopathies. InTech 2013.

[13] Hazebroek M, Moors S, Dennert R et al. Prognostic Relevance of Gene-Environment Interactions in Patients With Dilated Cardiomyopathy.J.JACC 2015; 66: 1013–1023.

[14] Walsh R, Buchan R, Wilk A et al. Defining the genetic architecture of hypertrophic cardiomyopathy: re-evaluating the role of non-sarcomeric gene. European Heart Journal 2017a; 38, 3461–3468.

[15] Walsh R, Thomson K, Ware J et al. Reassessment of Mendelian gene pathogenicity using 7,855 cardiomyopathy cases and 60,706 reference samples. Genet Med. 2017b; 19:192–203.

[16] Elkilany G. New Classification of Cardiomyopathy: Who are at Risk? Integrative Clinical Cardiology 2017; 1 (1): 001e.

[17] Richard P, Charron P, Carrier L, et al. Hypertrophic cardiomyopathy: distribution of disease genes, spectrum of mutations, and implications for a molecular diagnosis strategy. Circulation. 2003; 107:2227–2232.

[18] Ommen, SR, Mital S, Burke MA, Day SM, Deswal A, Elliott P, Evanovich LL, Hung J, Joglar JA, Kantor P, Kimmelstiel C, Kittleson M, Link MS, Maron MS, Martinez MW, Miyake CY, Schaff HV, Semsarian C, Sorajja P. 2020 AHA/ACC Guideline for the diagnosis and treatment hypertrophic cardiomyopathy executive summary. Circ 2020; 142:e533–e557

[19] Lorenzini M, Norrish G, Field E et al. Penetrance of hypertrophic cardiomyopathy in sarcomere protein mutation carriers. J Am Coll Cardiol. 2020; 76: 550–559

[20] Elliott P, Anastasakis A, Borger M et al. 2014 ESC Guidelines on diagnosis and management of hypertrophic cardiomyopathy The Task Force for the Diagnosis and Management of Hypertrophic Cardiomyopathy of the European Society of Cardiology (ESC). European Heart Journal 2014; 35: 2733–2779.

[21] Branzi A, Romeo G, Specchia S et al. Genetic heterogeneity of hypertrophic cardiomyopathy. Int J Cardiol.1985; 7: 129–138.

[22] Niimura H, Bachinski L, Sangwatanaroj S et al. Mutations in the gene for cardiac myosin-binding protein C and late-onset familial hypertrophic cardiomyopathy. N Engl J Med 1998; 338:1248–1257.

[23] Seidman CE, Seidman JG. Identifying sarcomere gene mutations in hypertrophic cardiomyopathy: a personal history. Circ Res 2011; 108: 743–750.

[24] Wang, Y., Wang, Z., Yang, Q. et al. Autosomal recessive transmission of MYBPC3 mutation results in malignant phenotype of hypertrophic cardiomyopathy. PLoS One 8: e67087, 2013. Note: Electronic Article

[25] Hartmannova H; Kubanek M, Sramko M et al. Isolated X-Linked Hypertrophic Cardiomyopathy Caused by a Novel Mutation of the Four-and-a-Half LIM Domain 1 Gene. Circ Cardiovasc Genet. 2013; 6: 543-551.

[26] Lipshultz S, MD, Law Y, Asante-Korang A. Cardiomyopathy in Children: Classification and Diagnosis. A Scientific Statement From the American Heart Association. Circulation. 2019; 140: e9–e68.

[27] Bos JM, Towbin JA, Ackerman MJ. Diagnostic, prognostic, and therapeutic implications of genetic testing for hypertrophic cardiomyopathy. J Am Coll Cardiol 2009; 54:201–211.

[28] Maron BJ, Gardin JM, Flack JM et al. Prevalence of hypertrophic cardiomyopathy in a general population of young adults. Echocardiographic analysis of 4111 subjects in the CARDIA Study. Coronary Artery Risk Development in (Young) Adults. Circulation. 1995; 92: 785–789.

[29] Maron BJ, Shirani J, Poliac LC et al. Sudden death in young competitive athletes. JAMA 1996: 276; 199–204.

[30] Mavrogeni SI, Tsarouhas K, Spandidos DA et al. Sudden cardiac death in football players: Towards a new pre-participation algorithm. Exp Ther Med. (2019); 17:1143–1148.

[31] Maron BJ, Maron MS, Semsarian C. Genetics of hypertrophic cardiomyopathy after 20 years: clinical

perspectives. J Am Coll Cardiol 2012; 60: 705–715.

[32] Semsarian C, Ingles J, Maron M & Maron B. New Perspectives on the Prevalence of Hypertrophic Cardiomyopathy. JACC 2015; 65 : 1249 – 1254.

[33] Sarkar S, Trivedi D, Morck M. et al. The hypertrophic cardiomyopathy mutations R403Q and R663H increase the number of myosin heads available to interact with actin. Sci. Adv. 2020; 6 : eaax0069

[34] Frank D & Frey N. Cardiac Z-disc Signaling Network. JBC 2011 286; 12: 9897–9904

[35] Hayashi T, Arimura T, Itoh-Satoh M, et al. Tcap gene mutations in hypertrophic cardiomyopathy and dilated cardiomyopathy. J Am Coll Cardiol. 2004;44:2192–2201.

[36] Marian A & Braunwald E. Hypertrophic Cardiomyopathy Genetics, Pathogenesis, Clinical Manifestations, Diagnosis, and Therapy. Circ Res. 2017;121:749-770.

[37] Das KJ, Ingles J, Bagnall R et al. Determining pathogenicity of genetic variants in hypertrophic cardiomyopathy: importance of periodic reassessment. GenetMed. 2014; 16: 286–293.

[38] Furqan A, Arscot P, Girolami F et al. Care in specialized centers and data sharing increase agreement in hypertrophic cardiomyopathy genetic test interpretation. Circ Cardiovasc Genet. 2017; 10:e001700.

[39] Ga Overeem S, Schelhaas H, Blijham P et al. Symptomatic distal myopathy with cardiomyopathy due to a MYH7 mutation. Neuromuscul Disord 2007;17: 490–493.

[40] Ingles J, Goldstein J, Thaxton C et al. Evaluating the Clinical Validity of Hypertrophic Cardiomyopathy Genes. Circ Genom Precis Med. 2019;12; 57–64.

[41] Kelly MA, Caleshu C, Morales et al. Adaptation and validation of the ACMG/AMP variant classification framework for MYH7-associated inherited cardiomyopathies: recommendations by ClinGen's Inherited Cardiomyopathy Expert Panel. Genet Med. 2018; 20: 351–359.

[42] Marian A, Roberts R. The molecular genetic basis for hypertrophic cardiomyopathy. J Mol Cell Cardiol 2001; 33:655.

[43] Rehm HL, Berg J, Brooks L et al; ClinGen. ClinGen–the Clinical Genome Resource. N Engl JMed. 2015; 372: 2235–2242.

[44] Moolman J, Corfield V, Posen B et al. Sudden death due to troponin T mutations. J Am Coll Cardiol 1997b;29: 549.

[45] Strande NT,Riggs E, Buchanan A et al. Evaluating the clinical validity of gene-disease associations: an evidence-based framework developed by the clinical genome resource. Am J Hum Genet. 2017;100: 895–906.

[46] Erdmann J, Daehmlow S, Wischke S et al. Mutation spectrum in a large cohort of unrelated consecutive patients with hypertrophic cardiomyopathy. Clin Genet. 2003 ; 64:339–349.

[47] Millat G, Bouvagnet P, Chevalier P. et al. Prevalence and spectrum of mutations in a cohort of 192 unrelated patients with hypertrophic cardiomyopathy. Eur J Med Genet. 2010; 53:261–267.

[48] Lilienbaum A & Vernengo L. Cardiomyopathies associated with myofibrillar myopathies. In Joseph Veselka, editor.: Cardiomyopathies – from basic research to clinical management InTech 2012; p.353–382.

[49] Miyamoto L. Molecular Pathogenesis of Familial Wolff-Parkinson-White Syndrome. ~Molecular Mechanisms of Cardiac Glycogen Regulation by AMPK~. J Med Invest 2018; 65 : 1 -8.

[50] Elliott, P. Cardiomyopathy. Diagnosis and management of dilated cardiomyopathy. *Heart* 2000 84; 1; 106–112.

[51] Hershberger R, Givertz M, Ho C et al; ACMG Professional Practice and Guidelines Committee.Genetic evaluation of cardiomyopathy: a clinical practice resource of the American College of Medical Genetics and Genomics (ACMG). GenetMed. 2018; 20: 899–909.

[52] Jefferies, J & Towbin, J. (2010). Dilated cardiomyopathy. Lancet 2010; 375:752–762.

[53] McNally E & Mestroni L. Dilated Cardiomyopathy: Genetic Determinants and Mechanisms. Circ Res. 2017; 121;: 731–748.

[54] Park HY. Hereditary Dilated Cardiomyopathy: Recent Advances in Genetic Diagnostic. Korean Circ J 2017; 47: 291–298.

[55] Sugrue DD, Rodeheffer RJ, Codd MB, et al. The clinical course of idiopathic dilated cardiomyopathy: a population-based study. Ann Intern Med 1992;117:117–123.

[56] Paldino A, De Angelis G, Merlo M et al. Genetics of Dilated Cardiomyopathy: Clinical Implications. Curr Cardiol Rep 2018; 20: 83.

[57] Baig M, Goldman J, Caforio A et al. Familial dilated cardiomyopathy: cardiac abnormalities are common in asymptomatic relatives and may represent early disease. J Am Coll Cardiol 1998; 3:195–201.

[58] Lennermann D, Backs J, van den Hoogenhof MMG. New Insights in RBM20 Cardiomyopathy. Current Heart Failure Reports 2020; 17:234–246.

[59] Hershberger R, Lndenfeld J, Mestroni L et al Genetic evaluation of cardiomyopathy-A Heart Failure Society of America Practice Guideline J Cardiac Fail 2009;15:83–97

[60] Mangin L, Charron P, Tesson F et al. Familial dilated cardiomyopathy: clinical features in French families. Eur J Heart Fail 1999; 14: 353–361.

[61] Aernout Somsen, Kees Hovingh G, Tulevski I. Familial dilated cardiomyopathy. In Baars H, van der Smagt, J, Doevendans P, editors. Clinical Cardiogenetics: Springer 2011; p. 63–78.

[62] Ortiz-Genga MF et al.Truncating FLNC Mutations Are Associated With High-Risk Dilated and Arrhythmogenic Cardiomyopathies. J Am Coll Cardiol. 2016; 68:2440–2451.

[63] Van den Hoogenhof M , Beqqali A, Amin A et al. RBM20 Mutations Induce an Arrhythmogenic Dilated Cardiomyopathy Related to Disturbed Calcium Handling. Circulation 2018; 138: 1330–1342.

[64] Dek GW & Arbustini, E. Utilizing the MOGE(S) classification for predicting prognosis in dilated cardiomyopathy. J.JACC 2015; 66: 1324–1326.

[65] Katritsis D, Wilmshurst P, Wendon J et al. Primary restrictive cardiomyopathy: clinical and pathologic characteristics. J Am Coll Cardiol 1991; 18:1230–1235 .

[66] Kaski J, Syrris P, Burch M, Tomé-Esteban M et al. Idiopathic restrictive cardiomyopathy in children is caused by mutations in cardiac sarcomere protein genes. Heart 2008a; 94:1478–1484.

[67] Kaski J, Syrris P, Burch M, Tomé-Esteban M et al. Idiopathic restrictive cardiomyopathy in children is caused by mutations in cardiac sarcomere protein genes. Heart 2008b; 94:1478–1484.

[68] Bahl A, Saikia U & Khullar Madhu. Idiopathic restrictive cardiomyopathy-perspectives from genetics studies. Is it time to Redefine these disorders. Cardiogenetics 2012: 2e4.

[69] Kushwaha S, Narula J, Narula N et al.Pattern of changes over time in myocardial blood flow and microvascular dilator capacity in patients with normally functioning cardiac allografts. Am J Cardiol. 1998; 82:1377-1381.

[70] Albakri A. Restrictive cardiomyopathy: A review of literature on clinical status and meta-analysis of diagnosis and clinical management. Pediatr Dimensions. 2018, 3: 1-14.

[71] Altmann HM, Tester DJ, Will ML, Middha S, Evans JM, Eckloff BW, Ackerman MJ. Homozygous/compound heterozygous triadin mutations associated with autosomal-recessive long-QT syndrome and pediatric sudden cardiac arrest: elucidation of the triadin knockout syndrome. Circulation. 2015; 131:2051–2060.

[72] Kamisago M, Sharma S, DePalma S et al. Mutations in sarcomere protein genes as a cause of dilated cardiomyopathy. New Eng. J. Med. 2000; 343: 1688–1696.

[73] Kirkels J & de Jonge N. Restrictive cardiomyopathy. In In Baars H, van der Smagt, J, Doevendans P, editors. Clinical Cardiogenetics: Springer 2011b; p130–139.

[74] Olson T; Illenberger S, Kishimoto N et al. Metavinculin mutations alter actin interaction in dilated cardiomyopathy. Circulation. 2002; 105: **431–437**.

[75] Zhang J, Kumar A, Kaplan L et al. Genetic linkage of a novel autosomal dominant restrictive cardiomyopathy locus. J Med Genet 2005; 42: 663-665.

[76] Brodehl A., Ferrier, R, Hamilton S et al. Mutations in FLNC are associated with familial restrictive cardiomyopathy. Hum. Mutat. 2016; 37: 269–279.

[77] James C, Syrris P, van Tintelen J, Calkins H.The role of genetics in cardiovascular disease: arrhythmogenic cardiomyopathy. European Heart Journal, 2020; 41, 1393–1400.

[78] Patel V, Asatryan B, Siripanthong B et al. State of the Art Review on Genetics and Precision Medicine in Arrhythmogenic Cardiomyopathy. Int. J. Mol. Sci. 2020, 21, 6615–6762.

[79] Brun F,. Barnes C, Sinagra G et al. Titin and desmosomal genes in the natural history of arrhythmogenic right ventricular cardiomyopaty. J Med Genet. 2014; 51: 669–676.

[80] Cox M & Hauer R. Arrhythmogenic right ventricular dysplasia/ cardiomyopathy from desmosome to disease. In Baars H, van der Smagt, J, Doevendans P, editors. Clinical Cardiogenetics: Springer 2011; p 80–96.

[81] Hamid M, Norman M, Quraishi A, et al. Prospective evaluation of relatives for familial arrhythmogenic right ventricular cardiomyopathy/dysplasia reveals a need to broaden diagnostic criteria. J Am Coll Cardiol. 2002;40: 1445–1450.

[82] Klauke B, Kossmann S, Gaertner A et al. De novo desmin-mutation N116S is associated with arrhythmogenic right ventricular cardiomyopathy. Hum Mol Genet 2010; 19; 4595–4607.

[83] Peters S. Advances in the diagnostic management of arrhythmogenic right

ventricular dysplasia-cardiomyopathy. Int J Cardiol. 2006;113:4–11.

[84] Awad M, Calkins H, Judge D. Mechanisms of disease: molecular genetics of arrhyth- mogenic right ventricular dysplasia/cardiomyopathy. Nat Clin Pract Cardiovasc 2008;5:258-267.

[85] Norgett E, Hatsell S, Carvajal-Huerta L et al. Recessive mutation in desmoplakin disrupts desmoplakin-intermediate filament interactions and causes dilated cardiomyopathy, woolly hair and keratoderma. Hum. Mol. Genet 2000; 9:2761–2766.

[86] Protonotarios N, Tsatsopoulou A, Patsourakos P et al. **Cardiac abnormalities in familial palmoplantar keratosis.** Brit. Heart J. 1986; 56: 321–326,.

[87] Schonberger J, Seidman CE. **Many roads lead to a broken heart: the genetics of dilated cardiomyopathy.** Am. J. Hum. Genet. 69: 249–260, 2001.

[88] McKoy G, Protonotarios N, Crosby A et al. Identification of a deletion in plakoglobin in arrhythmogenic right ventricular cardiomyopathy with palmoplantar keratoder- ma and woolly hair (Naxos disease). Lancet 2000; 355: 2119-2124.

[89] Al-Jassar C, Knowles T, Jeeves M et al. The nonlinear structure of the desmoplakin plakin domain and the effects of cardiomyopathy-linked mutations. J Mol Biol. 2011 411:1049–1061.

[90] James C, Syrris P, van Tintelen JP & Calkins H. The role of genetics in cardiovascular disease: arrhythmogenic cardiomyopathy. Euro Heart Journal 2008; 41:1393–1400.

[91] Tintelen J,, Entius M, Bhuiyan Z et al. Plakophilin-2 Mutations Are the Major Determinant of Familial Arrhythmogenic Right Ventricular Dysplasia/Cardiomyopathy. **Circulation** 2006; 113: 1650–1658.

[92] Van Tintelen J, Van Gelder I, Asimaki A et al. Severe cardiac phenotype with right ventricular predominance in a large cohort of patients with a single missense mutation in the DES gene. Heart Rhythm 2009; 6: 1574–1583.

[93] Vernengo L, Choubargi O, Panuncio A et al. Desmin myopathy with severe cardiomyopathy in a Uruguayan family due to a codon deletion in a new location within the desmin 1A rod domain. Neuromuscul Disord 2010; 20:178–187.

[94] Hedberg C, Melberg A, Kuhl A et al. Autosomal dominant myofibrillar myopathy with arrhythmogenic right ventricular cardiomyopathy 7 is caused by a DES mutation. Eur J Hum Genet 2012; 20:984–985.

[95] Melberg A, Oldfors, A, Blomstrom-Lundqvist C et al. Autosomal dominant myofibrillar myopathy with arrhythmogenic right ventricular cardiomyopathy linked to chromosome 10q .Ann. Neurol. 46: 684–692, 1999.

[96] Budde B, Binner P, Waldmuller S et al. Noncompaction of the ventricular myocardium is associated with a de novo mutation in the beta-myosin heavy chain gene. PLoS One.2007; 2:e1362.

[97] Freedom, R, Yoo, S, Perrin D et al. The morphological spectrum of ventricular noncompaction. Cardiology in the Young 2005;15:345–364.

[98] Hermida-Prieto MML, Castro-Beiras A, Laredo R et al. Familial dilated cardiomyopathy and isolated left ventricular noncompaction associated with Lamin A/C gene mutations. Am J Cardiol. 2004; 94:50–54.

[99] Klaassen S, Probst S, Oechslin E et al. Thierfelder L. Mutations in

sarcomere protein genes in left ventricular noncompaction. Circulation 2008; 117:2893–2901.

[100] Monserrat L, Hermida-Prieto M, Fernandez X et al. Mutation in the alpha-cardiac actin gene associated with apical hypertrophic cardiomyopathy, left ventricular noncompaction, and septal defects. Eur Heart J. 2007a; 28: 1953–1961.

[101] Monserrat L, Hermida-Prieto M, Fernandez X et al. Mutation in the alpha-cardiac actin gene associated with apical hypertrophic cardiomyopathy, left ventricular noncompaction, and septal defects. Eur Heart J. 2007b; 28: 1953–1961.

[102] Van Waning J, Caliskan K, Hoedemaekers Y et al. Genetics, Clinical Features, and Long-Term Outcome of Noncompaction Cardiomyopathy. JACC 2018: 7; 711-722.

[103] Dooijes D, Hoedemaekers Y, Michels M et al. Left ventricular noncompaction cardiomyopathy: disease genes, mutation spectrum and diagnostic implications. *Submitted.* 2009.

[104] Ichida F, Tsubata S, Bowles KR et al. Novel gene mutations in patients with left ventricular noncompaction or Barth syndrome.Circulation. 2001;103: 1256–1263.

[105] Shan L, Makita N, Xing Y et al. SCN5A variants in Japanese patients with left ventricular noncompaction and arrhythmia. Mol Genet Metab. 2008;93: 468–474.

[106] Vatta M, Mohapatra B, Jimenez S et al. Mutations in Cypher/ZASP in patients with dilated cardiomyopathy and left ventricular noncompaction. J Am Coll Cardiol 2003;42:2014–2027.

[107] Li S, Zhang C, Liu N et al. Clinical implications of sarcomere and nonsarcomere gene variants in patients with left ventricular noncompaction cardiomyopathy. Mol Genet Genomic Med. 2019;7:e874.

[108] Akashi Y, Goldstein D, Barbaro, G; Ueyama T. Takotsubo Cardiomyopathy A New Form of Acute, Reversible Heart Failure. Circulation. 2008;118:2754–2762.

[109] Borchert T, Hübscher D, Guessoum C et al. Catecholamine-Dependent β-Adrenergic Signaling in a Pluripotent Stem Cell Model of Takotsubo Cardiomyopathy. JACC 2017, 20: 975–991.

[110] Limongelli G, Masarone D, Maddaloni V et al. Genetics of Takotsubo Syndrome. Heart Fail Clin 2016; 12: 499–506.

[111] Sealove B, Tiyyagura S, & Fuster, V. Takotsubo cardiomyopathy. J of Gen Intern Med, 2008; 23; 1904–1908.

[112] Sharkey S., Lesser J, Zenovich et al.. Acute and reversible cardiomyopathy provoked by stress in women from the United States. Circulation 2005; 111: 472–479

[113] Aleong, R.G., Milan, D.J. & Ellinor, P. The diagnosis and treatment of cardiac ion channelopathies: congenital long QT syndrome and Brugada syndrome. Cur Treat Opt in Cardio Med 2007; 9; 5:364–371.

[114] Garcia-Elias A & Benito B. Ion Channel Disorders and Sudden Cardiac Death. Int. J. Mol. Sci. 2018; 19, 692.

[115] Modell, S.M. & Lehmann, M.H. (2006).The long QT syndrome family of cardiac ion channelopathies: a HuGE review. . Genet in Med 2006; 8; 143–155.

[116] Nakano Y & Shimizu W. Genetics of long-QT syndrome. J Hum Genet 2016; 61:51–55.

[117] Ackerman M, Priori S, Willems Set al. HRS/EHRA Expert Consensus Statement on the State of Genetic Testing for the Channelopathies and Cardiomyopathies. Europace 2011; 13: 1077–1109.

[118] Mizusawa Y, Horie M, Wilde A. Genetic and Clinical Advances in Congenital Long QT Syndrome. Circ J 2014; 78: 2827–2283

[119] Schulze-Bahr E, Wang Q, Wedekind H, Haverkamp W, Chen Q, Sun Y, et al. KCNE1 mutations cause Jervell and Lange-Nielsen syndrome. Nat Genet 1997 17:267–268.

[120] Splawski I, Timothy K, Sharpe L et al. Ca(V)1.2 calcium channel dysfunction causes a multisystem disorder including arrhythmia and autism. Cell 2004; 119:19-31.

[121] Splawski I, Timothy KW, Decher N et al. Severe arrhythmia disorder caused by cardiac L-type calcium channel mutations. Proc Natl Acad Sci 2005; 102: 8089– 8096.

[122] Etheridge S, Bowles N., Arrington C et al. Somatic mosaicism contributes to phenotypic variation in Timothy syndrome. **Am.** J. Med. Genet. 155A: 2578–2583, 2011.

[123] Plaster N, Tawil R, Tristani-Firouzi M et al. Mutations in Kir2.1 cause the developmental and episodic electrical phenotypes of Andersen's syndrome. Cell 2001 18;105: 511–519.

[124] Schwartz PJ, Stramba-Badiale M, Crotti et al. Prevalence of the congenital long-QT syndrome. Circulation 2009; 120:1761–1767.

[125] Marks M, Trippel D, Keating M. Long QT syndrome associated with syndactyly identified in females. Am J Cardiol. 1995a; 76:744–745.

[126] Marks ML, Whisler SL, Clericuzio C, Keating M. A new form of long QT syndrome associated with syndactyly. J Am Coll Cardiol. 1995b; 25:59–64.

[127] Lo-A-Njoe SM, Wilde AA et al. Syndactyly and long QT syndrome (CaV1.2 missense mutation G640R) is associated with hypertrophic cardiomyopathy. Heart Rhythm. 2005; 2:1365–1368.

[128] Nguyen HL, Pieper GH, Wilders R. Andersen-Tawil syndrome: clinical and molecular aspects. Int J Cardiol. 2013; 170: 1-16.

[129] Pérez-Riera A, Barbosa-Barros R, Samesina N et al. Andersen-Tawil Syndrome: A Comprehensive Review. Cardiol Rev. 2020.

[130] Campuzano O, Fernandez-Falgueras A, Lemus X. Short QT Syndrome: A Comprehensive Genetic Interpretation and Clinical Translation of Rare Variants. J. Clin. Med. 2015;8, 1035.

[131] Giustetto C, Scrocco C, Giachino D et al. Short QT syndrome. *Cardiogenetics* 2011;*1(s1)*, 21–27.

[132] Rudic B, Schimpf R, Borggrefe M. Short QT Syndrome – Review of Diagnosis and Treatment. Arrhythmia & Electrophysiology Review 2011; 3:76–79.

[133] Al-Khatib S, Stevenson W, Ackerman et al. 2017 AHA/ACC/HRS Guideline for Management of Patients With Ventricular Arrhythmias and the Prevention of Sudden Cardiac Death: A Report of the American College of Cardiology/American Heart Association Task Force on Clinical Practice Guidelines and the Heart Rhythm Society. J Am Coll Cardiol . 2018; 72:e91-e220.

[134] Begoña B, Brugada J et al. The Brugada syndrome. In Baars H, van der Smagt, J, Doevendans P, editors.

Clinical Cardiogenetics: Springer 2011; p.165–188.

[135] Brugada R, Hong K, Dumaine R, Cordeiro J et al. Sudden death associated with short-QT syndrome linked to mutations in HERG. Circulation. 2004; 109:30–35.

[136] Gourraud J, Barc J, A. Thollet A The Brugada Syndrome: A Rare Arrhythmia Disorder with Complex Inheritance, Front. Cardiovasc. Med. 3 2016 9.

[137] Li K , Lee S , Yin C et al. Brugada syndrome: A comprehensive review of pathophysiological mechanisms and risk stratification strategies. IJC Heart & Vasculature 2020a; 26: 1–10.

[138] Monasky M , Micaglio E , Ciconte G et al. Brugada Syndrome: Oligogenic or Mendelian Disease? Int. J. Mol. Sci. 2020, 21, 1687

[139] Ohno S, Zankov D, Ding W et al. KCNE5 (KCNE1L) Variants Are Novel Modulators of Brugada Syndrome and Idiopathic Ventricular Fibrillation. Circ Arrhythm Electrophysiol 2011; 4: 352–361.

[140] Li KHC, Lee S, Yin C et al. Brugada syndrome: A comprehensive review of pathophysiological mechanisms and risk stratification strategies IJC Heart & Vasculature 2020b 26; 100468.

[141] Juang JM & Huang SK. Brugada syndrome-an under-recognized electrical disease in patients with sudden cardiac death. Cardiology 2004; 101: 157-169.

[142] Al-Hassnan ZN, Tulbah S, Al-Manea W et al. The phenotype of a CASQ2 mutation in a Saudi family with catecholaminergic polymorphic ventricular tachycardia. Pacing Clin Electrophysiol. 2013; 36:140–142

[143] Behere S & Weindling S. Catecholaminergic polymorphic ventricular tachycardia: An exciting new era. 2016 Annals of Pediatric Cardiology. Annals of Pediatric Cardiology 2016; 136–147.

[144] Jensen HH, Brohus M, Nyegaard Met al Human calmodulin mutations. Front Mol Neurosci. 2018;11:396.

[145] Rooryck C, Kyndt F, Bozon D, et al. New family with catecholaminergic polymorphic ventricular tachycardia linked to the triadin gene. J Cardiovasc Electrophysiol. 2015 ; 26:1146–1150.

[146] Van der Zwaag, P, Jongbloed J, van den Berg M et al. A genetic variants database for arrhythmogenic right ventricular dysplasia/cardiomyopathy. Hum Mutat 2009; 30:1278–1283.

[147] Hermans M, Pinto Y, Merkies et al. Hereditary muscular dystrophies and the heart Neuromusc Disord 2010; 20: 479–492.

[148] Finsterer J, Stöllberger C , Wahb K. Cardiomyopathy in neurological disorders. Cardiovasc Pathol. 2013: 5¸389-400.

[149] Meola G, Cardani R. Myotonic dystrophies: An update on clinical aspects, genetic, pathology, and molecular pathomechanisms. Biochim Biophys Acta. 2015; 1852: 594-606.

[150] Barresi R, Di Blasi C, Negri T, et al. Disruption of heart sarcoglycan complex and severe cardiomyopathy caused by beta sarcoglycan mutations. J Med Genet 2000; 37:102–107.

[151] Connuck D, Sleeper L, Colan S et al. Characteristics and outcomes of cardiomyopathy in children with Duchenne or Becker muscular dystrophy: a comparative study from the Pediatric Cardiomyopathy Registry. Am Heart J 2008; 155:998–1005.

[152] De Ambroggi L, Raisaro A, Marchiano V, Radice S, Meola G.

Cardiac involvement in patients with myotonic dystrophy: characteristic features of magnetic resonance imaging. Eur Heart J 1995;16:1007–1010.

[153] Fanin M, Melacini P, Boito C et al. LGMD2E patients risk developing dilated cardiomyopathy. Neuromuscul Disord 2003;13:303–309.

[154] Goldfarb L, Dalakas M. Tragedy in a heartbeat: malfunctioning desmin causes skeletal and cardiac muscle disease. J Clin Invest 2009; 119:1806–1813.

[155] Jefferies J, Eidem B, Belmont J et al. Genetic predictors and remodeling of dilated cardiomyopathy in muscular dystrophy. Circulation 2005; 112:2799–2804.

[156] Kaspar R, Allen H, Ray W et al. Alvarez CE, Kissel JT, Pestronk A, et al. Analysis of dystrophin deletion mutations predicts age of cardiomyopathy onset in Becker muscular dystrophy. Circ Cardiovasc Genet 2009a; 2:544–451.

[157] Kaspar R, Allen H, Ray W et al. Alvarez CE, Kissel JT, Pestronk A, et al. Analysis of dystrophin deletion mutations predicts age of cardiomyopathy onset in Becker muscular dystrophy. Circ Cardiovasc Genet 2009b; 2:544–551.

[158] Lazarus A, Varin J, Ounnoughene Z et al. Relationships among electrophysiological findings and clinical status, heart function, and extent of DNA mutation in myotonic dystrophy. Circulation 1999; 99:1041–1046.

[159] Melacini P, Fanin M, Duggan D et al. Heart involvement in muscular dystrophies due to sarcoglycan gene mutations. Muscle Nerve 1999; 22: 473–479.

[160] Nakanishi T, Sakauchi M, Kaneda Y et al. Cardiac involvement in Fukuyama-type congenital muscular dystrophy. Pediatrics 2006a;117:1187–1119.

[161] Nguyen H, Wolfe 3rd J, Holmes Jr D, Edwards W. Pathology of the cardiac conduction system in myotonic dystrophy: a study of 12 cases. J Am Coll Cardiol 1988a; 11:662–671.

[162] Nakanishi T, Sakauchi M, Kaneda Y et al. Cardiac involvement in Fukuyama-type congenital muscular dystrophy. Pediatrics 2006b;117:e1187–e1119.

[163] Nguyen H, Wolfe 3rd J, Holmes Jr D, Edwards W. Pathology of the cardiac conduction system in myotonic dystrophy: a study of 12 cases. J Am Coll Cardiol 1988b; 11:662–671.

[164] Politano L, Nigro V, Passamano L et al. Evaluation of cardiac and respiratory involvement in sarcoglycanopathies. Neuromuscul Disord 2001;11:178–185.

[165] Schoser B, Ricker, K, Schneider-Gold C et al. Sudden cardiac death in myotonic dystrophy type 2. Neurology 2004; 63: 2402–2404.

[166] Selcen D, Engel AG. Myofibrillar myopathy caused by novel dominant negative alpha B-crystallin mutations. Ann Neurol 2003; 54:804–810.

[167] Vicart P, Caron A, Guicheney P et al. A missense mutation in the alphaB-crystallin chaperone gene causes a desmin-related myopathy. Nat Genet 1998; 20:92–95.

[168] Lehman S, Tal-Grinspan L, Lynn M et alChronic Calmodulin-Kinase II Activation Drives Disease Progression in Mutation-Specific Hypertrophic Cardiomyopathy. Circulation 2019; 139: 1517-1529.

[169] Harris S, de Tombe P. Sarcomeric mutations in cardiac diseases. Pflugers Arch. 2019 ; 471: 659-660.

[170] Carrasco L, Vernengo L, Mesa R et al. Síndrome de Kearns-Sayre. Presentación de un caso clínico y revisión de la bibliografía. Arch. Inst. Neurol. 2005; 8(2):31–35. [Article in Spanish. Abstract in English].

[171] De Jonge N & Kirkels J. Restrictive cardiomyopathy. In Baars H, van der Smagt, J, Doevendans P, editors. Clinical Cardiogenetics: Springer 2011; p.123–128.

[172] Walter L, Nogueira V, Leverve X et al. Three classes of ubiquinone analogs regulate the mitochondrial permeability transition pore through a common site. J Biol Chem 2000; 275: 29521-29527.

[173] Behjati M, Sabri M, Far M et al. Cardiac complications in inherited mitochondrial diseases. Heart Fail Rev. 2021; 26: 391-403.

[174] Holgrem D, Wahlander H, Eriksson, B et al. Cardiomyopathy in children with mitochondrial disease: clinical course and cardiologigal findings. Eur Heart J 2003; 24:280–288.

[175] Annan R, Nakagawa M, Miyata M et al. Cardiac involvement in mitocondrial disease. A study of 17 patients with documental mitochondrial DNA defects. Circulation 1995; 91: 955–961.

[176] Roberts N, Perloff J, Kark R. A follow up study of myocardial involvement in pa- tients with mitochondrial encephalomyopathy, lactic acidosis, and stroke-like episodes (MELAS). Heart 1998a; 80: 292-2955.

[177] Roberts N, Perloff J, Kark R. A follow up study of myocardial involvement in patients with mitochondrial encephalomyopathy, lactic acidosis, and stroke-like episodes (MELAS). Heart 1998b; 80:292-2955.

[178] Hirano M & Pavlakis S. Mitochondrial myopathy, encephalopathy, lactic acidosis, and strokelike episodes (MELAS): current concepts. J Child Neurol. 1994; 9: 4-13

[179] Vydt T, de Coo R, Soliman O et al. Cardiac involvement in adults with m.3243A>G MELAS gene mutation. Am J Cardiol. 2007; 99: 264-269.

[180] Wortmann S, Rodenburg R, Backx A et al. Early cardiac involvement in children carrying the A3243G mtDNA mutation. Acta Paediatr. 2007; 96: 450-451.

[181] Kirkels J & de Jonge N. Mitochondrial cardiomyopathy. In Baars H, van der Smagt, J, Doevendans P, editors. Clinical Cardiogenetics: Springer 2011a; p123–128.

[182] Okajima Y, Tanabe Y, Takayanagi M & Aotsuka H. A follow up study of myocardial involvement in patients with mitochondrial encephalomyopathy, lactic acidosis, and stroke-like episodes (MELAS). Heart 1998; 80: 292-295.

[183] Spencer C, Bryant R, Day J et al. Cardiac and clinical phenotype in Barth syndrome. Pediatrics 2006;118:337–346.

[184] Jacoby D & McKenna W. Genetics of inherited cardiomyopathies. European Heart Journal 2012; 33: 296–304.

[185] Towbin JA. Inherited cardiomyopathies. Circ J. 2014;78:2347-2356.

[186] Ingles J, Doolan A, Chiu C et al. Compound and double mutations in patients with hypertrophic cardiomyopathy: implications for genetic testing and counselling. J Med Genet. 2005;42:e59.

[187] Richard P, Isnard R, Carrier L, et al. Double heterozygosity for mutations in the beta-myosin heavy chain and in the cardiac myosin binding protein C genes

in a family with hypertrophic cardiomyopathy. J Med Genet. 1999; 36: 542–545.

[188] Van Driest SL, Vasile VC, Ommen SR, Will ML, Jamil Tajik A, Gersh BJ, Ackerman MJ. Myosin binding protein C mutations and compoundheterozygosity in hypertrophic cardiomyopathy. J Am Coll Cardiol2004;44:1903–1016 ;

[189] Ho C, Lever H, DeSanctis R, Farver C et al. Homozygous mutation in cardiac troponin T: implications for hypertrophic cardiomyopathy. Circulation 2000;102:1950–1955.

[190] Ingles J, Sarina T, Yeates L, et al. Clinical predictors of genetic testing outcomes in hypertrophic cardiomyopathy. Genet Med 2013; 15: 972–977.

[191] Uro-Coste E, Arne-Bes M, Pellissier J et al. Striking phenotypic variability in two familial cases of myosin storage myopathy with a MYH7 Leu1793pro mutation. Neuromuscul Disord 2009;19: 163–1636.

[192] Watkins H, McKenna W, Thierfelder L et al. Mutations in the genes for cardiac troponin T and alpha-tropomyosin in hypertrophic cardiomyopathy. N Engl J Med 1995; 332: 1058-1064.

[193] Landstrom, A. & Ackerman M. Mutation type is not clinically useful in predicting prognosis in hypertrophic cardiomyopathy. Circulation 2010; 22: 2441–2451.

[194] Tardiff JC. Sarcomeric proteins and familial hypertrophic cardiomyopathy: linking mutations in structural proteins to complex cardiovascular phenotypes. Heart Fail Rev 2005;10:237

[195] Fourey D, Care M, Siminovitch M et al. Prevalence and clinical implication in double mutation in hypertrophic cardiomyopathy: revisiting the gene dose effect. Circ Cardiovasc Genet . 2017;10: e001685.

[196] Maron B, Maron M, Semsarian C. Double or compound sarcomere mutations in hypertrophic cardiomyopathy: A potential link to sudden death in the absence of conventional risk. Heart Rhythm 2012b; 9: 57-63

[197] Crilley J, Boehm E, Blair E et al. Hypertrophic cardiomyopathy due to sarcomeric gene mutations is characterized by impaired energy metabolism irrespective of the degree of hypertrophy. J Am Coll Cardiol 2003;41: 1776–1787.

[198] Mestroni L, Rocco C, Gregori D, et al. Familial dilated cardiomyopathy: evidence for genetic and phenotypic heterogeneity. Heart Muscle Disease Study Group. J Am Coll Cardiol 1999; 34:181–190.

[199] Michels V, Moll P, Miller F et al. The frequency of familial dilated cardiomyopathy in a series of patients with idiopathic dilated cardiomyopathy. N Engl J Med 1992; 326:77–82.

[200] MacArthur DG, Manolio TA, Dimmock DP et al. Nature 2014. Guidelines for investigating causality of sequence variants in human disease. Nature 508, 469–476.

[201] Manrai AK, et al. Genetic misdiagnoses and the potential for health disparities.N Engl J Med. 2016; 375: 655–665.

[202] Moolman J, Corfield V, Posen B et al. Sudden death due to troponin T mutations. J Am Coll Cardiol 1997a;29: 549..

[203] Menon S., Michels V, Pellikka et al. Cardiac troponin T mutation in familial cardiomyopathy with variable

remodeling and restrictive physiology. Clin. Genet. 2008; 74: 445–454.

[204] Peddy S, Vricella L, Crosson J et al. Infantile restrictive cardiomyopathy resulting from a mutation in the cardiac troponin T gene. Pediatrics 2006; 117: 1830–1833.

[205] Hoedemaekers Y, Caliskan K, Michels M. The importanceof genetic counseling, DNA diagnostics and cardiologic family screening in left ventricular noncompaction cardiomyopathy. Circ Cardiovasc Genet. 2010; 3:232–239.

[206] Becane H, Bonne G, Varnous S et al. High incidence of sudden death with conduction system and myocardial disease due to lamins A and C gene mutation. Pacing Clin Electrophysiol 2000; 23:1661–1666.

[207] Brodsky G, Muntoni F, Miocic S et al. Lamin A/C gene mutation associated with dilated cardiomyopathy with variable skeletal muscle involvement. Circulation 2000; 101:473–476.

[208] Emmanuele V, Silvers DS, Sotiriou E, Tanji K, DiMauro S, Hirano M. MERRF and Kearns-Sayre overlap syndrome due to the mitochondrial DNA m.3291T>C mutation. Muscle Nerve. 2011; 44:448-451.

[209] Pitceathly R, Fassone E, Taanman J et al. Kearns-Sayre syndrome caused by defective R1/p53R2 assembly. J Med Genet. 2011; 48: 610-617.

[210] Di Mauro S, Bonilla E, Zeviani M et al. Mitochondrial myopathies. Ann Neurol 1985; 17:521–538.

[211] Baltogiannis G, Lysitsas D; Di Giovanni G e al. CPVT: Arrhythmogenesis, therapeutic management, and future perspectives. A brief review of the literature.Front. Cardiovasc. Med. 12 July 2019.

[212] Hoedemaekers Y, Caliskan K, Majoor-Krakauer D. Non-compaction cardiomyopathy. In Baars H, van der Smagt, J, Doevendans P, editors. Clinical Cardiogenetics: Springer 2011; P.98–122.

[213] Hsu, YH.R., Yogasundaram, H., Parajuli, N. *et al.* MELAS syndrome and cardiomyopathy: linking mitochondrial function to heart failure pathogenesis. Heart Fail Rev 2016; 21: 103–116

[214] Kumar Singh B, Kolappa Pilla K et al. Classification and definitions of cardiomyopathies. In Joseph Veselka, editor.: Cardiomyopathies –from basic research to clinical management InTech 2012; p.3–20.

[215] Nimura H, Bachinski LL, Sangwatanaroj S, et al. Mutations in the gene for cardiac myosin binding protein C and late-onset familial hypertrophic cardiomyopathy. N Engl J Med 1998; 338: 1248 1257.

[216] Thierfelder, L., Watkins, H., MacRae, C et al .Alpha-tropomyosin and cardiac troponin T mutations cause familial hypertrophic cardiomyopathy: a disease of the sarcomere, Cell 1994; 77: 701–712.

[217] Van der Werf C & Wilde A. Catecholaminergic polymorphic ventricular tachycardia. In Baars H, van der Smagt, J, Doevendans P, editors. Clinical Cardiogenetics: Springer 2011; p.197–206.

Chapter 7

The Z-Disk Final Common Pathway in Cardiomyopathies

Enkhsaikhan Purevjav and Jeffrey A. Towbin

Abstract

The sarcomeres represent the essential contractile units of the cardiac myocyte and are bordered by two Z-lines (disks) that are made by various proteins. The cardiac Z-disk is recognized as one of the nodal points in cardiomyocyte structural organization, mechano-sensation and signal transduction. Rapid progress in molecular and cellular biology has significantly improved the knowledge about pathogenic mechanisms and signaling pathways involved in the development of inherited cardiomyopathies. Genetic insult resulting in expression of mutated proteins that maintain the structure of the heart can perturb cardiac function. The primary mutation in the cardiac contractile apparatus or other subcellular complexes can lead to cardiac pathology on a tissue level, resulting in organ and organism level pathophysiology. The "final common pathway" hypothesis interpreting the genetic basis and molecular mechanisms involved in the development of cardiomyopathies suggests that mutations in cardiac genes encoding proteins with similar structure, function, or location and operating in the same pathway, are responsible for a particular phenotype of cardiomyopathy with unique morpho-histological remodeling of the heart. This chapter will describe genetic abnormalities of cardiac Z-disk and related "final common pathways" that are triggered by a Z-disk genetic insult leading to heart muscle diseases. In addition, animal models carrying mutations in Z-disk proteins will be described.

Keywords: cardiomyopathy, final common pathway, Z-disk, sarcomere, mutation, animal models

1. Introduction

In comparison to skeletal muscle fibers that are organized in parallel arrangements, cardiac muscle fibers create an interlaced three-dimensional network comprised of bifurcating and recombining myocytes connected with adjacent myocytes at each end in particular series [1]. These specialized areas, the intercalated discs, are interdigitating cell membranes that play essential roles in transmitting signals between myocytes. Cardiac intercalated discs contain mechanical junctions that consists of adherens junctions, desmosomes, and gap junctions [2]. Adherens junctions contain N-cadherin, catenins and vinculin, desmosomes comprise desmin, desmoplakin, plakophilin, junctional plakoglobin, desmocollin, desmoglein and gap junctions mainly include connexins. A thin cell membrane or sarcolemma surrounds the lateral sides of cardiac myocytes enveloping the interior (sarcoplasm) of each myocyte. The sarcoplasm contains the myofibril bundles arranged in a longitudinal manner and appears as parallel lines with visible striations similar to that of skeletal muscle formed by repeating sarcomeres. Sarcomeres, the fundamental structural and functional elements of striated muscle composed of thick and thin filaments, are bound by two Z lines (**Figure 1**) [3, 4]. The thick filaments are comprised primarily of myosin but additionally contain myosin binding proteins C, H and X. Cardiac actin, α-tropomyosin (α-TM), and troponins T, I, and C (cTnT, cTnI, cTnC) compose the thin filaments that interdigitate with the thick filaments. On electron micrograph, each sarcomere flanked by two Z-lines has an A band corresponding to the overlap of thick filaments and thin filaments, I bands comprised of thin filaments only, and M band is comprised of thick filaments only [3–7]. The sarcomeric cytoskeleton, assembled by titin, myomesins and nebulin, provides a scaffolding for the thick and thin filaments. The extra-sarcomeric cytoskeleton is a complex network of intermyofibrillar and subsarcolemmal proteins which connects the sarcomere with the sarcolemmal membrane and extracellular matrix (ECM). The extra-sarcomeric cytoskeleton provides universal structural support for subcellular components and transmits mechanical and biochemical signals within and between cells. The intermyofibrillar components of the extra-sarcomeric cytoskeleton are made up of intermediate filaments, microfilaments and microtubules [5–11]. Desmin intermediate filaments form a three-dimensional scaffold throughout the sarcoplasm, linking longitudinally extra-sarcomeric cytoskeleton and adjacent Z-disks as well as forming lateral connections between extra-sarcomeric cytoskeleton, surrounding Z-disks and sub-sarcolemmal costameres [10, 11]. Microfilaments composed of non-sarcomeric actin (mainly γ-actin) also form an additional mesh network linking α-actinin (expressed at the sarcomeric Z-disks) to the adjacent costameres. Costameres are subsarcolemmal components arranged in a periodic and grid-like pattern and are found at the sarcoplasmic side of the sarcolemma of

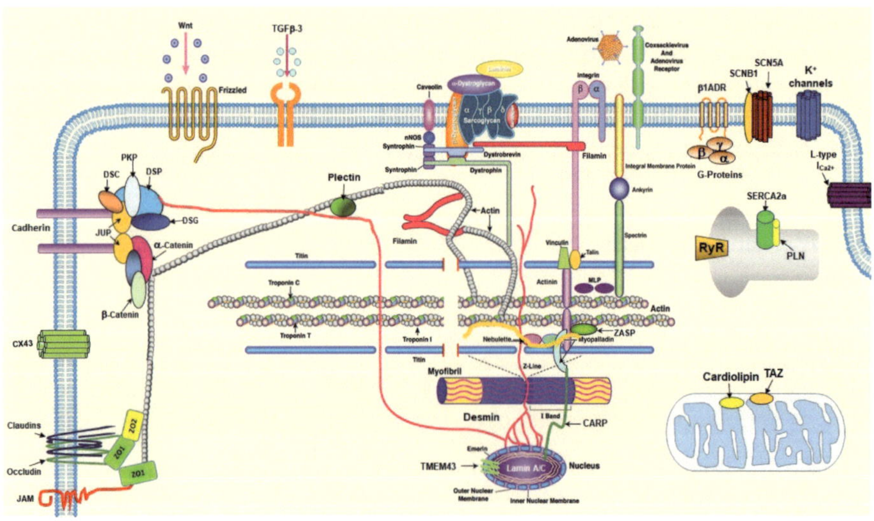

Figure 1.
Schema of cardiac myocyte cytoarchitecture. The key proteins of extracellular matrix (ECM), sarcolemma (cellular membrane), sarcoplasm containing sarcomeres (contractile units), mitochondria, endoplasmic reticulum and nuclei are depicted. Sarcolemmal proteins include ion channels such as SCN5A, L-type calcium channels and others, as well as the dystrophin-associated binding proteins that interact with dystrophin and other cytoplasmic cytoskeletal proteins (dystroglycans, sarcoglycans, syntrophins, dystrobrevin, sarcospan, caveolin), and cadherins that bind with desmosomal proteins (desmocollin, desmoglein, plakophilin, desmoplakin, plakoglobin). The integral membrane proteins interact with the ECM via α-dystroglycan-laminin α2 connections. The sarcomere includes thick and thin filament contractile proteins and Z-disk proteins (alpha-actinin, muscle LIM protein (MLP), nebulette, myopalladin, ZASP). The nucleus includes lamin A/C and emerin. Dystrophin binds actin and connects dystrophin with the sarcomere, sarcolemma and ECM. The intermediate filament protein, desmin, is another important and prominent linker protein.

cardiac myocytes adjoining the Z-lines and overlying the surrounding I-bands. Costameres contain three major components: the focal adhesion-type complex, the spectrin-based complex, and the dystrophin and dystrophin-associated protein complex (DAPC) [12, 13]. The focal adhesion-type complexes contain cytoplasmic proteins (i.e., vinculin, talin, tensin, paxillin, zyxin) that interact with cytoskeletal actin filaments connecting with the transmembrane proteins α-, and β- dystroglycan, α-, β-, γ-, δ--sarcoglycans, dystrobrevin, and syntrophin [8, 9]. Several actin-associated proteins are located at sites of attachment of cytoskeletal actin filaments with costameric complexes, including α-actinin and the muscle LIM protein (MLP) encoded by the cystein-serine rich protein 3 or *CSRP3* gene. Dystrophin C-terminus binds β-dystroglycan which interacts with α-dystroglycan to link to the ECM, while the N-terminus of dystrophin interacts with actin. Also notable, voltage-gated sodium channels co-localize with dystrophin, β-spectrin, ankyrin, and syntrophins while potassium channels interact with the sarcomeric Z-disks and intercalated disks [14–16]. Taken together, the sarcomeric Z-disk is an important structural component of cardiomyocytes.

2. Z-disk structure and function

In electron micrographs of cardiac muscle, the Z-lines are seen as a series of dark lines. The Z-disks (at the Z lines), lateral borders of the sarcomere, are formed by a lattice of interdigitating proteins that maintain myofilament organization by cross-linking antiparallel titin and thin actin filaments from adjoining sarcomeres. The backbone of the Z-disk contains layers of α-actinin aligned in an antiparallel pattern where α-actinin cross-links the interdigitating barbed ends of the actin thin filaments and connects the thin filaments to the sarcomere. Therefore, from each Z-disk, thin filaments extend to two neighboring sarcomeres. The Z-disk stretches when myosin heads pull actin filaments during systolic contraction and condenses when titin, a huge spring protein, develops elastic spring forces during diastolic sarcomere relaxation [17–19]. Numerous proteins (α-actinin, MLP, filamins, nebulette, telethonin, myotilin, myopalladin, nexilin, ZASP (ZO-2 associated speckle protein) and others listed in **Table 1**) are expressed in Z-disks that permit bidirectional force transmission with conformational changes [20].

In addition to structural and force transmission functions, the Z-disk is an important nodal point for cardiac mechano-sensation during mechanical stretch [21]. Cardiac myocytes respond to mechanical stretch *via* mechano-sensation, an ultimate conversion of a mechanical stimulus into a biochemical signal, and transmission of signals (namely mechano-transduction) which results in immediate increase in contractility, as well as long-term changes in gene expression, resulting in myocyte hypertrophy [22]. The immediate contractility changes are mediated through altered Ca^{2+} transients, while the gene expression changes seem to be mediated through induction of "immediate early genes" encoding transcription factors, such as *c-fos, c-jun, Egr-1,* and *c-myc.* The final response to stretch is established by an orchestrated response between multiple independent and cross-talking signaling pathways including MAPK, PI3K/Akt, FAK, RAS, JAK/STAT, and calcium signaling [23]. These signaling pathways control the hypertrophic response, the survival response and apoptotic response of the myocyte to mechanical stretch; the balance between these responses determines the final phenotype of the cardiomyocyte. There are multiple mechanosensitive signaling units: (a) Stretch activated ion channels [24]; (b) Integrin-based units which interact bundles with proteins from the extracellular matrix and the cytoskeleton [25]; (c) Titin-based units (titin-N2A, titin-telethonin, titin-calsarcin, titin-PEVK) [26];

Gene	Locus	Protein	Cardiomyopathy phenotype
ACTN2	1q43	α-Actinin 2	DCM, HCM, LVNC
CSRP3	11p15.1	Muscle LIM protein	DCM, HCM, LVNC
TCAP	17q12	Telethonin	HCM
NEBL	10p12.31	Nebulette	DCM
BAG3	10q26.11	BCL2-associated athanogene 3	DCM
FHL2	2q12.2	Four and a half LIM domain 2	
MYOT	5q31.2	Myotilin	
MYPN	10q21.3	Myopalladin	DCM, HCM, RCM
FLNC	7q32.1	Filamin C	HCM, RCM
ANKRD1	10q23.31	Cardiac ankyrin repeat, domain 1	DCM
NEXN	1p31.1	Nexilin	DCM, HCM
SYNPO2	4q26	Myopodin	
ZYX	7q34	Zyxin	
LMCD1	3p25.3	LIM and Cysteine-rich domains 1, Dyxin	
LDB3	10q23.2	LIM domain-binding 3, Cypher, ZASP	DCM, HCM, LVNC
ITGB1BP2	Xq13.1	Integrin, beta-1, binding protein of, melusin	
TTN	2q31.2	Titin	DCM, HCM
MYOZ2	4q26	Calsarcin/FATZ/Myozenin	HCM
DES	2q35	Desmin	DCM
PDLIM3	4q35.1	Actinin-associated LIM protein, ALP	
PDLIM7	5q35.3	Enigma	
PDLIM5	4q22.3	Enigma homolog, ENH	
PDLIM1	10q23.33	CLP36	
ILK	11p15.4	Integrin-linked kinase	
OBSCN	1q42.13	Obscurin	
PPP3CB	10q22.2	Calcineurin	

Table 1.
Cardiac Z-disk genes and associated cardiomyopathy phenotypes.

and (d) Cytoskeletal-nuclear connections (desmin, CARP, MLP, MYPN, zyxin, myopodin) [27]. The Z-disk linking all these mechanosensors, and the signaling pathways through α-actinin, desmin, MLP, filamin C, nebulette, myopalladin and CARP is involved in both, mechano-sensation and mechano-transduction [28]. This multifunctional role of the Z-disk places it in an ideal position to sense, integrate, and transduce biomechanical stretch and stress signals. Specifically, multiple upstream signals from the sarcomere as well as transmitted from the membrane converge on the Z-disk. Likewise, several components of downstream signaling, including *bona fide* signaling molecules such as kinases and phosphatases (including the phosphatase calcineurin and protein kinases like PKC) and their positive and negative modulators, are localized at or in immediate proximity of the Z-disk. Moreover, several Z-disk molecules (CARP, MLP, MYPN, zyxin) share the ability to shuttle to the nucleus, where they can act as transcriptional co-modulators [22].

3. The Z-disk "common final pathway" in cardiomyopathy

Cardiomyopathies are devastating diseases of the heart muscle with a significant percentage of inheritable cases, eventually resulting in congestive heart failure, transplant or sudden cardiac death [29]. Despite significant advances in the understanding of the major forms of cardiomyopathies and discovering the genetic causes of different forms of these disorders, in large part because of progresses in genetics, genomics and advanced cardiac imaging, over last 3 decades, no effective treatment has been established [30] with an increasing incidence and prevalence [31–33] and high cost [34, 35]. Types of CM are categorized by changes in cardiac chamber size, thickness ventricular walls and stiffness of the myocardium, and cardiac function [36, 37]. Dilated cardiomyopathy (DCM) is characterized by left ventricular (LV) chamber dilation and dysfunction in systolic performance; hypertrophic cardiomyopathy (HCM) is distinguished by ventricular myocardial hypertrophy and diastolic dysfunction. Restrictive cardiomyopathy (RCM) is distinguished by increased myocardial stiffness without significant ventricular myocardial hypertrophy and dilated atria as result of diastolic dysfunction [38]. Arrhythmogenic cardiomyopathy (ACM) is a subset of cardiomyopathies with a broad range of clinical presentations including early-onset arrhythmias including atrial fibrillation, conduction disturbances, and/or right ventricular (RV) and/or LV tachyarrhythmias with or without cardiac dysfunction [39, 40]. Left ventricular noncompaction cardiomyopathy (LVNC) is a heterogeneous group of disorders of ventricular myocardium characterized by presence of protuberant trabeculae and intra-trabecular recesses that are most noticeable in the LV apex, and compacted and noncompacted layers of the LV myocardium [37, 41, 42].

The "final common pathway" hypothesis first was described in the late 1990s aiming to elucidate the mechanisms of inherited cardiomyopathies and suggested that genes encoding proteins with similar functions and/or location or involved in the same pathway are responsible for a consistent cardiomyopathy phenotype with distinctive morpho/histological cardiac remodeling [43]. Further, disruption of a particular protein and related pathways may intersect with other intracellular and intercellular pathways, leading to an isolated or in an overlapping cardiomyopathy phenotype (**Figure 2**). The most common inheritance pattern in familial cardiomyopathies is autosomal dominant, whereas autosomal recessive, X-chromosome linked and mitochondrial inheritance is also reported, including in infantile cases [13, 20, 21].

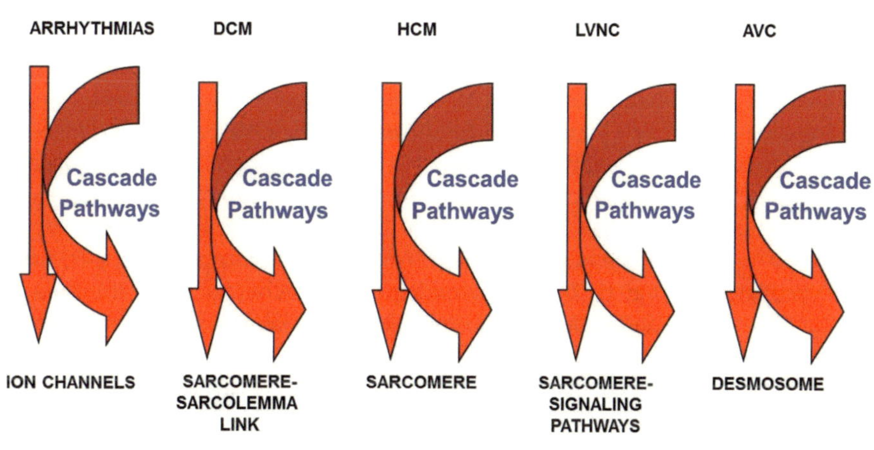

Figure 2.
"Final common pathway" hypothesis for arrhythmia disorders, dilated cardiomyopathy (DCM), hypertrophic cardiomyopathy (HCM) or restrictive cardiomyopathy, left ventricular noncompaction (LVNC), or arrhythmogenic ventricular cardiomyopathy (AVC or ACM).

Based on knowledge gained from genes encoding the proteins responsible for the functional myocardium, we can reasonably understand the physiology of the disease.

The sarcomere is the key unit for cardiac function. The Z-disk common pathway identified structure, function and pathway(s) involvement similarities of proteins encoded by genes affected by genetic insult and affects sarcomere function. The Z-disk genetic abnormalities appear to disturb the normal expression, structure, localization and function of their encoding proteins as well as the Z-disk structures in which it is integrated [3–7]. For instance, Z-disk mutations result in abnormal force generation and contractility resulting in HCM or RCM (*via* sarcomere disturbance), results in reduced force transmission causing DCM (*via* sarcolemmal-sarcomeric connections), in cardiac rhythm disorders (*via* connections with ion channels), and cell–cell contact disorders or ACMs (*via* desmosomal/intercalated disk connections). Therefore, the critical links between Z-disks are responsible for heterogeneous cardiomyopathy phenotypes originated from Z-disk abnormalities when the Z-disk link is disturbed. For instance, the Z-disk link most commonly disrupts sarcomeres (eg, the sarcomere in HCM when the mutated gene encodes a sarcomeric protein), but, in some instances, may disrupt its binding partner protein(s), which cause downstream disturbance of the "final common pathway" (eg, a Z-disk protein mutation may cause ACM as result of disrupted the cell–cell junction *via* an abnormal binding to desmin, which in turn interacts with desmoplakin at the desmosomes of the intercalated disks) (**Figure 1**).

While our classic "final common pathway" hypothesis led to a somewhat predictable gross clinical phenotype, it has become clear over the last decade that genes and proteins do not work in isolation. Gene expression is constructed on a complex combinations genes with other genes and their encoding proteins as well as the environment. Therefore, a genetic abnormality in a single causal gene does not completely determine a disease course; rather interactions of multiple genes, causal and modifiers (and their encoded proteins), may be required to explain diverse cardiomyopathy phenotypes [44, 45]. In particular, the modifier genes that alter the effect of causal gene(s) can influence the clinical and pathological variation in cardiomyopathies [44, 46, 47]. Thus, it is critical to recognize genetic and genomic networks rather than individual gene or individual pathway for complex diseases, such as cardiomyopathies, using systems genetics approaches [48].

4. Animal models of cardiac Z-disk pathology

Translational and comparative research involving animal modeling provides considerable and important benefits in inherited cardiomyopathies, because animal models enable not only the exploration and investigation of the pathological consequences on cellular, sub-cellular and molecular levels originating from the initial genetic defect, but also may closely simulate the specific cardiomyopathy phenotype seen in humans as the result of pathological cardiac remodeling. The complexity of disease-causing mechanisms and modulators of genetic cardiomyopathies [49] has been investigated by a variety of genetic modeling approaches including transgenic (TG), knockout (KO) and knock-in (KI) murine models [50]. In particular, with recent advances in CRISPR/Cas9 (clustered regularly interspaced short palindromic repeats/CRISPR associated 9) system approaches, researchers are able to achieve more effective and precise genome editing for animal modeling. This approach has been successfully used over other traditional methods for genetic editing such as transgenesis and homologous recombination targeting techniques because of its simplicity, design and efficiency in developing novel animal models [51–53]. Animal models

Z-disk gene	Human phenotype	Animal model	Animal phenotype	Pathogenesis/pathway/ proteins
Titin	DCM, HCM	zebrafish [54, 55]	cardiac edema, poor contraction	blockage of sarcomere assembly
Myopalladin	DCM, HCM, RCM	murine TG Y20C [56]	HCM and heart failure	desmin, DPS, Cx43 and vinculin disruption
MYPN	RCM	murine KI Q529X [57]	disrupted intercalated discs, heart failure	desmin, DSP, connexin43 and vinculin disruption
CARP	HCM, DCM	murine TG αMHC [58]	HCM in response to pressure overload stress	reduced TGF-β, ERK1/2, MEK and Smad3
CARP	HCM, DCM	murine KO [59]	No cardiac phenotype	
CSRP3 (MLP)	HCM	murine KI C58G [60]	HCM	protein depletion *via* Bag3 and proteasomal overload
MLP	DCM	murine KO [61]	DCM with hypertrophy and heart failure	altered mechano-sensation
MLP x MYBPC3	Varied CMs	Double KO [62]	DCM	increased Ca2+ sensitivity
Nebulette	DCM	murine TG [63]	DCM, mitochondrial abnormalities	stretch induced alteration of Z-disk assembly
Nexilin	DCM	zebrafish [64]	Z-disk damage, heart failure	stretch induced Z-disk destabilization
NEXN	DCM	KO [65]	DCM, EFE	collagen and elastin deposits
Telethonin	DCM	murine KO [66]	heart failure following biomechanical stress	modulation of nuclear p53 turnover after biomechanical stress
Telethonin	DCM	zebrafish [67]	deformed muscle structure and impaired swimming ability	disruption of sarcomere-T-tubules ILK
Cypher/ ZASP	DCM	murine KO [68]	DCM, Z disk disruption, muscle weakness	α-actinin or other Z-line components disruption
Filamin C	DCM, HCM	medaka zacrofish K1680X [69]	DCM, myocardial wall rupture	Disrupted structure of cardiac and skeletal muscles
ERBB2		murine Tg [70]	HCM, diastolic dysfunction	ErbB2 signaling
Calcineurin		*CnAβ* deficient mouse [71]	Impaired HCM response	NFATc4, ANF signaling to pressure overload

Table 2.
Animal models of Z-disk pathologies.

of Z-disk pathologies, summarized in **Table 2**, demonstrate that the prime Z-disk genetic defect can lead to perturbed cardiac function with heterogeneous cardiomyopathy phenotypes *via* different binding partners and pathways involved in the "final common pathway". The disturbed pathways include blockage of sarcomere assembly (titin), desmin, DPS, Cx43 and vinculin disruption (MYPN), reduced TGF-β signaling, downregulation in ERK1/2, MEK and Smad3 pathways (CARP), protein depletion *via* Bag3 and proteasomal overload, altered mechano-sensation and increased Ca2+ sensitivity (MLP), alteration of Z-disk assembly due to abnormal stretch and Z-disk destabilization (nebulette, nexilin), collagen and elastin deposits and biomechanical stress induced modulation of nuclear p53 turnover (telethonin), disruption of sarcomere-T-tubules connections and disturbance of ILK signaling (ZASP), or α-actinin or other Z-line and costamere component disruption (filamin C).

5. Conclusion

Cardiomyopathies are a group of complex multifaceted diseases that can originate from genetic insult to the heart muscle. The "final common pathway" hypothesis reviewed in this chapter provides the mechanisms in the development of cardiomyopathy phenotypes originated from cardiac Z-disk abnormalities. As the boundaries of the sarcomere, the Z-disk, is linked mechanically with many cellular compartments and the extracellular matrix *via* its multiple proteins and acts not only as a structural unit, but also is involved in contractile and mechanosensing signaling in the heart. Therefore, the nature of disturbed critical links of the Z-disks determine the cardiomyopathy phenotypes that develop.

Conflict of interest

The authors declare no conflict of interest.

Author details

Enkhsaikhan Purevjav* and Jeffrey A. Towbin
University of Tennessee Heart Science Center, Memphis, TN, USA

*Address all correspondence to: epurevja@uthsc.edu

References

[1] Schwartz SM, Duffy JY, Pearl JM, Nelson DP. Cellular and molecular aspects of myocardial dysfunction. Crit Care Med. 2001;29(10 Suppl): S214-9.

[2] Saffitz JE. Dependence of electrical coupling on mechanical coupling in cardiac myocytes. In: Thiene G, A.C. P, editors. Advances in Cardiovascular Medicine. Padova, Italy: Universita degli Studi di Padova Press; 2002.

[3] Squire JM. Architecture and function in the muscle sarcomere. Curr Opin Struct Biol. 1997;7(2):247-57.

[4] Gregorio CC, Antin PB. To the heart of myofibril assembly. Trends Cell Biol. 2000;10(9):355-62.

[5] Vigoreaux JO. The muscle Z band: lessons in stress management. J Muscle Res Cell Motil. 1994;15(3):237-55.

[6] Franzini-Armstrong C. The structure of a simple Z line. J Cell Biol. 1973;58(3):630-42.

[7] Clark KA, McElhinny AS, Beckerle MC, Gregorio CC. Striated Muscle Cytoarchitecture: An Intricate Web of Form and Function. Annu Rev Cell Dev Biol. 2002;18:637-706.

[8] Barth AI, Nathke IS, Nelson WJ. Cadherins, catenins and APC protein: interplay between cytoskeletal complexes and signaling pathways. Curr Opin Cell Biol. 1997;9(5):683-90.

[9] Burridge K, Chrzanowska-Wodnicka M. Focal adhesions, contractility, and signaling. Annu Rev Cell Dev Biol. 1996;12:463-518.

[10] Capetanaki Y. Desmin cytoskeleton in healthy and failing hearts. Heart Failure Reviews. 5. Amsterdam: Kluwer Academic Publishers; 2000. p. 203-20.

[11] Stewart M. Intermediate filament structure and assembly. Curr Opin Cell Biol. 1993;5(1):3-11.

[12] Straub V, Campbell KP. Muscular dystrophies and the dystrophin-glycoprotein complex. Curr Opin Neurol. 1997;10(2):168-75.

[13] Cohn RD, Campbell KP. Molecular basis of muscular dystrophies. Muscle Nerve. 2000;23(10):1456-71.

[14] Kucera JP, Rohr S, Rudy Y. Localization of sodium channels in intercalated disks modulates cardiac conduction. Circ Res. 2002;91(12):1176-82.

[15] Ribaux P, Bleicher F, Couble ML, Amsellem J, Cohen SA, Berthier C, et al. Voltage-gated sodium channel (SkM1) content in dystrophin-deficient muscle. Pflugers Arch. 2001;441(6):746-55.

[16] Furukawa T, Ono Y, Tsuchiya H, Katayama Y, Bang ML, Labeit D, et al. Specific interaction of the potassium channel beta-subunit minK with the sarcomeric protein T-cap suggests a T-tubule-myofibril linking system. J Mol Biol. 2001;313(4):775-84.

[17] Pyle WG, Solaro RJ. At the crossroads of myocardial signaling: the role of Z-discs in intracellular signaling and cardiac function. Circulation research. 2004;94(3):296-305.

[18] Luther PK. Three-dimensional structure of a vertebrate muscle Z-band: implications for titin and alpha-actinin binding. J Struct Biol. 2000;129(1):1-16.

[19] Luther PK. The vertebrate muscle Z-disc: sarcomere anchor for structure and signalling. Journal of muscle research and cell motility. 2009;30(5-6):171-85.

[20] Hoshijima M. Mechanical stress-strain sensors embedded in cardiac

cytoskeleton: Z disk, titin, and associated structures. AJP: Heart and Circulatory Physiology. 2005;290(4):H1313-H25.

[21] Hoshijima M. Mechanical stress-strain sensors embedded in cardiac cytoskeleton: Z disk, titin, and associated structures. Am J Physiol Heart Circ Physiol. 2006;290(4): H1313-25.

[22] Buyandelger B, Ng KE, Miocic S, Gunkel S, Piotrowska I, Ku CH, et al. Genetics of mechanosensation in the heart. J Cardiovasc Transl Res. 2011;4(3):238-44.

[23] Dostal DE, Feng H, Nizamutdinov D, Golden HB, Afroze SH, Dostal JD, et al. Mechanosensing and Regulation of Cardiac Function. J Clin Exp Cardiolog. 2014;5(6):314.

[24] Ward ML, Williams IA, Chu Y, Cooper PJ, Ju YK, Allen DG. Stretch-activated channels in the heart: contributions to length-dependence and to cardiomyopathy. Prog Biophys Mol Biol. 2008;97(2-3):232-49.

[25] Valencik ML, Zhang D, Punske B, Hu P, McDonald JA, Litwin SE. Integrin activation in the heart: a link between electrical and contractile dysfunction? Circ Res. 2006;99(12):1403-10.

[26] Miller MK, Granzier H, Ehler E, Gregorio CC. The sensitive giant: the role of titin-based stretch sensing complexes in the heart. Trends Cell Biol. 2004;14(3):119-26.

[27] Wilson KL. Cytoskeletal and nuclear ("nucleoskeletal") intermediate filaments and disease. Mol Biol Cell. 2011;22(6):725.

[28] Frank D, Frey N. Cardiac Z-disc signaling network. J Biol Chem. 2011;286(12):9897-904.

[29] Towbin JA. Inherited cardiomyopathies. Circ J. 2014;78(10):2347-56.

[30] Cahill TJ, Ashrafian H, Watkins H. Genetic cardiomyopathies causing heart failure. Circ Res. 2013;113(6):660-75.

[31] Arola A, Jokinen E, Ruuskanen O, Saraste M, Pesonen E, Kuusela AL, et al. Epidemiology of idiopathic cardiomyopathies in children and adolescents. A nationwide study in Finland. Am J Epidemiol. 1997;146(5):385-93.

[32] Arola A, Tuominen J, Ruuskanen O, Jokinen E. Idiopathic dilated cardiomyopathy in children: prognostic indicators and outcome. Pediatrics. 1998;101(3 Pt 1):369-76.

[33] Lipshultz SE, Sleeper LA, Towbin JA, Lower AM, Orav EJ, Cox GF, et al. The incidence of pediatric cardiomyopathy in two geographic regions of the United States: The prospective Pediatric Cardiomyopaty Registry. New England Journal of Medicine. 2003;In Press.

[34] Evans RW. Socioeconomic aspects of heart transplantation. Curr Opin Cardiol. 1995;10(2):169-79.

[35] O'Connell JB, Bristow MR. Economic impact of heart failure in the United States: time for a different approach. J Heart Lung Transplant. 1994;13(4):S107-12.

[36] Towbin JA, Bowles NE. The failing heart. Nature. 2002;415(6868):227-33.

[37] Maron BJ, Towbin JA, Thiene G, Antzelevitch C, Corrado D, Arnett D, et al. Contemporary definitions and classification of the cardiomyopathies: an American Heart Association Scientific Statement from the Council on Clinical Cardiology, Heart Failure and Transplantation Committee; Quality of Care and Outcomes Research

and Functional Genomics and Translational Biology Interdisciplinary Working Groups; and Council on Epidemiology and Prevention. Circulation. 2006;113(14):1807-16.

[38] Hershberger RE, Cowan J, Morales A, Siegfried JD. Progress with genetic cardiomyopathies: screening, counseling, and testing in dilated, hypertrophic, and arrhythmogenic right ventricular dysplasia/cardiomyopathy. Circ Heart Fail. 2009;2(3):253-61.

[39] Towbin JA, McKenna WJ, Abrams DJ, Ackerman MJ, Calkins H, Darrieux FCC, et al. 2019 HRS expert consensus statement on evaluation, risk stratification, and management of arrhythmogenic cardiomyopathy. Heart Rhythm. 2019.

[40] Marcus FI, Fontaine GH, Guiraudon G, Frank R, Laurenceau JL, Malergue C, et al. Right ventricular dysplasia: a report of 24 adult cases. Circulation. 1982;65(2):384-98.

[41] Ichida F. Left ventricular noncompaction - Risk stratification and genetic consideration. J Cardiol. 2020;75(1):1-9.

[42] Towbin JA. Left ventricular noncompaction: a new form of heart failure. Heart Fail Clin. 2010;6(4): 453-69, viii.

[43] Bowles NE, Bowles KR, Towbin JA. The "final common pathway" hypothesis and inherited cardiovascular disease. The role of cytoskeletal proteins in dilated cardiomyopathy. Herz. 2000;25(3):168-75.

[44] Marian AJ. Modifier genes for hypertrophic cardiomyopathy. Curr Opin Cardiol. 2002;17(3):242-52.

[45] Sweet M, Taylor MR, Mestroni L. Diagnosis, prevalence, and screening of familial dilated cardiomyopathy. Expert Opin Orphan Drugs. 2015;3(8):869-76.

[46] Brugada R, Kelsey W, Lechin M, Zhao G, Yu QT, Zoghbi W, et al. Role of candidate modifier genes on the phenotypic expression of hypertrophy in patients with hypertrophic cardiomyopathy. J Investig Med. 1997;45(9):542-51.

[47] Chung MW, Tsoutsman T, Semsarian C. Hypertrophic cardiomyopathy: from gene defect to clinical disease. Cell Res. 2003;13(1):9-20.

[48] Gu Q, Mendsaikhan U, Khuchua Z, Jones BC, Lu L, Towbin JA, et al. Dissection of Z-disc myopalladin gene network involved in the development of restrictive cardiomyopathy using system genetics approach. World J Cardiol. 2017;9(4):320-31.

[49] Houser SR, Margulies KB, Murphy AM, Spinale FG, Francis GS, Prabhu SD, et al. Animal models of heart failure: a scientific statement from the American Heart Association. Circ Res. 2012;111(1):131-50.

[50] Duncker DJ, Bakkers J, Brundel BJ, Robbins J, Tardiff JC, Carrier L. Animal and in silico models for the study of sarcomeric cardiomyopathies. Cardiovasc Res. 2015;105(4):439-48.

[51] Doudna JA, Charpentier E. Genome editing. The new frontier of genome engineering with CRISPR-Cas9. Science. 2014;346(6213):1258096.

[52] Hsu PD, Lander ES, Zhang F. Development and applications of CRISPR-Cas9 for genome engineering. Cell. 2014;157(6):1262-78.

[53] Suzuki K, Tsunekawa Y, Hernandez-Benitez R, Wu J, Zhu J, Kim EJ, et al. In vivo genome editing via CRISPR/Cas9 mediated homology-independent targeted integration. Nature. 2016;540(7631):144-9.

[54] Song Y, Xu J, Li Y, Jia C, Ma X, Zhang L, et al. Cardiac ankyrin repeat

protein attenuates cardiac hypertrophy by inhibition of ERK1/2 and TGF-beta signaling pathways. PLoS One. 2012;7(12):e50436.

[55] Xu X, Meiler SE, Zhong TP, Mohideen M, Crossley DA, Burggren WW, et al. Cardiomyopathy in zebrafish due to mutation in an alternatively spliced exon of titin. Nat Genet. 2002;30(2):205-9.

[56] Bang ML, Gu Y, Dalton ND, Peterson KL, Chien KR, Chen J. The muscle ankyrin repeat proteins CARP, Ankrd2, and DARP are not essential for normal cardiac development and function at basal conditions and in response to pressure overload. PLoS One. 2014;9(4):e93638.

[57] Ehsan M, Kelly M, Hooper C, Yavari A, Beglov J, Bellahcene M, et al. Mutant Muscle LIM Protein C58G causes cardiomyopathy through protein depletion. Journal of molecular and cellular cardiology. 2018;121:287-96.

[58] Zhou Q, Chu PH, Huang C, Cheng CF, Martone ME, Knoll G, et al. Ablation of Cypher, a PDZ-LIM domain Z-line protein, causes a severe form of congenital myopathy. J Cell Biol. 2001;155(4):605-12.

[59] LL Sr, Bedja D, Sysa-Shah P, Liu H, Maxwell A, Yi X, et al. Echo cardiographic Characterization of a Murine Model of Hypertrophic Obstructive Cardiomyopathy Induced by Cardiac-specific Overexpression of Epidermal Growth Factor Receptor 2. Comparative medicine. 2016;66(4):268-77.

[60] Fujita M, Mitsuhashi H, Isogai S, Nakata T, Kawakami A, Nonaka I, et al. Filamin C plays an essential role in the maintenance of the structural integrity of cardiac and skeletal muscles, revealed by the medaka mutant zacro. Dev Biol. 2012;361(1):79-89.

[61] Purevjav E, Arimura T, Augustin S, Huby AC, Takagi K, Nunoda S, et al. Molecular basis for clinical heterogeneity in inherited cardiomyopathies due to myopalladin mutations. Hum Mol Genet. 2012;21(9):2039-53.

[62] Huby AC, Mendsaikhan U, Takagi K, Martherus R, Wansapura J, Gong N, et al. Disturbance in Z-disk mechanosensitive proteins induced by a persistent mutant myopalladin causes familial restrictive cardiomyopathy. J Am Coll Cardiol. 2014;64(25):2765-76.

[63] Arber S, Hunter JJ, Ross J, Jr., Hongo M, Sansig G, Borg J, et al. MLP-deficient mice exhibit a disruption of cardiac cytoarchitectural organization, dilated cardiomyopathy, and heart failure. Cell. 1997;88(3): 393-403.

[64] Li J, Gresham KS, Mamidi R, Doh CY, Wan X, Deschenes I, et al. Sarcomere-based genetic enhancement of systolic cardiac function in a murine model of dilated cardiomyopathy. International journal of cardiology. 2018;273:168-76.

[65] Purevjav E, Varela J, Morgado M, Kearney DL, Li H, Taylor MD, et al. Nebulette mutations are associated with dilated cardiomyopathy and endocardial fibroelastosis. J Am Coll Cardiol. 2010;56(18):1493-502.

[66] Maiellaro-Rafferty K, Wansapura JP, Mendsaikhan U, Osinska H, James JF, Taylor MD, et al. Altered regional cardiac wall mechanics are associated with differential cardiomyocyte calcium handling due to nebulette mutations in preclinical inherited dilated cardiomyopathy. J Mol Cell Cardiol. 2013;60:151-60.

[67] Hassel D, Dahme T, Erdmann J, Meder B, Huge A, Stoll M, et al. Nexilin

mutations destabilize cardiac Z-disks and lead to dilated cardiomyopathy. Nat Med. 2009;15(11):1281-8.

[68] Aherrahrou Z, Schlossarek S, Stoelting S, Klinger M, Geertz B, Weinberger F, et al. Knock-out of nexilin in mice leads to dilated cardiomyopathy and endomyocardial fibroelastosis. Basic research in cardiology. 2016;111(1):6.

[69] Bueno OF, Wilkins BJ, Tymitz KM, Glascock BJ, Kimball TF, Lorenz JN, et al. Impaired cardiac hypertrophic response in Calcineurin Abeta -deficient mice. Proc Natl Acad Sci U S A. 2002;99(7):4586-91.

[70] Knoll R, Linke WA, Zou P, Miocic S, Kostin S, Buyandelger B, et al. Telethonin deficiency is associated with maladaptation to biomechanical stress in the mammalian heart. Circ Res. 2011;109(7):758-69.

[71] Zhang R, Yang J, Zhu J, Xu X. Depletion of zebrafish Tcap leads to muscular dystrophy via disrupting sarcomere-membrane interaction, not sarcomere assembly. Hum Mol Genet. 2009;18(21):4130-40.

Section 3

Arrhythmogenic Cardiomyopathy

Chapter 8

Update on Genes Associated with Arrhythmogenic Cardiomyopathy

Marta Vallverdú-Prats, Mireia Alcalde, Georgia Sarquella-Brugada, Sergi Cesar, Elena Arbelo, Josep Brugada, Ramon Brugada and Oscar Campuzano

Abstract

Arrhythmogenic cardiomyopathy is a rare genetic entity characterized by progressive fibro-fatty replacement of myocardium leading to malignant arrhythmias, syncope, and sudden cardiac death. Mostly it affects the right ventricle, but cases have also been described with biventricular and even isolated left ventricular involvement. The disease affects mainly young males and arrhythmias are usually induced by exercise. Arrhythmogenic cardiomyopathy has a genetic origin and is basically caused by deleterious alterations in genes encoding desmosomal proteins, especially plakophilin-2. To date, more than 400 rare genetic alterations have been identified in 18 genes, mainly with autosomal dominant inheritance, but some recessive forms have also been reported (Naxos disease and Carvajal syndrome). A comprehensive genetic analysis identifies a rare variant as potential cause of the disease in around 60% of patients, suggesting the existence of unknown genes as well as other genome alterations not yet discovered. Genetic interpretation classifies some of these rare variants as ambiguous, playing an uncertain role in arrhythmogenic cardiomyopathy. This makes a proper translation of genetic data into clinical practice difficult. Moreover, incomplete penetrance and variable phenotypic expression makes it difficult to arrive at the correct diagnosis. In the present chapter, we focus on recent advances in the knowledge regarding the genetic basis of arrhythmogenic cardiomyopathy.

Keywords: sudden cardiac death, Arrhythmogenic cardiomyopathy, arrhythmias, genetics, desmosome

1. Introduction

Arrhythmogenic cardiomyopathy (ACM), (Online Mendelian Inheritance in Man -OMIM- 107970) is a rare (prevalence 1:2500–5000) inheritable structural heart disease first described by Fontaine *et al* in 1978 [1]. ACM is characterized by progressive replacement of myocardium by fibro-fatty infiltrates, predominantly of the right ventricle (RV) [2], but biventricular forms have also been reported in nearly 50% of cases [3, 4]. Moreover, isolated forms affecting only the left ventricle have been reported in 15% of cases [5, 6]. The name of this disease has been changed over the last years as the knowledge of it has been increased. First, it was called arrhythmogenic right ventricular dysplasia (ARVD), but some studies revealed that patients had normal hearts at birth and the disease was progressive and genetically determined [4]. For this reason, from that moment on, it was called arrhythmogenic right ventricular cardiomyopathy (ARVC). However, when it was obvious that this disease not only affects the RV but that it also can affect the LV or even both ventricles, it was necessary to modify its name to ACM. The heart tissue affected in ACM patients shows localized/diffuse atrophy with progressive fibro-fatty infiltration. These structural alterations are assessed by echocardiography, cardiac magnetic resonance, angiography, and biopsy of the myocardial wall, if necessary. Structural alterations in the myocardium are responsible for electrical abnormalities, with or without impaired mechanical function, subsequent ventricular arrhythmias, syncope and even sudden cardiac death (SCD) [7, 8]. Unfortunately, SCD is often the first symptom of the disease, usually during exercise in young males (less than 35-year-old). Despite both genders being affected, males are the main affected population (the ratio of men to women is 3:1) [9].

ACM is a cardiac disease with a clearly genetic implication, and pathogenic alterations in genes encoding desmosomal proteins are the main cause of the disease. In recent years, continuous advances in the genetic and molecular basis of ACM are occurring despite some pathophysiological mechanisms involved in ACM being not yet completely understood [10]. For example, it has been shown that myocardial inflammation is a common trait in ACM patients, but it is not clear if it is a primary phenomenon or reactive to ACM pathology [4, 11, 12]. The fibrosis mechanism is another characteristic hallmark poorly understood so far. It has been described a complex network of interactions between cytokines, growth factors, and hormones that promote cardiac fibrosis [12, 13]. One thing that seems certain is that canonical and non-canonical TGFβ signaling pathway are both involved in the induction of myocardial fibrosis in ACM [12]. The origin of adipocytes in the myocardium of ACM patients is not yet resolved today. Thus, it is not clear if the signals for adipogenesis are autonomous to desmosome-expressing cells (intracellular signal) or non-autonomous from desmosome-expressing cells to adipogenic cell (paracrine signal) [12]. However, several signaling pathways have been described that are involved in the adipogenic phenotype of ACM such as WNT, Hippo–Yes-associated protein (YAP), peroxisome proliferator-activated receptor-γ (PPARγ) and microRNA (miRNA) signaling [12].

Currently, clinical diagnosis is based on the presence of a series of diagnostic items (major and minor) called Task Force criteria. It was firstly proposed in 1994 [14], but it was revised in 2010 to improve diagnostic sensitivity maintaining its specificity and included genetics as a diagnostic item [15]. Nowadays it takes into account structural assessment (echocardiography, magnetic resonance, RV angiography), histological (endomyocardial biopsy), electrocardiographic (12-lead ECG and Signal-Averaged ECG, Holter monitoring, exercise testing, electrophysiological study), and familial factors (genetic study according to the Rhythm Society/European Heart Rhythm Association Consensus Statement) [16]. Recently, it has been proposed "The Padua Criteria", a new diagnostic criteria based on 2010 TFC multi-parametric approach to include biventricular and arrhythmogenic left ventricular cardiomyopathy (ALVC) involvement [4, 17]. However, it has to be validated by future clinical studies in large cohorts of ACM patients. The diagnosis of ACM is confirmed if 2 major, 1 major and 2 minor, or 4 minor criteria from different categories are present. A borderline diagnosis is considered with 1 major and 1 minor or 3 minor criterions from different categories and a possible diagnosis with only 1 major or 2 minor criterions. The disease can be classified into four phases:

- The early "*silent phase*" that can manifest as SCD because arrhythmias occur without structural abnormalities;

- The "*overt electrical disorder*" in which RV arrhythmias are associated with structural abnormalities;
- The "*phase of right ventricular failure*" with extension of the fibro-fatty substitution that leads to RV dysfunction; and,
- The phase of "*biventricular failure*" which is often indistinguishable from dilated cardiomyopathy (DCM).

The diagnostic tools are evolving together with the knowledge of the disease because detecting ACM at an early stage is crucial for the patient. All the treatment approaches are focused on preventing life-threatening arrhythmias, delay the course of the heart failure, and relieve symptoms [12]. The different options include pharmacological treatment, the placement of an implantable cardioverter-defibrillator (ICD), radiofrequency ablation, and even heart transplantation in severe cases at high risk of death. To date, ICD is the only proven lifesaving therapy; other treatment options may reduce the arrhythmic burden and alleviate symptoms, without evident impact on prevention of SCD [18]. There are some studies that have demonstrated the efficacy of ICD therapy in the prevention of SCD in patients affected by ACM [19–22]. However, it is associated with a significant morbidity due to device-related complications and inappropriate ICD interventions [1]. Decisions about the placement of an ICD are based on an estimated patient risk of SCD that is determined by several parameters including electrical instability, proband status, extent of structural disease, cardiac syncope, male gender, exercise practice, and deleterious genetic alterations. Unfortunately, there are no conclusive data concerning risk stratification or the best approach in patients with ACM, so treatment should be personalized [23].

2. Genetic basis

ACM can be caused by deleterious alterations located in genes encoding mainly desmosomal proteins but also proteins implicated in electric signal transmission. A comprehensive genetic analysis of all genes reported so far identify at least one rare variant as a potential cause of ACM in around 60% of the patients [24]. Genetic testing allows cascade screening of relatives identifying other genetic carriers in the family, which may be at risk of developing the disease and suffer SCD [25]. Predominantly, ACM follows an autosomal dominant pattern of inheritance, with incomplete and age-related penetrance [26] as well as polymorphic phenotypic expression [9, 27]. Autosomal recessive forms have also been reported although in a reduced number of cases (Naxos disease and Carvajal syndrome) [28–30]. In recent years, compound and/or digenic variants have been identified associated with ACM [31, 32]. In addition, alterations in number of copies (Copy Number Variation, CNV) were also associated with ACM [33]. Despite these recent advances, around 35–50% of ACM patients remain without an identified disease-associated variant [12]. For this reason, the interpretation of rare variants found in ACM patients has to be extremely careful. The "American College of Medical Genetics and Genomics (ACMG) standards and guidelines" structured a standard terminology for classifying sequence variants using available evidence weighted according to a system developed through expert opinion, work-group consensus, and community input [34]. This classification of the variants is composed of 5 terms: "pathogenic", "likely pathogenic", "uncertain significance", "likely benign", and "benign" and the classification depends on several different criteria: the variant frequency in population database, computational (*in silico*) predictive programs, biological factors (levels of expression in the tissue, function of the gene,...), localization of the variant in conserved regions or hotspots, type of mutation, functional studies and segregation analyses. It is important to remark that a large part of the rare genetic variants identified as potentially disease-causing remains of inconclusive significance after a comprehensive genetic interpretation. It is crucial to clarify their clinical role whether definitive risk stratification can be based on genetics. Even if a conclusive pathogenic variation associated with ACM is identified, it does not indicate that the patient is going to be affected because of the variable expressivity and incomplete penetrance [4]. This represents an additional challenge to perform a genetic interpretation of rare variants. Moreover, it is known that genes associated with ACM have nearly 50% of genetic variation rate [35]. Therefore, clinical translation should be done carefully after a comprehensive personalized interpretation of all data obtained. A group of experts should discuss all data concerning each family, performing an exhaustive interpretation and translation into clinical practice helping to adopt personalized measures to reduce risk of lethal events.

In the human myocardium, three different structures are involved in cell-to-cell adhesion: desmosomes, adherens junctions (*fascia adherens*), and gap junctions. The majority of ACM patients present alterations in genes encoding desmosomal proteins. Currently, more than 1000 rare genetic variants have been identified in 18 genes, but only around 400 rare genetic alterations have been classified as definitely pathogenic [36]. All other rare variants remain with an ambiguous role and further data is needed to conclude if they play a decisive role in ACM. **Table 1** shows information related to the genetic role and ventricular involvement of the ACM causal genes (plakophilin-2 -*PKP2*-, desmocollin-2 -*DSC2*-, desmoglein-2 -*DSG2*-, desmoplakin -*DSP*-, plakoglobin -*JUP*-, desmin -*DES*-, transforming growth factor beta-3 -*TGFβ3*-, transmembrane protein 43 -*TMEM43*-, lamin A/C -*LMNA*-, titin -*TTN*-, phospholamban -*PLN*-, αT-catenin -*CTNNA3*-, voltage-gated sodium channel -*SCN5A*-, Cadherin 2 -*CDH2*-, Filamin C -*FLNC*-, Ryanodine Receptor 2 -*RYR2*-, RNA-Binding Motif Protein 20 -*RBM20*-, Tight Junction Protein ZO-1 -*TJP1*-) [4, 11]. **Figure 1** presents the intracellular localization of proteins codified by ACM-associated genes and their prevalence in causing the disease.

2.1 Desmosomal genes

Desmosomes are classified as a calcium-dependent anchoring junction that tethers cells together through its extracellular contacts and internally links to the intermediate filament (IF) cytoskeleton [37]. This cell union provide structural resilience that allows heart tissue to resist mechanical stress. Moreover, it has been described that desmosomal proteins have a role in the regulation of transcription of genes involved in adipogenesis and apoptosis, and play a major role in myocardial electrical conduction through regulation of gap junctions and calcium homeostasis [4]. Deleterious alterations are mainly located in genes encoding desmosomal proteins that are responsible for around 60% of all ACM cases [4, 17]. Concretely, the main gene associated with ACM is *PKP2*, being responsible for approximately 35–40% of cases [35, 38, 39]. Pathogenic variants in *PKP2* are found in around 75% of genotype-positive ACM cases in American cohorts, and nearly 60% of genotype-positive index cases in European cohorts [4, 40]. In general, rare variants in genes encoding desmosomal proteins are more associated with right ventricular involvement. However, rare deleterious alterations in *DSP* are often associated with left ventricular involvement, and *DSG2* and *PKP2* with biventricular ACM, although the latter is observed in all gene groups at later stages of disease progression [4, 9].

Gene	Protein	Frequency (%)*	Inheritance Pattern	Ventricular Disease**
Desmosome				
PKP2	plakophilin-2	19–46	AD/AR	RV, BIV
DSP	desmoplakin	1–16	AD/AR	LV, BIV
DSG2	desmoglein-2	2.5–10	AD/AR	RV, LV, BIV
DSC2	desmocollin-2	1–8	AD	RV, BIV
JUP	plakoglobin	Rare	AD/AR	RV, BIV
Adherens junction				
CTNNA3	αT-catenin	Rare	AD	RV, BIV
CDH2	cadherin 2	Rare	AD	RV, BIV
TJP1	tight Junction Protein ZO-1	Rare	AD	?
Cytoskeletal structure				
LMNA	lamin A/C	Rare	AD	LV, BIV
DES	desmin	Rare	AD	LV, BIV
FLNC	filamin C	Rare	AD	LV, BIV
TMEM43	transmembrane protein 43	Rare	AD	RV, BIV
TTN	titin	Rare	AD	RV, LV, BIV
Ion transport				
SCN5A	voltage-gated sodium channel	Rare	AD	LV, BIV
RYR2	ryanodine Receptor 2	Rare	AD	?
PLN	phospholamban	Rare	AD	LV, BIV
Cytokine				
TGFB3	transforming growth factor, beta-3	Rare	AD	RV
Slicing factor				
RBM20	RNA-Binding Motif Protein 20	Rare	AD	LV

Taken from Austin et al. (2019) [51].
**Taken from Patel et al. (2020) [4].*
? = Not conclusive association with ACM. AD = autosomal dominant; AR = autosomal recessive; BIV = biventricular disease; LV = left ventricle; RV = right ventricle.

Table 1.
Genes associated with ACM.

2.1.1 Plakophilin-2

The most prevalent form of ACM is caused by rare pathogenic alterations in the *PKP2* gene (ENSG00000057294), which encode plakophilin-2 protein (PKP2, ENSP00000070846). It is an essential armadillo repeat protein located in the outer dense plaque of cardiac desmosomes that interacts with multiple other cell adhesion proteins [41]. To date, more than 300 rare genetic variants potentially pathogenic have been identified in *PKP2* [42]. Most of the ACM-linked pathogenic variants in the *PKP2* gene have an autosomal dominant pattern of inheritance, even though recessive form was also described in 2006 [30]. Lately, calcium handling dysregulation caused by disruption of *PKP2 has been described* [43]. It seems that *PKP2* is necessary to maintain transcription of genes that control intracellular calcium cycling. This could be the cause of life-threatening arrhythmias even in the absence of structural disease in those patients that present alterations in *PKP2*, which are the majority of ACM patients.

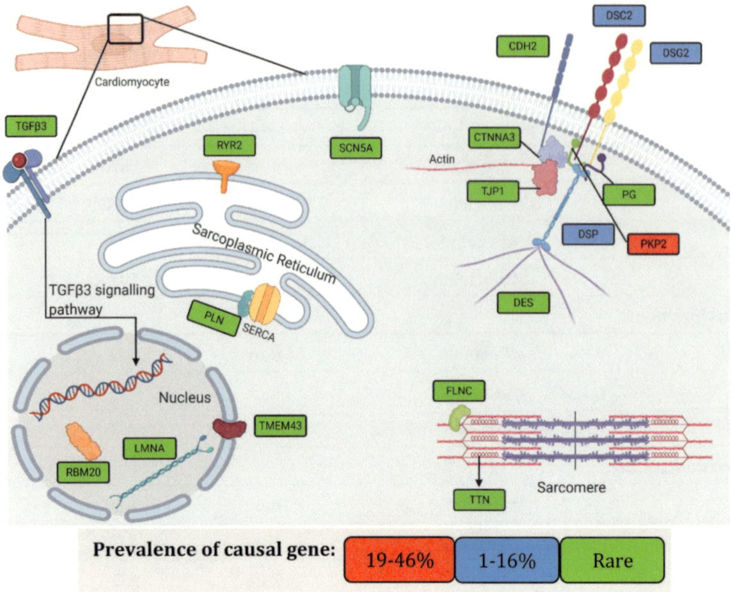

Figure 1.
Schematic representation of the intracellular localization of proteins codified by genes associated with ACM. Created with BioRender.com

2.1.2 Desmoplakin

Desmoplakin is the most abundant protein of the desmosomes, encoded by the *DSP* gene (ENSG00000096696). Desmoplakin has two isoforms produced by alternative splicing: the longest desmoplakin I isoform (ENSP00000369129) and the shorter desmoplakin II (ENSP00000396591). Desmoplakin isoform I has been reported to be a force constituent of desmosomes and the major isoform present in cardiac tissue, even though expression of isoform II (DSPII) occurs in different heart compartments [44]. Nowadays, almost 250 rare variations in the *DSP* gene have been linked to ACM [42], mainly with autosomal dominant pattern of inheritance. The *DSP* gene was also implicated in Carvajal syndrome, an autosomal recessive cardiocutaneous form of ACM that was described as a variant of Naxos disease (see below, plakoglobin section) [45].

2.1.3 Desmocollin-2 and Desmoglein-2

The desmosomal cadherins proteins, such as desmocollin and desmoglein are the major constituents of the desmosomal plaque. The *DSG2* gene (ENSG0000046604) encodes Desmoglein-2 protein (DSG2, ENSP00000261590) that has four extracellular cadherin domains and a transmembrane domain. Currently, more than 150 rare variants have been associated to ACM [42]. Despite the fact that most of the identified *DSG2* mutations have a dominant pattern of inheritance, a recessive pattern has been also suggested in ACM patients [46]. The *DSC2* gene (ENSG00000134755) encodes the desmocollin protein type 2 (DSC2, ENSP00000280904), the most widely distributed form of desmocollin proteins [47]. It is a type I integral membrane glycoprotein with four conserved extracellular subdomains, variable extracellular anchor domain, a single transmembrane domain, an intracellular anchor domain, and additional cytoplasmatic subdomains. It participates in calcium-dependent cell adhesion, regulation of tissue morphogenesis and intracellular signaling processes [48]. To date, nearly 120 genetic alterations have been identified in *DSC2* associated with ACM following an autosomal pattern of inheritance [42].

2.1.4 Plakoglobin

The plakoglobin protein (PG, ENSP00000311113) is codified by the *JUP* gene (ENSG00000173801). PG is a major protein component of cell adhesion junctions, and the only constituent common to submembranous plaques of both desmosomes and adherens junctions. It plays a crucial role in linking the desmosomal cadherins to the cytoskeleton via desmoplakin. The first genetic alteration associated with ACM was an homozygous deletion in the *JUP* gene, with an autosomal recessive pattern of inheritance [28]. In later years, it was referred to as "Naxos disease" [49]. To date, more than 30 rare genetic variants have been identified in *JUP* [42], including homozygous variants [50].

2.2 Non-desmosomal genes

This group includes genes encoding proteins of cytoskeletal architecture, calcium handling, sodium transport, and cytokine signaling among others. All of them have a diverse range of biological functions, but a pathogenic alterations in them can converge into similar phenotypes [51]. Genetic defects in non-desmosomal genes are thought to be more frequently associated with involvement of the left ventricle compared with rare variants in desmosomal genes that, in general, are more often associated with RV involvement [4]. There are several rare deleterious alterations in non-desmosomal genes that cause ACM that are also involved in other cardiac diseases such as DCM, Brugada syndrome (BrS), Long QT syndrome (LQTS) or Catecholaminergic Polymorphic Ventricular Tachycardia (CPVT). Thereby, in some cases, there is an overlap of symptoms that makes it challenging to determine the correct diagnosis. For this reason, it is necessary to perform more studies of genotype–phenotype correlation to increase the reliability of the diagnosis.

2.2.1 Desmin

The *DES* gene (ENSG00000175084) encodes the protein desmin (DES, ENSP00000363071) that is the main intermediate filament in mature skeletal and heart muscle cells. It forms a scaffold around the Z-disc and links whole contractile structure with subsarcolemmal cytoskeleton, intercalated disc, nucleus, and other components of the cytoplasm. Currently, less than 10 rare variants in this gene have been associated with ACM [42, 52, 53].

2.2.2 Transforming growth factor, beta-3

The *TGFβ3* gene (ENSG00000119699) encodes the transforming growth factor, beta-3 protein (TGFβ3, ENSP00000238682), a cytokine that stimulates fibrosis and modulates cell adhesion and expression of desmosomal genes [54]. To date, there are only 4 rare alterations located in *TGFβ3* as potential causes of ACM.

2.2.3 Transmembrane protein 43

The *TMEM43* gene (ENSG00000170876) encodes the transmembrane protein 43 (TMEM43, ENSP00000303992). It has an important role in maintaining nuclear envelope structure by organizing protein complexes at the inner nuclear membrane. Moreover, it has been suggested to have a role in an adipogenic pathway [55]. To date, around 15 ACM associated rare variants in *TMEM43* has been identified [42], one of them (p.S358L) exhibits an aggressive phenotype presenting with a fully penetrant, biventricular ACM with LV predominance and a high predilection for SCD in males [4, 55–57].

2.2.4 Lamin A/C

The *LMNA* gene (ENSG00000160789) encodes lamin A (ENSP00000357283) and lamin C (ENSP00000357284), by alternative splicing. Both of them belong to the family of type V intermediate filaments that take part in the constitution of the nuclear lamina, a complex of proteins below the inner part of the nuclear membrane [58]. Genetic alterations in *LMNA* are associated with an heterogeneous group of disorders commonly named "laminopathies" [59], including cardiac disorders with DCM as the main disease. In 2012, the first association between this gene and ACM was reported [60]. To date, nearly 25 rare variants have been described in *LMNA* associated with ACM [42].

2.2.5 Titin

The *TTN* gene (ENSG00000155657) encodes the titin protein (TTN, ENSP00000343764) that is a giantic and the third most abundant protein in the muscle after actin and myosin. It is an essential component of the sarcomere linking myosin and the Z-disc, providing structural support, flexibility, and stability [4]. This gene has been associated with cardiac diseases, mainly DCM. In 2011 the first variant associated with ACM was reported [61]. To date, more than 20 rare variants have been associated with ACM [42]. Most of these variants remain as potentially pathogenic, with doubtful role due to lack of conclusive genotype–phenotype studies.

2.2.6 Phospholamban

The *PLN* gene (ENSG00000198523) encodes the protein phospholamban (PLN, ENSP00000350132), a small phosphoprotein closely associated with the cardiac sarcoplasmic reticulum. It is a regulator of the sarcoplasmic reticulum Ca^{2+} (SERCA2a) pump in cardiac muscle and therefore important for maintaining Ca^{2+} homeostasis [62]. Consequently, the PLN protein is one of the major determinants of cardiac contractility and relaxation [63]. To date, only one rare pathogenic variant associated with ACM has been identified in this gene [42, 64].

2.2.7 Alpha T-catenin

The *CTNNA3* gene (ENSG00000183230) encodes the protein αT-catenin (CTNNA3, ENSP00000389714). Alpha T-catenin protein is located within the area composite of intercalated discs of cardiomyocytes. It is a key element for dynamic maintenance of tissue morphogenesis by integrating in the cadherin–catenin complex. In 2013, genetic variants of potentially pathogenic significance were identified in two unrelated patients suffering from ACM [42, 65]. Moreover, it has been shown that *CTNNA3* knockout mice exhibit a progressive cardiomyopathy with increased incidence of ventricular arrhythmias after acute ischemia [4, 66]. To date, no other rare variants associated with ACM have been identified in this gene.

2.2.8 Voltage-gated sodium channel

The *SCN5A* gene (ENSG00000183873) encodes for the cardiac sodium channel, voltage-gated, type V, alpha subunit (SCN5A, ENSP00000410257). This gene is mainly associated with BrS and LQTS but it was also reported in patients diagnosed with ACM [67]. Recently, a study suggested that almost 2% of ACM patients harbor rare *SCN5A* variants [68]. In total, for the moment, no more than 10 *SCN5A* rare variants associated with ACM have been described.

2.2.9 Cadherin 2

The *CDH2* gene (ENSG00000170558) encodes the protein cadherin type 2 (CDH2, ENSP00000269141) that is a large transmembrane adherens junction protein that connects actin filaments in neighboring cardiomyocyte sarcomeres [4, 69]. It is a member of the cadherin superfamily and provides strength and stability to cardiac tissue and calcium-ion-dependent adhesion among other functions. In 2017 data were published regarding the firsts cadherin variants associated with ACM in this gene [70, 71]. To date, only 3 rare variants have been associated with ACM [42, 72].

2.2.10 Filamin C

The *FLNC* gene (ENSG00000128591) encodes for the protein filamin C (FLNC, ENSP00000327145) that is an actin cross-linking protein associated with Z-discs found only in striated muscle, important for structural cell stability and membrane-triggered signal transduction [4, 51]. Pathogenic alterations in *FLNC* have been linked to skeletal myopathies as well as DCM and restrictive cardiomyopathies and possibly hypertrophic cardiomyopathy. Recently, this gene, particularly truncating variants, have been associated with ventricular arrhythmias and a high SCD risk [73, 74]. To date, it has been described that nearly 30 *FLNC* rare variants are associated with ACM [42].

2.2.11 Ryanodine receptor 2

The *RYR2* gene (ENSG00000198626) encodes for the protein Ryanodine Receptor 2 (RYR2, ENSP00000355533) that is a sarcoplasmic reticulum calcium release channel that mediates the release of Ca^{2+} from the sarcoplasmic reticulum into the cytoplasm which generates calcium transients to trigger sarcomere contraction. The majority of *RYR2* deleterious alterations are associated with CPVT, but there are some studies that have been shown that rare variants in *RYR2* can also cause ACM [75, 76]. For the moment, there are nearly 20 rare variants associated with ACM [42]. However, it is necessary to continue investigating the relationship between *RYR2* and ACM to clarify the overlapping in diagnosis. There has even been described a case where the causal genetic alteration could not be identified, but the patient presented with phenotypes of both disorders [77].

2.2.12 RNA-binding motif protein 20

The *RBM20* gene (ENSG00000203867) encodes for the protein RNA-Binding Motif Protein 20 (RBM20, ENSP00000358532) that acts as a regulator of mRNA splicing of a subset of genes involved in cardiac development (sarcomeric, calcium regulation and ion regulation genes). There have been identified several rare alterations in *RBM20* implicated in DCM and ACM and that causes severe arrhythmia and SCD [78–81]. Therefore, pathogenic alterations in *RMB20* are associated with a high propensity for malignant arrhythmias usually with minor structural abnormalities [4, 80].

2.2.13 Tight junction protein ZO-1

The *TJP1* gene (ENSG00000104067) encodes for the protein tight junction protein Zona Occludens-1 (TJP ZO-1, ENSP00000281537), a multi-functional scaffolding protein that localizes to the intercalated discs of cardiomyocytes and interacts with proteins of gap junctions and area composita including connexin43, N-cadherin, αT-catenin, and actin [4]. Recently, it has been identified that 4 rare variants in ACM patients could be deleterious according to *in silico* tools predictions [42, 82]. Case–control studies provided evidence for enrichment with *TJP1* variants in ACM patients compared with controls, supporting the causality role of *TJP1* in ACM. Further evidence from larger cohorts for the role of *TJP1* as a disease causing in ACM is still needed [4, 82].

3. Conclusion

Arrhythmogenic cardiomyopathy is an inherited rare cardiac disease characterized by progressive replacement of myocardium by fibrofatty tissue, leading to ventricular arrhythmias and sudden cardiac death. Structural abnormalities mainly occur in the right ventricle, but it is well recognized that also sole left ventricular involvement and even biventricular substitution is common, particularly in advanced stages of the disease. Several molecular mechanisms are involved in the phenotype of ACM such as myocardial inflammation and signaling pathways that cause fibrosis and adipogenesis. Today, most of these mechanisms are not completely understood. Task Force Criteria for the diagnosis of arrhythmogenic cardiomyopathy include several clinical tests and also genetic data. Despite progressive improvement in diagnosis, it is difficult to obtain conclusive risk stratification in families suffering from arrhythmogenic cardiomyopathy. Hundreds of rare alterations are reported in mainly genes encoding desmosomal proteins, but there are also other causal genes with several functions within the cardiac tissue. A comprehensive genetic analysis may identify the potential genetic cause of the disease in nearly 60% of cases. Genetic testing is especially useful in families with at least one affected member that carries a potential deleterious alteration because it allows early identification and adoption of therapeutic measures among relatives at risk of malignant arrhythmias. Currently, one of main challenges is the genetic interpretation and clinical translation of amount of genetic data generated by new genetic technologies.

Acknowledgements

This work was supported by Obra Social “La Caixa Foundation” (LCF/PR/GN16/50290001 and LCF/PR/GN19/50320002), and Sociedad Española Cardiología, Proyecto Investigación Básica Cardiología 2020. CIBERCV is an initiative of the ISCIII, Spanish Ministry of Economy and Competitiveness. Funders had no role in study design, data collection, data analysis, interpretation, or writing of the report.

Author details

Marta Vallverdú-Prats[1†], Mireia Alcalde[1,2,3†], Georgia Sarquella-Brugada[3,4], Sergi Cesar[4], Elena Arbelo[2,5], Josep Brugada[2,5], Ramon Brugada[1,2,3,6*‡] and Oscar Campuzano[1,2,3*‡]

1 Cardiovascular Genetics Center, University of Girona – IDIBGi, Girona, Spain

2 Centro Investigación Biomédica en Red de Enfermedades Cardiovasculares (CIBERCV), Spain

3 Medical Science Department, School of Medicine, University of Girona, Girona, Spain

4 Arrhythmias Unit, Hospital Sant Joan de Déu, University of Barcelona, Barcelona, Spain

5 Arrhythmias Unit, Hospital Clinic de Barcelona, University of Barcelona, Barcelona, Spain

6 Cardiology Service, Hospital Josep Trueta, University of Girona, Girona, Spain

*Address all correspondence to: ramon@brugada.org and oscar@brugada.org

† Both authors equally contributed as first author.

‡ Both authors equally contributed as senior author.

References

[1] Frank R, Fontaine G, Vedel J et al. Electrocardiology of 4 cases of right ventricular dysplasia inducing arrhythmia.

[2] Marcus FI, Abidov A. Arrhythmogenic Right Ventricular Cardiomyopathy 2012: Diagnostic Challenges and Treatment. J Cardiovasc Electrophysiol. 2012 Oct;23(10):1149-53.

[3] Berte B, Denis A, Amraoui S, Yamashita S, Komatsu Y, Pillois X, et al. Characterization of the Left-Sided Substrate in Arrhythmogenic Right Ventricular Cardiomyopathy. Circ Arrhythm Electrophysiol. 2015 Dec;8(6):1403-12.

[4] Patel V, Asatryan B, Siripanthong B, Munroe PB, Tiku-Owens A, Lopes LR, et al. State of the Art Review on Genetics and Precision Medicine in Arrhythmogenic Cardiomyopathy. Int J Mol Sci. 2020;47.

[5] Sen-Chowdhry S, McKenna WJ. Left ventricular noncompaction and cardiomyopathy: cause, contributor, or epiphenomenon?: Curr Opin Cardiol. 2008 May;23(3):171-5.

[6] Norman M, Simpson M, Mogensen J, Shaw A, Hughes S, Syrris P, et al. Novel Mutation in Desmoplakin Causes Arrhythmogenic Left Ventricular Cardiomyopathy. Circulation. 2005 Aug 2;112(5):636-42.

[7] Li C-H, Lin Y-J, Huang J-L, Wu T-J, Cheng C-C, Lin W-S, et al. Long-Term Follow-Up in Patients with Arrhythmogenic Right Ventricular Cardiomyopathy. J Cardiovasc Electrophysiol. 2012 Jul;23(7):750-6.

[8] Battipaglia I, Scalone G, Macchione A, Pinnacchio G, Laurito M, Milo M, et al. Association of Heart Rate Variability With Arrhythmic Events in Patients With Arrhythmogenic Right Ventricular Cardiomyopathy/Dysplasia. Circ J. 2012;76(3):618-23.

[9] Sen-Chowdhry S, Syrris P, Ward D, Asimaki A, Sevdalis E, McKenna WJ. Clinical and Genetic Characterization of Families With Arrhythmogenic Right Ventricular Dysplasia/Cardiomyopathy Provides Novel Insights Into Patterns of Disease Expression. Circulation. 2007 Apr 3;115(13):1710-20.

[10] Stadiotti I, Catto V, Casella M, Tondo C, Pompilio G, Sommariva E. Arrhythmogenic Cardiomyopathy: the Guilty Party in Adipogenesis. J Cardiovasc Transl Res. 2017 Dec;10(5-6):446-54.

[11] Elliott PM, Anastasakis A, Asimaki A, Basso C, Bauce B, Brooke MA, et al. Definition and treatment of arrhythmogenic cardiomyopathy: an updated expert panel report. Eur J Heart Fail. 2019 Aug;21(8):955-64.

[12] Austin KM, Trembley MA, Chandler SF, Sanders SP, Saffitz JE, Abrams DJ, et al. Molecular mechanisms of arrhythmogenic cardiomyopathy. Nat Rev Cardiol. 2019 Sep;16(9):519-37.

[13] Leask A. Getting to the Heart of the Matter. :8.

[14] McKenna WJ, Thiene G, Nava A, Fontaliran F, Blomstrom-Lundqvist C, Fontaine G. Diagnosis of arrhythmogenic right ventricular dysplasia/cardiomyopathy. :4.

[15] Marcus FI, McKenna WJ, Sherrill D, Basso C, Bauce B, Bluemke DA, et al. Diagnosis of arrhythmogenic right ventricular cardiomyopathy/dysplasia: Proposed Modification of the Task Force Criteria. Eur Heart J. 2010 Apr 1;31(7):806-14.

[16] CardioPulse Articles2015 European Society of Cardiology Guidelines for the management of patients with ventricular arrhythmias and the prevention of sudden cardiac death summarized by co-chairs'Ten Commandments' of 2015 European Society of Cardiology Guidelines for the management of patients with ventricular arrhythmias and the prevention of sudden cardiac deathAdolfo J. de Bold PhD OC FRSC: a pioneer in cardiovascular medicineNatriuretic peptides in 2015Teachable moment or missed opportunity? Eur Heart J. 2015 Nov 1;36(41):2757-62.

[17] Corrado D, Beffagna G, Cipriani A, Lazzari MD, Migliore F, Pilichou K, et al. DIAGNOSIS OF ARRHYTHMOGENIC CARDIOMYOPATHY: THE PADUA CRITERIA. :30.

[18] Corrado D, Wichter T, Link MS, Hauer RNW, Marchlinski FE, Anastasakis A, et al. Treatment of Arrhythmogenic Right Ventricular Cardiomyopathy/Dysplasia. :13.

[19] Corrado D, Leoni L, Link MS, Bella PD, Gaita F, Curnis A, et al. Implantable Cardioverter-Defibrillator Therapy for Prevention of Sudden Death in Patients With Arrhythmogenic Right Ventricular Cardiomyopathy/ Dysplasia. Circulation. 2003 Dec 23;108(25):3084-91.

[20] Wichter T, Paul M, Wollmann C, Acil T, Gerdes P, Ashraf O, et al. Implantable Cardioverter/Defibrillator Therapy in Arrhythmogenic Right Ventricular Cardiomyopathy. :6.

[21] Bhonsale A, James CA, Tichnell C, Murray B, Gagarin D, Philips B, et al. Incidence and Predictors of Implantable Cardioverter-Defibrillator Therapy in Patients With Arrhythmogenic Right Ventricular Dysplasia/Cardiomyopathy Undergoing Implantable Cardioverter-Defibrillator Implantation for Primary Prevention. J Am Coll Cardiol. 2011 Sep;58(14):1485-96.

[22] Corrado D, Calkins H, Link MS, Leoni L, Favale S, Bevilacqua M, et al. Prophylactic Implantable Defibrillator in Patients With Arrhythmogenic Right Ventricular Cardiomyopathy/ Dysplasia and No Prior Ventricular Fibrillation or Sustained Ventricular Tachycardia. Circulation. 2010 Sep 21;122(12):1144-52.

[23] Risk Stratification in Arrhythmogenic Right Ventricular Cardiomyopathy. :16.

[24] Groeneweg JA, Bhonsale A, James CA, te Riele AS, Dooijes D, Tichnell C, et al. Clinical Presentation, Long-Term Follow-Up, and Outcomes of 1001 Arrhythmogenic Right Ventricular Dysplasia/Cardiomyopathy Patients and Family Members. Circ Cardiovasc Genet. 2015 Jun;8(3):437-46.

[25] Oliva A, Brugada R, D'Aloja E, Boschi I, Partemi S, Brugada J, et al. State of the Art in Forensic Investigation of Sudden Cardiac Death. Am J Forensic Med Pathol. 2011 Mar;32(1):1-16.

[26] Quarta G, Muir A, Pantazis A, Syrris P, Gehmlich K, Garcia-Pavia P, et al. Familial Evaluation in Arrhythmogenic Right Ventricular Cardiomyopathy: Impact of Genetics and Revised Task Force Criteria. Circulation. 2011 Jun 14;123(23):2701-9.

[27] Sen-Chowdhry S, Syrris P, Pantazis A, Quarta G, McKenna WJ, Chambers JC. Mutational Heterogeneity, Modifier Genes, and Environmental Influences Contribute to Phenotypic Diversity of Arrhythmogenic Cardiomyopathy. Circ Cardiovasc Genet. 2010 Aug;3(4):323-30.

[28] McKoy G, Protonotarios N, Crosby A, Tsatsopoulou A, Anastasakis A, Coonar A, et al.

Identification of a deletion in plakoglobin in arrhythmogenic right ventricular cardiomyopathy with palmoplantar keratoderma and woolly hair (Naxos disease). The Lancet. 2000 Jun;355(9221):2119-24.

[29] Norgett EE. Recessive mutation in desmoplakin disrupts desmoplakin-intermediate filament interactions and causes dilated cardiomyopathy, woolly hair and keratoderma. Hum Mol Genet. 2000 Nov 1;9(18):2761-6.

[30] Awad MM, Dalal D, Tichnell C, James C, Tucker A, Abraham T, et al. Recessive arrhythmogenic right ventricular dysplasia due to novel cryptic splice mutation in *PKP2*. Hum Mutat. 2006 Nov;27(11):1157-1157.

[31] Nakajima T, Kaneko Y, Irie T, Takahashi R, Kato T, Iijima T, et al. Compound and Digenic Heterozygosity in Desmosome Genes as a Cause of Arrhythmogenic Right Ventricular Cardiomyopathy in Japanese Patients. Circ J. 2012;76(3):737-43.

[32] Rigato I, Bauce B, Rampazzo A, Zorzi A, Pilichou K, Mazzotti E, et al. Compound and Digenic Heterozygosity Predicts Lifetime Arrhythmic Outcome and Sudden Cardiac Death in Desmosomal Gene–Related Arrhythmogenic Right Ventricular Cardiomyopathy. :10.

[33] Roberts J, Herkert J, Rutberg J, Nikkel S, Wiesfeld A, Dooijes D, et al. Detection of genomic deletions of *PKP2* in arrhythmogenic right ventricular cardiomyopathy: Detection of genomic deletions of *PKP2*. Clin Genet. 2013 May;83(5):452-6.

[34] Richards S, Aziz N, Bale S, Bick D, Das S, Gastier-Foster J, et al. Standards and guidelines for the interpretation of sequence variants: a joint consensus recommendation of the American College of Medical Genetics and Genomics and the Association for Molecular Pathology. Genet Med. 2015 May;17(5):405-23.

[35] Kapplinger JD, Landstrom AP, Salisbury BA, Callis TE, Pollevick GD, Tester DJ, et al. Distinguishing Arrhythmogenic Right Ventricular Cardiomyopathy/Dysplasia–Associated Mutations From Background Genetic Noise. J Am Coll Cardiol. 2011 Jun;57(23):2317-27.

[36] Lazzarini E, Jongbloed JDH, Pilichou K, Thiene G, Basso C, Bikker H, et al. The ARVD/C Genetic Variants Database: 2014 Update. Hum Mutat. 2015 Apr;36(4):403-10.

[37] Najor NA. Desmosomes in Human Disease. Annu Rev Pathol Mech Dis. 2018 Jan 24;13(1):51-70.

[38] Bauce B, Rampazzo A, Basso C, Mazzotti E, Rigato I, Steriotis A, et al. Clinical phenotype and diagnosis of arrhythmogenic right ventricular cardiomyopathy in pediatric patients carrying desmosomal gene mutations. Heart Rhythm. 2011 Nov;8(11):1686-95.

[39] Christensen AH, Benn M, Bundgaard H, Tybj A, Svendsen JH. Wide spectrum of desmosomal mutations in Danish patients with arrhythmogenic right ventricular cardiomyopathy. J Med Genet. :10.

[40] Bhonsale A, Groeneweg JA, James CA, Dooijes D, Tichnell C, Jongbloed JDH, et al. Impact of genotype on clinical course in arrhythmogenic right ventricular dysplasia/cardiomyopathy-associated mutation carriers. Eur Heart J. 2015 Apr 7;36(14):847-55.

[41] Grossmann KS, Grund C, Huelsken J, Behrend M, Erdmann B, Franke WW, et al. Requirement of plakophilin 2 for heart morphogenesis and cardiac junction formation. J Cell Biol. 2004 Oct 11;167(1):149-60.

[42] HGMD [Internet]. [cited 2020 Nov 3]. Available from: https://my.qiagendigitalinsights.com/bbp/home.jsp

[43] Cerrone M, Montnach J, Lin X, Zhao Y-T, Zhang M, Agullo-Pascual E, et al. Plakophilin-2 is required for transcription of genes that control calcium cycling and cardiac rhythm. Nat Commun. 2017 Dec;8(1):106.

[44] Uzumcu A. Loss of desmoplakin isoform I causes early onset cardiomyopathy and heart failure in a Naxos-like syndrome. J Med Genet. 2005 Jun 17;43(2):e05–e05.

[45] Carvajal-Huerta L. Epidermolytic palmoplantar keratoderma with woolly hair and dilated cardiomyopathy. J Am Acad Dermatol. 1998 Sep;39(3):418-21.

[46] Awad MM, Dalal D, Cho E, Amat-Alarcon N, James C, Tichnell C, et al. DSG2 Mutations Contribute to Arrhythmogenic Right Ventricular Dysplasia/Cardiomyopathy. Am J Hum Genet. 2006 Jul;79(1):136-42.

[47] Greenwood MD, Marsden MD, Cowley CME, Sahota VK, Buxton RS. Exon-Intron Organization of the Human Type 2 Desmocollin Gene (DSC2): Desmocollin Gene Structure Is Closer to ``Classical" Cadherins Than to Desmogleins. :6.

[48] Saito M, Tucker DK, Kohlhorst D, Niessen CM, Kowalczyk AP. Classical and desmosomal cadherins at a glance. J Cell Sci. 2012 Jun 1;125(11):2547-52.

[49] Protonotarios NI, Gatzoulis KA. Arrhythmogenic Right Ventricular Cardiomyopathy Caused by a Deletion in Plakoglobin (Naxos Disease). 6(1):9.

[50] van der Zwaag PA, Jongbloed JDH, van den Berg MP, van der Smagt JJ, Jongbloed R, Bikker H, et al. A genetic variants database for arrhythmogenic right ventricular dysplasia/cardiomyopathy. Hum Mutat. 2009 Sep;30(9):1278-83.

[51] Austin KM, Trembley MA, Chandler SF, Sanders SP, Saffitz JE, Abrams DJ, et al. Molecular mechanisms of arrhythmogenic cardiomyopathy. Nat Rev Cardiol. 2019 Sep;16(9):519-37.

[52] van Tintelen JP, Van Gelder IC, Asimaki A, Suurmeijer AJH, Wiesfeld ACP, Jongbloed JDH, et al. Severe cardiac phenotype with right ventricular predominance in a large cohort of patients with a single missense mutation in the DES gene. Heart Rhythm. 2009 Nov;6(11):1574-83.

[53] Lorenzon A, Beffagna G, Bauce B, De Bortoli M, Li Mura IEA, Calore M, et al. Desmin Mutations and Arrhythmogenic Right Ventricular Cardiomyopathy. Am J Cardiol. 2013 Feb;111(3):400-5.

[54] Doetschman T, Barnett JV, Runyan RB, Camenisch TD, Heimark RL, Granzier HL, et al. Transforming growth factor beta signaling in adult cardiovascular diseases and repair. Cell Tissue Res. 2012 Jan;347(1):203-23.

[55] Merner ND, Hodgkinson KA, Haywood AFM, Connors S, French VM, Drenckhahn J-D, et al. Arrhythmogenic Right Ventricular Cardiomyopathy Type 5 Is a Fully Penetrant, Lethal Arrhythmic Disorder Caused by a Missense Mutation in the TMEM43 Gene. Am J Hum Genet. 2008 Apr;82(4):809-21.

[56] Dominguez F, Zorio E, Jimenez-Jaimez J, Salguero-Bodes R, Zwart R, Gonzalez-Lopez E, et al. Clinical characteristics and determinants of the phenotype in TMEM43 arrhythmogenic right ventricular cardiomyopathy type 5. Heart Rhythm. 2020 Jun;17(6):945-54.

[57] Baskin B, Skinner JR, Sanatani S, Terespolsky D, Krahn AD, Ray PN,

et al. TMEM43 mutations associated with arrhythmogenic right ventricular cardiomyopathy in non-Newfoundland populations. Hum Genet. 2013 Nov;132(11):1245-52.

[58] Burke B, Stewart CL. Life at the edge: the nuclear envelope and human disease. Nat Rev Mol Cell Biol. 2002 Aug;3(8):575-85.

[59] Carboni N, Sardu C, Cocco E, Marrosu G, Manzi RC, Nissardi V, et al. Cardiac involvement in patients with lamin A/C gene mutations: A cohort observation. Muscle Nerve. 2012 Aug;46(2):187-92.

[60] Quarta G, Syrris P, Ashworth M, Jenkins S, Zuborne Alapi K, Morgan J, et al. Mutations in the Lamin A/C gene mimic arrhythmogenic right ventricular cardiomyopathy. Eur Heart J. 2012 May;33(9):1128-36.

[61] Taylor M, Graw S, Sinagra G, Barnes C, Slavov D, Brun F, et al. Genetic Variation in Titin in Arrhythmogenic Right Ventricular Cardiomyopathy–Overlap Syndromes. :13.

[62] MacLENNAN DH, Asahi M, Tupling AR. The Regulation of SERCA-Type Pumps by Phospholamban and Sarcolipin. Ann N Y Acad Sci. 2003 Apr;986(1):472-80.

[63] Cerra MC, Imbrogno S. Phospholamban and cardiac function: a comparative perspective in vertebrates. Acta Physiol. 2012 Jan;n/a-n/a.

[64] van der Zwaag PA, van Rijsingen IAW, Asimaki A, Jongbloed JDH, van Veldhuisen DJ, Wiesfeld ACP, et al. Phospholamban R14del mutation in patients diagnosed with dilated cardiomyopathy or arrhythmogenic right ventricular cardiomyopathy: evidence supporting the concept of arrhythmogenic cardiomyopathy. Eur J Heart Fail. 2012 Nov;14(11):1199-207.

[65] van Hengel J, Calore M, Bauce B, Dazzo E, Mazzotti E, De Bortoli M, et al. Mutations in the area composita protein αT-catenin are associated with arrhythmogenic right ventricular cardiomyopathy. Eur Heart J. 2013 Jan 14;34(3):201-10.

[66] Li J, Goossens S, van Hengel J, Gao E, Cheng L, Tyberghein K, et al. Loss of αT-catenin alters the hybrid adhering junctions in the heart and leads to dilated cardiomyopathy and ventricular arrhythmia following acute ischemia. J Cell Sci. 2012 Feb 15;125(4):1058-67.

[67] Yu J, Hu J, Dai X, Cao Q, Xiong Q, Liu X, et al. SCN5A mutation in Chinese patients with arrhythmogenic right ventricular dysplasia. Herz. 2014 Mar;39(2):271-5.

[68] te Riele ASJM, Agullo-Pascual E, James CA, Leo-Macias A, Cerrone M, Zhang M, et al. Multilevel analyses of SCN5A mutations in arrhythmogenic right ventricular dysplasia/cardiomyopathy suggest non-canonical mechanisms for disease pathogenesis. Cardiovasc Res. 2017 Jan 1;113(1):102-11.

[69] Vermij SH, Abriel H, van Veen TAB. Refining the molecular organization of the cardiac intercalated disc. Cardiovasc Res. 2017 Jan 8;cvw259.

[70] Turkowski KL, Tester DJ, Bos JM, Haugaa KH, Ackerman MJ. Whole exome sequencing with genomic triangulation implicates *CDH2* -encoded N-cadherin as a novel pathogenic substrate for arrhythmogenic cardiomyopathy: Turkowski et al. Congenit Heart Dis. 2017 Mar;12(2):226-35.

[71] Mayosi BM, Fish M, Shaboodien G, Mastantuono E, Kraus S, Wieland T, et al. Identification of Cadherin 2 (*CDH2*) Mutations in Arrhythmogenic Right Ventricular Cardiomyopathy.

Circ Cardiovasc Genet [Internet]. 2017 Apr [cited 2020 Oct 30];10(2). Available from: https://www.ahajournals.org/doi/10.1161/CIRCGENETICS.116.001605

[72] Poloni G, Calore M, Rigato I, Marras E, Minervini G, Mazzotti E, et al. A targeted next-generation gene panel reveals a novel heterozygous nonsense variant in the TP63 gene in patients with arrhythmogenic cardiomyopathy. Heart Rhythm. 2019 May;16(5):773-80.

[73] Begay RL, Graw SL, Sinagra G, Asimaki A, Rowland TJ, Slavov DB, et al. Filamin C Truncation Mutations Are Associated With Arrhythmogenic Dilated Cardiomyopathy and Changes in the Cell–Cell Adhesion Structures. JACC Clin Electrophysiol. 2018 Apr;4(4):504-14.

[74] Ortiz-Genga MF, Cuenca S, Dal Ferro M, Zorio E, Salgado-Aranda R, Climent V, et al. Truncating FLNC Mutations Are Associated With High-Risk Dilated and Arrhythmogenic Cardiomyopathies. J Am Coll Cardiol. 2016 Dec;68(22):2440-51.

[75] Tiso N. Identification of mutations in the cardiac ryanodine receptor gene in families affected with arrhythmogenic right ventricular cardiomyopathy type 2 (ARVD2). Hum Mol Genet. 2001 Feb 1;10(3):189-94.

[76] Kannankeril PJ, Mitchell BM, Goonasekera SA, Chelu MG, Zhang W, Sood S, et al. Mice with the R176Q cardiac ryanodine receptor mutation exhibit catecholamine-induced ventricular tachycardia and cardiomyopathy. Proc Natl Acad Sci. 2006 Aug 8;103(32):12179-84.

[77] Patel H, Shah P, Rampal U, Shamoon F, Tiyyagura S. Arrythmogenic right ventricular dysplasia/cardiomyopathy (ARVD/C) and cathecholaminergic polymorphic ventricular tachycardia (CPVT): A phenotypic spectrum seen in same patient. J Electrocardiol. 2015 Sep;48(5):874-8.

[78] van den Hoogenhof MMG, Beqqali A, Amin AS, van der Made I, Aufiero S, Khan MAF, et al. RBM20 Mutations Induce an Arrhythmogenic Dilated Cardiomyopathy Related to Disturbed Calcium Handling. Circulation. 2018 Sep 25;138(13):1330-42.

[79] Hey TM, Rasmussen TB, Madsen T, Aagaard MM, Harbo M, Mølgaard H, et al. Pathogenic *RBM20* -Variants Are Associated With a Severe Disease Expression in Male Patients With Dilated Cardiomyopathy. Circ Heart Fail [Internet]. 2019 Mar [cited 2020 Oct 28];12(3). Available from: https://www.ahajournals.org/doi/10.1161/CIRCHEARTFAILURE.118.005700

[80] Parikh VN, Caleshu C, Reuter C, Lazzeroni LC, Ingles J, Garcia J, et al. Regional Variation in *RBM20* Causes a Highly Penetrant Arrhythmogenic Cardiomyopathy. Circ Heart Fail [Internet]. 2019 Mar [cited 2020 Oct 28];12(3). Available from: https://www.ahajournals.org/doi/10.1161/CIRCHEARTFAILURE.118.005371

[81] Peters S, Kumar S, Elliott P, Kalman JM, Fatkin D. Arrhythmic Genotypes in Familial Dilated Cardiomyopathy: Implications for Genetic Testing and Clinical Management. Heart Lung Circ. 2019 Jan;28(1):31-8.

[82] De Bortoli M, Postma AV, Poloni G, Calore M, Minervini G, Mazzotti E, et al. Whole-Exome Sequencing Identifies Pathogenic Variants in *TJP1* Gene Associated With Arrhythmogenic Cardiomyopathy. Circ Genomic Precis Med [Internet]. 2018 Oct [cited 2020 Oct 28];11(10). Available from: https://www.ahajournals.org/doi/10.1161/CIRCGEN.118.002123

Chapter 9

Naxos Disease: Current Knowledge and Future Advances

Marianna Leopoulou, Gustav Mattsson, Ida Kåks and Peter Magnusson

Abstract

Naxos disease is a genetic cardiocutaneous syndrome manifesting with a cardiomyopathy that belongs in the arrhythmogenic right ventricular cardiomyopathy (ARVC) spectrum and follows an autosomal recessive pattern. It manifests with wooly hair, keratosis of the extremities and right ventricular dysfunction. It is accompanied by risk of arrhythmias as well as sudden cardiac death (SCD), even at a young age. Furthermore, the disease often progresses to right ventricular heart failure, but can also affect the left ventricle. Patient management follows current guidelines on ARVC and principles for heart failure management. Bioengineering and research about pluripotent stem cells seem to have potential to improve future management of the disease. This chapter covers current knowledge on Naxos disease regarding clinical features, epidemiology, pathogenesis, guidelines on patient management and provides insights in research frontlines.

Keywords: arrhythmias, cardiomyopathy, genetics, heart failure, Naxos disease, sudden cardiac death

1. Introduction

Naxos disease is an arrhythmogenic cardiomyopathy, considered to represent a form of ARVC [1]. It is of genetic origin and two main proteins have been associated with the disease. The clinical manifestations include wooly hair, keratosis of the extremities, and right ventricular dysfunction. Albeit rare, the disease can cause advanced heart failure and life-threatening arrhythmias, even in the young [2]. Data on Naxos disease are limited, and current patient management follows the guidelines for heart failure and ARVC. In recent years, research has focused on the field of bioengineering, illuminating some of the aspects of the disease and cultivating future perspectives regarding its management. In this chapter we present current knowledge regarding the clinical presentation, epidemiology, genetic substrate, pathophysiology, current guidelines for patient management, and future paths for Naxos disease.

2. Clinical presentation of Naxos disease

Naxos disease manifests with a typical phenotype including both cardiac and extracardiac characteristics. The extracardiac manifestation of the disease involves tight, wooly and rough hair, commonly present from birth [3]. In addition, Naxos patients exhibit diffuse palmoplantar non-epidermolytic keratosis, with clear borders, manifesting as soon as the child starts using hands and feet [3, 4]. Small arms and hands, short fingers, curved nails and hypo/oligodontia have also been reported in some cases [5, 6]. Notably, heterozygous carriers do not display certain aspects of the disease, such as palmoplantar keratoderma but wooly hair may manifest [7].

Regarding the cardiac characteristics, the disease resembles the ARVC phenotype. Echocardiography frequently portrays right ventricular dysfunction. In more detail, prominent dilation is often present along with hypokinesia and aneurysms that affect mainly the outflow tract, apex, and inferior wall of the right ventricle [3, 7]. In a quarter of the cases, the left ventricle is also affected, exhibiting the same characteristics as seen in dilated cardiomyopathy [4]. The term 'triangle of dysplasia' has been suggested in Naxos disease, which refers to aneurysms of the outflow tract, apex, and posterior wall of the right ventricle [8]. The disease prognosis is generally adverse [8]. The annual cardiac mortality reaches 3.0% [7].

While the extra-cardiac manifestations are prominent from a young age, symptoms suggestive of cardiac involvement usually occur in adolescence and in young adulthood. Heart failure and life-threatening ventricular arrhythmias may occur in adolescence [4]. Palpitations, syncope, and atrial arrhythmias are frequently encountered [5]. Arrhythmic events involve a wide range of patterns, from numerous premature ventricular complexes to sustained ventricular tachycardia (VT) and are present in half of the patients [7]. Events of VT, most commonly of a left bundle branch block (LBBB) pattern suggestive of right ventricular origin [9], have been documented in Naxos disease, even being drug-refractory in some cases [5]. Symptomatic patients tend to exhibit inducible VT in electrophysiology studies [3].

Symptoms suggestive of right ventricular dysfunction occur in advanced heart failure [8], while heart failure, either right- or bi-ventricular affects half of the patients after 10-year follow-up after diagnosis [7]. When severe hypokinesia is present in the context of progression of heart failure, intra-cardiac thrombi may occur [10]. Heterozygous carriers do not display ventricular arrhythmias or late potentials on signal-averaged electrocardiography (ECG), but atypical ECG or echocardiographic discrepancies may occur [7]. Similarly, they did not display symptoms or echocardiographic abnormalities in follow-up, in a paper by Protonotarios et al. [7].

3. Epidemiology and genetic substrate

Naxos disease has been identified as a form of ARVC inherited in an autosomal recessive pattern by the World Health Organization since 1995 [11]. However, the disease was first described in 1986, when Protonotarios and associates first documented the disease manifestations and clinical course [5]. The name "Naxos" originates from this original description of the disease; nine patients, aged 7 to 41 years, from four families of Naxos island in Greece, were presented. All these patients had wooly hair and palmoplantar keratosis as well as a range of arrhythmic events, including VT. Interestingly, all patients had echocardiographic signs of right ventricular (RV) dysfunction, while in some the left ventricle (LV) was also affected [5]. Since then, more patients have been found not only in Greece, but in Israel, Saudi Arabia, Italy, and Turkey [12]. Sporadic cases of the disease have also been identified in Bangladesh and in Canada [13, 14]. The prevalence of the disease in the Greek islands has been calculated to 1:1000 [3]. Officially, the disease was first named "Naxos disease" in a 1994 abstract [15]. Of interest, since ARVC and its clinical spectrum has been found to manifest with biventricular or mainly LV dysfunction, the term arrhythmogenic cardiomyopathy (ACM) has been proposed as more accurate [1]. Prevalence of heterozygous carriers is up to 5% in the Naxos population [8].

The proposed recessive hereditary pattern and the resemblance of the disease to ARVC [5, 16], was confirmed in 1998, when its locus was identified in chromosome 17 in position q21 [17], and in 2000 when plakoglobin was identified as the mutated protein attributed to the disease [18]. Since then, research has concluded that the causative mutation (Pk2157del2TG) is in the gene truncating the C-terminal of the protein plakoglobin [3, 12]. In addition, another mutation, the homozygous 2-bp deletion (c.2157delTG) (also in the protein plakoglobin) has been associated with the disease [18]. Furthermore, mutations of the protein desmoplakin have been identified to cause cardiocutaneous ARVC [19, 20]. Early data suggested that Naxos disease was a more severe form of ARVC [12], while a more recent comparison between the two entities indicates a similar cardiac phenotype, easily identified through non-invasive screening [2, 21]. In 2017, a novel homozygous mutation was discovered to cause Naxos disease, in unrelated patients of French-Canadian families. This is a mutation of the exon 5 of the JUP gene (p.Glu301 Gly) [14]. Two mutations of the desmoplakin gene have been implicated; Dsp7901del1G and DspG2375R [19, 20]. All aforementioned mutations follow an autosomal recessive pattern [2]. However, in 2011 a mutation (c.1790 C > T, p.Ser597Leu) was reported to be causative of the disease associated with hypo/oligodontia, that follows an autosomal dominant pattern [6].

A syndrome resembling Naxos disease, known as Carvajal syndrome, has been described in families from Ecuador and India as well as in Arab-Palestinian families [8, 22, 23]. Truncated proteins of desmoplakin, plakoglobin and desmocollin-2 have been implemented in the genetic substrate [23]. This syndrome was first described by Carvajal-Huerta [22]. Patients present with epidermolytic keratoderma while the disease usually manifests at a younger age and the LV is commonly affected [3, 8]. Notably, the replacement of the myocytes by fatty tissue is not apparent in Carvajal syndrome [24].

4. Pathophysiology and diagnostic criteria

Both plakoglobin (γ-catenin) and desmoplakin, that are linked with Naxos disease are associated with myocardial cell adhesion [3, 25]. Plakoglobin has a two-fold role in both mechanical contraction and electrical signal conduction; it is a component of the desmosomes, interconnecting with the intermediate filaments of desmin, and constitutes a component of the adherens junctions where it is connected to the actin skeleton [3, 26]. Similarly, desmoplakin is a cytoplasmic protein that links plakoglobin to the intermediate filaments of desmin [3]. The defective cell adhesion in the case of the truncated plakoglobin protein, also causes a reduction in the connexin-43 levels, a major gap junction protein. The associated myocardial gap-junction remodeling, creates a substrate for arrhythmogenic events [27]. Furthermore, the defective cell adhesion of the cardiomyocytes leads to their apoptosis which is then followed by fibrofatty replacement in the affected ventricles [18]. The associated conduction disturbances created can induce arrhythmogenic events and sustain re-entry circuits [3].

In the landmark paper Protonotarios et al., all patients were reported to have signs of intra-ventricular conduction delay ECG as well as echocardiographic findings of right- or bi-ventricular dysfunction. In more detail, the ECG abnormalities that were reported include a wide QRS ≥120 ms and abnormal T-wave inversions in seven out of nine patients [5]. The most common abnormalities documented

Category	Criteria

Global or regional dysfunction and structural alterations	**Major**
	By 2-D echocardiography:
	• Regional RV akinesia, dyskinesia, or aneurysm
	• and 1 of the following (measured in end diastole):
	  o PLAX RVOT ≥32 mm (corrected for body size PLAX/BSA ≥19 mm/m2)
	  o PSAX RVOT ≥36 mm (corrected for body size PSAX/BSA ≥21 mm/m2)
	  o or fractional area change ≤33%
	By CMR:
	• Regional RV akinesia, dyskinesia or dyssynchronous RV contraction
	• and 1 of the following:
	  o Ratio of RV end-diastolic volume to BSA ≥110 mL/m2 (male) or ≥100 mL/m2 (female)
	  o or RV ejection fraction ≤40%
	By RV angiography:
	• Regional RV akinesia, dyskinesia or aneurysm
	Minor
	By 2-D echocardiography:
	• Regional RV akinesia or dyskinesia
	• and 1 of the following (measured in end diastole):
	  o PLAX RVOT ≥29 to <32 mm (corrected for body size PLAX/BSA ≥ 16 to <19 mm/m2)
	  o PSAX RVOT 32 to 36 mm (corrected for body size PSAX/BSA ≥18 to <21 mm/m2)
	  o or fractional area change 33–40%
	By CMR:
	• Regional RV akinesia or dyskinesia or dyssynchronous RV contraction
	• and 1 of the following:
	  o Ratio of RV end-diastolic volume to BSA ≥100 to <110 mL/m2 (male) or ≥ 90 to <100 mL/m2 (female)
	  o or RV ejection fraction >40% to ≤45%

Wall tissue characterization	**Major** Residual myocytes <60% by morphometric analysis (or < 50% if estimated), with fibrous replacement of the RV free wall myocardium in ≥1 sample, with or without fatty replacement of tissue on endomyocardial biopsy **Minor** Residual myocytes 60–75% by morphometric analysis (or 50–65% if estimated), with fibrous replacement of the RV free wall myocardium in ≥1 sample, with or without fatty replacement of tissue on endomyocardial biopsy
Repolarization abnormalities	**Major** Inverted T waves in right precordial leads (V1, V2, and V3), or beyond in individuals >14 years old (in the absence of complete RBBB ≥QRS 120 ms) **Minor** • Inverted T waves in leads V1 and V2 in individuals >14 years old (in the absence of complete RBBB) or in V4, V5 or V6 • Inverted T waves in leads V1, V2, V3, and V4 in individuals >14 years old in the presence of complete RBBB

Category	Criteria
Depolarization/ conduction abnormalities	**Major** Epsilon wave (reproducible low-amplitude signals between end of QRS complex to onset of the T wave) in the right precordial leads (V1 to V3) **Minor** • Late potentials by SAECG in ≥1 of 3 parameters in the absence of QRS ≥110 ms on the standard ECG • Filtered QRS duration (fQRS) ≥114 ms • Duration of terminal QRS <40 μV (low-amplitude signal duration) ≥38 ms • Root-mean-square voltage of terminal 40 ms ≤20 μV • Terminal activation duration of QRS ≥55 ms measured from the nadir of the S wave to the end of the QRS, including R', in V1, V2, or V3, in the absence of complete RBBB
Arrhythmias	**Major** Nonsustained or sustained ventricular tachycardia of LBBB morphology with superior axis (negative or indeterminate QRS in leads II, III, and aVF and positive in lead aVL) **Minor** • Nonsustained or sustained ventricular tachycardia of RV outflow configuration, LBBB morphology with inferior axis (positive QRS in leads II, III, and aVF and negative in lead aVL) or of unknown axis • >500 ventricular extrasystoles per 24 hours (Holter monitoring)
Family history	**Major** • ARVC confirmed in a first-degree relative who meets current Task Force criteria • ARVC confirmed pathologically at autopsy or surgery in a first degree relative • Identification of a pathogenic mutation categorized as associated or probably associated with ARVC in the patient under evaluation **Minor** • History of ARVC in a first-degree relative in whom it is not possible or practical to determine whether the family member meets current Task Force criteria • Premature sudden death (<35 years of age) due to suspected ARVC in a first-degree relative • ARVC confirmed pathologically or by current Task Force Criteria in a second-degree relative

Required for definite diagnosis: 2 major or 1 major and 2 minor criteria or 4 minor from different categories; borderline: 1 major and 1 minor or 3 minor criteria from different categories
Possible diagnosis: 1 major or 2 minor criteria from different categories.
ARVC, arrhythmogenic right ventricular cardiomyopathy; BSA, body surface area; CMR, cardiac magnetic resonance imaging; LBBB, left bundle branch block; PLAX, parasternal long-axis view; PSAX, parasternal short-axis view; RBBB, right bundle branch block; RV, right ventricular; RVOT, RV outflow tract; SAEG, signal averaged ECG.
Adapted from Marcus et al. [31].

Table 1.
Revised task force criteria for arrhythmogenic right ventricular cardiomyopathy.

in Naxos patients are wide QRS and inverted T-waves in V1-V3 or in all precordial leads, while epsilon waves may also be present [3]. An incomplete right bundle branch block may also be apparent, while the extrasystoles tend to manifest with an LBBB morphology [7]. Flattened T-waves appear in the case of biventricular involvement [3]. Late potentials in Naxos disease are more often abnormal than in other forms of cardiomyopathies [28]. In echocardiography, dysfunction, hypokinesia and aneurysms are prominent [3, 7]. In histological specimens fibrofatty patterns are prominent, while focal myocarditis has also been reported in follow-up histology specimens [4]. Both the subepicardial and the mediomural myocardium of the involved ventricles is replaced by fibrofatty tissue, while healthy myocytes are surrounded by fatty tissue [3, 29]. In immunohistochemical specimens the signal of plakoglobin and connexin-43 in the intracellular junctions is diminished [24, 27].

Since the disease belongs in the ARVC spectrum and there are currently no specific diagnostic criteria for the cardiac manifestations of Naxos disease, the diagnostic criteria of ARVC are widely used [30, 31]. However, while the specificity of the revised task force criteria is high, sensitivity has been shown to be as low as 13–20% [32]. Since then, progress has been made regarding tissue characterization through cardiac magnetic resonance (CMR), possibly providing a tool of higher diagnostic accuracy, high specificity and high sensitivity [32, 33]. The revised task force criteria for ARVC are depicted in **Table 1**. In November 2020 the Padua criteria for the diagnosis of ACM was published. The Padua diagnostic criteria introduce tissue characterization by contrast enhanced cardiac magnetic resonance for detection of fibro-fatty myocardial replacement of both ventricles. It also adds new ECG criteria, including depolarization/ repolarization abnormalities and ventricular arrhythmias, specific for the LV involvement [34]. The proposed Padua diagnostic criteria need to be validated by further clinical studies in large cohorts of patients.

5. Therapeutic management

5.1 Heart failure

Naxos disease is predominantly a condition affecting the right ventricle, causing right ventricular failure. Unlike for LV failure, less is known regarding the optimal pharmacological therapy. However, the expert consensus regarding the management of ACMs suggests that when treating left or right ventricular dysfunction, angiotensin-converting enzyme (ACE) inhibitors, angiotensin receptor blockers, beta-blockers, mineralocorticoid receptor antagonists, and diuretics, in the case of fluid overload, should be considered [35]. Despite the lack of Naxos-specific guidelines, ACE inhibitors, betablockers, and diuretics are reasonable prescribing choices [2]. Dapagliflozine and empagliflozine have been introduced in the treatment of heart failure, even in non-diabetic patients [36, 37], while sacubitril/valsartan is indicated for patients with left ventricular ejection fraction (EF) $\leq$35% [38]. Anticoagulation treatment is indicated in the case of atrial fibrillation/flutter, in the event of intra-cardiac thrombi and can also be considered in patients with ventricular aneurysms, either left or right [35, 39]. In the case of advanced heart failure, patients may benefit from devices such as cardiac resynchronization therapy (CRT), often combined with an implantable cardioverter-defibrillator (ICD), left ventricular assist devices (LVAD) and assist devices for the right ventricle (RVAD or BiVAD) in the setting of an LVAD implantation and considered as bridge to transplant [38].

5.2 Arrhythmias and sudden cardiac death

The prognosis of the disease is adverse, especially in the young and annual SCD mortality is 2.3% [7, 8]. As risk factors for SCD, the following have been identified: history of syncope, onset of symptoms before the age of 35, structural progression before the age of 35, and left-ventricular involvement [7]. However, risk stratification of SCD constitutes a challenge. ARVC guidelines and position papers on ICD implantation, guide the same decisions in the management of Naxos disease [35, 40]. Criteria for risk stratification for SCD is presented in **Table 2**. A clear indication for an ICD implantation is aborted SCD and VT with haemodynamic instability, while in the case of VT without haemodynamic compromise it should also be considered [35, 40]. An ICD protects from SCD in ARVC either in secondary prevention or is justified as primary prevention based on careful judgment of risk factors [40–42]. However, the clinical presentation should play a major part in the decision making; unexplained syncope, risk markers associated with medical history, family history and severity of clinical presentation and deterioration should be considered [40]. An ICD is indicated for ACM patients with low ejection fraction ≤35% and New York Heart Association (NYHA) class II or III, provided that the patient's estimated survival exceeds one year [35]. The same guidelines apply for Naxos patients. The first implantation of an ICD in a Naxos patient was reported in 2000 [43]. Naxos-specific guidelines are rare. Among those, an ICD is indicated for patients who are symptomatic or present structural progression especially before the age of 35 [8, 44]. Naxos patients, like ARVC patients, should abstain from competitive sports as myocardial stress can exacerbate the dysplasia [40]. Regarding drug therapy, beta-blockers (Class I), and possibly amiodarone (Class IIb) and sotalol (Class IIb) in special cases have been suggested for patients with ACMs for the control of arrhythmias and the reduction of ICD shocks [35, 45]. Specifically for Naxos patients with recurrent sustained VTs, anti-arrhythmic drugs should be prescribed as per the general guidelines of arrhythmias, while amiodarone or sotalol alone or in combination with beta-blockers have been suggested [8, 40, 45]. As far as catheter ablation is concerned, it should be considered in ACM cases with amiodarone-refractory recurrent monomorphic VT, recurrent symptomatic drug-refractory

Estimated Risk	Parameters
High risk (>10% / year)	*Major arrhythmic events* • Cardiac arrest due to ventricular arrhythmia • Sustained ventricular tachycardia
Intermediate risk (1–10% / year)	*Major risk factors* • Non-sustained ventricular tachycardia • Unexplained syncope • Severe right or left ventricular dysfunction *Minor risk factors* • Male sex, proband • Frequent ectopic beats (≥1000 premature ventricular beats per day) • Extent of negative T-waves (beyond V3) • Inducibility on electrophysiological study • Extent of right ventricular fibrofatty scarring • Multiple associated desmosomal mutations
Low risk (<1% / year)	*No events/no risk factor* • Healthy gene carriers • Patients with definite ARVC

Adapted from Corrado et al. [46].

Table 2.
Risk stratification for sudden cardiac death in ARVC.

sustained VT, symptomatic nonsustained VT or a high ectopic burden (≥1000 premature ventricular contractions/day) refractory to beta-blockers [35]. Beta-blockers are also recommended for patients without an ICD (Class IIa) [35].

5.3 Bioengineering

On the front of cellular and molecular engineering, advances have been made that may create a substrate with therapeutic potentials in the future. The pharmaceutical substance SB216763 (SB21) (an inhibitor of the glycogen synthase kinase GSK-3β) prevented heart failure and reduced mortality when administered early on to zebrafish models with induced plakoglobin mutations that resulted in Naxos disease. The effect could possibly be attributed to the prevention of the formation of an arrhythmic substrate on the intercalated disk level [47]. Further data on mammalian models are, however, needed [2, 48].

On the front of induced pluripotent stem cells (iPSCs) that enable the in-vitro study of human genetic disorders like ARVC through the induction of mutant cardiomyocytes, albeit a challenging field, promising results have been reported [49–51]. Researchers have been able to re-create the ARVC phenotype using adult-like metabolic energetics, proving that adultlike metabolism plays a crucial role in establishing ARVC models through iPSCs [49]. Furthermore, cultured ARVC cardiomyocytes manifest with adipogenic phenotype and reduced cell surface localization of desmosomal proteins, characteristic features of ARVC [50]. Also Naxos-ARVC has been created in mice models through a homozygous mutation of the plakoglobin gene [52] and of the desmoplakin gene, the latter causing human-like cardiac arrhythmias, palmoplantar keratosis, and alopecia [53]. Interestingly, cardiac function was restored in mice through the normalization of Naxos plakoglobin levels, indicating that it is the downregulation of the protein that causes the cardiac dysfunction, rather than the mutation itself [54]. This conclusion, if further supported, could have clinical applications in Naxos disease [2]. The article suggests that an approach to this would be to use antisense technology to specifically block nonsense-mediated decay of mutant plakoglobin mRNA, enabling the expression of the truncated protein at increased levels [54, 55].

6. Conclusion

In this chapter key aspects of Naxos disease are presented. Due to its rarity, the condition follows the general guidelines for arrhythmias and heart failure, as disease-specific criteria is lacking. However, due to its uniqueness, larger Naxos registries are needed, as they would illuminate the individual characteristics of the disease as well as guide the way to designated guidelines for the management of Naxos patients. Possibly, the thorough study of the origins of the disease, the genetic substrate and pathogenesis, can offer insights with therapeutic potential.

Conflict of interest

IK and ML reports no conflicts of interest. GM has received speaker's fee from Alnylam, MSD, and Internetmedicin. PM is on the advisory board of Coala Life and has received speaker's fees or grants from Abbott, Alnylam, Amicus Therapeutics, AstraZeneca, Bayer, Boehringer-Ingelheim, Internetmedicin, Lilly, MSD, Novo Nordisk, Octopus Medical, OrionPharma, Pfizer, Vifor Pharma, and Zoll.

DOI: http://dx.doi.org/10.5772/intechopen.96020

Acronyms and abbreviations

ACE	angiotensin-converting enzyme
ACM	arrhythmogenic cardiomyopathy
ARVC	arrhythmogenic right ventricular cardiomyopathy
CMR	cardiac magnetic resonance
CRT	cardiac resynchronization therapy
ECG	electrocardiography
iPSC	induced pluripotent stem cell
ICD	implantable cardioverter-defibrillator
LBBB	left bundle branch block
LV	left ventricle
LVAD	left ventricular assist device
NYHA	New York Heart Association
SCD	sudden cardiac death
VT	ventricular tachycardia

Author details

Marianna Leopoulou[1]*, Gustav Mattsson[2], Ida Kåks[2] and Peter Magnusson[2,3]

1 Cardiology Department, Athens General Hospital 'Elpis', Athens, Greece

2 Centre for Research and Development, Uppsala University/Region Gävleborg, Gävle, Sweden

3 Cardiology Research Unit, Department of Medicine, Solna, Karolinska Institutet, Stockholm, Sweden

*Address all correspondence to: mariannina.leo@gmail.com

References

[1] Elliott PM, Anastasakis A, Asimaki A, Basso C, Bauce B, Brooke MA, et al. Definition and treatment of arrhythmogenic cardiomyopathy: an updated expert panel report. Eur J Heart Fail. 2019;21(8):955-964

[2] Leopoulou M, Mattsson G, LeQuang JA, Pergolizzi JV, Varrassi G, Wallhagen M, et al. Naxos disease–a narrative review. Expert Rev Cardiovasc Ther. 2020;1-8 Epub ahead of print

[3] Protonotarios N, Tsatsopoulou A. Naxos Disease. Indian Pacing Electrophysiol J. 2005;5(2):76-80

[4] Protonotarios N, Tsatsopoulou A, Fontaine G. Naxos disease: Keratoderma, scalp modifications, and cardiomyopathy [3 J Am Acad Dermatol. 2001; 44(2):309-311

[5] Protonotarios N, Tsatsopoulou A, Patsourakos P, Alexopoulos D, Gezerlis P, Simitsis S, et al. Cardiac abnormalities in familial palmoplantar keratosis. Br Heart J. 1986;56(4):321-326

[6] Chalabreysse L, Senni F, Bruyère P, Aime B, Ollagnier C, Bozio A, et al. A new hypo/oligodontia syndrome: Carvajal/Naxos syndrome secondary to desmoplakin-dominant mutations. J Dent Res. 2011;90(1):58-64

[7] Protonotarios N, Tsatsopoulou A, Anastasakis A, Sevdalis E, McKoy G, Stratos K, et al. Genotype-phenotype assessment in autosomal recessive arrhythmogenic right ventricular cardiomyopathy (Naxos Disease) caused by a deletion in plakoglobin. J Am Coll Cardiol. 2001;38(5):1477-1484.

[8] Protonotarios N, Tsatsopoulou A. Naxos disease: Cardiocutaneous syndrome due to cell adhesion defect. Orphanet J Rare Dis. 2006;1:4

[9] Protonotarios NI, Tsatsopoulou AA, Gatzoulis KA. Arrhythmogenic right ventricular cardiomyopathy caused by a deletion in plakoglobin (Naxos disease). Card Electrophysiol Rev. 2002;6(1-2):72-80

[10] Baykan A, Olgar Ş, Argun M, Özyurt A, Pamukçu Ö, Üzüm K, et al. Different clinical presentations of Naxos disease and Carvajal syndrome: Case series from a single tertiary center and review of the literature. Anadolu Kardiyol Derg. 2015;15(5):404-408

[11] Richardson P, McKenna RW, Bristow M, Maisch B, Mautner B, O'Connell J, et al. Report of the 1995 World Health Organization/ International Society and Federation of Cardiology Task Force on the definition and classification of cardiomyopathies. Circulation. 1996;93(5):841-842

[12] Protonotarios N, Tsatsopoulou A. Naxos disease and Carvajal syndrome: Cardiocutaneous disorders that highlight the pathogenesis and broaden the spectrum of arrhythmogenic right ventricular cardiomyopathy. Cardiovasc Pathol. 2004;13(4):185-194

[13] Islam AKMM, Rahman MT, Chowdhury AH. Cardiocutaneous syndrome (Naxos disease) in a bangladeshi boy. Cardiovasc Diagn Ther. 2016;6(5):462-465

[14] Marino TC, Maranda B, Leblanc J, Pratte A, Barabas M, Dupéré A, et al. Novel founder mutation in French-Canadian families with Naxos disease. Clin Genet. 2017;92(4):451-453

[15] Fontaine G, Protonotarios N, Tsatsopoulou A, Tsezana R, Fontaliran F FR. Comparisons between Naxos disease and arrhythmogenic right ventricular dysplasia by electrocardiography and biopsy. Circulation. 1994;90:3233

[16] Protonotarios N, Tsatsopoulou A, Scampardonis G. Right ventricular cardiomyopathy and sudden death in young people. N Engl J Med. 1988;319:175

[17] Coonar AS, Protonotarios N, Tsatsopoulou A, Needham EWA, Houlston RS, Cliff S, et al. Gene for arrhythmogenic right ventricular cardiomyopathy with diffuse nonepidermolytic palmoplantar keratoderma and woolly hair (Naxos disease) maps to 17q21. Circulation. 1998;97(20):2049-2058

[18] McKoy G, Protonotarios N, Crosby A, Tsatsopoulou A, Anastasakis A, Coonar A, et al. Identification of a deletioninplakoglobininarrhythmogenic right ventricular cardiomyopathy with palmoplantar keratoderma and woolly hair (Naxos disease). Lancet. 2000;355(9221):2119-2124

[19] Norgett EE. Recessive mutation in desmoplakin disrupts desmoplakin-intermediate filament interactions and causes dilated cardiomyopathy, woolly hair and keratoderma. Hum Mol Genet. 2000;9(18):2761-2766

[20] Alcalai R, Metzger S, Rosenheck S, Meiner V, Chajek-Shaul T. A recessive mutation in desmoplakin causes arrhythmogenic right ventricular dysplasia, skin disorder, and woolly hair. J Am Coll Cardiol. 2003;42(2):319-327

[21] Antoniades L, Tsatsopoulou A, Anastasakis A, Syrris P, Asimaki A, Panagiotakos D, et al. Arrhythmogenic right ventricular cardiomyopathy caused by deletions in plakophilin-2 and plakoglobin (Naxos disease) in families from Greece and Cyprus: Genotype-phenotype relations, diagnostic features and prognosis. Eur Heart J. 2006;27(18):2208-2216

[22] Carvajal-Huerta L. Epidermolytic palmoplantar keratoderma with woolly hair and dilated cardiomyopathy. J Am Acad Dermatol. 1998;39(3):418-421

[23] Molho-Pessach V, Sheffer S, Siam R, Tams S, Siam I, Awwad R, et al. Two Novel Homozygous Desmoplakin Mutations in Carvajal Syndrome. Pediatr Dermatol. 2015;32(5):641-646

[24] Kaplan SR, Gard JJ, Carvajal-Huerta L, Ruiz-Cabezas JC, Thiene G, Saffitz JE. Structural and molecular pathology of the heart in Carvajal syndrome. Cardiovasc Pathol. 2004;13(1):26-32

[25] Li GL, Saguner AM, Fontaine GH. Naxos disease: From the origin to today. Orphanet J Rare Dis. 2018;13(1):74

[26] Zhurinsky J, Shtutman M, Ben-Ze'ev A. Plakoglobin and β-catenin: Protein interactions, regulation and biological roles. J Cell Sci. 2000;113(Pt 18):3127-3139

[27] Kaplan SR, Gard JJ, Protonotarios N, Tsatsopoulou A, Spiliopoulou C, Anastasakis A, et al. Remodeling of myocytegapjunctionsinarrhythmogenic right ventricular cardiomyopathy due to a deletion in plakoglobin (Naxos disease). Hear Rhythm. 2004;1(1):3-11

[28] Gatzoulis KA, Arsenos P, Trachanas K, Dilaveris P, Antoniou C, Tsiachris D, et al. Signal-averaged electrocardiography: Past, present, and future. Journal of Arrhythmia. 2018;34(3):222-229

[29] Basso C, Tsatsopoulou A, Thiene G, Anastasakis A, Valente M, Protonotarios N. "Petrified" right ventricle in long-standing naxos arrhythmogenic right ventricular cardiomyopathy. Circulation. 2001;104(23):E132-3

[30] Protonotarios N, Anastasakis A, Antoniades L, Chlouverakis G, Syrris P, Basso C, et al. Arrhythmogenic right

ventricular cardiomyopathy/dysplasia on the basis of the revised diagnostic criteria in affected families with desmosomal mutations. Eur Heart J. 2011;32(9):1097-1104

[31] Marcus FI, McKenna WJ, Sherrill D, Basso C, Bauce B, Bluemke DA, et al. Diagnosis of arrhythmogenic right ventricular cardiomyopathy/ Dysplasia: Proposed modification of the task force criteria. Circulation. 2010;121(13):1533-1541

[32] Aquaro GD, Barison A, Todiere G, Grigoratos C, Ait Ali L, Di Bella G, et al. Usefulness of Combined Functional Assessment by Cardiac Magnetic Resonance and Tissue Characterization Versus Task Force Criteria for Diagnosis of Arrhythmogenic Right Ventricular Cardiomyopathy. Am J Cardiol. 2016;118(11):1730-1736

[33] Corrado D, Van Tintelen PJ, McKenna WJ, Hauer RNW, Anastastakis A, Asimaki A, et al. Arrhythmogenic right ventricular cardiomyopathy: Evaluation of the current diagnostic criteria and differential diagnosis. Eur Heart J. 2020;41(14):1414-1429

[34] Corrado D, Perazzolo Marra M, Zorzi A, Beffagna G, Cipriani A, Lazzari M De, et al. Diagnosis of arrhythmogenic cardiomyopathy: The Padua criteria. Int J Cardiol. 2020;319:106-114

[35] Towbin JA, McKenna WJ, Abrams DJ, Ackerman MJ, Calkins H, Darrieux FCC, et al. 2019 HRS expert consensus statement on evaluation, risk stratification, and management of arrhythmogenic cardiomyopathy. Heart Rhythm. 2019;16(11):e301–e372

[36] McMurray JJV, Solomon SD, Inzucchi SE, Kober L, Kosiborod MN, Martinez FA, et al. Dapagliflozin in patients with heart failure and reduced ejection fraction. N Engl J Med. 2019;381(21):1995-2008

[37] PackerM, Anker SD, Butler J, et al. Cardiovascular and Renal Outcomes with Empagliflozin in Heart Failure. N Engl J Med. 2020;383(15):1413-1424

[38] Ponikowski P, Voors AA, Anker SD, Bueno H, Cleland JGF, Coats AJS, et al. 2016 ESC guidelines for the diagnosis and treatment of acute and chronic heart failure: the task force for the diagnosis and treatment of acute and chronic heart failure of the European Society Of Cardiology (ESC). Developed with the special contribution of the Heart Failure Association (HFA) of the ESC. Eur Heart J. 2016;18(8):891-975

[39] Kirchhof P, Benussi S, Kotecha D, Ahlsson A, Atar D, Casadei B, et al. 2016 ESC Guidelines for the management of atrial fibrillation developed in collaboration with EACTS. Eur Heart J. 2016;37(38):2893-2962

[40] Priori SG, Blomstrom-Lundqvist C, Mazzanti A, Bloma N, Borggrefe M, Camm J, et al. 2015 ESC Guidelines for the management of patients with ventricular arrhythmias and the prevention of sudden cardiac death the Task Force for the Management of Patients with Ventricular Arrhythmias and the Prevention of Sudden Cardiac Death of the European Society of Cardiology (ESC) endorsed by: association for European Paediatric and Congenital Cardiology (AEPC). Eur Heart J. 2015;(41):2793-2867

[41] Corrado D, Calkins H, Link MS, Leoni L, Favale S, Bevilacqua M, et al. Prophylactic implantable defibrillator in patients with arrhythmogenic right ventricular cardiomyopathy/dysplasia and no prior ventricular fibrillation or sustained ventricular tachycardia. Circulation. 2010;122(12):1144-1152

[42] Bhonsale A, James CA, Tichnell C, Murray B, Gagarin D, Philips B, et al. Incidence and predictors of implantable cardioverter-defibrillator therapy in

patients with arrhythmogenic right ventricular dysplasia/cardiomyopathy undergoing implantable cardioverter-defibrillator implantation for primary prevention. J Am Coll Cardiol. 2011;58(14):1485-1496

[43] Gatzoulis KA, Protonotarios N, Anastasakis A, Tsatsopoulou A, Vlasseros J, Gialafos J, et al. Implantable defibrillator therapy in Naxos disease. PACE - Pacing Clin Electrophysiol. 2000;23(7):1176-1178

[44] Noain JAG, Golet AC, Calzada JN, Mellado AM, Duarte JM. Living after sudden death: A case report of Naxos disease. Indian J Crit Care Med. 2012;16(4):207-209

[45] Dan GA, Martinez-Rubio A, Agewall S, Boriani G, Borggrefe M, Gaita F, et al. Antiarrhythmic drugs-clinical use and clinical decision making: A consensus document from the European Heart Rhythm Association (EHRA) and European Society of Cardiology (ESC) Working Group on Cardiovascular Pharmacology, endorsed by the Heart Rhythm Society (HRS), Asia-Pacific Heart Rhythm Society (APHRS) and International Society of Cardiovascular Pharmacotherapy (ISCP). Europace. 2018;20(5):731-732an

[46] Domenico Corrado, Mark S. Link HC. Arrhythmogenic Right Ventricular Cardiomyopathy. N Engl J Med. 2017;376(1):61-72

[47] Asimaki A, Kapoor S, Plovie E, Arndt AK, Adams E, Liu ZZ, et al. Identification of a new modulator of the intercalated disc in a zebrafish model of arrhythmogenic cardiomyopathy. Sci Transl Med. 2014;6(240):240ra74

[48] Kessler EL, van Veen TAB. A fishing trip to cure arrhythmogenic cardiomyopathy? Annals of Translational Medicine. 2015;3(7):90

[49] Kim C, Wong J, Wen J, Wang S, Wang C, Spiering S, et al. Studying arrhythmogenic right ventricular dysplasia with patient-specific iPSCs. Nature. 2013;494(7435):105-110

[50] Ma D, Wei H, Lu J, Ho S, Zhang G, Sun X, et al. Generation of patient-specific induced pluripotent stem cell-derived cardiomyocytes as a cellular model of arrhythmogenic right ventricular cardiomyopathy. Eur Heart J. 2013;34(15):1122-1133

[51] Caspi O, Huber I, Gepstein A, Arbel G, Maizels L, Boulos M, et al. Modeling of arrhythmogenic right ventricular cardiomyopathy with human induced pluripotent stem cells. Circ Cardiovasc Genet. 2013;6(6):557-568

[52] Li D, Liu Y, Maruyama M, Zhu W, Chen H, Zhang W, et al. Restrictive loss of plakoglobin in cardiomyocytes leads to arrhythmogenic cardiomyopathy. Hum Mol Genet. 2011;20(23):4582-4596

[53] Karmouch J, Zhou QQ, Miyake CY, Lombardi R, Kretzschmar K, Bannier-Hélaouët M, et al. Distinct Cellular Basis for Early Cardiac Arrhythmias, the Cardinal Manifestation of Arrhythmogenic Cardiomyopathy, and the Skin Phenotype of Cardiocutaneous Syndromes. Circ Res. 2017;121(12):1346-1359

[54] Zhang Z, Stroud MJ, Zhang J, Fang X, Ouyang K, Kimura K, et al. Normalization of Naxos plakoglobin levels restores cardiac function in mice. J Clin Invest. 2015;125(4):1708-1712

[55] Kole R, Krainer AR, Altman S. RNA therapeutics: Beyond RNA interference and antisense oligonucleotides. Nature Reviews Drug Discovery. 2012;11(2):125-140

Chapter 10

Arrhythmogenic Right Ventricular Cardiomyopathy

Sukanya Ghosh

Abstract

Arrythmogenic right ventricular cardiomyopathy (ARVC) is a genetic form of cardiomyopathy causing fibro-fatty replacement of the myocardium. Although usually transmission is autosomal dominant, 12 genes encoding cardiac desmosomes have been found to be closely linked to this disease process shifting the congenital disease theory to a genetic one. The categorisation of ARVC as a myocyte adhesion disorder was first suggested by a molecular genetic study involving patients with Naxos disease. Misnomeric to only affect the right ventricle, ARVC also affects the left ventricle - culminating into biventricular failure as a long term prognosis. Epidemiology is well established with a male to female preponderance. It is currently the second most common cause of sudden cardiac death (SCD) in population < 35 yrs. Pathological basis of the varied clinical presentation is explained at the molecular level with myocardial atrophy, fibro fatty replacement and chamber dilatation. Diagnosing the condition by ruling out the pitfall differentials is an enormous challenge due to the broad phenotypic spectrum including syncope on one end and SCD on the other. Task Force Criteria combines electrocardiography (ECG), echocardiography (ECHO), cardiac magnetic resonance imaging (CMRI), myocardial biopsy for diagnosis; early detection, family screening and risk stratification being the cornerstones. Therapeutic options although limited due to the progressive nature of the disease is based on preventing life threatening arrhythmias encompassing primary and secondary prevention - Implantable cardioverter -defibrillator (ICD) implantation, radiofrequency ablation and heart transplantation are the main ones.

Keywords: Arrythmogenic right ventricular cardiomyopathy (ARVC), Arrythmogenic right ventricular dysplasia (ARVD), sudden cardiac death, cardiomyopathy, genetic cardiomyopathy, cardiac desmosomes, plakophilin-2 (PKP-2), pathophysiology, diagnosis, treatment

1. Introduction

Arrhythmogenic right ventricular cardiomyopathy/dysplasia (ARVC/D) is a genetic form of cardiomyopathy and was initially known to primarily affect only the right ventricle (RV). It has now been found out that this disease process also may involve the left ventricle (LV) and culminate in life-threatening ventricular arrhythmias prompting sudden cardiac death (SCD) and/or biventricular heart failure [1]. ARVC is one of the leading causes of arrhythmic cardiac arrest in young people and athletes [2, 3]. The pathological hallmark of the disease is progressive loss of right ventricular myocardium and its replacement by fibrofatty tissue (**Figure 1**) [2, 4].

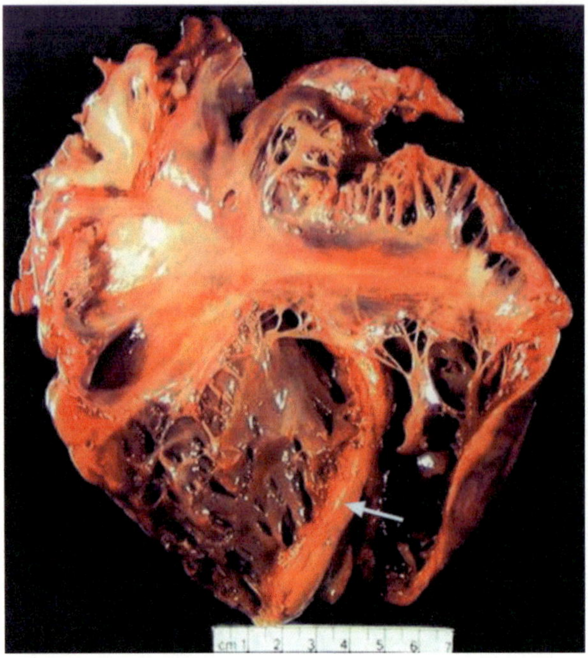

Figure 1.
Heart of a 37-year-old woman admitted with heart failure who suffered a subsequent cardiac arrest. The arrow identifies fatty infiltration of the right ventricle [9].

2. Epidemiology

The estimated prevalence of ARVC in the general population is approximately 1:5000 but in some European countries like Italy and Germany, it can be almost 1:2000, affecting men more frequently than women with a ratio of 3:1 [2] and can be explained either by a direct influence of sex hormones on the mechanisims involved in the phenotypic expression of the disease [2] or by sex based differences in the amount or intensity of exercise [2].

The exact prevalence, however, is unknown and could be higher than the estimated value because of the existence of many undiagnosed or missed diagnosed cases.

Approximately 50% of affected patients have a positive family history, but both incomplete penetrance and limited phenotypic expression are common and probably account for underestimation of the prevalence of familial disease. The disease is typically transmitted with an autosomal dominant pattern of inheritance, although rare autosomal recessive forms have been described [3].

3. History

This disease was first described in 1736 by the Pope's physician, Giovanni Maria Lancisi in his book *De Motu Cordis et Aneurysmatibus* where he mentions about a family where the affected members of the family had presented with palpitations, heart failure dilation and aneurysms of RV and SCD [4].

Dalla Volta *et al.* Reported a patient having "auricularization" the RV pressure curve, in 1961, emphasising on the peculiar haemodynamic picture of this non-ischaemic heart muscle disease where the RV was behaving like an atrium [5]. It was only in the 1980's when Drs Marcus, Nava, and Thiene found out the first clinical and pathologic series of patients with ARVC [6].

In 1982, Marcus *et al.* reported the disease in 24 adults, emphasising the origin of arrhythmias from the RV and the histopathological substrate consisting of fibrofatty replacement of the RV free wall. He also accounted for the ventricular arrhythmias of RV origin with left bundle branch block (LBBB) morphology. However, it was not until 1984 that the electrocardiographic features of ARVC were first elaborately described including the epsilon wave [6].

In 1988, Thiene *et al.* mentioned a significant series of sudden deaths in the young (< 35 years). It was noted that the pathology consisting of ARVC mostly occurred during effort and were characterised by ventricular arrhythmias of LBBB morphology and inverted T- waves in the right precordial leads in electrocardiogram (ECG). At the time this accounted for 20% of all sudden deaths in the young and this was the first time when ARVC was acknowledged as an important cause of sudden deaths in the young population [6].

ARVD1 is the first gene locus that was found by Rampazzo *et al.* in 1994 at chromosome 14q23 [5]. Basso *et al.* described the pathological profile in detail in 1996. He emphasised the frequent left ventricular (LV) involvement and the presence of an inflammatory component [6].

ARVC was included among cardiomyopathies in the revised World Health Organisation (WHO) classification in 1995 and progressive cell death (apoptosis) in myocyte was proven [6].

The need of an International Registry of the disease arose and two research programs where implemented on both sides of the Atlantic Ocean [6].

The first gene defect was discovered in the recessive variant of the disease which was originally identified in 1985 from the Naxos island and consisted of a cardiocutaneous syndrome presenting with ARVC, palmoplantar keratosis and woolly hair. A deletion was detected in the gene encoding plakoglobin which is the cell function protein [6].

Thereafter, other genes which encode cell junction proteins were found defective in the dominant, classical form of ARVC. Some of them were desmoplakin, plakophilin, desmoglein-2, desmocollin-2. These mutations accounted for intercalated disc remodelling at the ultrastructural level. The other variants of the disease were explained by mutation of ryanodine- 2 receptor and transforming growth factor beta 3 gene [6].

4. Genetics

ARVC is typically inherited as a dominant Mendelian disease, although recessive variants exist and the involvement of family members often can only be detected by directed screening. Human genetic studies in the past have offered insight into the potential causes of ARVC. Early work demonstrated substantial genetic heterogenetic T cells, and at least 9 independent loci have now been identified [7].

The genetic hypothesis has been thoroughly studied. The first chromosomal locus identified was published by Rampazzo [8] *et al.* in 1994 in Italy as previously mentioned. Linkage analysis supported the evidence for genetic heterogeneity for several ARVC loci on chromosomes (1, 2,3,6,10,12 and 14) [1, 8]. Similarly, he reported the desmoplakin gene (DSP), the first desmosomal protein gene to be associated with a major form of the disease, with autosomal dominant inheritance, also called ARVC type 8 [1].

In addition, the gene for Naxos disease was mapped on chromosome 17 (locus 17q21), by McCoy *et al.* [1]. This is the first disease causing gene, also named junction plakoglobin (JUP) gene (autosomal recessive variant of ARVC) [1].

The discovery of cutaneous and hair follicle involvement in recessive forms of ARVC led to the identification of mutations in the desmosomal proteins plakoglobin and desmoplakin [7]. These findings also implicated other desmosomal proteins or their partner proteins as candidate causes of the disorder. Subsequent work has revealed desmosomal mutations in a small proportion of dominantly inherited ARVC cases and in arrhythmogenic cardiomyopathy localised to the left ventricle [7]. The description of mutations in the cardiac ryanodine receptor in families with an exercise-related arrhythmia known as catecholaminergic, a polymorphic ventricular tachycardia has highlighted phenotypic distinctions from typical ARVC [7]. ARVC genetics took a significant step forward when it was discovered that mice null for the Armadillo protein plakophilin 2 (PKP 2), another desmosomal component, die at around E 11 with profound cardiac abnormalities [7]. These mice fail to form normal cardiac desmosomes, and desmoplakin disassociates from the abnormal junctions accumulating in cytoplasmic aggregates. These findings led in turn to the discovery of dominant mutations in the PKP2 gene in a large proportion of probands with ARVC and not only established mutant desmosomal proteins as a major cause of the syndrome but also raise the possibility of genetic testing as a diagnostic tool [7]. The initial report in a series of 120 and selected European probands identified PKP2 mutations in almost 1/3 of these individuals. Data from more selected cohorts of index patients with evidence of familial involvement have suggested that as many as 70% of such kindreds may have mutations in PKP2. Of note, these investigators also described evidence of founder effects for several PKP2 to mutations in remote kindreds, implying less dramatic effects on survival than are seen in other forms of ARVC [7].

A recessive mutation of DSP has been reported and associated with Carvajal syndrome, another cardiocutaneous disease [1]. PKP2 is the most frequent targeted protein with more than 25 different mutations identified in the gene encoding it. Thus, ARVC was found to be mainly a disease of the cardiomyocyte junction [2].

Furthermore, extra-desmosomal gene, unrelated to the cell adhesion complex, have been implicated as autosomal dominant forms of ARVC, such as (1). the cardiac ryanodine-2 receptor gene, responsible for the release of calcium from the sarcoplasmic reticulum; (2). the transforming growth factor beta3 gene (TGF beta3) implicated in the regulation of production of extracellular matrix and expression of genes encoding desmosomal proteins and the TMEM43 genes [1].

The cardiac ryanodine receptor gene (RyR2) has also recently been implicated in ARVC and office potential insight into the Association of Edren it adrenergically mediated ventricular arrhythmias with this disease. The ryanodine receptor induces calcium released from the sarcoplasmic reticulum into the cytosol. The cardiac ryanodine receptor has also been identified as being responsible for catecholamine-induced ventricular tachycardia. Its skeletal muscle counterpart has been implicated in malignant hyperthermia and central core disease, a congenital myopathy but the mechanisms by which mutations in the cardiac ryanodine receptor might mediate fibrofatty myocardial changes are not clear and will likely be the focus of future studies [9].

The discovery of these gene mutations allowed preliminary genotype–phenotype correlations to be made.

5. Histopathology

Characteristically, the RV in ARVC is replaced with a fibrofatty tissue. Morphologic alterations of ARVC usually begin in the subepicardium or mediomural layers of the RV and progress to the endocardium with fibrofatty replacement of myocytes and thinning of the wall (**Figure 2**). The regions of RV most frequently involved are the RV inflow area, the apex and the infundibulum. These three areas form "the triangle of dysplasia" [9]. However, small amounts of fat are present in the epicardial layer and within the RV myocardium in normal subjects. Fontaine *et al.* examined the hearts at necropsy in 140 individuals with no history of heart disorders. Over 50% of the subjects had fat within their RV myocardial fibres, and the presence of intramyocardial fat increased with age. Therefore, histologic diagnosis of ARVC may be difficult in borderline cases. To avoid overdiagnosing ARVC, Angeline *et al.* have proposed that the presence in biopsy sections of more than 3% of fibrous tissue and more than 40% of fatty tissue is highly suggestive of ARVC. These authors also emphasised the importance of identifying coexisting myocardial fibrosis in making the diagnosis. In a forensic autopsy study of 20 patients with ARVC who died suddenly, the fatty replacement involved the outer half of the RV free wall in 27%, the other 2/3 in 28% and the entire wall thickness in 45% of the cases [9]. Interestingly, the endocardial muscular trabeculae are generally spared but may occasionally also be atrophied. The LV was involved in 40% of cases in this report, although other reports have the identified LV involvement in up to 76% of individuals with ARVC examined at necropsy. When the LV is involved, the fibrofatty replacement can affect both the septum and LV free wall, either diffusely or, more often, regionally with a predilection for the posteroseptal and posterolateral areas. In the LV, fatty replacement of the myocardium has a predilection for the subepicardial and midventricular wall [9].

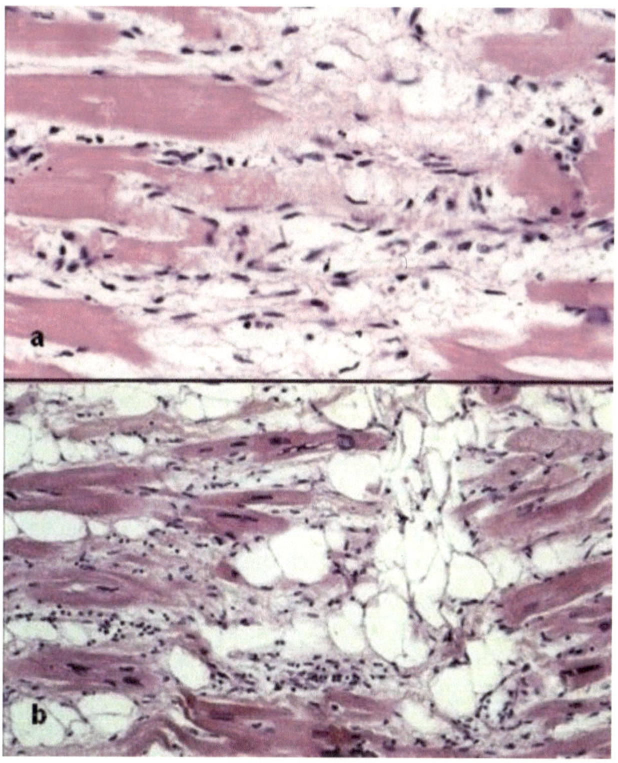

Figure 2.
Typical histologic features of ARVC/D. ongoing myocyte death (a) with early fibrosis and adipocytes infiltration (b) [6].

6. Pathogenesis

ARVC was initially believed to be secondary to a developmental defect of the RV myocardium, leading to the original designation of "dysplasia", similar to Uhl's anomaly [1]. Nonetheless, this process differs from ARVC/D based on the fact that Uhl's anomaly has not been documented to have a genetic basis, and it is not recognised as a desmosomal disease. In addition, myocardial atrophy is the consequence of cell death after birth and its progressive postnatal development has been definitely assessed. This concept has evolved over the last 30 years and based on its clinical characteristics, pathophysiology, postnatal development and genetic background, its inclusion in the World Health Organisation (WHO) classification of cardiomyopathies was finally achieved [1].

Several studies have been performed to determine the aetiology and pathogenesis of ARVC. However, there is still conflicting evidence. Different courses have been suggested as congenital defects, genetics and acquired factors [1]. In approximately 30–50% of cases it is transmitted with an autosomal dominant pattern of inheritance, with incomplete penetrance and variable expression [1].

Acquired factors have also been suggested as the cause of ARVC. The strongest association has been made with viral myocarditis inducing arrhythmogenic cardiomyopathy due to histopathological similarity between the two of lymphocytic infiltrate with disappearance of myocytes and fibrofatty replacement [1].

How do the mutant junctional proteins result in a unique, predominantly right ventricular cardiac phenotype? Desmosomal proteins are widely expressed, so the focal nature of apparent pathology in both dominant and recessive ARVC led to initial speculation on the role of mechanical stresses. Impaired desmosome function under conditions of mechanical stress was proposed to predispose to cardiomyocyte detachment and death, with subsequent inflammatory reaction and fibrofatty replacement. However, consideration of the distribution of skin lesions in recessive variants infers that this mechanism alone is unlikely to be responsible. Several areas of the body subject to substantial physical stresses are not involved, while the hair follicles are uniformly affected. In addition, the prominent adipose replacement suggests not scarring and healing, but rather a more fundamental perturbation of primary tissue architecture [7].

Three different types of intercellular junction are distinguished at the cardiac intercalated disc: (a) adherens junctions, which anchor actin filaments; (b) desmosomes, which anchor intermediate filaments; and (c) gap junctions, which mediate ion transfer. Cardiac myocytes rely on these specialised structures for both mechanical and electrical coupling of the myocardial syncytium [7]. Desmosomes may protect other junctions from mechanical stress, but they also have been implicated in the structural organisation of the intercalated disc. Desmosome dependent orchestration of local membrane and cytoplasmic domains may be critical for many of the physiologic functions of the intercalated disc. For example, the destabilisation of cell adhesion complexes may perturb the kinetics of gap junction turnover, resulting in heterogeneous conduction, a potential contributor to arrhythmogenesis in ARVC [7].

Desmosomes also participate in intercellular signalling networks, of which the Wnt/beta-catenin pathway is the most extensively studied. In the archetypal pathway the cytoplasmic concentration of beta-catenin is exquisitely regulated by multiple inputs, including secreted ligands of the Wnt family and recruitment of beta-catenin to intercellular junctional complexes. Cytoplasmic accumulation of beta-catenin leads to its nuclear translocation, association with the T-cell factor/lymphoid enhancer factor (Tcf/Lef) family of transcription factors and subsequent changes in gene expression. This evolutionarily conserved pathway plays a central role in many of the most fundamental cellular behaviours and has been directly implicated in the regulation of cell fate, proliferation, and apoptosis. Importantly, the various pathway components are duplicated in higher organisms, and specific isoforms may even be employed serially for discrete functions at different times and at different sites. In addition, superimposed on the basic structure of the Wnt/beta-catenin signalling network are many subtle feedback loops and points of cross-talk that are only beginning to be uncovered [7].

Elegant immunohistochemical studies have shown that the mutant form of the plakoglobin protein fails to integrate into desmosomes and shifts from intercalated discs to site cytosol and nuclear pools, where it causes changes in nuclear signalling and the transcriptional activity, in particular through pathways regulated by the protein beta-catenin [2].

The fibrofatty tissue that replaces myocardium in ARVC is thought to contribute to the development of ventricular arrhythmias by slowing intraventricular conduction and acting as a substrate for arrhythmias through a scar related macroreentry mechanism, similar to that observed after myocardial infarction. Life-threatening ventricular arrhythmias in ARVC may also be the result of mechanisms operating at the molecular and cellular levels. Desmosomes, sodium channels, and gap junction proteins interact synergistically to regulate adhesion, excitability, and coupling of myocytes; this coordinated network of proteins located at the intercalated discs has been termed the "connexome" [2]. Loss of expression of desmosomal proteins may cause (or contribute to) potentially fatal arrhythmias by inducing gap junction remodelling, with reduction of total content and substantial redistribution of the gap-junction protein connexin 43, and decreasing the amplitude and kinetics of the sodium current [2].

The Brugada syndrome is a cardiac ion-channel disorder caused by a genetic deficiency in sodium channel function. There is some evidence that the Bruguda syndrome and ARVC may share clinical features and arrhythmic mechanisms as a result of their common origin from the connexome [2].

7. Clinical presentation

The onset occurs usually after childhood, with palpitations and/or syncope. The following clinical pictures have been observed [6]: **1. Subclinical face with concealed structural abnormalities**-the affected patient has no symptoms, and cardiac arrest may be the first and last manifestation of the disease. ARVC has been reported as one of the leading causes of sudden death in the young [6]. **2. Overt electrical disorder**-with palpitations and syncope. The most typical clinical presentation of the disease is symptomatic ventricular arrhythmias of RV origin, usually triggered by effort. Arrhythmias range from isolated premature ventricular beat to sustained ventricular tachycardia (VT) with LBBB morphology up to ventricular fibrillation leading to cardiac arrest. The QRS morphology and axis during VT reflect its site of origin. A LBBB with inferior axis suggests an origin from the RV outflow tract (RVOT), while a LBBB with superior axis suggests an origin from the RV inferior wall. However, VTs with LBBB morphology are not specific for ARVC. Basal ECG may disclose inverted T waves in the right precordial leads (a T wave inverted beyond V1 after 14 years of age is almost pathognomonic of ARVC/D) (**Figure 3**) [6]. QRS enlargement of more than 110 ms and epsilon waves are strongly indicated of intraventricular impulse conduction delay. Signal average ECG may help to disclose fragmented low amplitude late potentials at the end of the QRS complex [6].

3. Heart failure- The progressive loss of the RV myocardium may impair the mechanical function of the RV and account for severe pump failure [6].

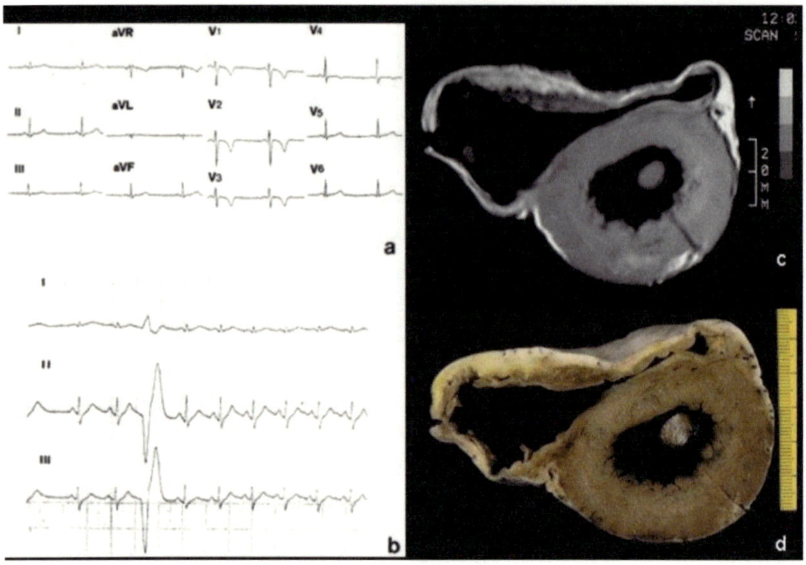

Figure 3.
A 17 year old asymptomatic male athlete who died suddenly during a soccer game. 12 lead ECG showing inverted T waves up to V4 (a) and isolated premature ventricular beats (b). In vitro MRI (c) and corresponding cross section of the heart (d) show RV dilatation with anterior and posterior aneurysms [6].

4. Biventricular failure- When the disease involves the ventricular septum and the LV, congestive heart failure occurs, mimicking dilated cardiomyopathy. Endocavitary mural thrombosis may occur, especially within aneurysms or in the atrial appendages when heart failure is complicated by atrial fibrillation, as to account for thromboembolism. In such conditions, contractile dysfunction may be so severe as to require cardiac transplantation. Clearly, when LV is affected ventricular arrhythmias may appear polymorphic, originating from different cardiac regions. The occurrence of fatal outcome, mostly sudden death varies between 0.1–3% per year in adults with diagnosed and treated ARVC, but it is unknown and may be higher in adolescents and young adults, in whom the disease is concealed and the first manifestation can be sudden death [6].

8. Diagnosis

To standardise the clinical diagnosis of ARVC, in 1994 an international task force proposed guidelines in the form of a qualitative scoring system with major and minor criteria [2]. In 2010, the task force revised the guidelines to improve diagnostic sensitivity, mostly for the clinical screening of family members, by providing quantitative criteria for diagnosing right ventricular abnormalities and adding molecular genetic criteria [1] (**Table 1**). However, the diagnosis remains problematic because of the low specificity of electrocardiographic abnormalities, multiple causes of right ventricular arrhythmias, difficulties in the use of imaging to assess right ventricular structure and function, and the sometimes puzzling results of genetic testing.

The diagnosis is particularly challenging in children, because clinical manifestations of earlier ARVC are subtle [2]. Cardiac Magnetic Resonance Imaging (MRI) is an attractive imaging toolBecause it is non-invasive and has the ability to characterise tissue by distinguishing fat from muscle [6] (**Figure 4**) and has proved to be more sensitive than electrocardiography for detecting early ventricular dilatation and dysfunction in children [2].

I. Global or regional dysfunction/structural alterations	
Major	2D TTE
	Regional RV akinesia, dyskinesia or aneurysm
	and 1 of the following criteria (end diastole):
	• PLAX RVOT ≥32 mm (PLAX/BSA] ≥19 mm/m^2)
	• PSAX RVOT ≥36 mm (PSAX/BSA] ≥21 mm/m^2)
	or RV fractional area change ≤33 %
	CMR
	Regional RV akinesia, dyskinesia, or dyssynchronous RV contraction
	and 1 of the following criteria (end diastole):
	• RV end-diastolic volume /BSA ≥110 mL/m^2 (male) or ≥100 mL/m^2 (female)
	or RV ejection fraction ≤40 %
	RV Angiography
	Regional RV akinesia, dyskinesia or aneurysm
Minor	2D TTE
	Regional RV akinesia, or dyskinesia
	and 1 of the following criteria (end diastole):
	• PLAX RVOT ≥29–31 mm ([PLAX/BSA] ≥16–18 mm/m^2)
	• PSAX RVOT ≥32–35 mm ([PSAX/BSA] ≥18–20 mm/m^2)
	• RV fractional area change >33–39 %
	CMR
	Regional RV akinesia, dyskinesia or dyssynchronous RV contraction
	and 1 of the following criteria (end diastolic):
	• RV end-diastolic volume/BSA ≥100–109 mL/'m^2 (male) or ≥90–99 mL/m^2 (female)
	or RV ejection fraction >40–44 %
II. Histopathology (endomyocardial biopsy)	
Major	Residual myocytes <60 % by morphometric analysis (or <50 % if estimated), with fibrous replacement of the RV free wall myocardium
	≥1 sample, with or without fatty replacement
Minor	Residual myocytes 60–75 % by morphometric analysis (or 50–65 % if estimated), with fibrous replacement of the RV free wall
	≥1 sample, with or without fatty replacement
III. Repolarisation abnormalities (14 years of age)	
Major	T-wave inversions V1–3 or beyond (in absence of complete RBBB)
Minor	T-wave inversions V1–2 or V4–6 (in absence of complete RBBB)
	T-wave inversions VI–4, if complete RBBB present

IV. Depolarisation abnormalities	
Major	ε wave (reproducible low-amplitude signals between end of QRS complex to onset of the T wave) in V1–3
Minor	Signal-averaged ECG with late potentials (if QRS on standard surface ECG <110 ms)
V. Arrhythmias	
Major	Non-sustained or sustained ventricular tachycardia (VT) of LBBB morphology with superior axis
Minor	Non-sustained or sustained VT of RVOT configuration, LBBB morphology with inferior axis or of unknown axis
	>500 VES per 24 h (Holter)
VI. Family history	
Major	ARVC/D in a first-degree relative who meets current Task Force Criteria
	ARVC/D confirmed pathologically at autopsy or surgery in a first-degree relative
	Identification of a pathogenic mutation categorised as associated with ARVC/D in index patient
Minor	Suspected ARVC/D in a first-degree relative (current Task Force criteria can not be determined)
	Premature SCD (<35 years of age) due to suspected ARVC/D in a first-degree relative
	ARVC/D confirmed pathologically or by current Task Force Criteria in second-degree relatives

Definite diagnosis: two major or one major and two minor criteria or four minor from different categories; Borderline diagnosis: one major and one minor or three minor criteria from different categories; Possible diagnosis: one major or two minor criteria from different categories BSA - body surface area; CMR - cardiac magnetic resonance tomography; ECG - electrocardiogram; LV - left ventricle; PLAX - parasternal long-axis view; PSAX - parasternal short-axis view; RBBB - right bundle branch block; RVOT - RV outflow tract; RV - right ventricle; TTE - transthoracic echocardiogram; VES - ventricular extrasystole; VT - ventricular tachycardia.[102]

Table 1.
Revised 2010 task force criteria for diagnosis of ARVC/D [1].

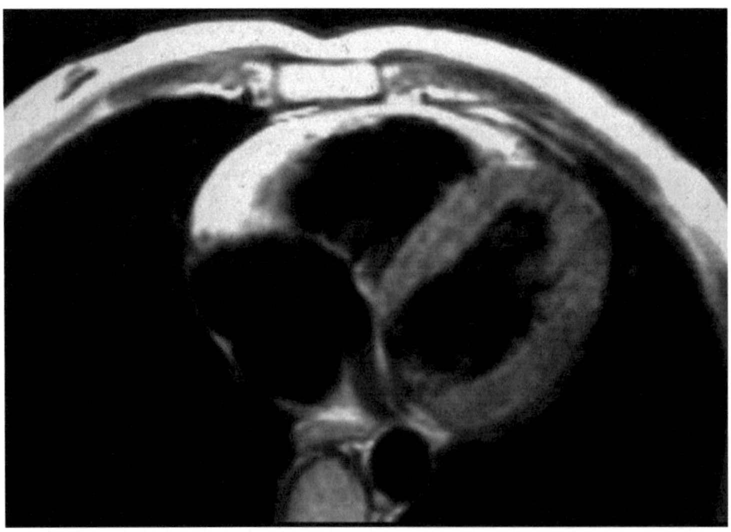

Figure 4.
MRI in a patient affected by ARVC/D (long axis view of the right ventricle): Note the transmural diffuse bright signal in the RV free wall on spin echo T1 (a) due to massive myocardial atrophy with fatty replacement (b) [6].

Conditions that may be difficult to differentiate from ARVC include idiopathic right ventricular outflow-tract tachycardia, cardiac sarcoidosis, and continental heart disease leading to right ventricular volume overload. Biventricular variants of the disease with severe left ventricular involvement may be indistinguishable from dilated cardiomyopathy. The difficult differential diagnosis, together with referral bias, may account for the discrepancies in the reported incidence of heart failure in patients with ARVC [2].

9. Risk stratification

The clinical course of ARVC is characterised by the occurrence of arrhythmic events, which can cause SCD, and the impairment of biventricular systolic function, which can lead to death from heart failure. The estimated overall mortality varies among studies, ranging from 0.08–3.6% per year [2]. The mortality was initially overestimated because it was based on studies at tertiary referral centres which predominantly included high-risk patients. Recent studies of community-based patient cohorts have shown that the long-term outcome for treated index patients and family members is favourable- annual mortality <1% [2].

The prognosis for patients with ARVC depends largely on the severity of arrhythmias and ventricular dysfunction. Prior cardiac arrest due to ventricular fibrillation and sustained VT are the most important predictors of life-threatening arrhythmic events during follow-up. Major risk factors include unexplained syncope, non-sustained VT on ambulatory monitoring or exercise testing, and severe systolic dysfunction of the RV, LV or both.

Although intracardiac electrophysiological testing has traditionally been used to assess the risk of ventricular arrhythmias, the prognostic value of VT or ventricular fibrillation induced by programmed ventricular stimulation in patients with asymptomatic ARVC remains unclear [2].

10. Management

The aims of clinical management of ARVC are to reduce the risk of sudden cardiac death and improve the quality of life by alleviating arrhythmic and heart failure symptoms. Restriction from intense sports activity (physical exercise may aggravate mechanical uncoupling of myocytes) is regarded as an important preventive tool for both healthy gene carriers and clinically affected persons in order to protect them from the risk of exercise-related malignant arrhythmic events and disease development or progression. The available evidence indicates that family members with a negative phenotype (either healthy gene carriers or those with an unknown genotype) do not need any specific treatment other than sports restriction; however, lifelong clinical assessment with the use of non-invasive tests at least every 2 years is warranted because of the age-related penetrance and progressive nature of ARVC [2].

Despite limited supportive data, beta-blockers are currently recommended for all clinically affected persons, for both prevention of arrhythmias and reduction of right ventricular wall stress. In patients with ventricular arrhythmias, antiarrhythmic drugs therapy offers the potential to ameliorate symptoms, although there is no proof that it confers protection against sudden cardiac death. Amiodarone, alone or in association with beta-blockers, and sotalol are the most effective drugs, combining the synergistic effects of class III antiarrhythmic properties and beta adrenergic blockade. The potential for serious cumulative toxic effects precludes long-term therapy with amiodarone, especially in younger patients [2].

Catheter ablation is a therapeutic option for patients who have episodes of sustained, monomorphic ventricular tachycardia. However, it should be regarded as a palliative rather than curative therapeutic approach because of the high frequency of subsequent recurrences of ventricular tachycardia and the unproven efficacy of ablation as a means of preventing sudden cardiac death. The poor long-term outcome has been attributed to the progressive nature of ARVC, which leads to the development of multiple arrhythmogenic foci over time. The epicardial location of some ventricular tachycardia reentry circuits, which reflects the propensity of ARVC lesions to originate and progress from the epicardium, may also explain the failure of conventional endocardial mapping and catheter ablation. Several studies have shown the feasibility and efficacy of epicardial catheter ablation for patients in whom one or more endocardial procedures have been unsuccessful [2].

Since surgical isolation of RV free wall (a therapeutic approach previously) risks postoperative RV failure, this procedure has been replaced by Implantable cardioverter-defibrillator (ICD) placement [1]. Although randomised trials of defibrillator therapy have not been performed, data from observational studies have consistently shown that it is effective and safe. Patients who benefit most from defibrillators (ICD) are those who have had an episode of ventricular fibrillation or sustained ventricular tachycardia. It remains uncertain whether defibrillator therapy is appropriate for primary prevention of sudden cardiac death among patients with one or more risk factors and no prior major arrhythmic events [2].

In asymptomatic patients with no risk factors and in healthy gene carriers, there is generally no indication for prophylactic defibrillator implantation because of the low risk of arrhythmias and the significant risk of device and electrode-related complications during long-term follow-up [2]. It has become apparent that defibrillators may be inappropriately implanted in patients with a false diagnosis of ARVC based on misinterpretation of cardiac MRI studies [2].

Patients in whom right or left heart failure develops are treated with a standard pharmacologic therapy, including angiotensin-converting enzyme inhibitors, angiotensin II receptor blockers, beta-blockers, and diuretics. Therapy with oral anticoagulants is reserved for patients with atrial fibrillation or thromboembolic complications. Cardiac transplantation is the ultimate therapy for patients with untreatable arrhythmias (e.g. incessant storms of ventricular tachycardia or fibrillation) or congestive heart failure that is refractory to pharmacologic and nonpharmacologic therapies [2].

In patients with late complications of the disease, who develop heart failure symptoms or life-threatening and untreatable VT, heart transplantation could be an option with good short and long-term survival. Heart transplantation is essentially the final therapeutic option for these patients [1].

Current therapeutic approaches to ARVC are palliative and partially alleviate symptoms and the risk of sudden cardiac death but do not prevent the development or progression of the disease process. A definitive curative treatment will require a deeper knowledge of the biologic mechanisms and environmental factors involved in the pathogenesis of ARVC. A recent observation concerns a small molecule designated SB216763, which is an activator of the Wnt signalling pathway. This molecule has been shown to prevent or reverse phenotypic manifestations of ARVC induced by overexpression of defective plakoglobin in a zebrafish model, as well as in rat cardiac myocytes. Although this drug is of interest as a potential mechanism-based therapy of ARVC, it has not yet been studied in humans [2].

11. Conclusion

ARVC is a progressive disease with life-threatening complications, which constitute a clinical diagnostic challenge for physicians, given the different genotype and phenotypic variations and the wide ranges of clinical manifestations. The main challenges to improve the risk stratification for better identification of high risk patients of SCD and heart failure, most benefit from early intervention with lifestyle changes, restriction of physical activity, antiarrhythmic drugs, ICD placement, new ablation approaches with simultaneous endocardial and epicardial ablation and, if necessary, heart transplantation. These interventions are available and life saving, with the potential to change the natural history of the disease by offering a good quality and better life expectancy [1].

ARVC at a quick glance

- Arrythmogenic right ventricular cardiomyopathy (ARVC) is a genetic form of cardiomyopathy causing fibro-fatty replacement of the myocardium.
- Transmission is usually autosomal dominant, with a male to female preponderance.
- The desmoplakin gene (DSP), the first desmosomal protein gene to be associated with a major form of the disease.
- ARVC is a myocyte adhesion disorder.
- ARVC is currently the second most common cause of SCD in the young population.
- Pathophysiology includes myocardial atrophy, fibrofatty replacement, and chamber dilatation.
- ARVC presents a diagnostic challenge- 2010 revised task force criteria for ARVC, ECG, echocardiogram, cardiac MRI, myocardial biopsy, family screening and risk stratification being the cornerstones.
- Therapeutic options are based on preventing life-threatening arrhythmia– both primary and secondary prevention – starting from ICD and radiofrequency ablation to heart transplantation in patients with late complications.

Acknowledgements

The author thanks her family and loved ones for their inspiration and unwavering support and faith.

Abbreviations

ARVC	Arrhythmogenic right ventricular cardiomyopathy
ARVC/D	Arrhythmogenic right ventricular cardiomyopathy/dysplasia
ICD	Implantable cardioverter-defibrillator
LBBB	Left bundle branch block
LV	Left ventricle
MRI	Magnetic Resonance Imaging
PKP2	Plakophilin 2
RV	Right ventricle
RVOT	Right ventricle outflow tract
SCD	Sudden cardiac death
TGF	Transforming growth factor
VT	Ventricular tachycardia
WHO	World Health Organisation

Author details

Sukanya Ghosh
Royal Preston Hospital, United Kingdom

*Address all correspondence to: sukanyaghosh18@gmail.com

References

[1] Jorge Romero; *et al.* "Arrhythmogenic right ventricular cardiomyopathy ARVC/D: A systemic literature review". *Clinical Medicine Insights: Cardiology* Libertas Academica 2013; 7(7):97-114.

[2] Domenico Corrado; *et al.* "Arrhythmogenic Right Ventricular Cardiomyopathy" *The New England Journal of Medicine* 2017; 376:61-72.

[3] Marcus FI;*et al.* *"Genetics of arrythmogenic right ventricular cardiomyopathy: a practical guide for physicians."* J Am Coll Cardiology 2013; 61:1945-8.

[4] Lancisi GM: "*De Motu Cordis et Aneurysmatibus.*" Naples. 1736

[5] Dalla Volta S,*et al.* *"'Auricularization' of right ventricular pressure curve."* Am Heart J. 1961, 61: 25-33.

[6] Thiene G,*et al."Arrhythmogenic right ventricular cardiomyopathy/dysplasia."* Orphanet J Rare Dis 2, 45 (2007).

[7] MacRae CA, *et al.* *"Arrhythmogenic right ventricular cardiomyopathy: moving toward mechanism."* J Clin Invest. 2006 Jul;116(7):1825-8.

[8] Rampazzo A,et al. *"A new locus for arrhythmogenic right ventricular cardiomyopathy (ARVD2) maps to chromosome 1q42-q43."* Hum Mol Genet. 1995;4(11):2151-4.

[9] Carol G *et al.* *" Arrhythmogenic right ventricular cardiomyopathy"* J Am Coll Cardiol. 2001 Dec, 38 (7) 1773-1781.

Section 4

Hypertrophic Cardiomyopathy

Chapter 11

Hypertrophic Cardiomyopathy: Genetics, Pathogenesis, Diagnosis, Clinical Course and Therapy

Davide Lazzeroni and Claudio Stefano Centorbi

Abstract

Hypertrophic cardiomyopathy (HCM) is a genetic disorder of cardiac myocytes that is characterized by cardiac hypertrophy, unexplained by the loading conditions, a non-dilated left ventricle and a normal or increased left ventricular ejection fraction (LV-EF). Prevalence of HCM has been estimated at 0.16% to 0.29% (≈ 1:625–1:344 individuals) in the general adult population. HCM represents the most common genetic heart disease and represent an archetypical single gene disorder with an autosomal dominant pattern of inheritance and historically termed a "disease of the sarcomere". The precise mechanisms by which sarcomere variants result in the clinical phenotype have not been fully understood. Mutant sarcomere genes trigger several myocardial changes, leading to hypertrophy and fibrosis, which ultimately result in a small, stiff ventricle with impaired systolic and diastolic performance despite a preserved LV-EF. The most common differential diagnosis challenges in the presence of hypertrophic heart disease are represented by: athlete's heart, hypertensive heart and other cardiomyopathies mimicking HCM. A multimodality approach using ECG, echocardiography, CMR, cardiac computed tomography (CCT) and cardiac nuclear imaging provides unique information about diagnosis, staging and clinical profiles, anatomical and functional assessment, metabolic evaluation, monitoring of treatment, follow-up, prognosis and risk stratification, as well as preclinical screening and differential diagnosis. HCM may be associated with a normal life expectancy and a very stable clinical course. However, about a third of patients develop heart failure (HF); in addition, 5–15% of cases show progression to either the restrictive or the dilated hypokinetic evolution of HCM, both of which may require evaluation for cardiac transplantation. The clinical course of HCM has been classified into four clinical stages: non-hypertrophic, classic, adverse remodeling and overt dysfunction phenotype. No evidence-based treatments are available for non-hypertrophic HCM patients (pre-hypertrophic stage), on the other hand in classic HCM, adverse remodeling and overt dysfunction phenotype, pharmacological or interventional strategies have the target to improve functional capacity, reduce symptoms, prevent disease progression. Therapeutic approach mainly differs on the basis of the presence or absence of significant obstructive HCM. Adult patients with HCM report an annual incidence for cardiovascular death of 1–2%, with sudden cardiac death (SCD), HF and thromboembolism being the main causes of death; the most commonly recorded fatal arrhythmic event is spontaneous ventricular fibrillation. For this reason, SCD risk estimation is an integral part of clinical management of HCM. International guidelines suggest the evaluation of several risk factor for SCD based on personal and family history, non-invasive testing including echocardiography, ambulatory electrocardiographic 24 hours monitoring and CMR imaging in order to identity those patients most likely to benefit implantable cardioverter-defibrillator (ICD) implantation. The present chapter summarize genetics, pathogenesis, diagnosis, clinical course and therapy of HCM as well as novel therapeutic options.

Keywords: hypertrophic cardiomyopathy, left ventricular hypertrophy, genetics, sudden cardiac death, heart failure, echocardiography, cardiac magnetic resonance, athlete's heart, hypertrophic phenocopies

1. Introduction

1.1 Definition and epidemiology

Cardiomyopathies are defined by structural and functional abnormalities of the ventricular myocardium that are unexplained by flow-limiting coronary artery disease or abnormal loading conditions [1]. Historically, cardiomyopathies has been subdivided into primary disease, in which the heart is the only involved organ, and secondary forms where the cardiomyopathy is a manifestation of a systemic disorder. Hypertrophic cardiomyopathy (HCM) is a genetic disorder of cardiac myocytes that is characterized by cardiac hypertrophy, unexplained by the loading conditions, a non-dilated left ventricle (LV) and a normal or increased left ventricular ejection fraction (LV-EF) [2]. HCM is a disorder without a distinct geographic, ethnic or gender pattern of distribution. Prevalence of HCM has been estimated at 0.16% to 0.29% ($\approx$ 1:625–1:344 individuals) in the general adult population [2–5]. HCM is characterized by highly variable genotype–phenotype relationship with intra- and inter-family expressivity and incomplete penetrance. Given the age-dependent expression of HCM mutations, its prevalence is expected to be higher in older subjects; in fact, HCM has been reported in 0.29% (1:333) of 60-year-old individuals undergoing echocardiography for cardiovascular evaluation. [2–5]. Moreover, a much higher estimate of 0.6% (1:167) has been suggested using more sensitive imaging methods, when family members are evaluated and when genetic testing is more widely used [6–8]. On the other hand, in children cardiac hypertrophy could result from the phenocopy conditions, which might account for 5% to 10% of the clinically diagnosed HCM cases [9–11].

2. Genetics

HCM represents the most common genetic heart disease reported in populations globally. HCM is an archetypical single gene disorder with an autosomal dominant pattern of inheritance, whereby a single mutation is usually sufficient to cause the disease, albeit with variable penetrance and expression [12]. Autosomal recessive and X-linked modes of inheritance have been described but are rare [13, 14]. Approximately 60% of patients with HCM have a clearly recognizable familial disease. On the other hand, despite the great advances of the research in the field of genetics in cardiomyopathies, to date about 40% of HCM shows negative genetic testing or variants of non-certain significance. These data suggest that even non-genetic factors could contribute to the development of HCM. Moreover, a substantial proportion of patients with HCM are currently without any evidence of a genetic etiology to their disease, including a subgroup who also have no other affected family members (named "non-familial" HCM) [15]. For these reasons, the absence of an identified causative mutation should not allow to exclude a diagnosis in the presence of diagnostic criteria for HCM. Historically, HCM was termed a

DOI: http://dx.doi.org/10.5772/intechopen.97033

"disease of the sarcomere" when the first three disease genes encoding components of the contractile apparatus of heart muscle were identified [16]. However, a wide variety of non-sarcomeric genes has been associated with HCM, thus suggesting that LV hypertrophy in HCM may not be a consequence of exclusive sarcomeric mutations. Among the known causal genes (**Figure 1**), thick myofilaments proteins such as MYH7 and MYBPC3 (myosin- binding protein C) are the 2 most common, together being responsible for approximately half of the patients with familial HCM [17–20]. On the other hand, mutations in thin myofilament proteins such as TNNT2, TNNI3 (cardiac troponin I) and TPM1 (α-tropomyosin) are relatively uncommon causes of HCM and together are responsible for less than 10% of cases [19–22]. Mutations in ACTC1 (cardiac α-actin), MYL2 (myosin light chain 2), MYL3 (myosin light chain 3), and CSRP3 (cysteine and glycine-rich protein 3) are also established, albeit uncommon, causes of HCM [23–25]. Moreover, mutations in TTN (titin), TCAP (telethonin), MYOZ2 (myozenin 2), TRIM63 (ubiquitin E3 ligase tripartite motif protein 63 or MuRF1), and FHL1 (four-and-a-half LIM domains 1) also have been implicated as causes of HCM but occur typically in sporadic cases and small families [26–33]. On the other hand, mutations in TNNC1 (cardiac troponin C), MYH6 (myosin heavy chain or α-myosin heavy chain), PLN (phospholamban), CAV3 (caveolin3), ALPK3 (α kinase 3), and JPH2 (junctophilin-2) have also been reported in patients with HCM [34–39] but their causal role in HCM is less certain and has not been established unambiguously. An X-linked inheritance typically raises the possibility of a phenocopy condition, such as Fabry disease [40]. A phenocopy condition also occurs in syndromic diseases, such as the Noonan syndrome and in storage diseases, such as Anderson–Fabry disease. [41, 42]. Finally, a subset of HCM patients (≈5%) exhibits 2 (digenic) or more (oligogenic) causal mutations in the same gene or causal mutations in different genes [20, 43–51] and the severity of LV hypertrophy in subjects with

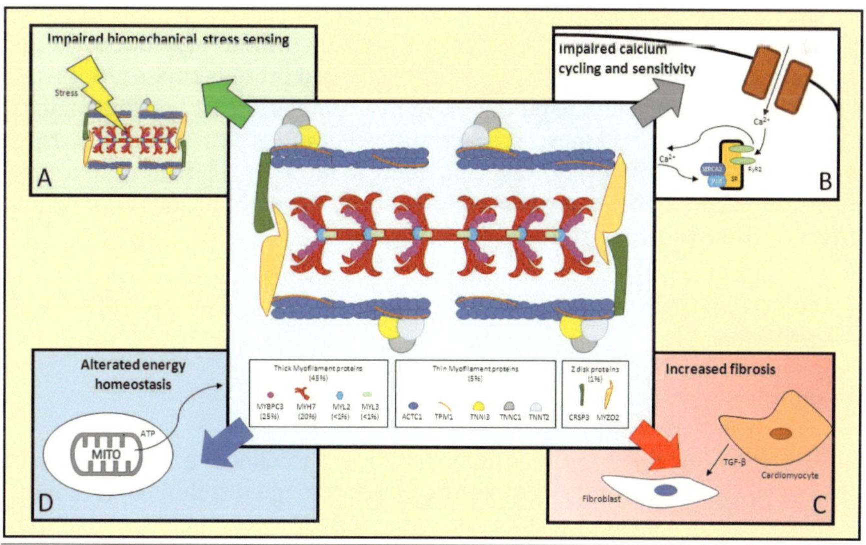

Figure 1.
HCM genetics and pathogenetic mechanisms. Center part: A schematic structure of a sarcomere composed of thick and thin filaments and Z discs is showed along with its protein constituents. Established causal genes for HCM and their relative population frequencies are listed. Panel A-D: HCM pathogenetic pathways (not be considered in isolation since they can act in concert). Panel a: Biomechanical stress sensing pathway. Panel B: Calcium cycling and sensitivity pathway. Panel C: Energy homeostasis pathway. Panel D: Fibrotic pathway. Abbreviations: LTCC, voltage-dependent L-type calcium channel; PLB, cardiac phospholamban; RyR2, ryanodine receptor 2; SERCA2, sarcoplasmic/endoplasmic reticulum calcium ATPase 2; SR, sarcoplasmic reticulum; TGF-β, transforming growth factor β; MITO, mitochondria.

such mutations seems to be more pronounced [44–48]. The majority of the causal mutations in HCM are missense mutations which may alter protein structure and function by changing the amino acid composition of the encoding protein. The insertion/deletion mutations induce a frameshift in the encoded protein. Likewise, the premature truncated proteins are subsequently degraded by the ubiquitin proteasome system, leading to haplo-insufficiency [19, 20, 52]. The missing causal gene in HCM might be in part because of the difficulty in ascertaining the causality of the genetic variants, in an unambiguous manner, in the sporadic cases and small families [53]. In general, genetic variants exert highly variable biological consequences, ranging from large and causal to clinically negligible [54–56]. The demonstration of an association between a candidate gene and the HCM phenotype in a discovery population is considered provisional (ie, hypothesis-generating) and requires testing for replication in an independent population.

3. Pathogenesis

The precise mechanisms by which sarcomere variants result in the clinical phenotype have not been fully understood. Mutant sarcomere genes trigger several myocardial changes, leading to hypertrophy and fibrosis, which ultimately result in a small, stiff ventricle with impaired systolic and diastolic performance despite a preserved LV-EF [57]. On the other hand, abnormal sarcomeric proteins may not be solely responsible for all of the clinical characteristics observed in patients with HCM. Diverse disease features including abnormal intramural coronary arteries, responsible for small vessel ischemia, elongated mitral valve leaflets, as well as congenital anomalies of the sub-mitral valve apparatus, appear to have no known direct association with sarcomere mutations. From a metabolic viewpoint, mutations in sarcomeric proteins generally increase myofilament activation and result in myocyte hypercontractility and excessive energy use [58] due to higher (disproportionate) mitochondrial activity (**Figure 1**). Mitochondrial impairments in the cardiac energy-sensing apparatus (e.g., AMP-activated protein kinase [AMPK]) as well as alterations in calcium handling result in a stimulation of signaling pathways (e.g., the Janus-associated kinase–signal transducers and activators of transcription [JAK–STAT] signaling pathway) that contribute to myocyte relaxation abnormalities and growth, with aberrant tissue architecture abnormalities such as myofibrillar disarray and myocardial fibrosis [59–62].

4. Diagnosis

4.1 Diagnostic criteria

In 2014 ESC Guidelines, HCM is defined by a wall thickness ≥ 15 mm in one or more LV myocardial segments - as measured by any imaging technique (echocardiography, cardiac magnetic resonance imaging (CMR) or computed tomography (CT) - that is not explained solely by loading conditions, thereby including both sarcomeric and non-sarcomeric mutations, such as other genetic disorders (inherited metabolic and neuromuscular diseases, chromosome abnormalities) genetic syndromes and non-genetic disorders (e.g. senile-TTR and AL amyloidosis) [2]. On the other hand, in 2020 AHA Guidelines, HCM is defined as a disease state in which morphologic expression is confined solely to the heart and characterized predominantly by LVH (wall thickness ≥ 15 mm) in the absence of another cardiac, systemic, or metabolic disease capable of producing the magnitude of hypertrophy evident in a given patient and for which a disease-causing sarcomere (or sarcomere-related) variant is identified, or genetic etiology remains unresolved [57].

Genetic and non-genetic disorders can present with lesser degrees of wall thickening (13–14 mm). In these cases, the diagnosis of HCM requires evaluation of other features including family history, non-cardiac symptoms and signs, electrocardiogram (ECG) abnormalities, laboratory tests and multi-modality cardiac imaging [2]. More limited LVH can be diagnostic in family members of HCM patients or with a positive genetic test [57]. Children, as in adults, the diagnosis of HCM requires an LV wall thickness more than two standard deviations greater than the predicted mean (z-score: defined as the number of standard deviations from the population mean) [63]. In first-degree relatives of HCM patients with unequivocal disease (LVH ≥15 mm) the diagnosis is based on the presence of otherwise unexplained increased LV wall thickness ≥ 13 mm in one or more LV myocardial segments, as measured using any cardiac imaging technique [echocardiography, cardiac magnetic resonance (CMR) or CT].

4.2 Differential diagnosis: *"from athlete's heart to HCM phenocopies"*

The most common differential diagnosis challenges in the presence of hypertrophic heart disease are represented by: athlete's heart, hypertensive heart and other cardiomyopathies mimicking HCM.

4.2.1 Athlete's heart

HCM is the most common cause of sudden cardiac death (SCD) among athletes [64]. Systematic and endurance training can lead to physiologic LV hypertrophy thereby mimicking mild forms of HCM [64]. Distinguishing between these two forms represents an important diagnostic dilemma during athlete cardiac evaluation, thus a combination of anamnestical, clinical and instrumental data is crucial to distinguish the physiological hypertrophy seen in athlete's heart from the pathological one seen in HCM. A positive family history of SCD represent an important factor that may point towards a genetic cardiomyopathy; similarly, ECG abnormalities such as ST depression, T wave inversion, abnormal Q waves or QRS axis increase the likelihood of HCM. On the other hand, isolated positive ECG criteria for hypertrophy are not enough to suspect HCM in the athlete [64]. Even in the presence of septal thickness values suspected for mild form of HCM (ranging form 14–16 mm), in the athlete's heart echocardiogram generally presents several characteristics that are uncommon in HCM such as: normal or dilated LV volumes or normal systolic and diastolic function evaluated both with traditional methods (M-Mode or 2D) and with tissue Doppler or strain echocardiography. Moreover, a reduction in LV wall thickness after a period of deconditioning points to physiological hypertrophy [65]. In some cases, further investigations such as exercise testing (arrhythmias or abnormal blood pressure response), 24 hours ECG monitoring (arrhythmias), CMR (fibrosis) or genetic testing (causative mutations) are needed to define the presence of HCM. **Table 1** summarizes the clinical-instrumental aspects most useful in the differential diagnosis between HCM and athlete's heart.

4.2.2 Hypertensive heart

Left ventricular hypertrophy secondary to arterial hypertension can be difficult to distinguish from mild forms of non-obstructive HCM caused by sarcomeric mutations; moreover an overlap between primary and secondary LV hypertrophy could be present in up to 25% of adult HCM patients with arterial hypertension [66].

	Inheritance	**Signs or symptoms *of multi-organ involvement***	**ECG abnormalities *beyond LVH criteria***	***Routine* laboratory tests**	**Echocardiography**	**CMR *(LGE)***
Athlete's heart.	None	Uncommon	Isolated LVH	Not specific	LVH symmetrical or eccentric (mild-to-moderate). Normal systolic and diastolic function	Negative
Hypertensive heart	None	Uncommon	ST and T abnormalities	Not specific	LVH: usually concentric (mild-to-moderate)	Mild degree No specific pattern
HCM	AD	Uncommon	High LVH ST and T abnormalities Giant T wave inversion. Q waves.	Not specific	Moderate-to-severe LVH (asymmetrical and septal but potentially found at any location). Diastolic dysfunction, the LVOT obstruction Mitral valve abnormalities (mitral SAM, leaflets elongation, dysplasia, prolapse, chordal elongation, laxity and hypermobility). Atrial enlargement. Apical aneurysm	Frequent RV insertion points and Intramural potentially found at any location
Anderson–Fabry disease	X-linked	Visual impairment Sensorineural deafness Paraesthesiae/ sensory abnormalities Angiokeratoma	Short P-R / preexcitation AV block	Proteinuria with/without glomerular filtration rate	Concentric LVH Increased atrioventricular valve thickness Increased RV free wall thickness Global hypokinesia (with/without LV dilatation)	Frequent Posterolateral LGE in concentric LVH
Familiar amyloidosis	AD	Visual impairment Paraesthesiae/ sensory abnormalities Carpal tunnel syndrome (bilateral)	Low QRS voltage AV block	Proteinuria with/without glomerular filtration rate	Increased interatrial septum thickness and atrioventricular valve thickness. Increased RV free wall thickness. Pericardial effusion. Ground-glass appearance of myocardium. Global hypokinesia (with/without LV dilatation)	Frequent Diffuse subendocardial LGE "zebra" pattern Intense myocardial 'avidity' for Gadolinium

DOI: http://dx.doi.org/10.5772/intechopen.97033

	Inheritance	**Signs or symptoms *of multi-organ involvement***	**ECG abnormalities *beyond LVH criteria***	***Routine* laboratory tests**	**Echocardiography**	**CMR *(LGE)***
Danon disease	X-linked	Learning difficulties, mental retardation Visual impairment	Short P-R / preexcitation AV block Extreme LVH (Sokolow >100)	↑Creatine kinase ↑ Transaminase	Extreme concentric LVH. Global hypokinesia (with/without LV dilatation)	Frequent Large amount subendocardial or transmural
Mitochondrial cardiomyopathy	X-linked or matrilinear	Sensorineural deafness Learning difficulties, mental retardation Visual impairment Muscle weakness	Short P-R / preexcitation	↑ Creatine kinase Transaminase Lactic acidosis	Global hypokinesia (with/without LV dilatation)	Frequent Large amount Non-ischemic LGE Intramural pattern mostly confined to the basal LV inferolateral wall

Table 1.
HCM diagnosiss and differential diagnosis: "from athlete's heart to HCM phenocopies". Inheritance, signs or symptoms of multi-organ involvement, ECG abnormalities beyond LVH criteria, routine laboratory tests, echocardiographic and CMR main findings are shown for HCM and each phenocopies.

Detailed arterial hypertension history and arterial blood pressure assessment as well as clinical evaluation of relatives may be crucial in distinguishing between hypertensive heart and HCM. Moreover, a multimodality imaging approach is crucial in the differential diagnosis of HCM in hypertensive patients. Echocardiographic tissue doppler shows more impairment of diastolic function as well as lower early diastolic velocities in HCM [67, 68]. Similarly, two-dimensional (2D) strain echocardiography in HCM reveals a mid and apical short axis segments reduced radial strain as well as a reduced longitudinal strain in HCM with sarcomeric mutations [67, 68]. Moreover, myocardial fibrosis in CMR imaging as well as natriuretic peptides and troponin levels tend to be higher in HCM than in hypertensive heart [69].

4.2.3 HCM phenocopies

Significant advances and widespread availability of genetic testing at the same time have improved detection of the sarcomeric mutations that cause HCM but have also highlighted the significance of inborn errors of metabolism or metabolic storage disorders that can mimic HCM, named "HCM phenocopies" [70]. Five to ten percent of adult cases of HCM are caused by other genetic disorders including inherited metabolic and neuromuscular diseases, chromosome abnormalities, genetic syndromes as well as non-genetic disorders (e.g. TTR or AL amyloidosis) [71–74]. Whilst HCM phenocopies are relatively rare, it is crucial to distinguish these conditions at an early stage as their natural history, management, therapy and prognosis vary significantly from that of HCM with sarcomeric mutations. **Table 1** illustrates the salient features (red flags) of HCM phenocopies.

4.3 Multimodality imaging in HCM

Imaging techniques play an essential role in the evaluation of patients with HCM. A multimodality approach using ECG, echocardiography, CMR, cardiac computed tomography (CCT) and cardiac nuclear imaging provides unique information about diagnosis, staging and clinical profiles, anatomical and functional assessment, metabolic evaluation, monitoring of treatment, follow-up, prognosis and risk stratification, as well as preclinical screening and differential diagnosis (**Figure 2**).

ECG: is recommended at the first clinic visit in all individuals with known or suspected HCM and should be repeated whenever there is a change in symptoms in patients with an established diagnosis. It can be normal at presentation but generally shows a variable combination of LV hypertrohy (LVH), ST- and T-wave abnormalities and pathological Q-wave; ECG abnormalities that could mimicks other conditions, such as myocardial ischaemia or infarction, when interpreted together with echocardiography and CMR imaging findings, can suggest an underlying diagnosis or provide clues to the distribution of LVH and myocardial scar [75]. Moreover, since ECG abnormalities generally precede the development of LVH, periodic clinical and instrumental evaluations as well as family screening are useful even in the absence of conclusive diagnostic criteria. The frequency of arrhythmias detected during ambulatory electrocardiographic monitoring is age-related; asymptomatic non-sustained ventricular tachycardia (NSVT) occurs in 25% of adults with HCM and for this reason a 24 or 48 hour Holter ECG represents a primary test for estimate the risk of SCD [2, 76–77].

Echocardiography: is the central imaging technique to the diagnosis and monitoring of HCM, given that identifies and quantify LVH that generally is asymmetric and involving the interventricular septum in the basal LV segments but often extends into the lateral wall, the posterior septum and LV apex [78]. In fact, increased ventricular wall thickness can be potentially found at any location.

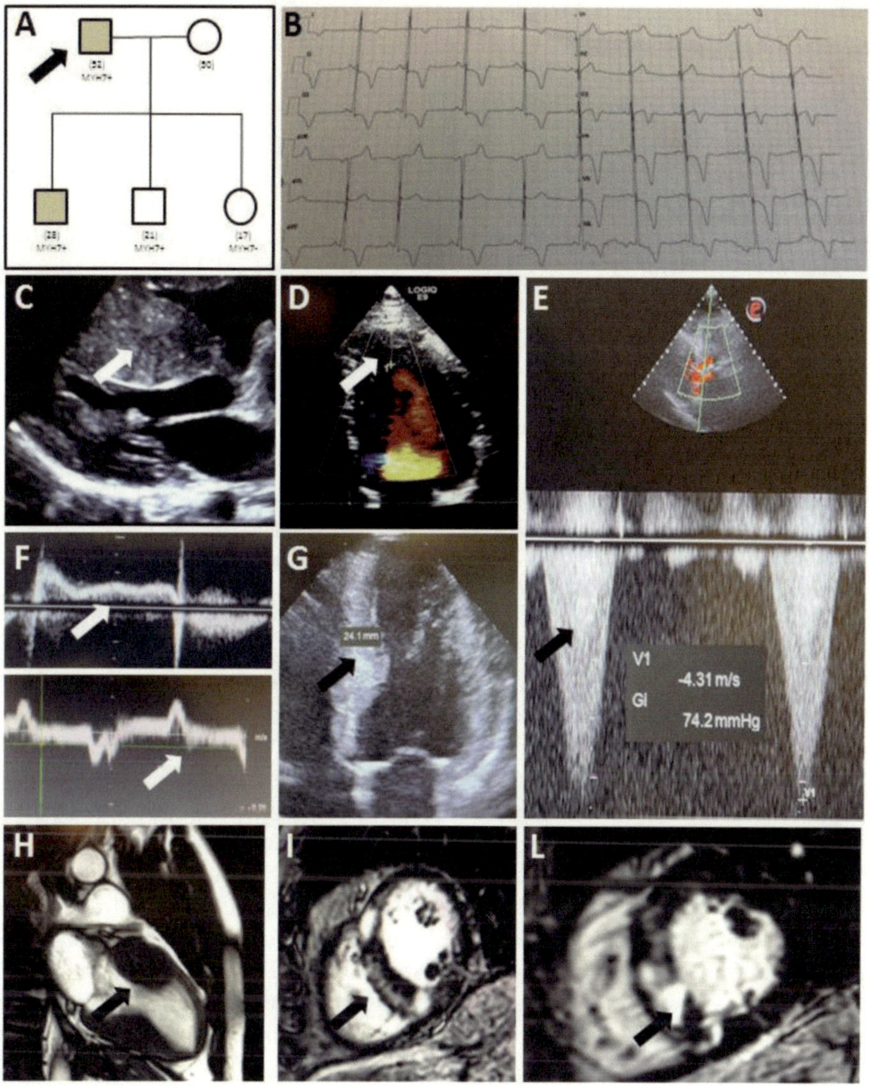

Figure 2.
*HCM: Inheritance and multimodality imaging. Panel A shows an HCM family pedigree with a MYH7+ mutation (autosomal dominant inheritance). The father and two of his children had HCM, another child was unaffected and was excluded from further clinical testing, and one child had a pathogenic mutation without LV hypertrophy. Black symbols denote affected family members, white symbols unaffected family members, squares male family members, and circles female family members; the arrow indicates the proband. The numbers under the symbols indicate age (in years) at the time of testing. Panel B shows ECG abnormalities in HCM characterized by: Short PR-interval, high QRS voltage, ST depression followed by diffuse giant T wave inversion. Panel C: HCM with extreme asymmetrical septal hypertrophy (45 mm – Echocardiography). Panel D: Apical HCM (echocardiography). Panel E shows HOCM with significant left ventricular outflow-tract obstruction (74 mmHg peak gradient at echocardiography). Panel F shows a triphasic doppler inflow velocities with restrictive pattern in addition to L wave (arrow) in HCM patients with thin myofilament associated mutation (upper side). Tissue Doppler showing severe diastolic dysfunction characterized by low e' (arrow) velocities (lower side). Panel G: Severe (24 mm) septal asymmetrical hypertrophy (arrow) in HCM (echocardiography). Panel H: Severe septal asymmetrical hypertrophy (arrow) in HCM (cardiac magnetic resonance). Panel I: HCM with fibrosis (cardiac magnetic resonance – LGE - arrow) at RV insertion points and intramural in the intraventricular septum. Panel L: HCM with diffuse and marked intramyocardial fibrosis (cardiac magnetic resonance – LGE - arrow) (**Figure 3**).*

Moreover, echocardiography estimates systolic and diastolic function, the presence of left ventricular outflow tract (LVOT) obstruction at rest and/or under provocative maneuvers such as Valsalva or standing, midventricular obstruction, mitral valve abnormalities (mitral SAM, leaflets elongation with excessive tissue, dysplasia and prolapse, chordal elongation, laxity and hypermobility), atrial enlargement, or apical aneurysm [79]. Stress echocardiography can be used to detect myocardial ischemia, significant misunderstood LVOT obstruction, symptoms and blood pressure response to exercise [80].

Cardiovascular magnetic resonance (CMR) imaging: provides detailed information on cardiac morphology, ventricular function and myocardial tissue characteristics [81]. CMR estimate left ventricle volumes, mass, ejection fraction as well as quantification, location, type and distribution of LVH but especially the visualization and quantification of myocardial fibrosis (LGE) [80].

In detection of myocardial ischaemia CCT is useful to evaluate the presence of epicardial coronary artery disease (CAD) in patients with HCM.

Single photon emission computed tomography/position emition tomography (SPECT/PET) myocardial perfusion imaging (using Thallium-201 and Tc-99 m labeled tracers) is useful to evaluate the presence of coronary microvascular dysfuntion showing reversible and fixed defects, thereby suggesting ischaemia and scar, with or without epicardial CAD detecting [82]. The assessment of myocardial metabolism can be performed through PET with F-18-fluorodeoxyglucose (FDG) or C-11-acetate, since an impairment in oxidative and glucose metabolism, mainly in the hypertrophic myocardium, has been found in HCM [83]. PET imaging has also been used to assess cardiac autonomic dysfunction, given that increased local catecholamine levels due to impaired neurotransmitter re-uptake into the cardiac nerve terminals, leading to decreased myocardial beta-adrenoceptor density, has been found in HCM [84].

Cardiopulmonary exercise testing (CPET): provides objective information about the severity of functional limitation, mechanisms responsible for symptoms during effort and plays a central role for cardiac transplantation indication [85]. CPET may be helpful in differentiating HCM from physiological ventricular hypertrophy since maximal oxygen consumption is normal or supra-normal in athlete's heart and reduced in HCM. Moreover, CPET or conventional treadmill- or bicycle ergometry may be used in several contests: initial clinical evaluation, change in symptoms, LVOT gradient evaluation during effort, blood pressure response during exercise, detecting signs of myocardial ischemia caused by epicardial CAD and/or microvascular dysfunction [86–90].

5. Clinical course and disease stanging

HCM may be associated with a normal life expectancy and a very stable clinical course. However, about a third of patients develop heart failure (HF); in addition, 5–15% of cases show progression to either the restrictive or the dilated hypokinetic evolution of HCM, both of which may require evaluation for cardiac transplantation [91, 92]. The clinical course of HCM has been masterfully classified by Olivotto et al. into four clinical stages: non-hypertrophic, classic, adverse remodeling and overt dysfunction phenotype [93] (**Figure 3**).

Non-hypertrophic HCM: is characterized by the absence of LVH in individuals with HCM-causing mutations identification during systematic family screenings. This stage of the disease is more frequent in newborn or very young children, while LVH tends to manifest during the second decade of life. However, due to incomplete penetrance and age-related onset, genotype-positive individuals can develop LVH as late as the 6th or 7th decade, and a significant minority seem to never develop the disease at all [94–96]. ECG, in this contest, is a fundamental tool to identify these patients since abnormalities can usually be evident even in the absence of LVH

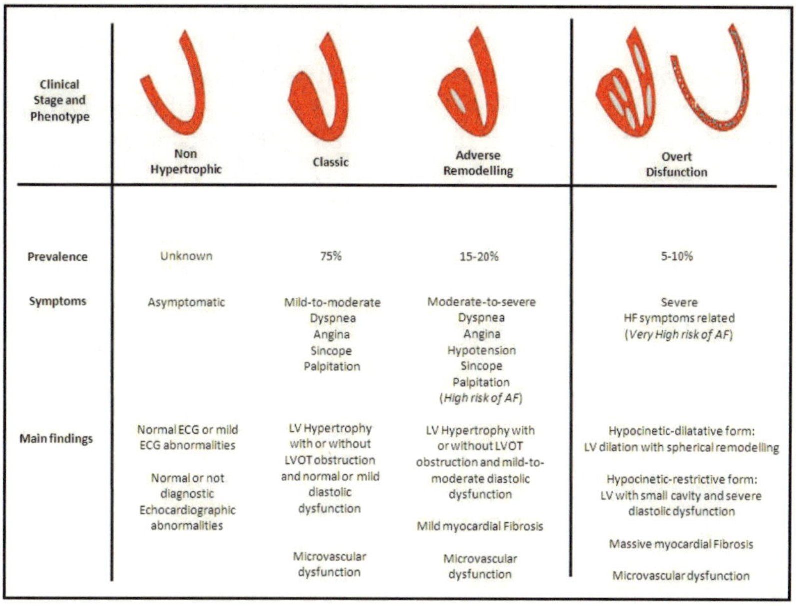

Figure 3.
Clinical stage and phenotypes of HCM: Prevalence, symptoms and main findings are separately shown for each stage of the disease.

on the echocardiogram [94]. Echocardiographic abnormalities may be found and includes impaired LV relaxation, mitral valve or subvalvar abnormalities, and mild degrees of left atrial enlargement. Although not diagnostic, these abnormalities may useful to suspect HCM in the context of familiar screening or ECG abnormalities context [79–94]. CMR shows some degree of LV hypertrophy in about 16% of genotype-positive subjects with negative echocardiography. Prognosis of genotype-positive individuals in this stage is unresolved, but presumed favorable [95, 96].

Classic HCM Phenotype: is defined as the phase in which the hypertrophic phenotype is fully expressed and the LV is hyperdynamic (as defined by an LV-EF >65%), without extensive fibrotic changes. LVH is typically regional and asymmetrical, generally involving the basal septum and anterior wall, but can potentially involve any part of myocardial muscle such as right ventricle or papillary muscles [94–97]. Moreover, a large number of mitral valve, sub-valvar, subaortic, midventricular abnormalities, atrial remodeling, coronary myocardial bridging, coronary microvascular dysfunction, crypts and autonomic nervous system abnormalities are present in this stage of the disease [79–99]. This stage is characterized by classic features such as myocardial disarray, microvascular remodeling, and interstitial fibrosis [95–101]. Most patients experience long periods of clinical stability without symptoms and may never undergo significant degrees of adverse remodeling or disease progression during their lifetime. Life expectancy is relatively favorable, with an annual cardiovascular mortality around 1% [94–102].

Adverse Remodeling Phenotype: is defined as the presence of structural modifications due to increasing LV fibrosis with worsening function (LV-EF 50%–65%) associated with relatively preserved clinical and hemodynamic balance (15% to 20% of patients) [103–105]. The definition of this intermediate stage of disease progression is based on a combination of several structural and functional features including an LV-EF in the low-normal range [106], moderate to severe diastolic dysfunction [107, 108], marked atrial enlargement [109], moderate areas of LV fibrosis [94, 106–111], severe microvascular dysfunction [112], thinning of the

LV walls [103], onset of atrial fibrillation (AF) [113], spontaneous reduction or loss of LVOT obstruction [103–114], LV apical aneurysms [115] and variable patterns of intramyocardial fibrosis [116] that is inversely related to LV-EF.

Overt dysfunction HCM Phenotype: (5% of patients) is characterized by severe functional deterioration of the LV (LV-EF < 50%) secondary by extreme degrees of fibrosis and remodeling and generally associated with hemodynamic decompensation and adverse outcome [103, 105, 110, 117–119] with accelerated clinical deterioration of clinical condition. The morpho-functional manifestation of this stage can be summarized in two distinct and opposite phenotypical patterns: the hypokinetic-dilated form (LV dilation with spherical remodeling) [95, 110, 118, 119], that often may be hard to distinguish from a primary dilated cardiomyopathy, and the hypokinetic restrictive form (LV with small cavity and extreme diastolic dysfunction), mimicking a primary restrictive cardiomyopathy [94, 118–122]. In both forms, overt dysfunction represents the extreme consequence of adverse remodeling and the outcome in this stage is severe, not only due to high rates of HF-related complications and mortality but also because of a considerable incidence of SCD [95, 118–123].

6. Management

No evidence-based treatments are available for non-hypertrophic HCM patients (pre-hypertrophic stage) and avoiding competitive activity may be considered in these individuals for the risk of development of HCM or SCD although this issue remains highly controversial [95, 124]. In classic HCM, adverse remodeling and overt dysfunction phenotype, pharmacological or interventional strategies have the target to improve functional capacity, reduce symptoms, prevent disease progression. Therapeutic approach mainly differs on the basis of the presence or absence of LVOT obstruction (HOCM). Patients with HCM who are asymptomatic and have no evidence of arrhythmias or LVOT obstruction at rest or on effort generally do not require medical treatment [125]. In symptomatic HOCM patients, the aim is to improve symptoms by using drugs, surgery, alcohol ablation or pacing. In symptomatic patients without LVOT obstruction, the target of therapy is to reduce arrhythmic risk, LV filling pressures as well as improve symptoms such as dyspnea and angina. Patients with progressive LV systolic or diastolic dysfunction refractory to medical therapy may be candidates for cardiac transplantation.

6.1 HOCM

LVOT obstruction is defined as a peak instantaneous Doppler gradient of ≥30 mm Hg and the threshold for invasive treatment is usually considered to be ≥50 mm Hg. In general, all HCOM patients should avoid dehydration and excess alcohol consumption, and weight loss should be encouraged. Arterial and venous dilators, such as nitrates and phosphodiesterase type 5 inhibitors, can exacerbate LVOT obstruction and should be avoided [126]. HOCM symptomatic patients can be treated initially with non-vasodilating ß-blockers titrated to maximum tolerated dose. If ß-blockers alone are ineffective, disopyramide can be added, titrated up to a maximum tolerated dose [127, 128] because can abolish basal LV outflow pressure gradients and improve exercise tolerance and functional capacity without pro-arrhythmic effects [129–131]. Verapamil or ditiazem can be used when ß-blockers are contraindicated or ineffective [132–135]. Patients with HOCM (gradient ≥50 mm Hg,) and drug-refractory symptoms benefit from septal reduction therapy (SRT). Both septal myectomy and alcohol septal ablation (ASA) are reasonable options when performed at experienced centres as part of a multidisciplinary team. Septal myectomy may be preferred when additional papillary muscle or mitral valve intervention can be performed, while ASA is favored for patients with elevated surgical risk [125]. Surgical myectomy has demonstrated excellent long-term efficacy and safety at selected high-volume centres with near-complete resolution of resting and inducible LVOT gradients. ASA showed similar perioperative mortality (about 1%) when compared to myectomy [136], although associated with a 10–15% rate of complete heart block, repeat procedures and increased risk of scar-related ventricular arrhythmias [137, 138]. Moreover, ASA is dependent on coronary anatomy since 15% of patients had unsuitable septal perforators [139]. In experienced centres, selective injection of alcohol into a septal perforator artery (or sometimes other branches of the left anterior descending coronary artery) to create a localized septal scar has outcomes similar to surgery in terms of gradient reduction, symptom improvement and exercise capacity [140–144]. Even in absence of randomized trials comparing surgery and ASA, several meta-analyses have shown that both procedures improve functional status with a similar procedural mortality [145–148].

6.2 Symptomatic patients without LVOT

In patients with normal LV-EF and no evidence of resting or provocable LVOT obstruction, aim of therapy is to reduce LV diastolic pressures and improve LV filling by slowing the heart rate with b-blockers, verapamil or diltiazem and cautious use of loop diuretics. Restoration of sinus rhythm or ventricular rate control is essential in patients who have permanent or frequent paroxysms of AF and digoxin is not recommended in patients with preserved EF because of the potentially adverse effects of positive inotropic stimulation [149]. ß-Blockers or calcium antagonists should be considered in patients with exertional or prolonged episodes of angina-like pain. Both classes improve diastolic function, reduce myocardial oxygen, thereby improving stress-induced sub-endocardial perfusion defects [150–154]. Patients with reduced LV-EF and HF symptoms should be treated with diuretics, ß-blockers, angiotensin-converting enzyme (ACE) inhibitors, angiotensin receptor blockers (ARB) and mineralocorticoid receptor antagonists (MRA) according to ESC guidelines for the management of chronic heart failure [155]. Moreover, CRT may be considered in individual patients with refractory symptoms, LV-EF < 35% and LBBB (QRS duration 120 ms) in accordance with current ESC Guidelines [156]. On the other hand, since LV-EF < 50%, rather than <35% as in primary or secondary dilated cardiomyopathies, is a strong discriminator of end-stage disease (associated with deteriorating HF and SCD) there is clear need for HCM disease-specific CRT and CRT-D criteria [57].

Orthotopic cardiac transplantation should be considered in patients with moderate-to-severe drug refractory symptoms (NYHA functional Class III–IV) and no LVOTO who meet standard eligibility criteria [157].

6.3 Management atrial fibrillation and anticoagulation therapy

Atrial fibrillation (AF) is the most frequent arrhythmia in HCM, affecting more than 20% of patients, and represents a marker of unfavorable prognosis, particularly when associated with LVOT obstruction and in patients younger than 50 years of age; moreover, the onset of AF worsens symptoms related to HF [158–160]. In haemodynamically stable patients, oral b-blockers or non-dihydropyridine calcium channel antagonists are recommended to slow the ventricular response to AF [161, 162]. Given the high incidence of stroke in patients with

HCM and paroxysmal, persistent or permanent AF, the current European Society of Cardiology (ESC) Guidelines of Atrial Fibrillation invite to do not use the CHA2DS2-VASc score to calculate stroke risk recommend that all patients with AF should receive treatment with OAC [163]. Similarly, the American Heart Association and American College of Cardiology (AHA/ACC) Guidelines recommended use direct-acting oral anticoagulants (NOAC) as first-line option and vitamin K antagonists as second-line option [57].

6.4 Prevention of sudden cardiac death

Adult patients with HCM report an annual incidence for cardiovascular death of 1–2%, with SCD, HF and thromboembolism being the main causes of death; the most commonly recorded fatal arrhythmic event is spontaneous ventricular fibrillation (VF), but asystole, AV block and pulseless electrical activity are described [2]. For this reason, SCD risk estimation is an integral part of clinical management of HCM [164]. Younger HCM patients are at higher risk for SCD than older patients [30, 165–171] since the 5-year cumulative proportion of SCD events is 8–10% from diagnosis in childhood HCM [172, 173]. In secondary prevention (patients which experiment cardiac arrest due to VT or VF or spontaneous sustained VT causing syncope or haemodynamic compromise), implantable cardioverter-defibrillator (ICD) implantation is indicated in all HCM patients. On the other hand, in primary prevention the best strategy to evaluated SCD risk seems to be a multiparametric approach. Recently, AHA/ACC guidelines suggest the evaluation of several risk factor for SCD based on personal and family history [165, 174–176], noninvasive testing including echocardiography [174, 177–179], ambulatory electrocardiographic 24 hours monitoring [180, 181] and CMR imaging [180–186] in order to identity those patients most likely to benefit ICD implantation [33, 168–170, 174, 187]. On the other hand, ESC guidelines [2] have proposed a risk score, named HCM Risk-SCD, that includes both clinical and instrumental data, thereby predicting annual risk of SCD and suggesting indication for ICD implantation (**Table 2**). Subcutaneous ICD (S-ICD) may be considered in HCM patients who have no indication for pacing especially in patients that have a long life expectancy. However, particular attention should be paid to ensuring optimal R-wave sensing to avoid inappropriate shocks [2].

6.5 New therapy prospective

Novel therapeutic options are being evaluated and validated with diversified targets in the context of the physiopathology of hypertrophic cardiomyopathy.

Myocardial Contractility and energetics: Hypercontractility appears to play a central role in the pathogenesis of HCM since the vast majority of known mutations affect sarcomeric proteins, and ~70% of identifiable mutations involving cardiac beta-myosin heavy chain (MYH7) and myosin-binding protein C (MYBPC) that contain the ATPase involved in actin–myosin cross bridging and muscle fiber shortening, thereby serving as the molecular motor for myocardial contraction [188–191]. It has been hypothesized that HCM mutations increase net power generation by the sarcomere resulting in LV hypercontractility and stiffening that is clinically observed. Mavacamten, a selective allosteric inhibitor of myosin ATPase capable of reducing the formation of bridges between actin and myosin at the sarcomere level and therefore of reducing contractility and improving the energy profile of the myocardium, helps ventricular hyper-contractility which has a pathophysiological role determinant in the genesis of the dynamic obstruction to the left ventricular outflow. It has been shown to improve exercise capacity, symptoms,

SCD risk factor		Definition	AHA/ ACC	ESC
Clinical and anamnestical data	**Family history of SCD**	Sudden death judged definitively or likely attributable to HCM in ≥first-degree or close relatives who are 50 years of age.	X	X
	Age	The effect of age on SCD is incremental. No data with age < 16 or > 80		X
	Unexplained syncope	≥1 Unexplained episodes involving acute transient loss of consciousness, judged by history unlikely to be of neurocardiogenic etiology, nor attributable to LVOTO, and especially when occurring within 6 months of evaluation (events beyond 5 years in the past do not appear to have relevance).	X	X
24 ECG monitoring	**NSVT**	NSVT with runs frequent (≥3), longer (≥10 beats), and faster (≥200 bpm) occurring usually over 24 to 48 hours of monitoring. For pediatric patients, a VT rate that exceeds the baseline sinus rate by >20%.	X	X
Echocardiographic data	**Massive LVH**	Wall thickness ≥ 30 mm in any segment within the chamber by echocardiography or CMR imaging; consideration for this morphologic marker is also given to borderline values of ≥28 mm in individual patients at the discretion of the treating cardiologist. For pediatric patients with HCM, an absolute or z-score threshold for wall thickness has not been established; however a maximal wall that corresponds to a z-score ≥ 20 (and > 10 in conjunction with other risk factors)	X	X
	LV systolic dysfunction	Systolic dysfunction with EF ≤ 50% by echocardiophy or CMR imaging	X	
	LV apical aneurism	Apical aneurysm defined as a discrete thin-walled dyskinetic or akinetic segment of the most distal portion of the LV chamber; independent of size.	X	
	Left atrial diameter	Left atrial diameter as determined by M-mode or 2D echocardiography in the parasternal long axis plane at the time of evaluation		X
	LVOT	Maximum LV outflow gradient determined at rest and with Valsalva provocation (irrespective of concurrent medical treatment)		X
Ergometric data	**Exercise blood pressure response**	A failureto increase systolic pressure by at least 20 mmHg from rest to peak exercise or a fall of > 20 mmHg from peak pressure.		X

SCD risk factor		Definition	AHA/ ACC	ESC
CMR	**Extensive LGE**	Diffuse and extensive LGE, representing fibrosis, either quantified or estimated by visual inspection, comprising ≥15% of LV mass (extent of LGE conferring risk has not been established in children).	X	
Recommendations for ICD implantation in primary prevention				
AHA/ACC		**ESC (HCM Risk-SCD score)**		
ICD is reasonable (2A) with at least one of the following: • Family history of SCD • Massive LVH • Unexplained syncope • Apical aneurism • LV-EF < 50% • NSVT (in children) **ICD may be considered (2B) with at least one of the following:** • NSVT in adults • Extensive LGE		• **LOW RISK (5-year risk < 4%):** ICD generally not indicated • **INTERMEDIATE RISK (5-year risk 4–6%):** ICD may be indicated • **HIGH RISK (5-YEAR RISK ≥ 6%):** ICDshould be indicated		

Table 2.
Sudden cardiac death risk factors: Type, definition, AHA/ACC and ESC guidelines criteria for SCD risk assessment in primary prevention (upper side). Recommendations for ICD implantation in primary prevention according to AHA/ACC and ESC guidelines, separately (lower side).

obstruction to the outflow and quality of life in patients with HOCM. Therefore, Mavacamten represents a valid new therapeutic option (but still not available) for patients with HCM and severe obstruction to the outflow tract despite maximal doses of beta-blocker, calcium channel blockers and disopyramide and before opting for a surgical approach [192].

Ion channels Regulation. HCM is associated with enhanced late sodium current (iNaL) activity due to enzyme-induced sodium-channel phosphorylation which results in increased intracellular sodium (Na+), and in turn, calcium (Ca2+) overload through ion exchange [193]. Dysregulated Ca2+ and Na + handling may contribute to altered cardiomyocyte mechanics (hyper-contractility and impaired relaxation) and predispose the myocardium to arrhythmias. Ranolazine is an inhibitor of iNaL with several potential beneficial effects in HCM, mainly related to the improvement in myocardial relaxation and both anti-ischemia and arrhythmia effects [193]. Although a open-label study (RHYME, NCT01721967) demonstrated positive effects on clinical outcomes, data from a phase II trial (RESTYLE-HCM) failed to demonstrate a significant effect on objective measures (peak VO2, serum B-type natriuretic peptide, diastolic function), while a reduction in premature ventricular complex burden [194] has been reported. For these reasons, ranolazine still remains an intriguing area of research in the field of HCM therapeutic options.

Fibrosis. *S*everal therapies have attempted to address fibrosis and disease progression in HCM, although nowadays no drug has shown convincing benefits, this target represents an interesting field of research in cardioyopathies. While losartan, valsartan and spironolactone was demonstrated to be ineffective [195–198], atorvastatin demonstrated effects on suppression of hypertrophy in pre-clinical models [199] but had no effect and poor treatment adherence in a small early feasibility study in humans [200].

Genome editing and gene silencing. Advances in genome editing technology have sparked excitement about the potential for therapeutic use in cardiovascular disease; however, there remain important hurdles prior to implementation in clinical practice [201, 202]. Current techniques including CRISPR/Cas9 cause a double-stranded DNA break at a desired genetic locus followed by intrinsic cellular repair that is virtually error-free and recently, high-fidelity gene repair in human embryos carrying HCM mutations was shown to be feasible [203]. Using sperm from a heterozygous MYBPC3 mutation carrying male patient, oocytes from healthy women were inseminated. Simultaneous injection of a mutation-specific CRISPR/Cas9 system during early metaphase resulted in editing of the mutation 100% of the time [204]. Allele-specific gene silencing is another gene-based therapeutic technology that holds promise for monogenic diseases. This typically involves the transduction of an adenovirus vector containing short-interfering ribonucleic acid segments designed to suppress expression of a specific pathogenic allele – a method more broadly defined as ribonucleic acid interference (RNAi). In pre-clinical models, RNAi was demonstrated to attenuate the phenotype of specific mutations causing catecholaminergic polymorphic ventricular tachycardia [205], HCM [206] and restrictive cardiomyopathy [207].

Author details

Davide Lazzeroni[1*] and Claudio Stefano Centorbi[2]

1 IRCCS Fondazione Don Gnocchi, Florence, Italy

2 Fondazione Don Gnocchi, Parma, Italy

*Address all correspondence to: davide.lazzeroni@gmail.com

References

[1] Elliott P, Andersson B, Arbustini E, Bilinska Z, Cecchi F, Charron P, Dubourg O, Kuhl U, Maisch B, McKenna WJ, Monserrat L, Pankuweit S, Rapezzi C, Seferovic P, Tavazzi L, Keren A. Classification of the cardiomyopathies: a position statement from the European Society Of Cardiology Working Group on Myocardial and Pericardial Diseases. Eur Heart J 2008; 29:270-276.

[2] Elliott PM, Anastasakis A, Borger MA, Borggrefe M, Cecchi F, Charron P, Hagege AA, Lafont A, Limongelli G, Mahrholdt H, McKenna WJ, Mogensen J, Nihoyannopoulos P, Nistri S, Pieper PG, Pieske B, Rapezzi C, Rutten FH, Tillmanns C, ns H. 2014 ESC Guidelines on diagnosis and management of hypertrophic cardiomyopathy: the Task Force for the Diagnosis and Management of Hypertrophic Cardiomyopathy of the European Society of Cardiology (ESC). Eur Heart J. 2014 Oct 14;35(39):2733-79. doi: 10.1093/eurheartj/ehu284. Epub 2014 Aug 29. PMID: 25173338

[3] Maron BJ, Rowin EJ, Casey SA, Maron MS. How hypertrophic cardiomyopathy became a contemporary treatable genetic disease with low mortality: shaped by 50 years of clinical research and practice. JAMA Cardiol2016;1:98-105.

[4] Maron BJ, Ommen SR, Semsarian C, Spirito P, Olivotto I, Maron MS. Hypertrophic cardiomyopathy: present and future, with translation into contemporary cardiovascular medicine. J Am Coll Cardiol2014;64:83-99.

[5] Braunwald E, Lambrew CT, Rockoff SD, Ross J Jr, Morrow AG. Idiopathic hypertrophic subaortic stenosis. I. A description of the disease based on an analysis of 64 patients. Circulation 1964;30:Suppl 4: 3-119.

[6] Maron BJ, Maron MS. The remarkable 50 years of imaging in HCM and how it has changed diagnosis and management: from M-mode echocardiography to CMR. JACC Cardiovasc Imaging 2016;9:858-72.

[7] Semsarian C, Ingles J, Maron MS, Maron BJ. New perspectives on the prevalence of hypertrophic cardiomyopathy. J Am Coll Cardiol2015;65:1249-54.

[8] Maron MS, Hellawell JL, Lucove JC, Farzaneh-Far R, Olivotto I. Occurrence of clinically diagnosed hypertrophic cardiomyopathy in the United States. Am J Cardiol2016;117:1651-4.

[9] Wells S, Rowin EJ, Bhatt V, Maron MS, Maron BJ. Association between race and clinical profile of patients referred for hypertrophic cardiomyopathy. Circulation 2018;137:1973-5

[10] Maron BJ. Importance and feasibility of creating hypertrophic cardiomyopathy centers in developing countries: the experience in India. Am J Cardiol 2015;116: 332-4.

[11] 4. Tang B, Song Y, Cui H, et al. Prediction of mid-term outcomes in adult obstructive hypertrophic cardiomyopathy after surgical ventricular septum myectomy. J Am Coll Cardiol2017;70:2092-4.

[12] Greaves SC, Roche AH, Neutze JM, Whitlock RM, Veale AM. Inheritance of hypertrophic cardiomyopathy: a cross sectional and M mode echocardiographic study of 50 families. *Br Heart J*. 1987;58:259-266)

[13] Burke MA, Cook SA, Seidman JG, Seidman CE. Clinical and mechanistic insights into the genetics of cardiomyopathy. J Am Coll Cardiol2016;68:2871-86

[14] Richards S, Aziz N, Bale S, et al. Standards and guidelines for the interpretation of sequence variants: a joint consensus recommendation of the American College of Medical Genetics and Genomics and the Association for Molecular Pathology. Genet Med 2015;17:405-24

[15] Ingles J, Burns C, Bagnall RD, et al. Nonfamilial hypertrophic cardiomyopathy: prevalence, natural history, and clinical implications. Circ Cardiovasc Genet. 2017;10:e001620.

[16] Thierfelder L, Watkins H, MacRae C, et al. Alpha-tropomyosin and cardiac tro-ponin T mutations cause familial hyper-trophic cardiomyopathy: a disease of the sarcomere. Cel l 1994;77:701-12.

[17] Valente AM, Lakdawala NK, Powell AJ, et al. Comparison of echocardiographic and cardiac magnetic resonance imaging in hypertrophic cardiomyopathy sarcomere mutation carriers without left ventricular hypertrophy. Circ Cardiovasc Genet 2013; 6:230-7

[18] Landry LG, Rehm HL. Association of racial/ethnic categories with the ability of genetic tests to detect a cause of cardiomyopathy. JAMA Cardiol2018;3:341-5

[19] Ingles J, Burns C, Bagnall RD, et al. Nonfamilial hypertrophic cardiomyopathy: prevalence, natural history, and clinical implications. Circ Cardiovasc Genet 2017; 10:e001620

[20] Chan RH, Maron BJ, Olivotto I, et al. Prognostic value of quantitative contrastenhanced cardiovascular magnetic resonance for the evaluation of sudden death risk in patients with hypertrophic cardiomyopathy. Circulation 2014;130:484-95.

[21] Weng Z, Yao J, Chan RH, et al. Prognostic value of LGE-CMR in HCM: a metaanalysis. JACC Cardiovasc Imaging 2016; 9:1392-402

[22] Spirito P, Bellone P, Harris KM, Bernabò P, Bruzzi P, Maron BJ. Magnitude of left ventricular hypertrophy and risk of sudden death in hypertrophic cardiomyopathy. N Engl J Med 2000;342:1778-85

[23] Klarich KW, AttenhoferJost CH, Binder J, et al. Risk of death in long-term follow-up of patients with apical hypertrophic cardiomyopathy. Am J Cardiol2013;111:1784-91.

[24] Maron MS, Olivotto I, Zenovich AG, et al. Hypertrophic cardiomyopathy is predominantly a disease of left ventricular outflow tract obstruction. Circulation 2006;114:2232-9.

[25] Sherrid MV, Balaram S, Kim B, Axel L, Swistel DG. The mitral valve in obstructive hypertrophic cardiomyopathy: a test in context. J Am Coll Cardiol 2016;67: 1846-58.

[26] Maron BJ, Shen W-K, Link MS, et al. Efficacy of implantable cardioverter–defibrillators for the prevention of sudden death in patients with hypertrophic cardiomyopathy. N Engl J Med 2000;342:365-73.

[27] Schinkel AF, Vriesendorp PA, Sijbrands EJ, Jordaens LJ, ten Cate FJ, Michels M. Outcome and complications after implantable cardioverter defibrillator therapy in hypertrophic cardiomyopathy: systematic review and meta-analysis. Circ Heart Fail 2012;5:552-9.

[28] Maron BJ, Maron MS. Contemporary strategies for risk stratification and prevention of sudden death with the implantable defibrillator in hypertrophic cardiomyopathy. Heart Rhythm 2016;13:1155-65.

[29] Vriesendorp PA, Schinkel AF, Van Cleemput J, et al. Implantable

cardioverterdefibrillators in hypertrophic cardiomyopathy: patient outcomes, rate of appropriate and inappropriate interventions, and complications. Am Heart J 2013;166:496-502.

[30] Maron BJ, Spirito P, Shen WK, et al. Implantable cardioverter-defibrillators and prevention of sudden cardiac death in hypertrophic cardiomyopathy. JAMA 2007; 298:405-12.

[31] Maron BJ, Rowin EJ, Casey SA, et al. Hypertrophic cardiomyopathy in adulthood associated with low cardiovascular mortality with contemporary management strategies. J Am Coll Cardiol 2015;65: 1915-28.

[32] Maron BJ, Rowin EJ, Casey SA, et al. Hypertrophic cardiomyopathy in children, adolescents, and young adults associated with low cardiovascular mortality with contemporary management strategies. Circulation 2016;133:62-73.

[33] Maron BJ, Spirito P, Ackerman MJ, et al. Prevention of sudden cardiac death with implantable cardioverter-defibrillators in children and adolescents with hypertrophic cardiomyopathy. J Am Coll Cardiol2013;61:1527-35.

[34] Rowin EJ, Maron BJ, Haas TS, et al. Hypertrophic cardiomyopathy with left ventricular apical aneurysm: implications for risk stratification and management. J Am Coll Cardiol2017;69:761-73

[35] Maron BJ, Udelson JE, Bonow RO, et al. Eligibility and disqualification recommendations for competitive athletes with cardiovascular abnormalities: Task Force 3: hypertrophic cardiomyopathy, arrhythmogenic right ventricular cardiomyopathy and other cardiomyopathies, and myocarditis: a scientific statement from the American Heart Association and American College of Cardiology. J Am Coll Cardiol 2015; 66:2362-71.

[36] Maron MS, Rowin EJ, Olivotto I, et al. Contemporary natural history and management of nonobstructive hypertrophic cardiomyopathy. J Am Coll Cardiol 2016; 67:1399-409.

[37] Galati G, Leone O, Pasquale F, et al. Histological and histometric characterization of myocardial fibrosis in end-stage hypertrophic cardiomyopathy: a clinicalpathological study of 30 explanted hearts. Circ Heart Fail 2016;9(9):e003090.

[38] Ho CY, López B, Coelho-Filho OR, et al. Myocardial fibrosis as an early manifestation of hypertrophic cardiomyopathy. N Engl J Med 2010;363:552-63.

[39] Maron BJ, Nishimura RA, Maron MS. Shared decision-making in HCM. Nat Rev Cardiol2017;14:125-6.

[40] Manrai AK, Funke BH, Rehm HL, et al. Genetic misdiagnoses and the potential for health disparities. N Engl J Med 2016; 375:655-65.

[41] Maron BJ, Maron MS, Semsarian C. Genetics of hypertrophic cardiomyopathy after 20 years: clinical perspectives. J Am Coll Cardiol2012;60:705-15.

[42] Biagini E, Olivotto I, Iascone M, et al. Significance of sarcomere gene mutations analysis in the end-stage phase of hypertrophic cardiomyopathy. Am J Cardiol 2014; 114:769-76.

[43] Geske JB, Ong KC, Siontis KC, et al. Women with hypertrophic cardiomyopathy have worse survival. Eur Heart J 2017; 38:3434-40.

[44] Olivotto I, Maron MS, Adabag AS, et al. Gender-related differences in the clinical presentation and outcome of

hypertrophic cardiomyopathy. J Am Coll Cardiol2005;46:480-7.

[45] Rastegar H, Boll G, Rowin EJ, et al. Results of surgical septal myectomy for obstructive hypertrophic cardiomyopathy: the Tufts experience. Ann CardiothoracSurg2017;6:353-63

[46] Ferrazzi P, Spirito P, Iacovoni A, et al. Transaortic chordal cutting: mitral valve repair for obstructive hypertrophic cardiomyopathy with mild septal hypertrophy. J Am Coll Cardiol2015;66:1687-96.

[47] Vriesendorp PA, Liebregts M, Steggerda RC, et al. Long-term outcomes after medical and invasive treatment in patients with hypertrophic cardiomyopathy. JACC Heart Fail 2014;2:630-6

[48] Desai MY, Bhonsale A, Smedira NG, et al. Predictors of long-term outcomes in symptomatic hypertrophic obstructive cardiomyopathy patients undergoing surgical relief of left ventricular outflow tract obstruction. Circulation 2013;128:209-16.

[49] Geske JB, Konecny T, Ommen SR, et al. Surgical myectomy improves pulmonary hypertension in obstructive hypertrophic cardiomyopathy. Eur Heart J 2014;35: 2032-9.

[50] Balaram SK, Ross RE, Sherrid MV, et al. Role of mitral valve plication in the surgical management of hypertrophic cardiomyopathy. Ann ThoracSurg 2012; 94:1990-7.

[51] Rowin EJ, Maron BJ, Olivotto I, Maron MS. Role of exercise testing in hypertrophic cardiomyopathy. JACC Cardiovasc Imaging 2017;10:1374-86.

[52] Valente AM, Lakdawala NK, Powell AJ, et al. Comparison of echocardiographic and cardiac magnetic resonance imaging in hypertrophic cardiomyopathy sarcomere mutation carriers without left ventricular hypertrophy. Circ Cardiovasc Genet 2013; 6:230-7.

[53] O'Mahony C, Jichi F, Ommen SR, et al. International external validation study of the 2014 European Society of Cardiology Guidelines on Sudden Cardiac Death Prevention in Hypertrophic Cardiomyopathy (EVIDENCE-HCM). Circulation 2018;137: 1015-23.

[54] Maron BJ, Rowin EJ, Casey SA, et al. Risk stratification and outcome of patients with hypertrophic cardiomyopathy ≥60 years of age. Circulation 2013;127: 585-93.

[55] Spirito P, Autore C, Formisano F, et al. Risk of sudden death and outcome in patients with hypertrophic cardiomyopathy with benign presentation and without risk factors. Am J Cardiol2014;113:1550-5.

[56] Kotkar KD, Said SM, Dearani JA, Schaff HV. Hypertrophic obstructive cardiomyopathy: theMayo Clinic experience. Ann CardiothoracSurg2017;6:329-36.

[57] Writing Committee Members, Ommen SR, Mital S, Burke MA, Day SM, Deswal A, Elliott P, Evanovich LL, Hung J, Joglar JA, Kantor P, Kimmelstiel C, Kittleson M, Link MS, Maron MS, Martinez MW, Miyake CY, Schaff HV, Semsarian C, Sorajja P. 2020 AHA/ACC Guideline for the Diagnosis and Treatment of Patients With Hypertrophic Cardiomyopathy: A Report of the American College of Cardiology/American Heart Association Joint Committee on Clinical Practice Guidelines. Circulation. 2020 Dec 22;142(25):e558-e631. doi: 10.1161/CIR.0000000000000937. Epub 2020 Nov 20. Erratum in: Circulation. 2020 Dec 22;142(25):e633. PMID: 33215931.

[58] Smith GA, Dixon HB, Kirschenlohr HL, Grace AA,

Metcalfe JC, Vandenberg JI. Ca2+ buffering in the heart: Ca2+ binding to and activation of cardiac myo-fibrils. Biochem J 2000;346:393-402.

[59] Knollmann BC, Kirchhof P, Sirenko SG, et al. Familial hypertrophic cardiomy-opathy-linked mutant troponin T causes stress-induced ventricular tachycardia and Ca2+–dependent action potential remod-eling. Circ Res 2003;92:428-36.14.

[60] Bers DM, Guo T. Calcium signaling in cardiac ventricular myocytes. Ann N Y Acad Sci 2005;1047:86-98.15.

[61] Huke S, Knollmann BC. Increased myofilament Ca2+–sensitivity and ar-rhythmia susceptibility. J Mol Cell Cardiol2010;48:824-33.16.

[62] Robinson P, Griffiths PJ, Watkins H, Redwood CS. Dilated and hypertrophic cardiomyopathy mutations in troponin and alpha-tropomyosin have opposing ef-fects on the calcium affinity of cardiac thin filaments. Circ Res 2007;101:1266-73

[63] Kampmann C, Wiethoff CM, Wenzel A, Stolz G, Betancor M, Wippermann CF, Huth RG, Habermehl P, Knuf M, Emschermann T, Stopfkuchen H. Normal values of M mode echocardiographic measurements of more than 2000 healthy infants and children in central Europe. Heart 2000;83:667-672

[64] Maron BJ. Distinguishing hypertrophic cardiomyopathy from athlete's heart: a clinical problem of increasing magnitude and significance. Heart 2005;91:1380-2.

[65] Gersh BJ, Maron BJ, Bonow RO, et al. 2011 ACCF/AHA Guideline for the Diagnosis and Treatment of Hypertrophic Cardiomyopathy: a report of the American College of Cardiology Foundation/American Heart Association Task Force on Practice Guidelines. Developed in collaboration with the American Association for Thoracic Surgery, American Society of Echocardiography, American Society of Nuclear Cardiology, Heart Failure Society of America, Heart Rhythm Society, Society for Cardiovascular Angiography and Interventions, and Society of Thoracic Surgeons. J Am Coll Cardiol 2011;58:e212-60.

[66] Li Y, Guo L. Clinical value of carotid wave intensity analysis for differentiating nonobstructive hypertrophic cardiomyopathy from left ventricular hypertrophy secondary to systemic hypertension. J Clin Ultrasound 2013;41:151-7.

[67] Kato TS, Noda A, Izawa H, et al. Discrimination of nonobstructive hypertrophic cardiomyopathy from hypertensive left ventricular hypertrophy on the basis of strain rate imaging by tissue Doppler ultrasonography. Circulation 2004;110:3808-14.

[68] Nagakura T, Takeuchi M, Yoshitani H, et al. Hypertrophic cardiomyopathy is associated with more severe left ventricular dyssynchrony than is hypertensive left ventricular hypertrophy. Echocardiography 2007;24:677-84.

[69] Ogino K, Ogura K, Kinugawa T, et al. Neurohumoral profiles in patients with hypertrophic cardiomyopathy: differences to hypertensive left ventricular hypertrophy. Circ J 2004;68:444-50.

[70] Rapezzi C, Arbustini E, Caforio AL, Charron P, Gimeno-Blanes J, Heliö T, Linhart A, Mogensen J, Pinto Y, Ristic A, Seggewiss H, Sinagra G, Tavazzi L, Elliott PM. Diagnostic work-up in cardiomyopathies: bridging the gap between clinical phenotypes and final diagnosis. A position statement from the ESC Working Group on Myocardial and Pericardial Diseases. Eur Heart J.

2013 May;34(19):1448-58. doi: 10.1093/eurheartj/ehs397. Epub 2012 Dec 4. PMID: 23211230.

[71] Van der Burgt I. Noonan syndrome. Orphanet J Rare Dis 2007;2:4

[72] Limongelli G, Pacileo G, Marino B, Digilio MC, Sarkozy A, Elliott P, Versacci P, Calabro P, De Zorzi A, Di Salvo G, Syrris P, Patton M, McKenna WJ, Dallapiccola B, Calabro R. Prevalence and clinical significance of cardiovascular abnormalities in patients with the LEOPARD syndrome. Am J Cardiol 2007;100: 736-741.

[73] Vergani V, Lazzeroni D, Peretto G. Bridging the gap between hypertrabeculation phenotype, noncompaction phenotype and left ventricular noncompaction cardiomyopathy. J Cardiovasc Med (Hagerstown). 2020 Mar;21(3):192-199. doi:10.2459/JCM.0000000000000924. PMID: 31895132.

[74] Mehta A, Ricci R, Widmer U, Dehout F, Garcia de Lorenzo A, Kampmann C, Linhart A, Sunder-Plassmann G, Ries M, Beck M. Fabry disease defined: baseline clinical manifestations of 366 patients in the Fabry Outcome Survey. Eur J Clin Invest 2004;34:236-242.

[75] McLeod CJ, Ackerman MJ, Nishimura RA, Tajik AJ, Gersh BJ, Ommen SR. Outcome of patients with hypertrophic cardiomyopathy and a normal electrocardiogram. J Am Coll Cardiol2009;54:229-233.

[76] Monserrat L, Elliott PM, Gimeno JR, Sharma S, Penas-Lado M, McKenna WJ. Nonsustained ventricular tachycardia in hypertrophic cardiomyopathy: an independent marker of sudden death risk in young patients. J Am Coll Cardiol2003;42:873-879. 70.

[77] Adabag AS, Casey SA, Kuskowski MA, Zenovich AG, MaronBJ. Spectrum and prognostic significance of arrhythmias on ambulatory Holter electrocardiogram in hypertrophic cardiomyopathy. J Am Coll Cardiol2005;45:697-704.

[78] Klues HG, Schiffers A, Maron BJ. Phenotypic spectrum and patterns of left ventricular hypertrophy in hypertrophic cardiomyopathy: morphologic observations and significance as assessed by two-dimensional echocardiography in 600 patients. J Am Coll Cardiol1995;26:1699-1708

[79] Cardim N, Galderisi M, Edvardsen T, Plein S, Popescu BA, D'Andrea A, Bruder O, Cosyns B, Davin L, Donal E, Freitas A, Habib G, Kitsiou A, Petersen SE, Schroeder S, Lancellotti P, Camici P, Dulgheru R, Hagendorff A, Lombardi M, Muraru D, Sicari R. Role of multimodality cardiac imaging in the management of patients with hypertrophic cardiomyopathy: an expert consensus of the European Association of Cardiovascular Imaging Endorsed by the Saudi Heart Association. Eur Heart J Cardiovasc Imaging. 2015 Mar;16(3):280. doi: 10.1093/ehjci/jeu291. Epub 2015 Feb 3. PMID: 25650407.

[80] DCiampi Q, Olivotto I, Gardini C, Mori F, Peteiro J, Monserrat L, Fernandez X, Cortigiani L, Rigo F, Lopes LR, Cruz I, Cotrim C, Losi M, Betocchi S, Beleslin B, Tesic M, Dikic AD, Lazzeroni E, Lazzeroni D, Sicari R, Picano E. Prognosticrole of stress echocardiography in hypertrophiccardiomyopathy: The International Stress EchoRegistry. Int J Cardiol. 2016 Sep 15;219:331-8. doi: 10.1016/j.ijcard.2016.06.044. Epub 2016 Jun 15. PMID: 27348413.

[81] O'Hanlon R, Assomull RG, Prasad SK. Use of cardiovascular magnetic resonance for diagnosis and management in hypertrophic cardiomyopathy. CurrCardiol Rep 2007;9:51-56.

[82] O'Gara PT, Bonow RO, Maron BJ, Damske BA, Van Lingen A, Bacharach SL et al. Myocardial perfusion abnormalities in patients with hypertrophic cardiomyopathy: assessment with thallium-201 emission computed tomography. Circulation 1987; 76:1214-23

[83] Shiba N, KagayaY, Ishide N, Otani H, Takeyama D, YamaneYet al. Heterogeneityof myocardial fluoro-18 2-deoxyglucose uptake in patients with apical hypertrophic cardiomyopathy. JpnCirc J 1997;61:223-30.

[84] Schafers MM, Dutka DD, Rhodes CGC, Lammertsma AAA, Hermansen FF, Schober OO et al.Myocardial presynaptic and postsynaptic autonomic dysfunction in hypertrophic cardiomyopathy. Circ Res 1998;82:57-62.

[85] Mehra MR, Kobashigawa J, Starling R, Russell S, Uber PA, Parameshwar J, Mohacsi P, Augustine S, Aaronson K, Barr M. Listing criteria for heart transplantation: International Society for Heart and Lung Transplantation guidelines for the care of cardiac transplant candidates - 2006. J Heart Lung Transplant 2006;25:1024-1042

[86] Elliott PM, Hanna MG, Ward SA, Chinnery PF, Turnbull DM, Wood NW, McKenna WJ. Diagnostic utility of metabolic exercise testing in a patient with cardiovascular disease. Heart 1999;81:441-443. 233.

[87] Sharma S, Elliott P, Whyte G, Jones S, Mahon N, Whipp B, McKenna WJ. Utility of cardiopulmonary exercise in the assessment of clinical determinants of functional capacity in hypertrophic cardiomyopathy. Am J Cardiol2000;86:162-168.

[88] Arena R, Owens DS, Arevalo J, Smith K, Mohiddin SA, McAreavey D, Ulisney KL, Tripodi D, Fananapazir L, Plehn JF. Ventilatoryefficiency and resting hemodynamics in hypertrophic cardiomyopathy. Med Sci Sports Exerc2008;40:799-805.

[89] Sharma S, Elliott PM, Whyte G, Mahon N, Virdee MS, Mist B, McKenna WJ. Utility of metabolic exercise testing in distinguishing hypertrophic cardiomyopathy from physiologic left ventricular hypertrophy in athletes. J Am Coll Cardiol 2000;36: 864-870. 232.

[90] Elliott PM, Hanna MG, Ward SA, Chinnery PF, Turnbull DM, Wood NW, McKenna WJ. Diagnostic utility of metabolic exercise testing in a patient with cardiovascular disease. Heart 1999;81:441-443.

[91] Olivotto I, Cecchi F, Poggesi C, Yacoub MH. Patterns of disease progression in hypertrophic cardiomyopathy: an individualized approach to clinical staging. Circ Heart Fail 2012;5:535-546. 14.

[92] Pasqualucci D, Fornaro A, Castelli G, Rossi A, Arretini A, Chiriatti C, Targetti M, Girolami F, Corda M, Orru P, Matta G, Stefano P, Cecchi F, Porcu M, Olivotto I. Clinical spectrum, therapeutic options, and outcome of advanced heart failure in hypertrophic cardiomyopathy. Circ Heart Fail 2015;8:1014-1021.

[93] Olivotto I, Cecchi F, Poggesi C, Yacoub MH. Patterns of disease progression in hypertrophic cardiomyopathy: an individualized approach to clinical staging. Circ Heart Fail. 2012 Jul 1;5(4):535-46. doi: 10.1161/ CIRCHEARTFAILURE.112.967026. PMID: 22811549.

[94] Olivotto I, Girolami F, Nistri S, Rossi A, Rega L, Garbini F, Grifoni C, Cecchi F, Yacoub MH. The many faces of hypertrophic cardiomyopathy: from developmental biology to clinical

practice. J Cardiovasc Transl Res. 2009;2:349-367.

[95] Gersh BJ, Maron BJ, Bonow RO, Dearani JA, Fifer MA, Link MS, Naidu SS, Nishimura RA, Ommen SR, Rakowski H, Seidman CE, Towbin JA, Udelson JE, Yancy CW. 2011 ACCF/AHA Guideline for the Diagnosis and Treatment of Hypertrophic Cardiomyopathy: a report of the American College of Cardiology Foundation/American Heart Association Task Force on Practice Guidelines. Circulation. 2011;124:2761-2796.

[96] Ho CY. Hypertrophic cardiomyopathy: preclinical and early phenotype. J Cardiovasc Trans Res. 2009;2:462-470

[97] Force T, Bonow RO, Houser SR, Solaro RJ, Hershberger RE, Adhikari B, Anderson ME, Boineau R, Byrne BJ, Cappola TP, Kalluri R, LeWinter MM, Maron MS, Molkentin JD, Ommen SR, RegnierM,TangWH,TianR,KonstamMA, Maron BJ, Seidman CE. Research priorities in hypertrophic cardiomyopathy: report of a Working Group of the National Heart, Lung, and Blood Institute Circulation. 2010;122:1130-1133.

[98] Maron BJ, Maron MS, Wigle ED, Braunwald E. The 50-year history, controversy, and clinical implications of left ventricular outflow tract obstruction in hypertrophic cardiomyopathy: from idiopathic hypertrophic subaortic stenosis to hypertrophic cardiomyopathy. J Am Coll Cardiol. 2009;54:191-200.

[99] Watkins H, Ashrafian H, Redwood C. Inherited cardiomyopathies. N Engl J Med. 2011;364:1643-1656

[100] Spoladore R, Fisicaro A, Faccini A, Camici PG. Coronary microvascular dysfunction in primary cardiomyopathies. Heart. 2014 May;100(10):806-13. doi: 10.1136/heartjnl-2013-304291. Epub 2013 Jul 31. PMID: 23904360.

[101] Lazzeroni D, Rimoldi O, Camici PG. From Left Ventricular Hypertrophy to Dysfunction and Failure. Circ J. 2016;80(3):555-64. doi: 10.1253/circj.CJ-16-0062. Epub 2016 Feb 5. PMID: 26853555.

[102] Maron BJ, McKenna WJ, Danielson GK, Kappenberger LJ, Kuhn HJ, Seidman CE, Shah PM, Spencer WH III, Spirito P, Ten Cate FJ, Wigle ED. American College of Cardiology/ European Society of Cardiology clinical expert consensus document on hypertrophic cardiomyopathy. J Am Coll Cardiol. 2003;42:1687-1713

[103] Maron BJ, Spirito P. Implications of left ventricular remodeling in hypertrophic cardiomyopathy. Am J Cardiol. 1998;81:1339-1344.

[104] Olivotto I, Maron BJ, Appelbaum E, Harrigan CJ, Salton C, Gibson CM, Udelson JE, O'Donnell C, Lesser JR, Manning WJ, Maron MS. Spectrum and clinical significance of systolic function and myocardial fibrosis assessed by cardiovascular magnetic resonance in hypertrophic cardiomyopathy. Am J Cardiol. 2010;106:261-267.

[105] Yacoub MH, Olivotto I, Cecchi F. 'End–stage' hypertrophic cardiomyopathy: from mystery to model. Nat Clin Pract Cardiovasc Med. 2007;4:232-233.

[106] Olivotto I, Maron BJ, Appelbaum E, Harrigan CJ, Salton C, Gibson CM, Udelson JE, O'Donnell C, Lesser JR, Manning WJ, Maron MS. Spectrum and clinical significance of systolic function and myocardial fibrosis assessed by cardiovascular magnetic resonance in hypertrophic cardiomyopathy. Am J Cardiol. 2010;106:261-267

[107] Biagini E, Spirito P, Rocchi G, Ferlito M, Rosmini S, Lai F, Lorenzini M, Terzi F, Bacchi-Reggiani L, Boriani G, Branzi A, Boni L, Rapezzi C. Prognostic implications of the Doppler restrictive filling pattern in hypertrophic cardiomyopathy. Am J Cardiol. 2009;104:1727-1731.

[108] Melacini P, Basso C, Angelini A, Calore C, Bobbo F, Tokajuk B, Bellini N, Smaniotto G, Zucchetto M, Iliceto S, Thiene G, Maron BJ. Clinicopathological profiles of progressive heart failure in hypertrophic cardiomyopathy. Eur Heart J. 2010;31:2111-2123

[109] Nistri S, Olivotto I, Betocchi S, Losi MA, Valsecchi G, Pinamonti B, Conte MR, Casazza F, Galderisi M, MaronBJ,CecchiF.Prognosticsignificance of left atrial size in patients with hypertrophic cardiomyopathy (from the Italian Registry for Hypertrophic Cardiomyopathy). Am J Cardiol. 2006;98:960-965.

[110] Girolami F, Ho CY, Semsarian C, Baldi M, Will ML, Baldini K, Torricelli F, Yeates L, Cecchi F, Ackerman MJ, Olivotto I. Clinical features and outcome of hypertrophic cardiomyopathy associated with triple sarcomere protein gene mutations. J Am Coll Cardiol. 2010;55:1444-1453.

[111] O'Hanlon R, Grasso A, Roughton M, Moon JC, Clark S, Wage R, Webb J, Kulkarni M, Dawson D, Sulaibeekh L, Chandrasekaran B, Bucciarelli-Ducci C, Pasquale F, Cowie MR, McKenna WJ, Sheppard MN, Elliott PM, Pennell DJ, Prasad SK. Prognostic significance of myocardial fibrosis in hypertrophic cardiomyopathy. J Am Coll Cardiol. 2010;56:867-874.

[112] Maron MS, Olivotto I, Maron BJ, Prasad SK, Cecchi F, Udelson JE, Camici PG. The case for myocardial ischemia in hypertrophic cardiomyopathy. J Am Coll Cardiol. 2009;54:866-875.

[113] Olivotto I, Cecchi F, Casey SA, Dolara A, Traverse JH, Maron BJ. Impact of atrial fibrillation on the clinical course of hypertrophic cardiomyopathy. Circulation. 2001;104:2517-2524.

[114] Ciró E, Maron BJ, Bonow RO, Cannon RO, Epstein SE. Relation between marked changes in left ventricular outflow tract gradient and disease progression in hypertrophic cardiomyopathy. Am J Cardiol. 1984;53:1103-1109.

[115] Maron MS, Finley JJ, Bos JM, Hauser TH, Manning WJ, Haas TS, Lesser JR, Udelson JE, Ackerman MJ, Maron BJ. Prevalence, clinical significance and natural history of left ventricular apical aneurysms in hypertrophic cardiomyopathy. Circulation. 2009;118:1541-1549.

[116] Maron MS, Appelbaum E, Harrigan CJ, Buros J, Gibson CM, Hanna C, Lesser JR, Udelson JE, Manning WJ, Maron BJ. Clinical profile and significance of delayed enhancement in hypertrophic cardiomyopathy. Circ Heart Failure. 2008;1:184-191.

[117] Kelly M, Semsarian C. Multiple mutations in genetic cardiovascular disease: a marker of disease severity. Circulation Cardiovasc Genet. 2009;2:182-190.

[118] Biagini E, Coccolo F, Ferlito M, Perugini E, Rocchi G, Bacchi-Reggiani L, Lofiego C, Boriani G, Prandstraller D, Picchio FM, Branzi A, Rapezzi C. Dilated-hypokinetic evolution of hypertrophic cardiomyopathy: prevalence, incidence, risk factors, and prognostic implications in pediatric and adult patients. J Am Coll Cardiol. 2005;46:1543-1550.

[119] Harris KM, Spirito P, Maron MS, Zenovich AG, Formisano F, Lesser JR, Mackey-Bojack S, Manning WJ, Udelson JE, Maron BJ. Prevalence, clinical profile, and significance of left ventricular remodeling in the end-stage

phase of hypertrophic cardiomyopathy. Circulation. 2006;114: 216-225.

[120] Biagini E, Spirito P, Leone O, Picchio FM, Coccolo F, Ragni L, Lofiego C, Grigioni F, Potena L, Rocchi G, Bacchi-Reggiani L, Boriani G, Prandstraller D, Arbustini E, Branzi A, Rapezzi C. Heart transplantation in hypertrophic cardiomyopathy. Am J Cardiol. 2008; 101:387-392.

[121] Kubo T, Gimeno JR, Bahl A, Steffensen U, Steffensen M, Osman E, Thaman R, Mogensen J, Elliott PM, Doi Y, McKenna WJ. Prevalence, clinical significance, and genetic basis of hypertrophic cardiomyopathy with restrictive phenotype. J Am Coll Cardiol. 2007;49:2419-2426

[122] Biagini E, Spirito P, Rocchi G, Ferlito M, Rosmini S, Lai F, Lorenzini M, Terzi F, Bacchi-Reggiani L, Boriani G, Branzi A, Boni L, Rapezzi C. Prognostic implications of the Doppler restrictive filling pattern in hypertrophic cardiomyopathy. Am J Cardiol. 2009;104:1727-1731

[123] Melacini P, Basso C, Angelini A, Calore C, Bobbo F, Tokajuk B, Bellini N, Smaniotto G, Zucchetto M, Iliceto S, Thiene G, Maron BJ. Clinicopathological profiles of progressive heart failure in hypertrophic cardiomyopathy. Eur Heart J. 2010;31:2111-2123.

[124] Day SM. Exercise in hypertrophic cardiomyopathy. J Cardiovasc Transl Res. 2009;2:407-414.

[125] Ammirati E, Contri R, Coppini R, Cecchi F, Frigerio M, Olivotto I. Pharmacological treatment of hypertrophic cardiomyopathy: current practice and novel perspectives. Eur J Heart Fail. 2016 Sep;18(9):1106-18. doi: 10.1002/ejhf.541. Epub 2016 Apr 24. PMID: 27109894.

[126] Stauffer JC, Ruiz V, MorardJD. Subaortic obstruction aftersildenafilina patient with hypertrophic cardiomyopathy. N Engl J Med 1999;341:700-701

[127] Sherrid MV, Barac I, McKenna WJ, Elliott PM, Dickie S, Chojnowska L, Casey S, Maron BJ. Multicenter study of the efficacy and safety of disopyramide in obstructive hypertrophic cardiomyopathy. J Am Coll Cardiol2005;45:1251-1258.

[128] Sherrid MV, Shetty A, Winson G, Kim B, Musat D, Alviar CL, Homel P, Balaram SK, Swistel DG. Treatment of obstructive hypertrophic cardiomyopathy symptoms and gradient resistant to first-line therapy with beta-blockade or verapamil. Circ Heart Fail 2013;6:694-702.

[129] Adelman AG, Shah PM, Gramiak R, Wigle ED. Long-term propranolol therapy in muscular subaortic stenosis. Br Heart J 1970;32:804-811.

[130] Stenson RE, Flamm MD Jr., Harrison DC, Hancock EW. Hypertrophic subaortic stenosis. Clinical and hemodynamic effects of long-term propranolol therapy. Am J Cardiol1973;31:763-773.

[131] Flamm MD, Harrison DC, HancockEW. Muscular subaortic stenosis. Prevention of outflow obstruction with propranolol. Circulation 1968;38:846-858.

[132] Rosing DR, Kent KM, Borer JS, Seides SF, Maron BJ, Epstein SE. Verapamil therapy: a new approach to the pharmacologic treatment of hypertrophic cardiomyopathy. I. Hemodynamic effects. Circulation 1979;60:1201-1207.

[133] Bonow RO, Rosing DR, Epstein SE. The acute and chronic effects of verapamil on left ventricular function in patients with hypertrophic cardiomyopathy. Eur Heart J 1983;4 Suppl F:57-65.

[134] Spicer RL, Rocchini AP, Crowley DC, Vasiliades J, Rosenthal A. Hemodynamic effectsof verapamil inchildrenandadolescentswith hypertrophiccardiomyopathy. Circulation 1983;67:413-420.

[135] Rosing DR, Idanpaan-Heikkila U, Maron BJ, Bonow RO, Epstein SE. Use of calciumchannel blocking drugs in hypertrophic cardiomyopathy. Am J Cardiol 1985;55: 185B–195B.

[136] Veselka J, Faber L, Liebregts M, Cooper R, Januska J, Kashtanov M, Dabrowski M, Hansen PR, Seggewiss H, Hansvenclova E, Bundgaard H, Ten Berg J, Stables RH, Jensen MK. Short- and long-term outcomes of alcohol septal ablation for hypertrophic obstructive cardiomyopathy in patients with mild left ventricular hypertrophy: a propensity score matching analysis. Eur Heart J 2019;40:1681-1687.

[137] Maron BJ, Nishimura RA. Surgical septal myectomy versus alcohol septal ablation: assessing the status of the controversy in 2014. Circulation 2014;130:1617-1624.

[138] Ten Cate FJ, Soliman OI, Michels M, Theuns DA, de Jong PL, Geleijnse ML, Serruys PW. Long-term outcome of alcohol septal ablation in patients with obstructive hypertrophic cardiomyopathy: a word of caution. Circ Heart Fail 2010;3:362-369

[139] Chan W, Williams L, Kotowycz MA, Woo A, Rakowski H, Schwartz L, Overgaard CB. Angiographic and echocardiographic correlates of suitable septal perforators for alcohol septal ablation in hypertrophic obstructive cardiomyopathy. Can J Cardiol2014;30:912-919.

[140] Sigwart U. Non-surgical myocardial reductionfor hypertrophic obstructivecardiomyopathy. Lancet 1995;346:211-214.

[141] Faber L, Welge D, Fassbender D, Schmidt HK, Horstkotte D, Seggewiss H. One-year follow-up of percutaneous septal ablation for symptomatic hypertrophic obstructive cardiomyopathy in 312 patients: predictors of hemodynamic and clinical response. Clin Res Cardiol2007;96:864-873.

[142] Fernandes VL, Nielsen C, Nagueh SF, Herrin AE, Slifka C, Franklin J, Spencer WH III. Follow-upof alcohol septal ablationfor symptomatic hypertrophic obstructive cardiomyopathy the Baylorand Medical University of South Carolina experience 1996 to 2007. JACC Cardiovasc Interv2008;1:561-570.

[143] Kuhn H, Lawrenz T, Lieder F, Leuner C, Strunk-Mueller C, Obergassel L, Bartelsmeier M, Stellbrink C. Survival aftertranscoronary ablation of septal hypertrophy in hypertrophic obstructive cardiomyopathy (TASH): a 10 year experience. Clin Res Cardiol2008;97:234-243.

[144] Sorajja P, Valeti U, Nishimura RA, Ommen SR, Rihal CS, Gersh BJ, Hodge DO, Schaff HV, Holmes DR Jr. Outcome of alcohol septal ablation for obstructive hypertrophic cardiomyopathy. Circulation 2008;118:131-139.

[145] Agarwal S, Tuzcu EM, Desai MY, Smedira N, Lever HM, Lytle BW, Kapadia SR. Updated meta-analysis of septal alcohol ablation versus myectomy for hypertrophic cardiomyopathy. J Am Coll Cardiol2010;55:823-834.

[146] Alam M, Dokainish H, Lakkis NM. Hypertrophic obstructive cardiomyopathyalcohol septal ablation vs. myectomy: a meta-analysis. Eur Heart J 2009;30: 1080-1087.

[147] Zeng Z, Wang F, Dou X, Zhang S, Pu J. Comparison of percutaneous

transluminal septal myocardial ablation versus septal myectomy for the treatment of patients with hypertrophic obstructive cardiomyopathy: a meta analysis. Int J Cardiol 2006; 112:80-84.

[148] Leonardi RA, Kransdorf EP, Simel DL, Wang A. Meta-analyses of septal reduction therapies for obstructive hypertrophic cardiomyopathy: comparative rates of overall mortality and sudden cardiac death after treatment. Circ Cardiovasc Interv2010;3:97-104.

[149] Braunwald E, BrockenbroughEC, FryeRL. Studies on digitalis. V. Comparison of the effects of ouabain on left ventricular dynamics in valvular aortic stenosis and hypertrophic subaortic stenosis. Circulation 1962;26:166-173.

[150] Bourmayan C, Razavi A, FournierC, Dussaule JC, Baragan J, Gerbaux A, GayJ. Effect of propranolol on left ventricular relaxation in hypertrophic cardiomyopathy: an echographic study. Am Heart J 1985;109:1311-1316.

[151] Alvares RF, Goodwin JF. Non-invasive assessment of diastolic function in hypertrophic cardiomyopathy on and off beta adrenergic blocking drugs. Br Heart J 1982;48:204-212.

[152] Wilmshurst PT, Thompson DS, Juul SM, Jenkins BS, Webb-Peploe MM. Effects of verapamil on haemodynamic function and myocardial metabolism in patients with hypertrophic cardiomyopathy. Br Heart J 1986;56:544-553.

[153] Udelson JE, Bonow RO, O'Gara PT, Maron BJ, Van Lingen A, Bacharach SL, Epstein SE. Verapamil prevents silent myocardial perfusion abnormalities during exercise in asymptomatic patients with hypertrophic cardiomyopathy. Circulation 1989;79:1052-1060.

[154] Pacileo G, De Cristofaro M, Russo MG, Sarubbi B, Pisacane C, Calabro R. Hypertrophic cardiomyopathy in pediatric patients: effect of verapamil on regional and global left ventricular diastolic function. Can J Cardiol2000;16:146-152.

[155] McMurray JJ, Adamopoulos S, Anker SD, Auricchio A, Bohm M, Dickstein K, Falk V, Filippatos G, Fonseca C, Gomez-Sanchez MA, Jaarsma T, Kober L, Lip GY, Maggioni AP, Parkhomenko A, Pieske BM, Popescu BA, Ronnevik PK, Rutten FH, Schwitter J, Seferovic P, Stepinska J, Trindade PT, Voors AA, Zannad F, Zeiher A. ESC Guidelines for the diagnosis and treatment of acute and chronic heart failure 2012: The Task Force for the Diagnosis and Treatment of Acute and Chronic Heart Failure 2012 of the European Society of Cardiology. Developed in collaboration with the Heart Failure Association (HFA) of the ESC. Eur Heart J 2012;33:1787-1847.

[156] Brignole M, Auricchio A, Baron-Esquivias G, Bordachar P, Boriani G,Breithardt OA, Cleland J, Deharo JC, Delgado V, Elliott PM, Gorenek B, Israel CW, Leclercq C, Linde C, Mont L, Padeletti L, Sutton R, Vardas PE, Zamorano JL, Achenbach S, Baumgartner H, Bax JJ, Bueno H, Dean V, Deaton C, Erol C, Fagard R, Ferrari R, Hasdai D, Hoes AW, Kirchhof P, Knuuti J, Kolh P, Lancellotti P, Linhart A, Nihoyannopoulos P, Piepoli MF, Ponikowski P, Sirnes PA, Tamargo JL, Tendera M, Torbicki A, Wijns W, Windecker S, Kirchhof P, Blomstrom-Lundqvist C, Badano LP, Aliyev F, Bansch D, Baumgartner H, Bsata W, Buser P, Charron P, Daubert JC, Dobreanu D, Faerestrand S, Hasdai D, Hoes AW, Le Heuzey JY, Mavrakis H, McDonagh T, Merino JL, Nawar MM, Nielsen JC, Pieske B, Poposka L, Ruschitzka F, Tendera M, Van Gelder IC, Wilson CM. 2013 ESC Guidelines on cardiac pacing and cardiac

resynchronization therapy: the Task Force on cardiac pacing and resynchronization therapy of the European Society of Cardiology (ESC). Developed in collaboration with the European Heart Rhythm Association (EHRA). Eur Heart J 2013;34:2281-2329.

[157] Ponikowski P, Voors AA, Anker SD, Bueno H, Cleland JG, Coats AJ, Falk V, González-Juanatey JR, Harjola VP, Jankowska EA, Jessup M, Linde C, Nihoyannopoulos P, Parissis JT, Pieske B, Riley JP, Rosano GM, Ruilope LM, Ruschitzka F, Rutten FH, van der Meer P; Authors/ Task Force Members; Document Reviewers. 2016 ESC Guidelines for the diagnosis and treatment of acute and chronic heart failure: The Task Force for the diagnosis and treatment of acute and chronic heart failure of the European Society of Cardiology (ESC). Developed with the special contribution of the Heart Failure Association (HFA) of the ESC. Eur J Heart Fail. 2016 Aug;18(8):891-975. doi: 10.1002/ejhf.592. Epub 2016 May 20. PMID: 27207191.

[158] Nistri S, Olivotto I, Betocchi S, Losi MA, Valsecchi G, Pinamonti B, Conte MR, Casazza F, Galderisi M, Maron BJ, Cecchi F. Prognostic significance of left atrial size in patients with hypertrophic cardiomyopathy (from the italian registry for hypertrophic cardiomyopathy). Am J Cardiol2006;98:960-965.

[159] Guttmann OP, Rahman MS, O'Mahony C, Anastasakis A, Elliott PM. Atrial fibrillation and thromboembolism in patients with hypertrophic cardiomyopathy: systematic review. Heart 2014;100:465-472.

[160] Siontis KC, Geske JB, Ong K, Nishimura RA, Ommen SR, Gersh BJ. Atrial fibrillation in hypertrophic cardiomyopathy: Prevalence, clinical correlations, and mortality in a large high-risk population. J Am Heart Assoc 2014;3:e001002.

[161] Camm AJ, Lip GY, De Caterina R, Savelieva I, Atar D, Hohnloser SH, Hindricks G, KirchhofP. 2012 focused updateof the ESC Guidelines for the management of atrial fibrillation: an update of the 2010 ESC Guidelines for the management of atrial fibrillation. Developed with the special contribution of the European Heart Rhythm Association. Eur Heart J 2012;33:2719-2747.

[162] Camm AJ, Kirchhof P, Lip GY, Schotten U, Savelieva I, Ernst S, Van Gelder IC, Al Attar N, Hindricks G, Prendergast B, Heidbuchel H, Alfieri O, Angelini A, Atar D, Colonna P, De Caterina R, De Sutter J, Goette A, Gorenek B, Heldal M, Hohloser SH, Kolh P, Le Heuzey JY, Ponikowski P, RuttenFH. Guidelinesforthemanagement of atrial fibrillation: the Task Force for the Management of Atrial Fibrillation of the European Society of Cardiology (ESC). Europace 2010;12: 1360-1420.

[163] Hindricks G, Potpara T, Dagres N, Arbelo E, Bax JJ, Blomström-Lundqvist C, Boriani G, Castella M, Dan GA, Dilaveris PE, Fauchier L, Filippatos G, Kalman JM, La Meir M, Lane DA, Lebeau JP, Lettino M, Lip GYH, Pinto FJ, Thomas GN, Valgimigli M, Van Gelder IC, Van Putte BP, Watkins CL; ESC Scientific Document Group. 2020 ESC Guidelines for the diagnosis and management of atrial fibrillation developed in collaboration with the European Association of Cardio-Thoracic Surgery (EACTS). Eur Heart J. 2020 Aug 29:ehaa612. doi: 10.1093/ eurheartj/ehaa612. Epub ahead of print. PMID: 32860505.

[164] Elliott PM, Gimeno JR, Thaman R, Shah J, Ward D, Dickie S, Tome Esteban MT, McKenna WJ. Historical trends in reported survival rates in patients with hypertrophic cardiomyopathy. Heart 2006;92:785-791.

[165] Dimitrow PP, Chojnowska L, Rudzinski T, et al. Sudden death in

hypertrophic cardiomyopathy: old risk factors re-assessed in a new model of maximalized follow-up. Eur Heart J. 2010;31:3084-93.

[166] Vriesendorp PA, Schinkel AF, Van Cleemput J, et al. Implantable cardioverter-defibrillators in hypertrophic cardiomyopathy: patient outcomes, rate of appropriate and inappropriate interventions, and complications. Am Heart J. 2013;166:496-502.

[167] Wells S, Rowin EJ, Bhatt V, et al. Association between race and clinical profile of patients referred for hypertrophic cardiomyopathy. Circulation. 2018;137: 1973-5.

[168] Olivotto I, Maron MS, Adabag AS, et al. Genderrelated differences in the clinical presentation and outcome of hypertrophic cardiomyopathy. J Am Coll Cardiol. 2005;46:480-7.

[169] Elliott PM, Poloniecki J, Dickie S, et al. Sudden death in hypertrophic cardiomyopathy: identification of high risk patients. J Am Coll Cardiol. 2000;36:2212-8.

[170] Ostman-Smith I, Wettrell G, Keeton B, et al. Ageand gender-specific mortality rates in childhood hypertrophic cardiomyopathy. Eur Heart J. 2008;29: 1160-7.

[171] Maron BJ. Risk stratification and role of implantable defibrillators for prevention of sudden death in patients with hypertrophic cardiomyopathy. Circulation. 2010;74:2271-82.

[172] Miron A, Lafreniere-Roula M, Fan CS, et al. A validated model for sudden cardiac death risk prediction in pediatric hypertrophic cardiomyopathy. Circulation. 2020;142:217-29.

[173] Norrish G, Ding T, Field E, et al. Development of a novel risk prediction model for sudden cardiac death in childhood hypertrophic cardiomyopathy (HCM RiskKids). JAMA Cardiol. 2019;4:918-27.

[174] Maron MS, Rowin EJ, Wessler BS, et al. Enhanced American College of Cardiology/American Heart Association strategy for prevention of sudden cardiac death in high-risk patients with hypertrophic cardiomyopathy. JAMA Cardiol. 2019;4:644-57.

[175] Elliott PM, Sharma S, Varnava A, et al. Survival after cardiac arrest or sustained ventricular tachycardia in patients with hypertrophic cardiomyopathy. J Am Coll Cardiol. 1999;33:1596-601.

[176] Bos JM, Maron BJ, Ackerman MJ, et al. Role of family history of sudden death in risk stratification and prevention of sudden death with implantable defibrillators in hypertrophic cardiomyopathy. Am J Cardiol. 2010;106:1481-6.

[177] Spirito P, Bellone P, Harris KM, et al. Magnitude of left ventricular hypertrophy and risk of sudden death in hypertrophic cardiomyopathy. N Engl J Med. 2000; 342:1778-85.

[178] Autore C, Bernabò P, Barillà CS, et al. The prognostic importance of left ventricular outflow obstruction in hypertrophic cardiomyopathy varies in relation to the severity of symptoms. J Am Coll Cardiol. 2005; 45:1076-80.

[179] Elliott PM, Gimeno Blanes JR, Mahon NG, et al. Relation between severity of left-ventricular hypertrophy and prognosis in patients with hypertrophic cardiomyopathy. Lancet. 2001;357:420-4.

[180] Monserrat L, Elliott PM, Gimeno JR, et al. Nonsustained ventricular tachycardia in hypertrophic cardiomyopathy: an independent marker of sudden death risk in young patients. J Am Coll Cardiol. 2003;42:873-9.

[181] Wang W, Lian Z, Rowin EJ, et al. Prognostic implications of nonsustained ventricular tachycardia in high-risk patients with hypertrophic cardiomyopathy. CircArrhythmElectrophysiol. 2017;10:e004604.

[182] Corona-Villalobos CP, Sorensen LL, Pozios I, et al. Left ventricular wall thickness in patients with hypertrophic cardiomyopathy: a comparison between cardiac magnetic resonance imaging and echocardiography. Int J Cardiovasc Imaging. 2016;32: 945-54.

[183] Bois JP, Geske JB, Foley TA, et al. Comparison of maximal wall thickness in hypertrophic cardiomyopathy differs between magnetic resonance imaging and transthoracic echocardiography. Am J Cardiol. 2017; 119:643-50.

[184] Maron MS, Lesser JR, Maron BJ. Management implications of massive left ventricular hypertrophy in hypertrophic cardiomyopathy significantly underestimated by echocardiography but identified by cardiovascular magnetic resonance. Am J Cardiol. 2010;105:1842-3.

[185] Weng Z, Yao J, Chan RH, et al. Prognostic value of LGE-CMR in HCM: a meta-analysis. J Am Coll CardiolImg. 2016;9:1392-402. 19. Chan RH, Maron BJ, Olivotto I, et al. Prognostic value of quantitative contrast-enhanced cardiovascular magnetic resonance for the evaluation of sudden death risk in patients with hypertrophic cardiomyopathy. Circulation. 2014;130:484-95.

[186] Mentias A, Raeisi-Giglou P, Smedira NG, et al. Late gadolinium enhancement in patients with hypertrophic cardiomyopathy and preserved systolic function. J Am Coll Cardiol. 2018;72:857-70.

[187] Maron BJ, Rowin EJ, Casey SA, et al. Hypertrophic cardiomyopathy in adulthood associated with low cardiovascular mortality with contemporary management strategies. J Am Coll Cardiol. 2015;65:1915-28. 32. Maron BJ, Rowin EJ, Casey SA, et al. Risk stratification and outcome of patients with hypertrophic cardiomyopathy $60 years of age. Circulation. 2013; 127:585-93.

[188] Spudich JA. Three perspectives on the molecular basis of hypercontractility caused by hypertrophic cardiomyopathy mutations. Pflugers Arch 2019;471:701-717.

[189] Spudich JA, Aksel T, Bartholomew SR, Nag S, Kawana M, Yu EC, Sarkar SS, Sung J, Sommese RF, Sutton S, Cho C, Adhikari AS, Taylor R, Liu C, Trivedi D, Ruppel KM. Effects of hypertrophic and dilated cardiomyopathy mutations on power output by human beta-cardiac myosin. J Exp Biol 2016,219(Pt 2):161-167

[190] Frey N, Luedde M, Katus HA. Mechanisms of disease: hypertrophic cardiomyopathy. Nat Rev Cardiol2011;9:91-100.

[191] Toepfer CN, Wakimoto H, Garfinkel AC, McDonough B, Liao D, Jiang J, Tai AC, Gorham JM, Lunde IG, Lun M, Lynch TL, McNamara JW, Sadayappan S, Redwood CS, Watkins HC, Seidman JG, Seidman CE. Hypertrophic cardiomyopathy mutations in MYBPC3 dysregulate myosin. Sci Transl Med 2019;11:eaat1199

[192] Olivotto I, Oreziak A, Barriales-Villa R, Abraham TP, Masri A, Garcia-Pavia P, Saberi S, Lakdawala NK, Wheeler MT, Owens A, Kubanek M, Wojakowski W, Jensen MK, Gimeno-Blanes J, Afshar K, Myers J, Hegde SM, Solomon SD, Sehnert AJ, ZhangD,LiW,BhattacharyaM,EdelbergJM, Waldman CB, Lester SJ, Wang A, Ho CY, Jacoby D; EXPLORER-HCM study investigators. Mavacamten for treatment of symptomatic obstructive

hypertrophic cardiomyopathy (EXPLORER-HCM): a randomised, double-blind, placebo-controlled, phase 3 trial. Lancet. 2020 Sep 12;396(10253):759-769. doi: 10.1016/S0140-6736(20)31792-X. Epub 2020 Aug 29. Erratum in: Lancet. 2020 Sep 12;396(10253):758. PMID: 32871100.

[193] Coppini R, Ferrantini C, Yao L, Fan P, Del Lungo M, Stillitano F, Sartiani L, Tosi B, Suffredini S, Tesi C, Yacoub M, Olivotto I, Belardinelli L, Poggesi C, Cerbai E, Mugelli A. Late sodium current inhibition reverses electromechanical dysfunction in human hypertrophic cardiomyopathy. Circulation 2013;127:575-584.

[194] Olivotto I, Camici PG, Merlini PA, Rapezzi C, Patten M, Climent V, Sinagra G, Tomberli B, Marin F, Ehlermann P, Maier LS, Fornaro A, Jacobshagen C, Ganau A, Moretti L, Hernandez Madrid A, Coppini R, Reggiardo G, Poggesi C, Fattirolli F, Belardinelli L, Gensini G, Mugelli A. Efficacy of ranolazine in patients with symptomatic hypertrophic cardiomyopathy: the RESTYLE-HCM randomized, double-blind, placebo-controlled study. Circ Heart Fail 2018;11:e004124.

[195] Shimada YJ, Passeri JJ, Baggish AL, O'Callaghan C, Lowry PA, Yannekis G, Abbara S, Ghoshhajra BB, Rothman RD, Ho CY, Januzzi JL, Seidman CE, Fifer MA. Effects of losartan on left ventricular hypertrophy and fibrosis in patients with nonobstructive hypertrophic cardiomyopathy. JACC Heart Fail 2013;1:480-487.

[196] Axelsson A, Iversen K, Vejlstrup N, Ho C, Norsk J, Langhoff L, Ahtarovski K, Corell P, Havndrup O, Jensen M, Bundgaard H. Efficacy and safety of the angiotensin II receptor blocker losartan for hypertrophic cardiomyopathy: the INHERIT randomised, double-blind, placebo-controlled trial. Lancet Diabetes Endocrinol 2015;3:123-131.

[197] Maron MS, Chan RH, Kapur NK, Jaffe IZ, McGraw AP, Kerur R, Maron BJ, Udelson JE. Effect of spironolactone on myocardial fibrosis and other clinical variables in patients with hypertrophic cardiomyopathy. Am J Med 2018;131:837-841.

[198] Axelsson A, Iversen K, Vejlstrup N, Ho CY, Havndrup O, Kofoed KF, Norsk J, Jensen M, Bundgaard H. Functional effects of losartan in hypertrophic cardiomyopathy – a randomised clinical trial. Heart 2016;102:285-291.

[199] Senthil V, Chen SN, Tsybouleva N, Halder T, Nagueh SF, Willerson JT, Roberts R, Marian AJ. Prevention of cardiac hypertrophy by atorvastatin in a transgenic rabbit model of human hypertrophic cardiomyopathy. Circ Res 2005;97:285-292.

[200] Nagueh SF, Lombardi R, Tan Y, Wang J, Willerson JT, Marian AJ. Atorvastatin and cardiac hypertrophy and function in hypertrophic cardiomyopathy: a pilot study. Eur J Clin Invest 2010;40:976-983.

[201] Musunuru K. Genome editing: the recent history and perspective in cardiovascular diseases. J Am Coll Cardiol2017;70:2808-2821.

[202] German DM, Mitalipov S, Mishra A, Kaul S. Therapeutic genome editing in cardiovascular diseases. JACC Basic Transl Sci 2019;4:122-131.

[203] Strong A, Musunuru K. Genome editing in cardiovascular diseases. Nat Rev Cardiol2017;14:11-20.

[204] Ma H, Marti-Gutierrez N, Park SW, Wu J, Lee Y, Suzuki K, Koski A, Ji D, Hayama T, Ahmed R, Darby H, Van Dyken C, Li Y, Kang E, Park AR, Kim D,

Kim ST, Gong J, Gu Y, Xu X, Battaglia D, Krieg SA, Lee DM, Wu DH, Wolf DP, Heitner SB, Belmonte JCI, Amato P, Kim JS, Kaul S, Mitalipov S. Correction of a pathogenic gene mutation in human embryos. Nature 2017;548:413-419.

[205] Bongianino R, Denegri M, Mazzanti A, Lodola F, Vollero A, Boncompagni S, Fasciano S, Rizzo G, Mangione D, Barbaro S, Di Fonso A, Napolitano C, Auricchio A, Protasi F, Priori SG. Allele-specific silencing of mutant mRNA rescues ultrastructural and arrhythmic phenotype in mice carriers of the R4496C mutation in the ryanodine receptor gene (RYR2). Circ Res 2017;121: 525-536

[206] Jiang J, Wakimoto H, Seidman JG, Seidman CE. Allele-specific silencing of mutant MYH6 transcripts in mice suppresses hypertrophic cardiomyopathy. Science 2013;342:111-114.

[207] Zaleta-Rivera K, Dainis A, Ribeiro AJS, Cordero P, Rubio G, Shang C, Liu J, Finsterbach T, Parikh VN, Sutton S, Seo K, Sinha N, Jain N, Huang Y, Hajjar RJ, Kay MA, Szczesna-Cordary D, Pruitt BL, Wheeler MT, Ashley EA. Allele-specific silencing ameliorates restrictive cardiomyopathy attributable to a human myosin regulatory light chain mutation. Circulation 2019;140:765-778.

Chapter 12

Fabry Disease

Ida Kåks and Peter Magnusson

Abstract

Fabry disease (FD) is a lysosomal storage disorder where deficient or completely absent activity of the enzyme α-galactosidas A leads to accumulation of globotriaosylceramide (Gb_3) and other glycosphingolipids in lysosomes. The condition is rare, approximately 1:50,000, although underdiagnosis seems frequent. The condition can affect multiple organ systems, including the skin, nervous system, kidneys, and heart. Early manifestations include skin lesions (angiokeratoma), neuropathic pain, and gastrointestinal symptoms. Later on, FD can result in cardiomyopathy, kidney failure, and stroke. Both lifespan and health-related quality of life are affected negatively by FD. Patients are divided into a classical or a non-classical phenotype based on presentation, where the diagnosis of classical FD requires that a set of specific criteria are met. Patients with non-classical FD often have a less severe disease course, sometimes limited to one organ. The hereditary pattern is X-linked. Thus, men are in general more severely affected than women, although there is an overlap in symptomatic burden. Two types of specific treatment options are available: enzyme replacement therapy and pharmacological chaperone therapy. In addition to this, management of each organ manifestation with usual treatment is indicated.

Keywords: Fabry disease, hypertrophic cardiomyopathy, left ventricular hypertrophy, lysosomal storage disorder

1. Introduction

Anderson-Fabry disease, generally referred to as Fabry disease (FD), is a lysosomal storage disorder where the activity of lysosomal enzyme α-galactosidas A is deficient or completely absent. This leads to accumulation of globotriaosylceramide (Gb_3) and related glycosphingolipids inside the lysosomes [1], organelles which, among other things, are responsible for degradation of cellular waste [2]. FD is a rare condition, and the reported incidence varies greatly between sources, with reported incidences in the ranges of 1 in 40,000 [3], 1 in 117,000 [4], and 1 in 476,000 [5]. However, when screening newborn males a prevalence of around 1 in 3,100 was found in Italy [6] and 1 in 1,250 in Taiwan [7], suggesting the true prevalence is higher than previously thought [1].

2. Historical overview

In 1898, the German physician Johannes Fabry and the British surgeon William Anderson independently of each other reported seeing patients with angiokeratoma, a classical skin lesion associated with the disease [8–10]. Back then, physicians lacked knowledge about the underlying causes for the dermatoses they were

IntechOpen

describing, and the meaning of additional symptoms were mostly unknown [11]. Hence, FD was initially considered a purely dermatological disorder. Anderson did, however, describe proteinuria. No one else in the patient's family was affected. Fabry's patient had a paternal grandfather who passed away from "kidney trouble" at an age of 49 years, and the patient himself died of lung disease at 44 years of age. The average life expectancy in the general population in the year 1900 was about 40 years [11]. In 1963 the mainly accumulated substance, Gb_3, was identified [12]. A few years later, deficient α-galactosidas activity was described, followed by the discovery of the gene coding for α-galactosidas A. To date, almost a 1,000 mutations have been identified in this gene, although many of the mutations still have an unknown significance and it is unclear whether they cause FD [8].

3. Disease manifestations

Symptoms generally appear between ages 3 and 10 in males, and a few years later in females [1]. Pain is among the first symptoms to manifest, and it can be either as episodic crises or as chronic pain. Most often, it presents as episodic sensations that radiate proximally from the extremities, which can be burning or shooting in character. The pain crises can consist of excruciating pain spreading all across the body. Physical exercise and thermal stimuli are triggers of the pain [13]. In addition to this, patients with FD can suffer from heat intolerance due to an- or hypohidrosis. In some patients, the pain decreases as they reach adulthood [1]. Other symptoms that may develop early are gastrointestinal problems (abdominal pain, diarrhea, vomiting), angiokeratoma (small spots on the skin, dark-red and raised), tinnitus and corneal changes (cornea verticillata, rarely affecting vision, **Figure 1**) [1].

For a definite diagnosis of FD, presence of an α-galactosidas A gene mutation needs to be present. Furthermore, in males an α-galactosidas A deficiency of ≤5% of mean reference value in leukocytes is an additional criterion, whilst in females α-galactosidas A in leukocytes may be normal or deficient. Additionally, one of the

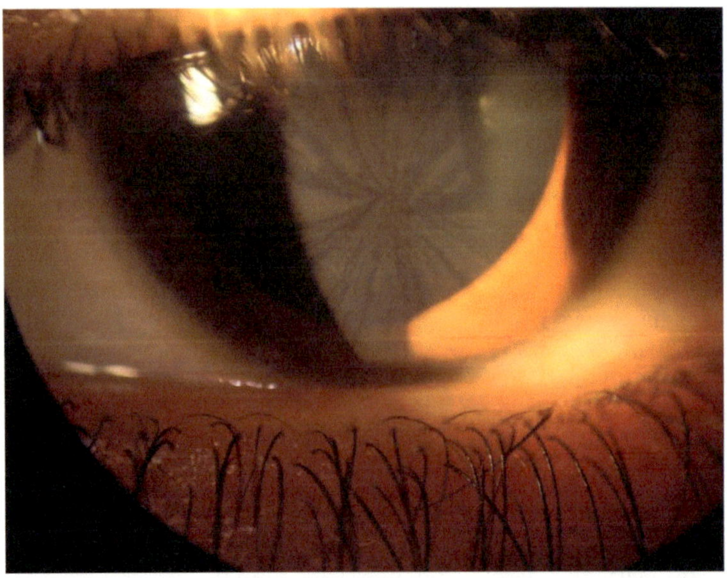

Figure 1.
Cornea verticillata, seen as sub-epithelial brown lines. From Germain [1]. Courtesy: Dr. Juan-Manuel POLITEI, Buenos-Aires, Argentina. Licensed under CC BY 2.0.

following must be present: at least one characteristic sign of FD (neuropathic pain, cornea verticillata, or clustered angiokeratoma), increased plasma Gb_3 (in the range of males with definite FD diagnosis), or a family member with definite FD with the same α-galactosidas A gene mutation [14].

FD is divided into a classical or a non-classical phenotype, where the diagnosis of classical phenotype in males is based on presence of an α-galactosidas A gene mutation, very low or completely absent enzyme activity, and one of the following signs: angiokeratoma, cornea verticillata, or very high Gb3-levels [15]. Hemizygous males are in general the ones most severely affected, although heterozygous females often have serious manifestations, which affect both quality of life and lifespan [16]. The varying severity of FD in females, where some are asymptomatic and others have a disease course comparable to that of males, is believed to be a result of skewed X-chromosome inactivation [17]. Females are considered to have classical FD when they present with angiokeratoma, cornea verticillata, or a very high Gb3-level [15]. Although the disease course is variable (more so in non-classical than in classical FD), patients with non-classical FD are less severely affected in general, sometimes with disease manifestation limited to one organ [18].

The heart, kidneys and brain may become affected as the disease progresses, and cardiovascular, renal and cerebrovascular disease represent the most common among the known and reported causes for mortality in patients with FD [16].

3.1 Cardiac involvement

Heart involvement is the main reason for impaired quality of life and death in patients with FD [19]. Between 40 and 60% report symptoms including left ventricular hypertrophy (LVH), angina, arrhythmia and dyspnea [1]. In most studies the prevalence of FD in adult patients with left ventricular hypertrophy is estimated at 0.5–1% [20]. For a suggestion on how to further investigate LVH that might be associated with FD, see **Figure 2**. Many patients have a cardiac variant of FD, meaning the disease manifests later in life, primarily as LVH or hypertrophic cardiomyopathy (HCM). This variant generally progresses slower because of

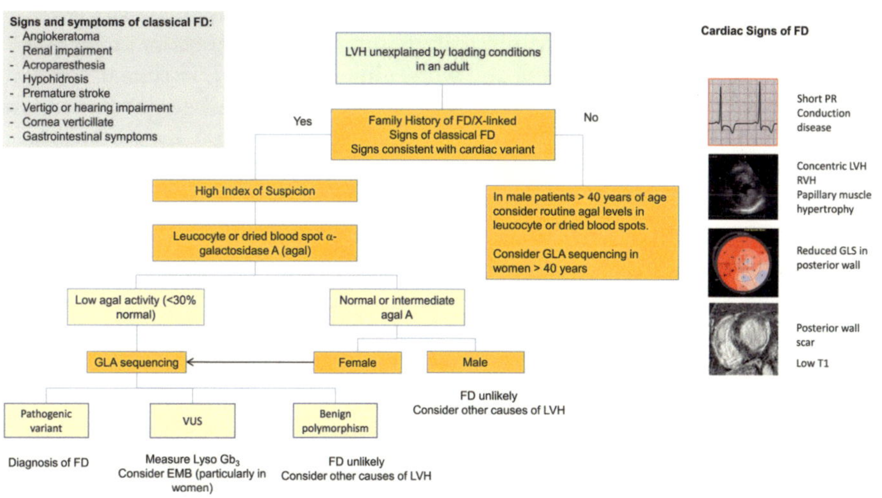

Figure 2.
Suggestion for further investigation of LVH when FD is suspected. Agal, α-galactosidas A; EMB, endomyocardial biopsy; GLA, α-galactosidas A gene; GLS, global longitudinal strain; RVH, right ventricular hypertrophy; VUS, variant of unknown significance. Image by Linhart A et al. [20] licensed under CC BY-NC 4.0.

residual α-galactosidas A-activity [20]. LVH manifests on average at age 32 in males, and at age 40 in women [21]. It is usually not accompanied by significantly impaired systolic function or restrictive diastolic dysfunction [22]. FD is considered a subgroup of HCM by the European Society of Cardiology (ESC), while the American Heart Association uses the term phenocopy to describe FD and other mimics of HCM [23, 24]. The prevalence of FD among patients with HCM above age 35–40 has been estimated to 0.5% [25].

In addition to LVH, cardiac involvement may lead to conduction defects and arrhythmia [8]. Since symptomatic bradycardia, AV block, chronotropic incompetence, supraventricular and ventricular arrhythmias are common, regular 24 h ECG monitoring is recommended [20]. The ESC recommend that patients with HCM who present with AV block or chronotropic incompetence should be suspected of having FD [23]. The arrhythmias in FD are a cause of significant morbidity. Atrial fibrillation is four times more common in patients with FD than in the general population, and twelve times more common in patients above the age of 50 [26]. Death from ventricular arrhythmia has been observed in a number of FD patients [26, 27]. Patients with FD can experience angina despite their coronary arteries being angiographically normal, which can be explained by microvascular dysfunction [28]. Valve disease occurs as a result of infiltrative changes in valvular fibroblasts, most clinically significant changes appear in the left heart valves. Valves become thickened which can lead to mild to moderate regurgitation, but disease requiring surgery is rare [29].

ECG changes associated with FD include shorter PQ interval, P-wave duration and QRS width, and increased QT and QTc duration [30]. As FD cardiomyopathy develops, voltage signs of LVH and inversed T-waves in precordial leads are usually seen [20].

Terminal stage cardiac FD leads to severe left ventricle dysfunction, associated with conduction disturbances and ventricular arrhythmia [27].

3.2 Renal involvement

The kidneys can be affected due to Gb_3 accumulating in renal cells (glomerular endothelial, mesangial, interstitial, podocytes), and the severity increases with age [1]. The first signs are usually microalbuminuria and proteinuria, presenting as early as the second decade of life and worsening with age [1]. In time, the glomerular filtration rate starts to decline, which might lead to end-stage renal failure [8]. Renal involvement is common; signs and symptoms of renal disease have been reported in half of patients in the Fabry Outcome Survey (a European database for all FD patients eligible for, or receiving, enzyme replacement therapy with agalsidase alfa). The most frequent sign was proteinuria, seen in 33% of females and 44% of males. End-stage renal failure affected 17% of males and 1% of females. Among the male patients 10% received a renal transplant and 7% were on dialysis [3].

3.3 Cerebrovascular involvement

Ischemic stroke and transient ischemic attacks are the most common cerebrovascular complications in FD, and occur at a younger age than in the general population [31]. Stroke can affect patients who have no other key signs of FD; data from the Fabry Registry showed that 46% suffered their first stroke prior to being diagnosed with FD [32]. The median age of first stroke was 39 in males and 46 in females. Approximately 87% of strokes were ischemic similar to the numbers in the general population. Among the strokes where vessel size was reported, most occurred in small vessels. The prevalence of stroke was 4.3% in females and 6.9%

in males, which by far exceeds the prevalence in the general population [1]. In men between ages 35 and 45, the risk of stroke is 12.2 times higher in patients with FD than in healthy subjects [31].

The pathological mechanisms for stroke in FD is not clear, but abnormalities in cerebral blood flow as well as in the walls of intracranial vessels have been seen [32]. A possible contributing factor is that formation of thrombi may be enhanced due to increased adhesion of neutrophils and monocytes to the endothelial wall [1, 33].

4. Pathophysiology

That Gb_3 is accumulated in lysosomes is well known, but the specifics regarding what causes cellular dysfunction is not [8]. Accumulation of substrate does lead to enlargement of the affected cells, in turn resulting in enlargement of entire organs. This is, however, not the only explanation [34]. One report presents a case where cardiac hypertrophy resulted in a heart weighing 1100 g, and Gb_3 only accounted for 3.5 g [35, 36]. Mitochondrial metabolism is affected by the substrate accumulation in FD, which is part of the explanation for the organ damage that occurs [37]. There may be dysfunction of the endoplasmic reticulum as well. Fibrosis, inflammation and oxidative stress appear to play important parts in pathogenesis [8].

5. Treatment

In 2001 enzyme replacement therapy (ERT) was introduced, human recombinant α-galactosidas A administered through bi-weekly intravenous infusions. Two recombinant enzyme preparations exist: agalsidase alfa and agalsidase beta. ERT has been shown to reduce pain, improve cardiac function [38], and stabilize kidney function [39]. Treatment is recommended for classically affected males and females and non-classically affected males who show early clinical signs of heart, kidney, or brain involvement. In classically affected males aged 16 or older without signs or symptoms of organ involvement and in non-classically affected females with early clinical signs, treatment should be considered [15]. ERT should be prescribed as early in the disease course as possible, since the benefit in advanced FD seems doubtful [40, 41]. Although the risk of developing a first or second complication is reduced by increased treatment duration, ERT does not seem to prevent disease progression [40].

Since 2016 another treatment option has become available: pharmacological chaperone therapy (PCT). The drug is taken orally, and can restore enzyme activity by promoting correct folding in patients with mutations responsive to the therapy (approximately 35–50% of patients) [8, 42]. Individual eligibility for treatment is tested through an in vitro enzyme activity assay [43]. During long-term therapy it has maintained renal function, and reduced cardiac mass more effectively than ERT [42].

Both ERT and PCT should always be combined with therapies to manage the different organ manifestations clinically [8].

Regarding implantable cardioverter-defibrillator therapy, the ESC state that their risk prediction model HCM Risk-SCD, used for calculating the risk of sudden cardiac death (SCD) in HCM patients, should not be used in patients with FD [23]. There are currently no guidelines for implantation of cardiac devices in FD, and data on risk predictors are scarce. One study showed a higher delivery of device therapy in FD than in HCM. The rates of asymptomatic non sustained ventricular tachycardia were similar, but FD patients experienced a higher rate of ventricular arrhythmia that required anti-tachycardia pacing or defibrillation [44].

6. Health-related quality of life

Patients with FD have a lower quality of life than the population in general; a systematic review found that they score lower in all domains in the SF-36 and EQ-5D questionnaires (the domains include aspects such as a physical and mental component summary score) [45]. However, no studies had examined the difference between classically and non-classically affected individuals. The effect of ERT on quality of life was not conclusive. A qualitative study using in-depth interviews with ten Norwegian women, heterozygous for FD, found that receiving the diagnosis can bring about feelings of relief as well as distress [46]. For symptomatic women the diagnosis can be an explanation of problems they have dealt with for years; many have been burdened by feeling like hypochondriacs because of health issues without an apparent cause. On the other hand, some women saw the diagnosis itself as stigmatizing. Almost every participant had negative feelings about passing the condition on to their children. Another qualitative study of 30 patients from the Netherlands, both male and female, found that many patients had experiences of being misdiagnosed and feeling misunderstood due to delayed correct diagnosis [47]. Others mentioned that presymptomatic diagnosis had drawbacks such as medicalization and labeling.

7. Prognosis

Before ERT, male patients died at a mean age of 50 [48], and a study of females showed a median cumulative survival of 70 years [49]. The long-term prognosis of FD in a modern setting needs to be further elucidated.

8. Future perspectives

There are current studies of gene therapy for FD, as well as substrate reduction therapy, second generation enzyme replacement therapies, and novel PCTs [8, 43]. The second generation enzyme replacement therapies currently in development are plant derived as opposed to agalsidase alfa (produced in human fibroblasts) and agalsidase beta (produced in hamster ovary cells), which could result in a different bio distribution. Substrate reduction therapy is an oral treatment, which aims to limit the formation of metabolites that FD patients cannot degrade. There are currently ongoing Phase I and II clinical trials in which haematopoetic stem cells are recruited from the patient and transduced with the lentivirus vector containing the human α-galactosidas A gene, then re-administered to the patient (NCT02800070 and NCT03454893) [43].

9. Conclusions

FD is a rare disease, generally underdiagnosed, with profound effects on morbidity and mortality. Symptoms, such as debilitating pain, can present themselves early in childhood and in time the disease may lead to severe cardiac, renal, and cerebrovascular complications. The available treatment with ERT has a doubtful effect in advanced FD, making it imperative that the diagnosis is made in time. The Fabry Registry has been used in several studies of FD patients, and registry data is a valuable resource when it comes to evaluating treatment options. In the future, different therapeutic approaches could be compared using the information this registry can provide regarding clinical and investigative findings. The suffering associated with living with unexplained symptoms for years is yet another reason why increased awareness of FD in the medical community is of great importance.

Conflict of interest

Ida Kåks reports no conflicts of interest. Peter Magnusson has received speaker's fees or grants from Abbott, Alnylam, Amicus Therapeutics, AstraZeneca, Bayer, BMS, Boehringer-Ingelheim, Coala Life, Internetmedicin, Lilly, MSD, Novo Nordisk, Octopus Medical, Orion Pharma, Pfizer, Sanofi, Vifor Pharma, and Zoll.

Abbreviations

ERT	enzyme replacement therapy
ESC	European Society of Cardiology
FD	Fabry disease
GB_3	globotriaosylceramide
HCM	hypertrophic cardiomyopathy
LVH	left ventricular hypertrophy
PCT	pharmacological chaperone therapy
SCD	sudden cardiac death

Author details

Ida Kåks[1*] and Peter Magnusson[1,2]

1 Centre for Research and Development, Uppsala University/Region Gävleborg, Gävle, Sweden

2 Cardiology Research Unit, Department of Medicine, Solna, Karolinska Institutet, Stockholm, Sweden

*Address all correspondence to: ida.kaks@regiongavleborg.se

References

[1] Germain DP. Fabry disease. Orphanet journal of rare diseases. 2010;5:30.

[2] Ballabio A. The awesome lysosome. EMBO molecular medicine. 2016;8(2):73-76.

[3] Mehta A, Ricci R, Widmer U, Dehout F, Garcia de Lorenzo A, Kampmann C, et al. Fabry disease defined: baseline clinical manifestations of 366 patients in the Fabry Outcome Survey. European Journal of Clinical Investigation. 2004;34(3):236-242.

[4] Meikle PJ, Hopwood JJ, Clague AE, Carey WF. Prevalence of lysosomal storage disorders. Jama. 1999;281(3): 249-254.

[5] Poorthuis BJ, Wevers RA, Kleijer WJ, Groener JE, de Jong JG, van Weely S, et al. The frequency of lysosomal storage diseases in The Netherlands. Human genetics. 1999;105(1-2):151-156.

[6] Spada M, Pagliardini S, Yasuda M, Tukel T, Thiagarajan G, Sakuraba H, et al. High incidence of later-onset fabry disease revealed by newborn screening. American journal of human genetics. 2006;79(1):31-40.

[7] Hwu WL, Chien YH, Lee NC, Chiang SC, Dobrovolny R, Huang AC, et al. Newborn screening for Fabry disease in Taiwan reveals a high incidence of the later-onset GLA mutation c.936+919G>A (IVS4+919G>A). Human mutation. 2009;30(10):1397-1405.

[8] Kok K, Zwiers KC, Boot RG, Overkleeft HS, Aerts J, Artola M. Fabry Disease: Molecular Basis, Pathophysiology, Diagnostics and Potential Therapeutic Directions. Biomolecules. 2021;11(2).

[9] ANDERSON W. A CASE OF "ANGEIO-KERATOMA."*. British Journal of Dermatology. 1898;10(4): 113-117.

[10] Fabry J. Ein Beitrag zur Kenntniss der Purpura haemorrhagica nodularis (Purpura papulosa haemorrhagica Hebrae). Arch f Dermat. 1898;43: 187-200.

[11] Fabry H. An historical overview of Fabry disease. Journal of inherited metabolic disease. 2001;24 Suppl 2:3-7.

[12] Sweeley CC, Klionsky B. FABRY'S DISEASE: CLASSIFICATION AS A SPHINGOLIPIDOSIS AND PARTIAL CHARACTERIZATION OF A NOVEL GLYCOLIPID. The Journal of biological chemistry. 1963;238:3148-3150.

[13] Politei JM, Bouhassira D, Germain DP, Goizet C, Guerrero-Sola A, Hilz MJ, et al. Pain in Fabry Disease: Practical Recommendations for Diagnosis and Treatment. CNS neuroscience & therapeutics. 2016;22(7):568-576.

[14] Smid BE, van der Tol L, Cecchi F, Elliott PM, Hughes DA, Linthorst GE, et al. Uncertain diagnosis of Fabry disease: consensus recommendation on diagnosis in adults with left ventricular hypertrophy and genetic variants of unknown significance. International journal of cardiology. 2014;177(2): 400-408.

[15] Biegstraaten M, Arngrímsson R, Barbey F, Boks L, Cecchi F, Deegan PB, et al. Recommendations for initiation and cessation of enzyme replacement therapy in patients with Fabry disease: the European Fabry Working Group consensus document. Orphanet journal of rare diseases. 2015;10:36.

[16] Waldek S, Patel MR, Banikazemi M, Lemay R, Lee P. Life expectancy and cause of death in males and females with Fabry disease: findings from the Fabry

Registry. Genetics in medicine : official journal of the American College of Medical Genetics. 2009;11(11):790-796.

[17] Echevarria L, Benistan K, Toussaint A, Dubourg O, Hagege AA, Eladari D, et al. X-chromosome inactivation in female patients with Fabry disease. Clinical genetics. 2016;89(1):44-54.

[18] Arends M, Wanner C, Hughes D, Mehta A, Oder D, Watkinson OT, et al. Characterization of Classical and Nonclassical Fabry Disease: A Multicenter Study. Journal of the American Society of Nephrology : JASN. 2017;28(5):1631-1641.

[19] Pieroni M, Moon JC, Arbustini E, Barriales-Villa R, Camporeale A, Vujkovac AC, et al. Cardiac Involvement in Fabry Disease: JACC Review Topic of the Week. Journal of the American College of Cardiology. 2021;77(7): 922-936.

[20] Linhart A, Germain DP, Olivotto I, Akhtar MM, Anastasakis A, Hughes D, et al. An expert consensus document on the management of cardiovascular manifestations of Fabry disease. European journal of heart failure. 2020;22(7):1076-1096.

[21] Linhart A, Kampmann C, Zamorano JL, Sunder-Plassmann G, Beck M, Mehta A, et al. Cardiac manifestations of Anderson-Fabry disease: results from the international Fabry outcome survey. European heart journal. 2007;28(10):1228-1235.

[22] Linhart A, Palecek T, Bultas J, Ferguson JJ, Hrudová J, Karetová D, et al. New insights in cardiac structural changes in patients with Fabry's disease. American heart journal. 2000;139(6): 1101-1108.

[23] Elliott PM, Anastasakis A, Borger MA, Borggrefe M, Cecchi F, Charron P, et al. 2014 ESC Guidelines on diagnosis and management of hypertrophic cardiomyopathy: the Task Force for the Diagnosis and Management of Hypertrophic Cardiomyopathy of the European Society of Cardiology (ESC). European heart journal. 2014;35(39):2733-79.

[24] Ommen SR, Mital S, Burke MA, Day SM, Deswal A, Elliott P, et al. 2020 AHA/ACC Guideline for the Diagnosis and Treatment of Patients With Hypertrophic Cardiomyopathy: A Report of the American College of Cardiology/American Heart Association Joint Committee on Clinical Practice Guidelines. Journal of the American College of Cardiology. 2020;76(25): e159-e240.

[25] Elliott P, Baker R, Pasquale F, Quarta G, Ebrahim H, Mehta AB, et al. Prevalence of Anderson-Fabry disease in patients with hypertrophic cardiomyopathy: the European Anderson-Fabry Disease survey. Heart (British Cardiac Society). 2011;97(23): 1957-1960.

[26] Shah JS, Hughes DA, Sachdev B, Tome M, Ward D, Lee P, et al. Prevalence and clinical significance of cardiac arrhythmia in Anderson-Fabry disease. The American journal of cardiology. 2005;96(6):842-846.

[27] Takenaka T, Teraguchi H, Yoshida A, Taguchi S, Ninomiya K, Umekita Y, et al. Terminal stage cardiac findings in patients with cardiac Fabry disease: an electrocardiographic, echocardiographic, and autopsy study. Journal of cardiology. 2008;51(1):50-59.

[28] Elliott PM, Kindler H, Shah JS, Sachdev B, Rimoldi OE, Thaman R, et al. Coronary microvascular dysfunction in male patients with Anderson-Fabry disease and the effect of treatment with alpha galactosidase A. Heart (British Cardiac Society). 2006;92(3):357-360.

[29] Linhart A, Elliott PM. The heart in Anderson-Fabry disease and other

lysosomal storage disorders. Heart (British Cardiac Society). 2007;93(4):528-535.

[30] Namdar M, Steffel J, Vidovic M, Brunckhorst CB, Holzmeister J, Lüscher TF, et al. Electrocardiographic changes in early recognition of Fabry disease. Heart (British Cardiac Society). 2011;97(6):485-490.

[31] Kolodny E, Fellgiebel A, Hilz MJ, Sims K, Caruso P, Phan TG, et al. Cerebrovascular Involvement in Fabry Disease. Stroke. 2015;46(1):302-313.

[32] Sims K, Politei J, Banikazemi M, Lee P. Stroke in Fabry Disease Frequently Occurs Before Diagnosis and in the Absence of Other Clinical Events. Stroke. 2009;40(3):788-794.

[33] DeGraba T, Azhar S, Dignat-George F, Brown E, Boutière B, Altarescu G, et al. Profile of endothelial and leukocyte activation in fabry patients. Annals of Neurology. 2000;47(2):229-233.

[34] Vellodi A. Lysosomal storage disorders. British journal of haematology. 2005;128(4):413-431.

[35] Elleder M, Bradová V, Smíd F, Budĕsínský M, Harzer K, Kustermann-Kuhn B, et al. Cardiocyte storage and hypertrophy as a sole manifestation of Fabry's disease. Report on a case simulating hypertrophic non-obstructive cardiomyopathy. Virchows Archiv A, Pathological anatomy and histopathology. 1990;417(5):449-455.

[36] Elleder M. Sequelae of storage in Fabry disease--pathology and comparison with other lysosomal storage diseases. Acta paediatrica (Oslo, Norway : 1992) Supplement. 2003;92 (443):46-53; discussion 45.

[37] Ivanova M. Altered Sphingolipids Metabolism Damaged Mitochondrial Functions: Lessons Learned From Gaucher and Fabry Diseases. Journal of clinical medicine. 2020;9(4).

[38] Schiffmann R, Kopp JB, Austin HA, 3rd, Sabnis S, Moore DF, Weibel T, et al. Enzyme replacement therapy in Fabry disease: a randomized controlled trial. Jama. 2001;285(21):2743-2749.

[39] Wilcox WR, Banikazemi M, Guffon N, Waldek S, Lee P, Linthorst GE, et al. Long-term safety and efficacy of enzyme replacement therapy for Fabry disease. American journal of human genetics. 2004;75(1):65-74.

[40] Rombach SM, Smid BE, Bouwman MG, Linthorst GE, Dijkgraaf MG, Hollak CE. Long term enzyme replacement therapy for Fabry disease: effectiveness on kidney, heart and brain. Orphanet journal of rare diseases. 2013;8:47.

[41] Weidemann F, Niemann M, Störk S, Breunig F, Beer M, Sommer C, et al. Long-term outcome of enzyme-replacement therapy in advanced Fabry disease: evidence for disease progression towards serious complications. Journal of internal medicine. 2013;274(4):331-341.

[42] McCafferty EH, Scott LJ. Migalastat: A Review in Fabry Disease. Drugs. 2019;79(5):543-554.

[43] van der Veen SJ, Hollak CEM, van Kuilenburg ABP, Langeveld M. Developments in the treatment of Fabry disease. Journal of inherited metabolic disease. 2020;43(5):908-921.

[44] Vijapurapu R, Zegard A, Leyva F, Bradlow W, Jovanovic A, Hughes D, et al. ICD implantation and device therapy: Fabry vs hypertrophic cardiomyopathy. European heart journal. 2020;41(Supplement_2).

[45] Arends M, Hollak CE, Biegstraaten M. Quality of life in

patients with Fabry disease: a systematic review of the literature. Orphanet journal of rare diseases. 2015;10:77.

[46] von der Lippe C, Frich JC, Harris A, Solbrække KN. Experiences of Being Heterozygous for Fabry Disease: a Qualitative Study. Journal of genetic counseling. 2016;25(5):1085-1092.

[47] Bouwman MG, de Ru MH, Linthorst GE, Hollak CE, Wijburg FA, van Zwieten MC. Fabry patients' experiences with the timing of diagnosis relevant for the discussion on newborn screening. Molecular genetics and metabolism. 2013;109(2):201-207.

[48] Schiffmann R, Warnock DG, Banikazemi M, Bultas J, Linthorst GE, Packman S, et al. Fabry disease: progression of nephropathy, and prevalence of cardiac and cerebrovascular events before enzyme replacement therapy. Nephrology, dialysis, transplantation : official publication of the European Dialysis and Transplant Association - European Renal Association. 2009;24(7): 2102-2111.

[49] MacDermot KD, Holmes A, Miners AH. Anderson-Fabry disease: clinical manifestations and impact of disease in a cohort of 60 obligate carrier females. Journal of medical genetics. 2001;38(11):769-775.

Chapter 13

Cardiomyopathy: Getting Bigger All the Time - Lessons Learned about Heart Disease from Tropomyosin

David F. Wieczorek

Abstract

In 1990, John and Christine Seidman uncovered the genetic association between mutations in sarcomeric contractile proteins and hypertrophic cardiomyopathy. Since then, the increase in knowledge and understanding of this disease has increased exponentially. Although pathologies associated with the various cardiomyopathies are vastly different, in some cases, the same proteins are causative, but with different genetic mutations. The focus of this article will be on hypertrophic and dilated cardiomyopathies, which are often caused by mutations in sarcomeric contractile proteins. Tropomyosin, a thin filament protein, serves as a paradigm to illustrate how different mutations within the same protein can generate the hypertrophic or dilated cardiomyopathic condition. As such, the significant advances in information derived from basic science investigations has led to the development of novel therapeutics in the treatment of these pathological diseases. This article will illustrate linkages which occur to bridge scientific advances to clinical treatments in cardiomyopathic patients.

Keywords: hypertrophic and dilated cardiomyopathy, tropomyosin

1. Introduction

Cardiomyopathies are diseases with primary defects associated with the structure and function of the heart. They are commonly classified into 5 different categories: hypertrophic cardiomyopathy (HCM), dilated cardiomyopathy (DCM), restrictive cardiomyopathy (RCM), arrhythmogenic right ventricular cardiomyopathy (ARVC), and left ventricular noncompaction (LVNC). HCM and DCM are the most common of the cardiomyopathies, with an incidence of 1:500 and 1:2500, respectively. Although there are variations in phenotypes and etiologies, there are also similar symptoms among the cardiomyopathies. For example, HCM, DCM, and RCM often present with signs and symptoms that are common in heart failure with reduced ejection fraction, including peripheral edema, fatigue, dyspnea on exertion, syncope, and cardiac ischemia [1, 2]. The focus of this article will be on HCM and DCM, the two most common cardiomyopathies.

2. Hypertrophic cardiomyopathy

Hypertrophic cardiomyopathy (HCM) is defined as left and/or right ventricle hypertrophy in the absence of external load, and without chamber dilation. Interventricular septal thickening predominates and may cause left ventricular outflow tract obstruction and/or mitral valve dysfunction. Other common features include myocyte disarray, fibrosis, alterations in calcium sensitivity of myofilaments, and cardiac arrhythmias that may lead to premature sudden death and/or heart failure. Phenotypic expression is variable, with some genetically-identified HCM individuals dying in their late teens/early twenties, whereas others have a normal life span with minimal disability dependent upon the specific mutation within the affected gene. In addition, modifier genes and environmental factors can influence disease progression and phenotype.

The genes associated with HCM can be roughly divided into several distinct categories: (1) genes definitively established as causing HCM via large family pedigrees; (2) genes likely causing HCM via small family pedigrees; and (3) genes associated with HCM via small families and sporadic cases [3]. However, as more genetic information is obtained on incidence of diseases, these categorizations may become blurred. Usually, HCM is inherited as an autosomal dominant disease where a single missense point mutation in the affected gene is sufficient to cause the disease, although there is variability in the phenotype. This variability in phenotype is also manifest by the numerous different point mutations that occur within a specific gene; for example, the myosin heavy chain 7 (*MYH7*) R403Q mutation is associated with a severe pathological phenotype, whereas other *MYH7* mutations, such as V606M, are relatively benign [4]. Studies also show that modifier genes and their polymorphisms, such as angiotensin II type 2 receptor and calmodulin, can influence the HCM pathology [4]. In addition, mutations that occur in different HCM-causing genes have dramatically different pathologies, with some being severe and others being relatively benign.

The genes primarily associated with the HCM phenotype are sarcomeric contractile protein genes associated with both thick and thin cardiac myofilaments, along with the Z discs (**Table 1**). There are over 1500 mutations in these genes that are associated with HCM. The pioneering studies that revealed the molecular genetic basis of HCM and its association with sarcomeric protein genes were conducted by Drs. Christine and Jonathan Seidman [5]. These initial studies led to the discovery that mutations within most of the thick and thin filament sarcomeric protein genes of the heart can cause HCM (**Table 1**). In the United States, the most common genes associated with HCM are β-myosin heavy chain (*MYH7*) and myosin-binding protein C (*MYBPC3*); other thick filament protein genes which cause HCM are the regulatory light chain (*MLC2*) and the essential light chains (*MLC 1/3*). Most *MYH7* mutations occur in the globular head and hinge region of the myosin heavy chain, although mutations in the rod domain also cause HCM. Although most HCM mutations in the contractile protein genes are missense mutations, there is a bias for insertion/deletion mutations and premature truncation mutations in the *MYBPC3* gene; these insertion/deletion mutations often result in translational reading frame shifts which lead to premature stop codons with subsequent degradation of the mRNA by nonsense mediated decay mechanisms or degradation of a truncated polypeptide. Thin filament protein genes associated with HCM are α-tropomyosin (*TPM1α*), troponin T, I, and C (*TNNT2, TNNI3, TNNC1*), and cardiac actin (*ACTC1*). The muscle LIM protein CSRP3, found in the Z-disc, also is a causal gene for HCM. Interestingly, HCM mutations in cardiac troponin T often have a relatively mild pathological phenotype but can lead to sudden cardiac

DOI: http://dx.doi.org/10.5772/intechopen.95509

Gene	Protein	Protein function	Cardiomyopathy
MYH7	β-Myosin heavy chain	ATPase activity and Force generation in sarcomere	HCM, DCM
MYH6	α-Myosin Heavy Chain	Principle protein of the thick filament with low expression in adult human ventricles	HCM, DCM
MYL2	Regulatory myosin light chain	Binds myosin heavy chain	HCM
MYL1/3	Essential myosin light chain	Binds myosin heavy chain	HCM
ACTC1	Cardiac α-actin	Principle component of the thin filament	HCM, DCM
TPM1	α-Tropomyosin	Blocks myosin interaction with actin in sarcomere	HCM, DCM
TNNT2	Cardiac troponin T	Holds troponin complex on tropomyosin	HCM, DCM
TNNI3	Cardiac troponin I	Inhibits actomyosin interaction	HCM, DCM
TNNC1	Cardiac troponin C	Binds calcium to regulate sarcomeric contraction	HCM, DCM
MYBPC3	Myosin binding protein C	Structure & Contraction in the sarcomere	HCM, DCM
TTN	TItin	Structural component of the sarcomere	HCM, DCM
CSRP3	Cysteine-and glycine-rich protein 3	Muscle LIM protein located in the Z disc	HCM, DCM
ACTN2	Actinin	Attaches actin filaments to the Z lines in muscle	HCM, DCM
TCAP	Tcap (telethonin)	Capping protein for titin	HCM, DCM
MYOZ2	Myozenin 2 (calsarcin 1)	Tethers calcineurin to the Z disc via actinin	HCM
PLN	Phospholamban	Regulates calcium entry into the sarcoplasmic reticulum	HCM, DCM
LDB3	Lim domain binding 3	Stabilizes the sarcomere during muscle contraction	HCM, DCM
FHL1	Four-and-a-half LIM domains 1	Muscle development and cardiac hypertrophy	HCM
MYLK2	Myosin light chain kinase 2	Phosphorylates myosin light chain 2	HCM
NEXN	Nexilin	Actin binding protein, part of T-tubule complex and Z discs	HCM, DCM
JPH2	Junctophilin-2	Structural protein linking the plasma membrane with the sarcoplasmic membrane.	HCM
CASQ2	Calsequestrin 2	Calcium binding protein	HCM
VCL	Vinculin	Cytoskeletal protein	HCM, DCM
ANKRD1	Ankyrin repeat domain 1	Transcriptional repressor of cardiac genes	HCM, DCM
TRM63	Muscle ring finger protein	Involved in proteasome-ubiquitin system for protein degradation	HCM,

Table 1.
Genes found to cause cardiomyopathies.

death. Over the years, the identification and verification of many of these sarcomeric genes with HCM has been primarily through large family pedigrees, and often confirmed through experimental animal systems.

In addition to those genes mentioned that have a strong association with causing HCM, there are other cardiac muscle protein genes that when mutated are likely candidates for HCM. These genes include four-and-a-half LIM domains 1 (*FHL1*), myozenin 2 (*MYOZ2*), phospholamban (*PLN*), titin (*TTN*), titin capping protein (*TCAP*), and muscle ring finger protein 1 (*TRM63*) (**Table 1**) [3, 6, 7]. Although some of these associated proteins are located in the sarcomere (titin, titin capping protein), others are found peripherally, such as phospholamban which is in the sarcoplasmic reticulum membrane, and myozenin 2, located in the Z disc. There are also genes that are associated with HCM but occur more sporadically [3, 6, 7]. Some of these proteins are associated with cardiac muscle, such as troponin C, myosin light chain kinase 2, actinin 2, vinculin, nexilin, α-myosin heavy chain, and Lim domain binding 3 protein; other proteins are found globally, such as caveolin, junctophilin-2, and calsequestrin (**Table 1**). The fact that a vast array of different genes encoding proteins with diverse functions can all trigger the HCM pathological response demonstrates a common end point in the development of cardiovascular disease. However, we must also consider HCM is a large phenotypic category and that with more detailed pathological and physiological analyses, an improved diagnostic system might be developed. This has already been demonstrated by the addition of other cardiomyopathic classifications, such as restrictive cardiomyopathy, storage and metabolic cardiomyopathies, dilated cardiomyopathy, arrhythmogenic right ventricular cardiomyopathy, and mitochondrial cardiomyopathy.

3. Dilated cardiomyopathy

Dilated cardiomyopathy (DCM) is defined as dilation of the left or both ventricles that is not explained by coronary artery disease or abnormal loading of the heart. The cardiac enlargement occurs with either normal thickness or thinning of the ventricular walls and varying amounts of fibrosis. Oftentimes, DCM leads to heart failure with reduced ejection fraction, tachyarrhythmias, and increased risk of sudden death. All four cardiac chambers may be dilated with increased end-systolic volumes in both ventricles. The incidence of DCM is less well defined, with numbers varying between 1/250 individuals to 1/2500 individuals [6, 7]. Some of this variability can be attributed to the increased number of causes associated with DCM which include familial, viral myocarditis, cardiac toxins (i.e. alcohol, cocaine, amphetamine, cancer chemotherapeutic agents), peripartum cardiomyopathy, and prolonged tachycardia-related cardiomyopathy.

The genes associated with familial DCM are numerous and varied in their function (**Table 1**); however, the most common mode of inheritance is autosomal dominant. Over 50 genes have been identified that are linked to familial DCM, which encode proteins in the sarcomeres, ion channels, cytoskeleton, nuclear envelope, and mitochondria [6, 7]. Familial DCM comprises 30–50% of the DCM population. There is also allelic heterogeneity with mutations occurring in multiple regions within a specific gene. In fact, many genes are associated with causing both DCM and HCM, dependent upon the specific mutation (**Table 1**).

Titin, lamin A/C, and β-myosin heavy chain account for >25% of genetically-inherited DCM [7, 8]. Titin, the longest human protein, is composed of 34,350 amino acids with a mass of 3,816,030 Da. This sarcomeric protein functions as a scaffold for both thick and thin filaments in striated muscle. Many of the DCM-associated mutations in titin encode premature stop codons, resulting in truncated forms of the protein. These truncations often map to the A band of the sarcomere, rather than the I band, and are associated with phenotypically mild DCM. Other titin mutations result in sarcomere instability, decreased binding to its cap-binding protein (TCAP), decreased binding to the Z-disc, and a decreased stretch response during sarcomere contraction.

Mutations in the *lamin A* gene account for approximately 6% of all DCM mutations, and is oftentimes associated with a high incidence of sudden cardiac death [8]. Lamin proteins are associated with intermediate filaments which support the nuclear membrane, along with a role in chromatin structure and possibly gene transcription. Mutations in the lamin gene often lead to nuclear membrane damage and/or chromatin disorganization and impaired gene transcription. Because of lamin's diverse function, mutations lead to a wide variety of disease conditions, including premature aging and various myopathies, including DCM. In the heart, *LMN A* mutations often lead to dysrhythmias including sinus node and AV node dysfunction, atrial and ventricular fibrillation, and sudden cardiac death [8].

Mutations in genes involved in calcium/sodium handling are also associated with the onset of DCM. Phospholamban (PLN), a regulator of the sarcoplasmic reticulum Ca^{2+}-ATPase pump, has several autosomal dominant mutations that result in DCM. In fact, the R14del mutation in PLN is associated with a founder effect in the Netherlands which results in a severe phenotype [9]. However, a milder DCM phenotype may also occur with the R14del mutation which demonstrates that modifying genes may play a role in the disease pathology. Another ion channel gene associated with DCM is *SCN5A*, a major sodium channel expressed in the heart. DCM mutations in this gene increase the risk for arrhythmias, whereas other *SCN5A* mutations result in channelopathies [6].

An examination of the genes associated with DCM and HCM clearly demonstrates commonality in causing cardiomyopathies (**Table 1**). A clear example of this are the numerous sarcomeric protein genes, including titin, α- and β-myosin heavy chains, troponin T, I, and C, α-tropomyosin, α-actin, and titin capping protein, vinculin, desmin, and nexin (**Table 1**). There are also genes which appear more specific in causing only a single phenotype; genes associated with HCM are myosin light chain 2 and 1/3, myosin light chain kinase, and myozenin, whereas genes associated with only DCM include laminin α4, presenilin 1 and 2, and numerous others [6, 7]. The multitude of mutated genes that can result in DCM and HCM would infer that a continuum of phenotypes may exist for these cardiomyopathies dependent upon when the diseased heart is examined, which gene is mutated, where the mutation occurs, the type of mutation, associated modifying genes, and environmental influences. In fact, there are many cases where HCM hearts transition to DCM and heart failure as the disease progresses.

4. Tropomyosin and HCM

Tropomyosin (TPM) is an essential component of the sarcomeric thin filament that regulates muscle contraction and relaxation through its interactions with actin and the troponin complex. More specifically, striated muscle TPM, along with the troponin complex, regulates Ca^{2+}-mediated actin-myosin crossbridges. As stated previously, the Seidman laboratory discovered through pedigree analysis and gene mapping that HCM was associated with mutations in myosin heavy chains [5]. The association of TPM with HCM was also reported by the Seidman laboratory in 1994 which confirmed that HCM was a disease of the sarcomere and not solely confined to the thick filament [10]. In the United States, the percentage of HCM attributed to mutations in TPM is ~5%, with most of these cases exhibiting benign symptoms, oftentimes first displayed in later years in life. However, in Japan, the phenotype is severe, but the incidence is low [11, 12]. Interestingly, TPM-associated cases are the most prevalent of all contractile proteins in causing HCM in Finland, with a severe pathological phenotype [13, 14]. The variability in incidence and pathology in the different populations is most likely due to allelic variants, modifier genes, founder effects, and environmental influences.

Mutations in the *TPM1α* gene are known to cause both HCM and DCM. There are at least 17 mutations that have been found to cause HCM and 11 mutations that can give rise to DCM (**Table 2**) [15, 16]. The striated muscle α-tropomyosin protein encodes 284 amino acids; this TPM isoform is the predominant TPM found in the adult human heart. The mutations that cause HCM are scattered throughout the

Amino Acid Mutation	Phenotype
Met8Arg	DCM
Lys15Asn	DCM
Arg21His	HCM
Ala22Ser	HCM
Glu23Gln	DCM
Glus40Lys	DCM
Glu54Lys	DCM
Asp58His	HCM
Glu62Gln	HCM
Ala63Val	HCM
Lys70Thr	HCM
Asp84Asn	DCM
Ile92Thr	DCM
Val95Ala	HCM
Ala107Thr	HCM
Ile172Thr	HCM
Asp175Asn	HCM
Glu180Gly	HCM
Glu180Val	HCM
Leu185Arg	HCM
Glu192Lys	HCM
Thr201Met	DCM
Ser215Leu	HCM
Asp230Asn	DCM
Ala239Thr	DCM
Ala277Val	DCM
Met281Thr	HCM
Ile284Val	HCM

Adapted from [15, 16].

Table 2.
TPM1α mutations that cause cardiomyopathy.

gene/protein with a significant number located in the troponin-T binding regions, around amino acids 170–190 (Ile172Thr; Asp175Asn; Glu180Gly; Glu180Val; Leu185Arg; Glu192Lys) and amino acids 270–284 (Met281Thr; Ile184Val). A number of these mutations lead to a change in amino acid charge which may disrupt the dimerization of TPM with itself, or TPM's interactions with actin and/or troponin T [17]. Also, most, if not all, of the HCM mutations occurring in thin filament sarcomeric proteins lead to increased calcium sensitivity of the myofilaments, coupled with decreased systolic and diastolic cardiac function which may be causative for the development of this cardiomyopathy.

To understand the role of TPM in the development of HCM, our laboratory generated animal models of HCM. We produced the first *in vivo* transgenic mouse models expressing TPM with known HCM human mutations (Asp175Asn; Glu180Gln) [18–20]. Since there is a 100% amino acid sequence identity and comparable expression in the heart between mouse and human TPM, the mutations used in these transgenic mice reflect mutations and expression found in HCM patients. In addition, the exogenous cardiac-specific TPM transgene expression leads to a reciprocal decrease in endogenous TPM levels so that the total amount of TPM protein expression is unchanged in the hearts of these transgenic mice. Histological analyses demonstrate that the Asp175Asn transgenic mouse hearts show a moderate hypertrophic response; in contrast, the Glu180Gln mice demonstrate a severe cardiac hypertrophy with significant fibrosis and atrial enlargement (**Figure 1**) [18–20]. Physiologically, mice from both models display significant systolic and diastolic dysfunction, coupled with increased sensitivity to Ca^{2+} in the myofilaments. The pathological and physiological disease state progresses rapidly in the HCM Glu180Gln mice, with the mice dying between 4 and 6 months postpartum.

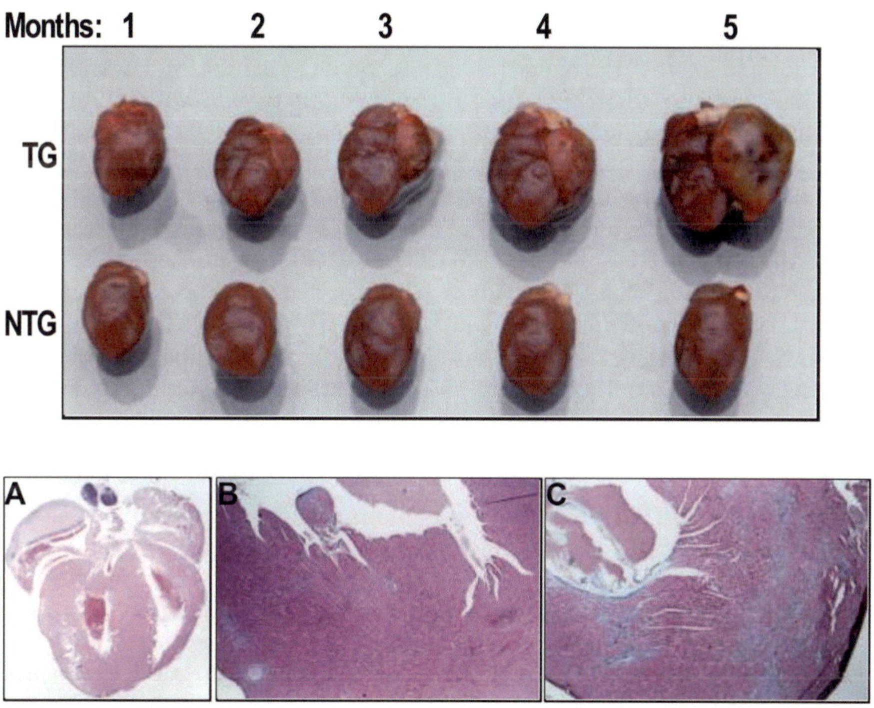

Figure 1.
HCM TPMα180 and NTG control hearts at the designated 1-month time intervals. (A) Cross-section of a three-month-old TPMα180 heart. (B and C) trichrome stain of left ventricular wall from control and TPMα180 hearts. B NTG control. C TPMα180. Note, blue fibrous staining in panel C.

To understand the molecular mechanisms associated with the development of cardiomyopathy, we conducted a detailed comparative microarray analyses of hearts obtained from mild and severe HCM mice [21]. Ventricular tissue was obtained from 2.5-month-old TPMα175 and TPMα180 hearts, along with control (NTG) samples. Results show 754 genes (from a total of 22,600) were differentially expressed between the NTG and HCM hearts; 178 between NTG and TPMα175, and 388 between NTG and TPMα180. There are 266 differentially expressed genes between HCM TPMα175 and TPMα180. The genes that exhibit the largest increase in expression are associated with "secreted/extracellular matrix" category, and the most significant decrease in expression are in the "metabolic enzyme" category. This work illustrates the diverse array of genes that are activated and repressed during the early signaling processes of mild and severe cardiac hypertrophy.

5. Rescue of HCM TPMα180 mice

The development of mouse models that mimic human HCM physiological and pathological conditions afford researchers the opportunity to examine various methods for rescuing these mice from cardiomyopathy. Studies demonstrate cardiac thin filaments with HCM mutations exhibit an increased sensitivity to calcium. As calcium is a prime regulator of muscle contraction, we hypothesized that by normalizing myofilament calcium sensitivity, we could phenotypically rescue the HCM phenotype in our TPMα180 mice. Previously, we generated transgenic mice that exchanged the carboxyl terminal region of TPMα with that of TPMβ (Chi 1) [22]; these mice exhibit a decreased myofilament calcium sensitivity. By mating mice from the HCM TPMα180 with the Chi 1 mice, we tested the hypothesis that attenuation of myofilament calcium sensitivity would modulate the severe physiological and pathological consequences of the HCM mutation. Results show the double-transgenic mice "rescue" the hypertrophic phenotype by exhibiting a normal morphology with no pathological abnormalities, improved cardiac function, and normal myofilament calcium sensitivity [23, 24]. These results demonstrate that alterations in calcium response by modification of contractile proteins can prevent the pathological and physiological effects of this disease.

To extend our studies on rescuing HCM TPMα180 mice by modulation of cytosolic calcium, we crossbred the TPMα180 mice with phospholamban knockout mice (PLNKO) [25]. PLN is a Ca^{2+}-handling protein that regulates calcium uptake into the sarcoplasmic reticulum. Previous studies show that PLNKO mice exhibit hypercontractility with no change in morphology or heart rate, no alterations in myofilament Ca^{2+} sensitivity, and myosin ATPase activity [26]. Results show that PLN ablation in the TPMα180 mice rescues cardiac function and morphological abnormalities for up to one year [25]. There was a reversal of the cardiac hypertrophy, fibrosis, and abnormal physiological function in these rescued mice. This work shows that by modulating sarcoplasmic reticulum calcium cycling, many of the deleterious aspects of HCM caused by a mutation in the thin filament protein TPM can be reversed.

We investigated whether oxidative myofilament modifications can reverse the diastolic dysfunction associated with HCM. The TPMα180 hearts display early signs of oxidative stress in the form of increased oxidative modifications of myosin binding protein C and activation of the MAPK signaling cascade. We hypothesized that treatment with the glutathione precursor N-acetylcysteine (NAC) may reverse the oxidative stress in the TPMα180 mice and improve the cardiomyopathic condition and diastolic dysfunction. To address this, NAC was administered for 30 days to control and TPMα180 mice. After NAC administration, the morphology, diastolic dysfunction, and myofilament Ca^{2+} sensitivity of the TPMα180 mice was similar to controls, indicating that NAC had reversed the abnormal pathology and physiology associated with HCM [27]. These studies indicate that oxidative myofilament modifications are an important mediator in diastolic function which can be of potential use in the treatment of HCM.

TPM is phosphorylated at a single site in the protein, located at the penultimate amino acid, serine 283. To address the significance of TPM phosphorylation, we generated transgenic mice where this serine residue is exchanged for alanine [28, 29]. These transgenic mice (S283A) exhibit a compensated hypertrophic response with significant increases in SERCA2a expression and phosphorylation of PLN. Having obtained these results, we postulated that decreasing TPMα phosphorylation may be beneficial in the context of a chronic, intrinsic stressor, such as HCM. To test this hypothesis, we generated mice expressing both the TPMα180 and S283A mutations and found the HCM phenotype was rescued [29, 30]. The double mutant transgenic mice exhibit no signs of HCM, displayed improved cardiac function, and have normal myofilament Ca^{2+} sensitivity. Changes in Ca^{2+} handling proteins may be responsible for the improved functional performance found in the double transgenic hearts. Also, changes in local flexibility of the TPM molecule conferred by the replacement of the Serine residue with an Ala residue in the S283A mice, and the significant loss of phosphorylation, may be responsible for the restoration of TPM to proper flexibility. Structural alterations in actin-TnT-TPM protein interactions could play a vital role, however, the precise mechanism whereby decreased TPM phosphorylation rescues the HCM phenotype remains to be elucidated.

6. TPM and DCM

DCM, a disease often associated with heart failure, is characterized by depressed systolic function, cardiomegaly, and ventricular dilation. As mentioned previously, DCM is caused by a variety of conditions, including idiopathic, viral and cardiotoxins. Mutations in genes associated with DCM include sarcomeric proteins, the cytoskeleton, and the sarcolemma. Sarcomeric protein genes that harbor DCM mutations include α- and β-myosin heavy chain, myosin binding protein C, actin, TPM, troponin T, I, and C, desmin, vinculin, and muscle LIM protein (**Table 1**).

TPM mutations known to cause DCM are located throughout the *TPM1* gene, from the 5′ to 3′ end of the associated transcript (**Table 2**). Some of the corresponding amino acid changes are positioned in the inner regions of the TPM coiled-coil dimer where electrostatic charge interactions between specific amino acids may alter the TPM dimerization and/or binding to actin [31]. These non-conserved amino acid substitutions are thought to disrupt force transmission through the sarcomere leading to DCM.

To investigate the structural and physiological consequences of known DCM mutations in TPM with cardiac morphology and performance, we generated the first mouse model of a sarcomeric thin filament protein that leads to DCM (TPMαGlu54Lys) [32]. As with the transgenic HCM mice that were generated, the increase in transgenic TPM protein expression led to a reciprocal decrease in endogenous wildtype TPMα levels, with the total myofilament TPM levels remaining unchanged. Also, since there is 100% amino acid identity between human and mouse TPM, the Glu54Lys DCM mutation is the same manifest in human DCM patients. Histological and morphological analyses of these transgenic mice revealed development of DCM with progression to heart failure, and death often ensuing by 6 months (**Figure 2**) [32]. Echocardiographic analyses confirmed the dilated phenotype of the heart with significant decreases in left ventricular fractional

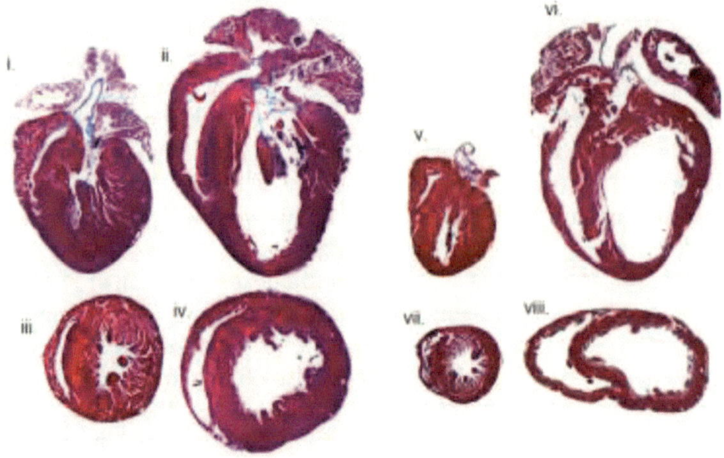

Figure 2.
Histopathology of DCM TPMα54 hearts. Masson trichrome staining of whole-heart longitudinal sections (i and ii) and cross sections (iii and iv) from 5-month-old NTG and moderate-copy TPMα54 mice; longitudinal sections (v and vi) and cross sections (vii and viii) from 1-month-old NTG and high-copy TPMα54 mice. Note the severe dilation of right and left ventricles in both the moderate and high-copy mice. Images in i through viii are all enlarged at the same magnification.

shortening. There was also impaired systolic and diastolic function, coupled with a decreased Ca^{2+} sensitivity and tension generation in cardiac myofilaments. Results indicate the Glu54Lys mutation decreases TPM flexibility, which may influence actin binding and myofilament Ca^{2+} sensitivity. In summary, the pathological and physiological phenotypes exhibited by these mice are consistent with those seen in human DCM and heart failure patients.

Phosphorylation of cardiac sarcomeric and non-sarcomeric proteins play a major role in the regulation of the physiological performance of the heart. Phosphorylation of the thin filament proteins, such as troponin T and I, dramatically affect myofilament Ca^{2+} sensitivity, along with systolic and diastolic function. Less is known about the physiological effect of TPM phosphorylation on cardiac performance. To address this issue, we generated transgenic mice having a phosphorylation mimetic substitution in the phosphorylation site of TPM (Ser283Asp) [33]. Previous work in our laboratory demonstrated that ablating the ability of TPM phosphorylation in transgenic mice (TPMαS283A) leads to a compensated physiological hypertrophy [28]. Our results show that high expression of the TPM Ser283Asp transgene leads to an increased heart:body weight ratio, coupled with a severe dilated cardiomyopathic phenotype resulting in death within 1 month of birth [33]. Moderate TPM Ser283Asp expression mice causes a mild myocyte hypertrophy and fibrosis, without affecting lifespan; physiological analysis revealed diastolic dysfunction, without changes in systolic performance. Surprisingly, there were no alterations in Ca^{2+} sensitivity of the myofibers, cooperativity, or calcium-ATPase activity in the myofibers. This work revealed for the first time that constitutive phosphorylation of TPM could result in a DCM phenotype with its severity dependent upon the extent of the posttranslational phosphorylation modification.

Studies demonstrate that during embryonic and fetal cardiogenesis, the murine heart expresses both TPMα and TPMβ isoforms, with the TPMα isoform being predominant in the adult heart [34–36]. During developmental, the ratio of TPMα:TPMβ changes from 5:1 to 60:1 in the embryonic to adult transition in the murine heart [36]. To address whether the TPMβ isoform could substitute for the TPMα protein, we generated transgenic mice that overexpressed TPMβ in the heart. Results show that with 60% TPMβ expression, there were no morphological changes in the heart [37]. However, there were physiological differences; although there were no systolic alterations, diastole was impaired in both the time and rate of relaxation, coupled with an increase in myofilament Ca^{2+} sensitivity. Additional studies demonstrated that when the TPMβ transgene was expressed at high levels (80% TPMβ, 20% TPMα) in the heart, the mice developed a severe DCM phenotype and die with 14 days postpartum [38]. In these high expression TPMβ hearts, there is significant chamber dilation, thrombus formation in the atria and ventricles, and diastolic dysfunction.

An extension of the research on the high expression TPMβ mice entailed treatment with cyclosporin and FK506, inhibitors of calcineurin. Calcineurin is a calcium-regulated phosphatase, which can initiate cardiac hypertrophy in hearts of transgenic mice that overexpress calcineurin [39]. Results show that treatment with cyclosporin or FK506 in various mouse models of cardiac hypertrophy, including the high expression TPMβ DCM mice, led to phenotypically rescued hearts [40]. This work suggests that in certain cases, inhibitors of calcineurin may play a potential therapeutic role in the treatment of heart disease.

There are 4 distinct tropomyosin genes, each one subject to alternative splicing which generates multiple isoforms of TPM. Our investigation into striated muscle TPM isoform content in the adult human heart found there is 92% TPMα1, 4% TPMβ, and 4% TPMα1κ [41]. TPMα1k is a unique human cardiac-specific TPM isoform which is normally not expressed in rodents [41, 42]. Additional studies show the associated protein is expressed and incorporated into organized myofibrils and that its level is increased in human dilated cardiomyopathy and heart failure patients [41]. To investigate the role of TPMα1κ in sarcomeric function, we generated transgenic mice overexpressing this cardiac-specific isoform. Incorporation of increased levels of TPMα1κ protein in myofilaments leads to DCM, coupled with systolic and diastolic dysfunction and decreased myofilament Ca^{2+} sensitivity [41, 43]. Additional biophysical studies demonstrate less structural stability and weaker actin-binding affinity of TPMα1κ protein compared with TPMα1. This functional analysis of TPMα1κ provides a possible mechanism for the consequences of the TPM isoform switch observed in DCM and heart failure patients.

7. Gene therapy approaches for repair of cardiomyopathies

Calcium plays a pivotal role in the regulation of muscle contraction and relaxation. As seen in the TPM mouse models, the HCM and DCM phenotypes all exhibit abnormalities in myofilament Ca^{2+} sensitivity and Ca^{2+} handling. As mentioned, when mice harboring a phospholamban (PLN) knockout are crossed with the HCM TPMα180 mice, the pathological phenotype is rescued from their offspring [25]. To extend our work, studies were conducted to more fully examine the role of calcium and calcium-handling proteins in the development of HCM. To test whether improvements in the hypertrophic phenotype can be achieved through increased Serca2 expression, the HCM TPMα180 mice were treated with exogenous Serca2a, the protein involved in sequestering calcium from the cytoplasmic space into the sarcoplasmic reticulum [44, 45]. We implemented a gene transfer approach using an adenoviral vector to express Serca2a in HCM TPMα180 hearts. Results showed that injection of a single dose improved heart morphology and cardiac function. As the mice aged, there was a significant decrease in heart:body weight ratio, and a decrease in fibrosis when compared with controls. Additional work demonstrated that parvalbumin, a calcium buffer, may also play a role in ameliorating HCM; when parvalbumin transgenic mice were crossed with HCM TPM1α180 mice, there was improvement in cardiovascular performance [45, 46].

With improvements in cardiac morphology and performance in the HCM and DCM mouse models that occur with modification in calcium handling proteins, therapeutic gene therapy trials in patients utilizing Serca2a expression as a potential treatment for cardiac disease were initiated. Using adeno-associated viruses to drive extended Serca2a expression, Phase 2 studies were conducted in patients with advanced heart failure [47, 48]. Results show there was a striking reduction in cardiovascular events that persisted through the 36 months of follow-up compared to patients who received the placebo. Additional work in this area is in progress.

Recently, investigators have examined the potential of the C-terminal end peptide of troponin I as a novel reagent to selectively facilitate cardiac muscle relaxation [49]. This is a highly conserved protein fragment across numerous vertebrate species. Protein binding studies found that this terminal fragment retains its binding affinity for TPM similar to intact cardiac troponin I. Addition of this fragment to skinned cardiac muscle preparations reduces myofibril Ca^{2+} sensitivity without decreasing maximum force production. Using this short peptide, studies were initiated to address whether it would be of therapeutic value in the treatment of HCM [50]. Recent work demonstrates that myofilament Ca^{2+} sensitivity isolated from TPMα180 hearts exhibit a more normalized decrease in myofilament Ca^{2+} sensitivity when treated with the C-terminal troponin I fragment. This demonstrates the C-terminal peptide of troponin I as a potential therapeutic reagent for the treatment of diastolic dysfunction in the heart.

There is no scientific doubt that CRISPR-Cas9-base targeting has revolutionized how research is being conducted. With the ability to modify genomes, there is the potential to conduct precise gene-editing in animal models along with correcting human disease mutations. With respect to cardiomyopathic diseases, Ma et al. corrected a human heterozygous germline HCM mutation in the myosin binding protein C gene using the CRISPR-Cas9 system [51]. This targeting strategy was employed on preimplantation human embryos; following targeting, the embryos were genetically analyzed for correctly targeted nucleotide changes and then allowed to develop to the 8-cell stage. Results show that over 50% of blastomeres were correctly targeted, but used the wildtype allele as the correcting genetic template. This work demonstrates that CRISPR has the potential for usage as a corrective therapeutic system of heritable mutations; however, additional research needs to be conducted and ethical considerations need to be addressed.

8. Lessons learned from TPM

Many lessons have been learned about HCM and DCM in the examination and usage of TPM and associated mouse model systems [52, 53]. Multiple mutations within the TPM1α gene lead to HCM and DCM. Surprisingly, for both disease conditions, the mutations are scattered throughout the gene, and are not confined to one or two specific regions or domains. The severity of the disease phenotype appears dependent upon the specific mutation, modifying genes, and environmental factors. The genetic animal models of HCM and DCM TPM mutations accurately reflect the disease process with respect to structural and functional abnormalities as they occur in humans. For HCM, the thickening of the left ventricular wall and interventricular septum with significant fibrosis is pronounced in these animal models. For DCM, the thinning of the ventricular walls and dilation of the ventricular cavities reflect the pathological features observed in patients. For both HCM and DCM, the functional abnormalities in systole and diastole are similar to those experienced by patients. More importantly, these basic research studies have been translated into potential therapeutic modalities, especially for investigations into the usage and modification of calcium-handling proteins as treatments of cardiovascular disease. Expansion of potential treatments utilizing phosphatases and kinases, along with sarcomeric protein peptides, may also prove beneficial for the treatment of specific cardiovascular conditions. An area of future expansion will be to focus on the identification and modification of protein expression for genes which are signaling agents for the development of cardiac HCM, DCM, and heart failure.

Acknowledgements

The author would like to gratefully recognize and thank the numerous members of the laboratory for their invaluable contributions to this research. The author also thanks the funding of this research provided by the NIH NHLBI, American Heart Association, and the University of Cincinnati College of Medicine.

Conflict of interest

There are no conflicts of interest to report.

Author details

David F. Wieczorek
Department of Molecular Genetics, Microbiology, and Biochemistry, University of Cincinnati College of Medicine, Cincinnati, Ohio, USA

*Address all correspondence to: david.wieczorek@uc.edu

References

[1] Braunwald E. Cardiomyopathies: an overview. Circ Res 2017; **121**:711-721

[2] Brieler J, Breeden M, Tucker J. Cardiomyopathy: an overview. Am Fam Physician 2017; **96**:641-646

[3] Marian A, Braunwald E. Hypertrophic cardiomyopathy: genetics, pathogenesis, clinical manifestations, diagnosis, and therapy. Circ Res 2017; **121**:749-770

[4] Marsiglia J, Pereira A. Hypertrophic Cardiomyopathy: how do mutations lead to disease? Arq Bras Cardiol. 2014; **102**:295-304

[5] Geistefer-Lowrance A, Kass F, Tanigawa G, Vosberg H, McKenna W, et al. A molecular basis for familial hypertrophic cardiomyopathy: a beta cardiac myosin heavy chain gene missense mutation. Cell 1990; **62**:999-1006

[6] Hershberger R, Hedges d, Morales A. Dilated cardiomyopathy: the complexity of a diverse genetic architecture. Nat. Rev. Cardiol 2013; **10**:531-547

[7] McNally E, Golbus J, Puckelwartz M. Genetics mutations and mechanisms in dilated cardiomyopathy. J Clin Invest. 2013; **123**:19-26

[8] McNally E, Mestroni L. Dilated cardiomyopathy: genetics determinants and mechanisms. Circ Res 2017; **121**:731-748

[9] van der Zwaag P, van Rijsingen I, Asimaki A, Jongbloed J, van Veldhuisen D, et al. Phospholamban r14del mutation in patients diagnosed with dilated cardiomyopathy or arrhythmogenic right ventricular cardiomyopathy: Evidence supporting the concept of arrhythmogenic cardiomyopathy. Eur J Heart Fail. 2012; **14**:1199-1207

[10] Thierfelder L, Watkins H, MacRae C, Lamas R, McKenna W, Vosberg H, et al. α-Tropomyosin and cardiac troponin T mutations cause familial hypertrophic cardiomyopathy: a disease of the sarcomere. Cell 1994; 77:701-712

[11] Nakajima-Taniguchi C, Matsui H, Nagata S, Kishimoto T, Yamauchi-Takihara Y. Novel missense mutation in α-tropomyosin gene found in Japanese patients with hypertrophic cardiomyopathy. J Mol Cell Cardiol 1995; **27**:2053-2058

[12] Yamauchi-Takihara K, Nakajima C, Matsue H, Fujio Y, Kunisada K, et al. Clinical implications of hypertrophic cardiomyopathy associated with mutations in the α-tropomyosin gene. Heart 1996; **76**:63-65.

[13] Jaaskelainen P, Soranta M, Miettinen R, Saarinen L, Philajamaki J, et al. The cardiac beta-myosin heavy chain gene is not the predominant gene for hypertrophic cardiomyopathy in the Finnish population. J Am Coll Cardiol 1998; **21**:1709-1716

[14] Jaaskelainen P, Helio T, Aalto-Setala K, Kaartinen M, Iliveskoski E, Hamalainen L, et al. Two founder mutations in the alpha-tropomyosin and the cardiac myosin-binding protein C genes are common causes of hypertrophic cardiomyopathy in the Finnish population. Annals of Medicine 2013; **45**:85-90

[15] Redwood C, Robinson P. Alpha-tropomyosin mutations in inherited cardiomyopathies. J Muscle Res Cell Motil 2013; **34**:285-294

[16] Wieczorek DF. Tropomyosin: an effector of cardiac remodeling. In: Sherman J, editor. Cardiac Remodeling. New York, USA: Nova Science Publishers, Inc; 2016. pp. 65-88

[17] Kremneva E, Boussouf S, Nikolaeva I, Maytum R, Geeves M, Levitsky V. Effects of two familial hypertrophic cardiomyopathy mutations in alpha-tropomyosin, Asp175Asn and Glu180Gly, on the thermal unfolding of actin-bound tropomyosin. BiophyJ 2004; **87**:3922-3933

[18] Muthuchamy M, Pieples K, Rethinasamy P, Hoit B, Grupp I, et al. Mouse model of a familial hypertrophic cardiomyopathy mutation in α-tropomyosin manifests cardiac dysfunction. Circ Res 1999; **85**:47-56.

[19] Prabhakar R, Boivin G, Grupp I, Hoit B, Arteaga G, Solaro RJ, Wieczorek DF. A familial hypertrophic cardiomyopathy α-tropomyosin mutation causes severe cardiac hypertrophy and death in mice. J. Mol. Cell. Card. 2001; **33**:1815-1828

[20] Prabhakar R, Petrashevskaya N, Schwartz A, Aronow B, Boivin G, et al. A mouse model of familial hypertrophic cardiomyopathy caused by a α-tropomyosin mutation. Mol Cell Biochem 2013; **251**:33-42

[21] Rajan S, Williams S, Jagatheesan G, Ahmed R, Fuller-Bicer F, et al. Microarray analysis of gene expression during early stages of mild and severe cardiac hypertrophy. Physiol Genomics 2006; **27**:309-317

[22] Jagatheesan G, Rajan S, Petrashevskaya N, Schwartz A, Boivin G, et al. Functional importance of the carboxyl-terminal region of striate muscle tropomyosin. J Biol Chem 2003; **278**:23204-23211

[23] Jagatheesan G, Rajan S, Petrashevskaya N, Schwartz A, Boivin G, et al. Rescue of tropomyosin-induced familial hypertrophic cardiomyopathy mice by transgenesis. Am J Physiol Heart Circ Physiol 2007; **293**:H949-H958

[24] Jagatheesan G, Rajan S, Wieczorek DF. Investigations into tropomyosin function using mouse models. J Mol Cell Cardiol. 2010; **48**:893-898

[25] Gaffin R, Pena J, Alves M, Dias F, Chowdhury S, et al. Long-term rescue of a familial hypertrophic cardiomyopathy caused by a mutation in the thin filament protein, tropomyosin, via modulation of a calcium cycling protein. J. Mol. Cell Cardiol. 2011; **51**:812-820

[26] Schwinger R, Brixius K, Savvidou-Zaroti P, Bolck B, Zobel C, et al. The enhanced contractility in phospholamban deficient mouse hearts is not associated with alterations in (Ca2+)-sensitivity or myosin ATPase-activity of the contractile proteins. Basic Res Cardiol 2000; **95**:12-18

[27] Wilder T, Ryba D, Wieczorek DF, Wolska B, Solaro RJ. *N*-acetylcysteine reverses diastolic dysfunction and hypertrophy in familial hypertrophic cardiomyopathy. Am J Physiol Heart Circ Physiol 2015; **309**:H1720-H1730

[28] Schulz E, Correll R, Sheikh H, Lofrano-Alves M, Engel P, et al. Tropomyosin dephosphorylation results in compensated cardiac hypertrophy. J. Biol. Chem. 2012; **287**:44478-44489

[29] Schulz E, Wieczorek DF. Tropomyosin de-phosphorylation in the heart: what are the consequences? J. Muscle Res. Cell Motil. 2013; **34**:239-246

[30] Schulz E, Wilder T, Chowdhury S, Sheikh H, Wolska B, et al. Decreasing tropomyosin phosphorylation rescues tropomyosin-induced familial hypertrophic cardiomyopathy. J. Biol. Chem. 2013; **288**:28925-28935

[31] Olson T, Kishimoto N, Whitby F, Michels V. Mutations that alter the surface charge of alpha-tropomyosin are

associated with dilated cardiomyopathy. J. Mol Cell Cardiol 2001; **33**:723-732

[32] Rajan S, Ahmed R, Ganapathy J, Petrashevskaya N, Boivin G, et al. Dilated cardiomyopathy mutant tropomyosin mice develop cardiac dysfunction with significantly decreased fractional shortening and myofilament calcium sensitivity. Circ Res 2007; **101**:205-214

[33] Rajan S, Jagatheesan G, Petrashevskaya N, Biesiadecki B, Warren C, et al. Tropomyosin pseudo-phosphorylation results in dilated cardiomyopathy. J Biol Chem. 2019; **294**:2913-2923

[34] Cummins P, Perry S. Chemical and immunochemical characteristics of tropomyosins from striated and smooth muscle. Biochem J. 1974; **141**:43-49

[35] Izumo S, Nadal-Ginard B, Mahdavi V. Protooncogene induction and reprogramming of cardiac gene expression produced by pressure overload. Proc Natl Acad Sci USA. 1988; **85**:339-343

[36] Muthuchamy M, Pajak L, Howles P, Doetschman, T, and Wieczorek, DF. Developmental analysis of tropomyosin gene expression in embryonic stem cells and mouse embryos. Mol. Cell. Biol. 1993; **13**:3311-3323

[37] Muthuchamy M, Grupp I, Grupp G, O'Toole B, Kier A, et al. Molecular and physiological effects of overexpressing striated muscle β-tropomyosin in the adult murine heart. J. Biol. Chem. 1995; **270**:30593-30603

[38] Muthuchamy M, Boivin G, Grupp I, Wieczorek DF. β-tropomyosin overexpression induces severe cardiac abnormalities. J Mol Cell Cardiol 1998; **30**:1545-1557

[39] Molkentin J, Lu J, Antos C, Markham B, Richardson J et al. A calcineurin-dependent transcriptional pathway for cardiac hypertrophy. Cell 1998; **93**:215-228

[40] Sussmann M, Lim H, Gude N, Taigen T, Olson E, et al. Prevention of cardiac hypertrophy in mice by calcineurin inhibition. Science 1998; **281**:1690-1693

[41] Rajan S, Jagatheesan G, Karam C, Alves M, Bodi I, et al. Molecular and functional characterization of a novel cardiac specific human tropomyosin isoform. Circulation. 2010; **121**:410-418

[42] Denz C, Narshi A, Zajdel R, Dube D. Expression of a novel cardiac-specific tropomyosin isoform in humans. Biochem. Biophys. Res. Commun. 2004; **320**:1291-1297

[43] Karam C, Warren C, Rajan S, de Tombe P, Wieczorek DF, Solaro RJ. Expression of tropomyosin-κ induces dilated cardiomyopathy and depresses cardiac myofilament tension by mechaniss involving cross-bridge dependent activation and altered tropomyosin phosphorylation. J Muscle Res Cell Motil 2011; **31**:315-322

[44] Pena J, Szkudlarek A, Warren C, Heinrich L, Gaffin R, et al. Neonatal gene transfer of Serca2a delays onset of hypertrophic remodeling and improves function in familial hypertrophic cardiomyopathy. J Mol Cell Cardiol 2010; **49**:993-1002

[45] Wieczorek DF, Wolska B. Rescue of familial hypertrophic cardiomyopathy by altering sarcomeric exposure and response to calcium. In: Kang C, editor. Gene Therapy Applications. Rijeka, Croatia: Intech. 2011. pp85-94.

[46] Coutu P, Bennett C, Favre E, Day S, Metzger J. Parvalbumin corrects slowed relaxation in adult cardiac myocytes expressing hypertrophic cardiomyopathy-linked a-tropomyosin mutations. Circ Res 2004; **94**:1235-1241

[47] Greenberg B. Gene therapy for heart failure. J. Cardiol 2015; **66**:195-200

[48] Gwathmey J, Yerevanian A, Hajjar R. Cardiac gene therapy with SERCA2a: from bench to bedside. J Mol Cell Cardiol 2011; **50**:803-812

[49] Wong S, Feng H-Z, Jin J-P. The evolutionary conserved C-terminal peptide of troponin I is an independently configured regulatory structure to function as a myofilament Ca^{2+}-desensitizer. J Mol Cell Cardiol 2019; **136**:42-52

[50] Hornos F, Feng H, Rizzuti B, Palomino-Schatzlein M, Wieczorek DF, et al. Isolated C-terminal peptide of troponin I populates a nascent helix forming a basis for binding tropomyosin as a therapeutic myofilament Ca^{2+}-desensitizer. J. Biol Chem. In revision.

[51] Ma H, Marti-Gutierrez N, Park S-W, Wu J, Lee Y, et al. Correction of a pathogenic gene mutation in human embryos. Nature 2017; **548**:413-419

[52] Wieczorek DF, Jagatheesan G, Rajan S. The role of tropomyosin in heart disease. In: Gunning P, editor. Tropomyosin. Landes Bioscience. 2008. pp132-142.

[53] Wieczorek DF. The role of tropomyosin in cardiac function and disease. In Karcioglu O, editor. Cardiac Diseases and Interventions in 21st Century. IntechOpen. 2019. pp9-22

Section 5

Dilated Cardiomyopathy

Chapter 14

Clinical Management of DMD-Associated Cardiomyopathy

Theo Lee-Gannon, Hannah Lehrenbaum, Rahul Sheth and Pradeep P.A. Mammen

Abstract

Over the past decade, cardiomyopathy has become the leading cause of mortality among patients with Duchenne muscular dystrophy (DMD). The majority of DMD patients over the age of 18 experience some degree of cardiac involvement. The primary cardiac manifestations of DMD include progressive left ventricular (LV) wall stress leading to LV dilatation and wall thinning, and the development of cardiac fibrosis, all of which culminate in decreased LV contractility and reduced cardiac output. Mortality in these patients is predominantly related to pump failure and fatal arrhythmias leading to sudden cardiac death. While basic guidelines for the management of cardiomyopathy in DMD patients exist, these recommendations are by no means comprehensive, and this chapter aims to provide further insight into appropriate clinical diagnosis and management of DMD-associated cardiomyopathy. Notably, earlier and more frequent cardiac assessment and care can allow for better outcomes for these patients. Pharmacological treatments typically include an angiotensin-converting enzyme inhibitor or angiotensin II receptor blocker, beta-adrenergic receptor blockers, mineralocorticoid receptor antagonists, and corticosteroids. Non-pharmacological therapies include automated implantable cardioverter defibrillators and left ventricular assist devices, as well as in rare cases cardiac transplantation. Additionally, many emerging therapies show great promise for improving standards of care. These novel therapies, based primarily on applied gene therapy and genome editing, have great potential to significantly alter the DMD care landscape in the near future.

Keywords: DMD-associated cardiomyopathy, Duchenne muscular dystrophy, dystrophinopathy, heart failure

1. Introduction

Duchenne muscular dystrophy (DMD) is a progressive neuromuscular disorder diagnosed during childhood and characterized by skeletal muscle wasting, diaphragmatic weakness and scoliosis resulting in chronic restrictive lung disease, and progressive cardiomyopathy. As an X-linked recessive disorder, DMD disproportionately impacts males compared to females and affects approximately 1 in every 3500 to 5000 live male births [1–3]. The disease is caused by mutations in the dystrophin gene located on the Xp21 chromosome, resulting in a lack of a functional dystrophin protein [4, 5]. While other dystrophinopathies result in a truncated but partially functional dystrophin protein, the total absence of functional dystrophin protein in DMD patients leads to a myriad of devastating clinical outcomes.

Over the past several decades, significant progress has been made in treating and managing many of the complications in DMD. Although respiratory failure was historically the leading cause of morbidity and mortality in this population, advancements in nocturnal ventilatory support and spinal stabilization therapy have dramatically improved clinical outcomes and increased the average life expectancy of DMD patients [6]. As a result, more patients are living into adulthood where cardiomyopathy begins to manifest and now accounts for the majority of deaths [1, 4, 6, 7]. Although there is ongoing research in gene therapy and genome editing techniques to improve skeletal muscle function in DMD patients, cardiomyopathy among DMD patients remains a problem of paramount clinical significance, with the current focus on reducing cardiac involvement and mitigating the effects of the cardiomyopathy. This chapter will highlight the genetic and molecular pathology underlying DMD and provide insight into the clinical manifestations, diagnosis, treatments, and therapies for DMD-associated cardiomyopathy.

2. Genetics and the molecular basis underlying cardiac dysfunction in Duchenne muscular dystrophy

The dystrophin gene is the largest protein-coding gene in the human genome at 2.5 Mb, located on chromosome Xp21.1 [1, 5, 8]. With 79 exons and a 14-kb encoding transcript, the gene has four promoters which produce different isoforms of the dystrophin protein in various organs, but primarily in skeletal muscle, cardiac muscle, and the brain (**Figure 1A**) [8]. Frame shift mutations resulting in deletions of one or more exons of the gene are the most common cause of DMD, accounting for at least 65-75% of DMD cases [9, 10]. Duplications, deep intronic changes, nonsense mutations, and missense mutations can also disrupt dystrophin expression and lead to DMD [9], though these mutations occur less commonly. The phenotypic manifestations of DMD occur when these mutations result in a complete lack of functional dystrophin protein. While most instances of DMD are inherited, around 30% of cases are caused by spontaneous mutations in the gene [1, 11].

The dystrophin protein plays an integral role in maintaining myocyte membrane stability, connecting the dystrophin-associated glycoprotein complex (DGC) to the intracellular contractile apparatus and extracellular matrix of the cell (**Figure 1B**) [1, 4, 12, 13]. An absence of dystrophin protein destabilizes this complex and promotes sarcolemmal fragility. In the skeletal muscle of DMD patients, this leads to the loss of the majority of the DGC. In contrast, cardiac muscle retains the remainder of the DGC despite the absence of dystrophin. Despite these pathophysiological differences, both skeletal and cardiac muscle are drastically impacted by the absence of dystrophin protein. Specifically, in cardiac muscle the absence of dystrophin impacts the ability of myocytes to function properly and leads to many secondary pathophysiological mechanisms of cell degradation [1, 4, 14].

One such mechanism contributing to myocyte degradation involves the disruption of ion gradients. As the myocyte membrane weakens due to the absence of dystrophin, calcium passively leaks through the membrane; the activation of sarcolemmal stretch-activated channels during myocyte contraction causes intracellular calcium levels to further increase [4, 15]. Additionally, transient receptor potential (TRP) channels and L-type calcium channels (LTCC) have been shown to contribute to increased intracellular calcium in DMD murine studies [16–18]. Increased intracellular calcium ultimately results in myocyte degradation through two distinct pathways. First, electrical and contractile activities of myocytes are interrupted by

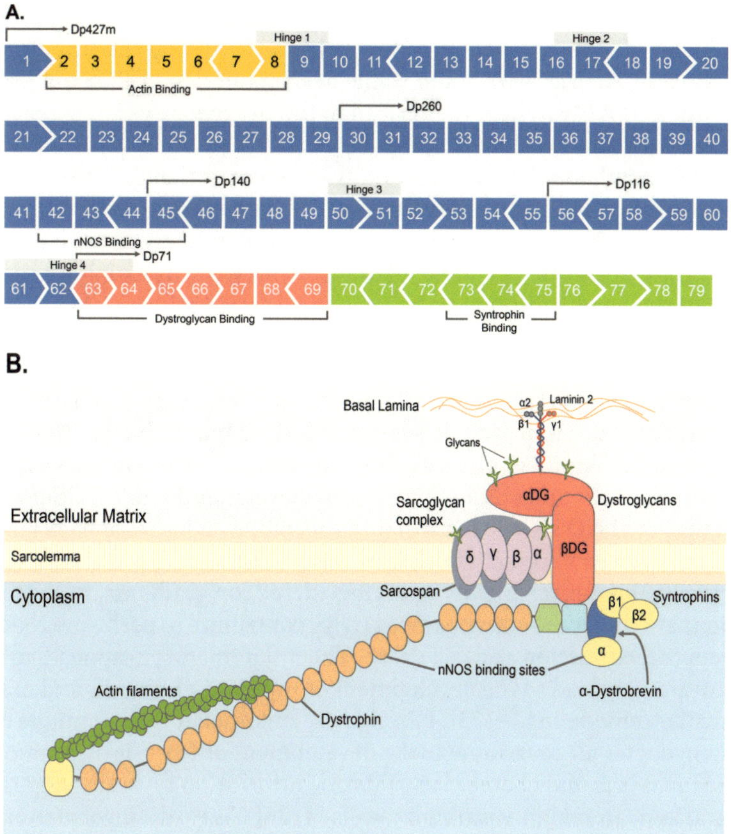

Figure 1.
Dystrophin structure and cellular location within a myocyte. (A) the dystrophin gene map composed of 79 exons and the essential regions highlighted in various colors. (B) Schematic of the dystrophin-associated glycoprotein complex (DGC). Adapted from Zhang et al. Physiolo. Rev 2018 98:1205-1240.

the inappropriate influx of calcium, promoting proteolytic activity via proteolytic enzymes and calpains, which eventually leads to cell death [15–17]. A secondary degradation pathway is triggered when excess cytosolic calcium begins to accumulate inside mitochondria, resulting in mitochondrial swelling and dysfunction that triggers separate apoptotic pathways [17]. Cardiac physiological studies on DMD^{mdx} mice have demonstrated elevated levels of mitochondrial calcium and mitochondrial swelling, leading to a disruption in mitochondrial ATP production in DMD^{mdx} hearts long before any fibrotic changes or reductions in left ventricular (LV) systolic function are detectable [4, 15–17].

In addition to calcium gradient disruption, increased generation of reactive oxygen species (ROS) and nitric oxide dysregulation also contribute to the development of DMD-associated cardiomyopathy. NADPH oxidase 2 (NOX2) is a membrane-bound isoform of the NOX enzyme, and it is the suspected source of increased ROS production in DMD patients. Elevated expression of NOX2 has been demonstrated in studies of both skeletal muscle and cardiomyocytes of DMD^{mdx} mice [19]. It has additionally been speculated that ROS produced by NOX2 may contribute to calcium leakage from the sarcoplasmic reticulum leading to mitochondrial dysfunction [4, 19, 20]. Activation of NOX2 leads to the production of an extracellular superoxide, which is then converted to hydrogen peroxide (H_2O_2). H_2O_2 is able to permeate through the myocyte membrane and results in the oxidation of various intracellular macromolecules, eventually leading to secondary pathways contributing to cell death [4, 21]. Finally, angiotensin II receptor type I (AT1R) is believed to be involved in redox pathways involving the stimulation of NADPH oxidases, such as NOX2, and so the overproduction of ROS can lead to the overstimulation of AT1R. These events lead to further oxidative stress resulting in increased cardiomyocyte cell death [21].

Nitric oxide synthases (NOS) are a family of enzymes that catalyze the production of nitric oxide. There are three isoforms of NOS: neuronal NOS, endothelial NOS, and inducible NOS. In skeletal muscle, dystrophin interacts with neuronal NOS to control vasculature [22]. The relationship between dystrophin and NOS is less clear in the myocardium, especially since all three isoforms of NOS are expressed within cardiomyocytes and the molecular mechanisms and interactions have not been well elucidated to date [4]. It is speculated that NOS may play a similar role in cardiomyocytes as in skeletal muscle, and that in affected DMD patients nitric oxide diffusion is impaired. Researchers believe that inducible NOS may play a key role in the development of cardiac dysfunction in DMD, since its expression is high in immune cells and studies have found elevated inducible NOS levels and decreased neuronal NOS levels in cardiac tissue, while endothelial NOS levels and activity were reported to remain fairly constant [4, 22].

Collectively, these mechanisms involving altered ion gradients, mitochondrial dysfunction, and impaired nitric oxide activity contribute to pathways that promote cardiomyocyte dysfunction and cell death. The inflammatory responses to these processes ultimately lead to the development of myocardial fibrosis and maladaptive ventricular remodeling [9, 23]. Fibroblasts, endothelial cells, immune cells, and cardiomyocytes all contribute to the development of fibrosis by promoting profibrotic cytokines and chemokines. Fibrotic infiltration typically begins in the posterobasal and lateral left ventricular walls [4, 23]. As cardiomyocytes undergo apoptosis, they are replaced by the extracellular matrix (ECM). Subsequently, matrix metalloproteinases promote the degradation of ECM proteins, including collagen [24]. The increase in cytokines, chemokines, and degraded ECM debris stimulates an immune response, attracting neutrophils and macrophages which eventually leads to myocardial scarring and fibrotic patches [4, 24]. In the heart, LV volume and wall stress progressively increase as fibrotic tissue causes thinning and stretching of the ventricular walls, decreasing contractility and cardiac output. These processes eventually lead to either clinically decompensated heart failure, pump failure, and/or sudden cardiac death due to ventricular arrhythmias [4, 9, 23].

3. Clinical manifestations and diagnosis

Initially, DMD presents very early in childhood and therefore it is paramount to diagnose and initiate treatment as early as possible. Symptoms of DMD can arise in patients as young as three years of age and typically involve progressive muscle weakness, often manifesting as difficulty with ambulation, gait instability, difficulty climbing stairs, and enlarged calf muscles (or calf pseudohypertrophy). Additional presenting symptoms include scoliosis with or without back pain, fatigue, dyspnea secondary to diaphragmatic muscle weakness and/or cardiomyopathy, and arrhythmias [4, 25, 26]. The Gower's sign, the act of a child using their hands to help prop themselves up into a standing position, is also a very common indicator of DMD [9, 25, 26]. These signs and symptoms suggest the possibility of underlying DMD and necessitate further diagnostic testing.

Key initial diagnostic tests include measurements of serum creatine kinase (CK) and liver transaminases (such as alanine aminotransferase, aspartate aminotransferase) [27]. When levels of these biomarkers are elevated, DMD should be suspected, and confirmatory genetic testing should be pursued. Genetic analysis via multiplex ligation-dependent probe amplification (MLPA) and genetic sequencing can help verify the presence and type of neuromuscular disorder [9, 27]. This is a critical step in diagnosis and is essential in informing which genetic therapies might be viable therapeutic options. On occasion, genetic testing yields no mutations in the DMD gene, or false negatives. In these instances of strong clinical suspicion of DMD with negative genetic test results, a muscle biopsy should be performed to assess for the absence of the dystrophin protein by immunohistochemistry [9]. Diagnosis of DMD occurs once genetic analysis and/or the biopsy confirms the absence of DMD.

However, diagnosing cardiac involvement in DMD is somewhat more challenging. Many of these patients are wheelchair-dependent and non-ambulatory well before adulthood, and as a result, patients are often asymptomatic until they have developed advanced disease [9, 28]. Studies report that approximately 25% of DMD patients develop cardiomyopathy by 6 years of age, and that percentage grows to almost 60% by age 10 [9, 29, 30]. Progression of cardiomyopathy often accelerates as patients age and nearly all DMD patients are expected to have clinical cardiac involvement by age 18 [7, 30]. Recognition and treatment of cardiomyopathy early in the disease course correlate with improved outcomes and more favorable ventricular remodeling, rendering it crucial to identify cardiac involvement as early as possible [1, 9, 23]. For this reason, guidelines strongly suggest including a cardiologist as a member of the care team from disease onset [4, 25, 31]. The 2018 DMD Care Considerations, presented by the Center for Disease Control and Prevention, recommends that cardiac care and assessment are essential at the time of diagnosis [25, 31]. While previous guidelines have recommended consulting with cardiologists every two years, it is now strongly recommended that DMD patients receive cardiac assessment and screening at least every year starting from diagnosis [25, 31].

Development of myocardial fibrosis along with ventricular dilation reflects myocyte destruction and progression in the underlying cardiomyopathy. Fatigue, nausea, dyspnea, palpitations, tachycardia, and chest discomfort may all represent symptomatic manifestations of DMD-associated cardiomyopathy, though many patients remain asymptomatic until later stages in life [31]. Therefore, the use of standard cardiac tools as well as high fidelity cardiac imaging are essential to accurately diagnose cardiac involvement in patients with subclinical disease [1, 25].

Electrocardiograms (ECG) should be among the first tests performed, and results are often abnormal in DMD patients, correlating with morphological changes in cardiac muscle [23]. Screening ECG usually reveals tall R waves and deep Q wave irregularities in the anterolateral leads, which typically suggest lateral wall scarring (**Figure 2A–C**) [29, 32].

The ECG may be suggestive of cardiac involvement; however, cardiac imaging is essential to diagnose and monitor progression of cardiac involvement in DMD patients. While echocardiography has been a mainstay in diagnostic cardiac imaging for years, studies in patients with DMD have demonstrated that echocardiograms often underestimate both LV cavity volume and function and are much less sensitive compared to cardiac magnetic resonance imaging (cMRI) in detecting wall motion abnormalities and overall cardiac function [9, 25, 32]. cMRI has been shown to be more accurate in assessing cardiac abnormalities in the setting of altered body habitus in DMD patients due to scoliosis, and it is considered the gold standard for cardiac imaging in DMD patients [25, 32]. The presence of late gadolinium enhancement (LGE) on cMRI indicates various degrees of myocardial inflammation, fibrotic scarring, and myocyte damage [25, 32]. In addition, LGE is often present before there is any clinically detectable deterioration in cardiac function or

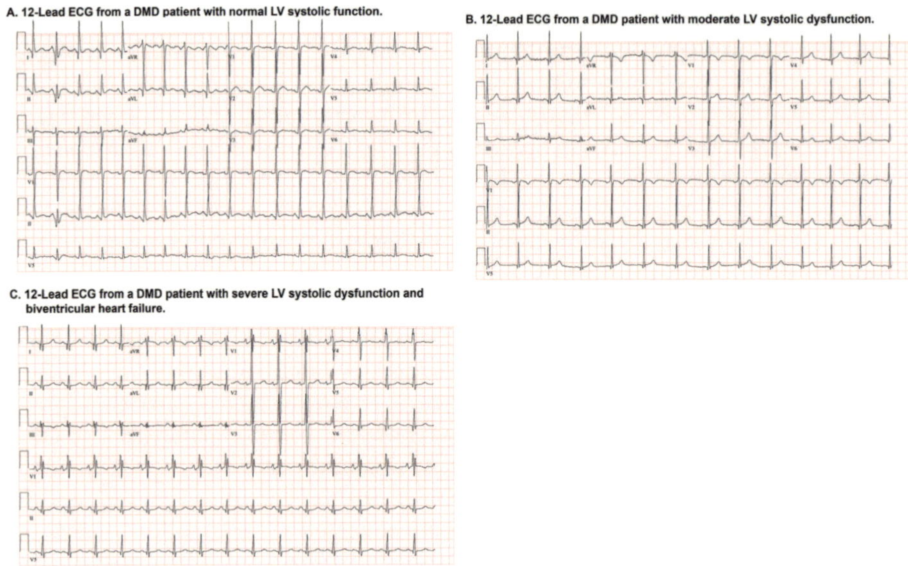

Figure 2.
ECG changes at various stages of DMD-associated cardiomyopathy. (A) DMD patient with normal cardiac function. (B) DMD patient with moderate LV systolic dysfunction. (C) DMD patient with severe LV systolic dysfunction and biventricular heart failure.

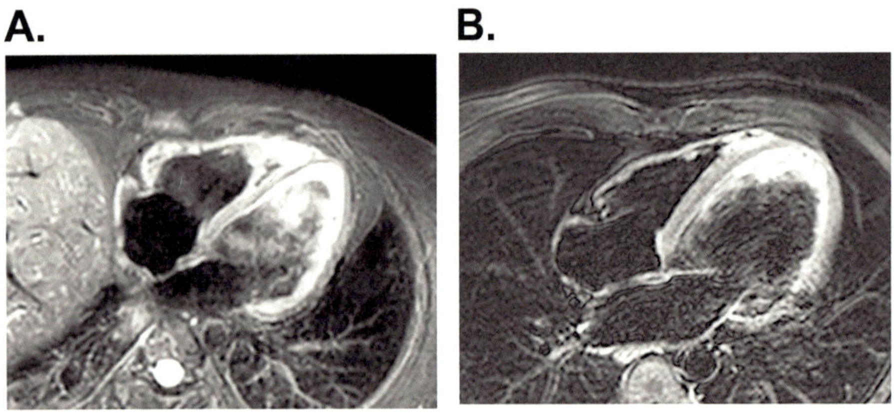

Figure 3.
Structural differences in DMD-associated cardiomyopathy. Representative 4-chamber cMRI images in (A) a DMD patient and (B) a healthy age-matched control patient.

symptoms of cardiomyopathy [25, 32]. When LGE is present, its distribution and change over time can be particularly effective in tracking cardiomyopathy progression [25, 32]. Finally, cMRI provides the most sensitive assessment of cardiac size, mass, and function, which can similarly be serially monitored to assess for progression of cardiac damage and response to medical therapy. Current DMD guidelines recommend a baseline cMRI to be performed between 8 and 10 years of age and repeated approximately every 2 years thereafter [25, 31]. **Figure 3** depicts representative cMRI images in a DMD patient and an age-matched healthy control patient.

In cMRI, the technique of strain imaging has also been shown to be highly sensitive in gauging LV ejection fraction (LVEF) and cardiac dysfunction, especially when circumferential strain imaging is used [33]. Deviations in strain imaging can be indicative of cardiac dysfunction, and these abnormalities are common in DMD patients, even when LVEF measures are normal. Use of cMRI strain imaging, along with the presence of LGE, can provide valuable diagnostic and prognostic information about a patient's cardiac condition beyond simple measurements of contractile function [9, 33].

While cMRI has become the preferred imaging modality in DMD patients, there are still barriers to widespread adoption and utilization of cMRI. High procedural cost limits accessibility of cMRI, and the procedure can be challenging for younger patients and patients with claustrophobia [1, 25]. Furthermore, muscular weakness, spinal abnormalities, and restrictive lung disease can often make it difficult to fully assess cardiac structure and function using any of the available imaging techniques, but especially echocardiogram (ECHO) [9, 25, 32]. Therefore, if a cMRI can not be obtained the next ideal cardiac imaging tool that can be used is a cardiac CT scan with IV contrast, followed by 3D-ECHO with contrast.

The need for comprehensive cardiovascular assessment in DMD patients is undisputed, but there is also a significant risk for cardiovascular disease in DMD carriers [9, 25]. Mothers and sisters of patients who have been diagnosed with DMD should undergo both genetic testing to determine carrier status and evaluation by a cardiologist, preferably a heart failure specialist, to determine presence of heart disease. Recent studies have shown an increased risk of cardiac involvement in approximately 50% of DMD carriers, despite the presence of a functional *DMD* gene [9, 23, 34, 35]. For this reason, mothers and sisters of patients who have been diagnosed with DMD should undergo both genetic testing to determine carrier status and evaluation by a cardiologist, preferably a heart failure specialist, to determine presence of heart disease.

4. Pathophysiology underlying DMD-associated cardiomyopathy

Prior studies of DMD patients have demonstrated early cardiac involvement, with cardiac manifestations present in approximately 25% of DMD patients by 6 years of age and nearly universal cardiac involvement by 18 years of age [29, 30, 36]. These DMD patients go on to develop progressive cardiomyopathy as loss of dystrophin within cardiomyocytes results in ongoing cell death, leading to cardiac fibrosis and impaired cardiac function.

The pathologic mechanism underlying heart failure in the DMD population has not been fully elucidated. It is proposed that pathologic remodeling of the heart occurs as a result of both structural and metabolic abnormalities [37]. The mechanism underlying both ischemic and non-ischemic cardiomyopathy is the development of pathological cardiac hypertrophy, which eventually leads to paradoxical maladaptive cardiac remodeling [38]. Overtime, this compensatory mechanism fails and leads to cardiac dilatation and clinical heart failure [38]. Today, significant strides have been made in treating congestive heart failure (CHF), particularly systolic heart failure. Blockade of the renin-angiotensin-aldosterone system and inhibition of sympathetic activation have largely been the primary modes of treating a cardiomyopathy and inducing reverse cardiac remodeling. At least in non-ischemic cardiomyopathy patients on optimal medical therapy, approximately one third of patients will achieve normalization of the LV ejection fraction (LVEF), one third of patients will have improvement in the LVEF and the latter one third of patients will have progression in the LVEF requiring assessment for advanced heart failure therapies [i.e. implantation of a LV assist device (LVAD) or a heart transplantation]. Thus, the standard of care for treatment of a cardiomyopathy is based on the development of pathological cardiac hypertrophy, which eventually leads to a dilated cardiomyopathy when left untreated. This approach to treating a cardiomyopathy has been extrapolated to the treatment of DMD-associated cardiomyopathy.

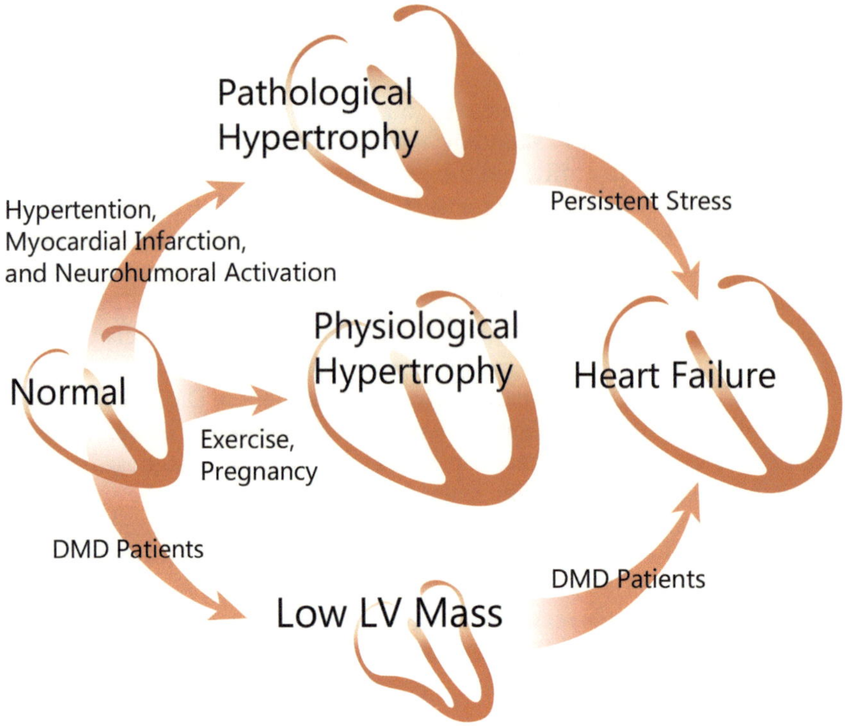

Figure 4.
Proposed mode of maladaptive cardiac remodeling leading to DMD-associated cardiomyopathy.

Although pathological cardiac hypertrophy has been assumed to be the primary mode of maladaptive cardiac remodeling in DMD-associated cardiomyopathy, clinical data suggests the use of guideline-directed medical therapy is not as effective in DMD-associated cardiomyopathy as it has been in other forms of cardiomyopathy with a reduced ejection fraction. Despite the increasing utilization of current standard of care heart failure therapies and device therapies, DMD-associated cardiomyopathy poses greater morbidity and mortality than other dilated cardiomyopathies and remains the leading cause of mortality in the DMD population [32]. Accordingly, the mechanism of maladaptive cardiac remodeling has been increasingly called into question. A cMRI study recently completed at UT Southwestern Medical Center suggests that adult DMD patients have small, atrophic hearts as compared to age-matched and weight-matched patients with non-ischemic cardiomyopathy or healthy patients enrolled in the Dallas Heart Study and this manuscript is currently under scientific review [39]. In an effort to further elucidate the mechanism leading to cardiac remodeling in DMD patients, the Mammen Laboratory at UT Southwestern Medical Center has discovered a proliferative defect in cardiomyocytes lacking dystrophin as early as four days postnatally in DMD^{mdx} mice. This work was presented at the 2019 American Heart Association Scientific Sessions meeting and the manuscript is also currently under scientific review [40]. The mechanism into how a proliferative defect within neonatal DMD cardiomyocytes leads to the eventual development of a DMD-associated cardiomyopathy in adult DMD patients is actively being investigated. These studies provide supportive data that the mode of maladaptive cardiac remodeling leading to DMD-associated cardiomyopathy, as illustrated in **Figure 4**, may be substantially different as compared to the mechanisms underlying non-ischemic cardiomyopathies. Once the signaling pathways governing these processes are better understood, appropriate targets for pharmacotherapy can be identified and allow for the development of novel drugs that can substantially improve the overall morbidity and mortality in the DMD population.

5. Management and treatment of DMD-associated cardiomyopathy

The majority of current therapies for DMD-associated cardiomyopathy collectively induce reverse cardiac remodeling and alleviate symptoms of the disease. Recent guideline documents have attempted to shift the focus of care to more proactive measures over the past decade [9, 25, 32, 41, 42]. These treatments include both pharmacological and non-pharmacological approaches.

5.1 Pharmacological treatments

The four major drug classes used to treat DMD-associated cardiomyopathy include angiotensin-converting-enzyme (ACE) inhibitors or angiotensin II receptor blockers (ARB), beta-adrenergic receptor blockers, mineralocorticoid receptor antagonists (MRA), and corticosteroids (**Table 1**).

ACE-inhibitors are a first line class of medications used to treat DMD-associated cardiomyopathy [1, 43]. Studies have shown that the use of ACE-inhibitors in DMD patients specifically can delay the onset and progression of DMD-associated cardiomyopathy [23, 43, 44]. In addition, teenage DMD patients started on a beta-blocker and an MRA along with an ACE-inhibitor have significantly increased LVEF compared to untreated control subjects [43, 45]. Therefore, as outlined in the 2017 scientific statement by the American Heart Association, as well as by the DMD Care Considerations Working Group in 2018, it is strongly recommended that all DMD patients should be treated with an ACE-inhibitor beginning by the age of 10, regardless of the presence of LV dysfunction [4, 41, 43, 46]. However, at the discretion of the physician and the family, an ACE inhibitor may be started earlier depending on the results of cMRI studies [25, 32, 46]. The most commonly prescribed ACE inhibitors in this population include enalapril and lisinopril [4, 43, 44].

Drug Class	Examples
Beta-Adrenergic Receptor Blockers	Carvedilol, Metoprolol Succinate, Bisoprolol
Angiotension-Converting-Enzyme Inhibitors	Perindopril, Enalapril, Lisinopril
Angiotension II Receptor Blockers	Candesartan, Losartan, Valsartan
Mineralocorticoid or Aldosterone Receptor Antagonists	Spironolactone, Eplerenone
Steroids	Prednisone, Deflazacort
Angiotension II Receptor-Neprilysin Inhibitor	Sacubitril/Valsartan
Vasodilators	Isosorbide Dinitrate/Hydralazine
Diuretics	Furosemide, Bumetanide, Torsemide
Cardiac Glycosides	Digoxin
Sodium-Glucose Co-Transporter-2 Inhibitors	Canagliflozin, Dapagliflozion, Empagliflozin
Hyperpolarization-Activated Cyclic Nucleotide-Gated Channel Blockers	Ivabradine

Table 1.
Pharmacological medications used in the treatment of DMD-associated cardiomyopathy.

While ACE-inhibitors are still widely prescribed, their use may be limited by side effects in certain patients, including dry cough and the development of hyperkalemia. The use of an ARB is an effective and safe alternative medication to an ACE-inhibitor and its mechanism of action is also mediated by inhibiting the renin-angiotensin aldosterone signaling pathway [4, 23]. Thus, ARBs are often prescribed as alternative cardioprotective class of medications in DMD patients who experience adverse reactions to ACE-inhibitors [1, 47, 48]. These data are in line with large double-blind randomized clinical trials looking at the efficacy of ARBs versus ACE-inhibitors in patients with either non-ischemic or ischemic cardiomyopathies [49].

MRAs are another class of medications that have been shown to have beneficial effects specifically in DMD-associated cardiomyopathy. The combined use of a MRA and an ACE-inhibitor has been shown to improve cardiac function in DMD patients in a randomized clinical trial [1, 4, 23]. In particular, eplerenone administered in conjunction with an ACE-inhibitor has been demonstrated in a clinical trial to significantly decrease ventricular circumferential strain in the treatment group compared to placebo [4, 50]. While spironolactone is a more potent MRA, eplerenone interferes less with the androgen receptor and has a more favorable side effect profile as compared to spironolactone [4].

Beta-adrenergic receptor blockers are another drug class frequently utilized in treating DMD-associated cardiomyopathy. Beta blockers, are commonly used in conjunction with ACE-inhibitors/ARBs and MRAs to improve clinical cardiac outcomes and induce reverse cardiac remodeling in DMD [4, 23]. Although there is no double blind clinical trial demonstrating the beneficial effects of combination therapy in DMD-associated cardiomyopathy, there are several non-randomized clinical studies in the DMD population supporting the use of combination therapy [51–54]. In one particular study, survival rates of those on carvedilol was found to be higher than the control group, data consistent with many large randomized clinical trials on the beneficial effects of beta-blockers [55]. The beneficial effects of this combinatorial therapy are both additive as well as synergistic in regards to inducing reverse cardiac remodeling and delaying cardiomyopathy progression in DMD-associated cardiomyopathy [23].

Corticosteroids are also very commonly used in DMD patients to improve ambulation, and are initiated early in the disease course, typically between 2 to 5 years of age [56–58]. Corticosteroids are primarily used to manage skeletal muscle wasting and are intended to improve muscle strength and ambulatory capacity in DMD patients [56]. However, long-term corticosteroid use is associated with significant adverse effects in DMD patients, including delayed puberty, decreased bone density, weight gain, development of type II diabetes, and risk of developing systemic infections [42, 59–61]. A recent retrospective study, revealed DMD patients on a corticosteroid had a higher LVEF and greater chance for survival, though study limitations prevent one from drawing a direct correlation between corticosteroid use alone and mortality benefit given the confounding effect of co-administration of ACE-inhibitors in this study [62]. Further research is warranted to determine whether the clinical benefit of continued corticosteroid therapy outweighs the known significant side effect profile. Current guidelines recommend continuation of corticosteroid therapy except in patients who develop severe systemic infections or clinically significant osteoporosis [42, 60, 61].

Digoxin, a cardiac glycoside, comprises another class of medications used to treat DMD-associated cardiomyopathy. Digoxin has been used in conjunction with beta-adrenergic receptor blockers, ACE-inhibitors/ARBs, MRAs, and corticosteroids to reduce morbidity associated with DMD-associated cardiomyopathy [23, 63]. However, digoxin has fallen out of favor recently due to its adverse side effect profile and the lack of available data demonstrating clear clinical mortality benefit of digoxin administration in DMD patients [23].

Other guideline directed therapies for heart failure (i.e. diuretics, isosorbide dinitrate/hydralazine, ivabradine, sacubitril/valsartan, and sodium-glucose co-transporter-2 inhibitors) have been shown to reduce morbidity and in some cases also mortality in patients with non-ischemic and ischemic cardiomyopathies (**Table 1**) [49, 64, 65]. The use of these medications in the treatment of DMD-associated cardiomyopathy have not yet been studied, so the impact on morbidity and mortality is unclear in the setting of DMD patients. However, some of these medications are being judiciously used in select DMD patients with progressive, refractory DMD-associated cardiomyopathy.

5.2 Non-pharmacological treatments

As is the case in the treatment of non-ischemic cardiomyopathy, a number of non-pharmacological therapies exist for the treatment of DMD-associated cardiomyopathy. These therapies include automated implantable cardioverter-defibrillators (AICD) with or without biventricular pacemaker capability, implantable left ventricular assist devices (LVAD) and heart transplantation. These treatments are most appropriate for DMD patients with end-stage heart failure who display signs of refractory disease, poor cardiac output, and/or severe conduction abnormalities. With the exception of AICDs, there is currently a lack of objective data regarding the benefits of LVAD implantation or heart transplantation in improving the morbidity or mortality in this unique patient population. As such, current guidelines do not recommend routine incorporation of these non-pharmacological therapies in treating DMD-associated cardiomyopathy.

In multiple large clinical trials, AICDs have demonstrated a mortality benefit by decreasing the incidence of sudden cardiac death in non-ischemic and ischemic cardiomyopathy patients with a LVEF less than 35% [49]. In addition, AICD implantation has been shown to reduce mortality rates in patients with sustained ventricular tachycardia or patients who have been resuscitated from sudden cardiac arrest [49]. The addition of cardiac resynchronization therapy to AICD implantation in patients with cardiomyopathy and a wide QRS complex has demonstrated improved morbidity and mortality in this patient population [66–68]. Therefore, the guidelines as set forth by the American College of Cardiology and the American Heart Association gave a Class I indication to the implantation of an AICD in patients with advanced heart failure and an LVEF less than 35% [49, 69]. These guidelines have been applied to DMD patients with cardiomyopathy and LVEF less than 35%, but in this unique population, special care and consideration must be taken into account when implanting an AICD given the high likelihood of significant muscle atrophy in the left upper portion of the chest [23, 25, 70]. It is generally recommended that these patients be referred to an electrophysiologist with extensive experience in implanting devices in muscular dystrophy patients.

A LVAD is a form of mechanical circulatory support device that can be implanted into patients with advanced DMD-associated cardiomyopathy, either as a destination therapy or as a bridge to heart transplantation. While LVADs have been demonstrated to improve mortality in patients with advanced end-stage non-ischemic and ischemic cardiomyopathy, approximately 20–30% of LVAD patients experience some complication within a year of implantation including infection, bleeding, and stroke [71–73]. Although LVADs have been implanted in DMD patients with advanced cardiomyopathy, the majority of these patients died within one year of LVAD implantation [74, 75]. As noted by Stoller et al., there are several essential or key factors that determine the long-term success of implanting a LVAD into DMD patients with advanced end-stage dilated cardiomyopathy (**Table 2**) [76].

Heart transplantation has been successfully undertaken in patients with muscular dystrophy. Both short and long term survival rates are very favorable

Key Factors Determining the Long-Term Success of a LVAD in a DMD Patient
Use of a multidisciplinary team pre- and post-LVAD implantation.
Appropriate candidate selection. While restrictive pulmonary physiology will be present, the DMD patient should not be on mechanical ventilatory support either pre-LVAD. In addition, the DMD patient should not have a GT-tube or PEG tube for supplemental feeding pre-LVAD.
Recognition of end organ dysfunction. DMD patients have very low baseline serum creatinine due to low muscle mass and even mild elevations are indicative of renal dysfunction. Conversely, liver function tests may be borderline elevated although further elevation, especially with evidence of volume overload, suggest right-sided heart failure in DMD patients.
An experienced cardiothoracic surgeon with significant expertise implanting LVADs into critically ill patients with advanced cardiomyopathy.
Selection of a LVAD that would not disrupt the diaphragm and thus further weaken the diaphragmatic muscle strength. This criteria is perhaps the most important factor that will determine the long-term success of a LVAD in a DMD patient and decrease the risk of any major medical complication.
Early extubation post-LVAD implantation with aggressive pulmonary toilet.
Aggressive care provided by physical, occupational, and respiratory therapy teams post-LVAD.
Very supportive and involved family.

Table 2.
Essential factors determining the long-term success of an LVAD in DMD-associated cardiomyopathy. Adapted from [76].

and comparable to age- and weight-matched cardiomyopathy patients without muscular dystrophy [77, 78]. However, there were only three DMD patients in both of these studies assessing the survival outcomes post-transplant. Due to significant skeletal muscle wasting in many DMD patients with advanced heart failure and restrictive lung disease, heart transplantation has only been undertaken in a limited number of DMD patients with advanced dilated cardiomyopathy, thus impairing the ability to draw conclusions regarding outcomes post-transplant specifically in this patient population.

6. Emerging therapies and future directions

Despite the many gaps that still exist in cardiac care in patients with DMD, much progress has been made over the past two decades, and recent developments have paved the way for future therapies. In particular, gene-replacement and genome-editing therapies hold significant promise due to the potentially corrective nature of these treatments by targeting the disease at the genetic level and restoring normal dystrophin levels.

Gene-replacement therapy using recombinant adenoviral virus vectors (rAVV) is one corrective method that has been proposed to treat DMD. This therapeutic approach is an especially promising therapy because this treatment modality has the potential to treat any underlying mutation within the dystrophin gene resulting in DMD disease and can therefore be applied to every DMD patient [4]. Since the full-length DMD gene is too large to package within a rAVV, micro-dystrophins, which contain only the most essential parts of the gene, can be successfully packaged into a rAVV [79]. While this approach has had some success in preclinical and early clinical trials, there are still several drawbacks that have been observed, including heightened immune responses to the rAVV [79, 80]. Additionally, it is uncertain if the truncated micro-dystrophin protein will sufficiently improve cardiac function and reduce the burden of cardiomyopathy in DMD patients [4].

Antisense-mediated exon skipping using antisense oligonucleotides (ASO) is one type of genome editing therapy, which strives to restore the open reading frame caused by a frame-shift mutation [4, 81]. The restoration of the open reading frame is accomplished by targeting a specific mutated exon via an ASO, and then removing the mutated exon with spliceosomes. By sacrificing the single exon, the remainder of the gene can be restored and a functional, truncated dystrophin protein is expressed, with a phenotype more similar to that of Becker muscular dystrophy (BMD) [4]. While preclinical and clinical studies have demonstrated promising results and have led to the FDA approval of some of these therapies, clinical trials have shown only minimal restoration of dystrophin and limited effects on cardiac physiology due to inadequate delivery to and correction of cardiomyocyte dysfunction [81, 82]. However, recent research suggests that optimizing dosage and personalizing treatment may yield more promising results for treating DMD-associated cardiomyopathy, so it remains a potential option [23, 81]. As of March 2021, there are four ASO therapies (eteplirsen targeting exon 51, golodirsen targeting exon 53, viltolarsen targeting exon 50, and casimersen targeting exon 45) that have received FDA approval for the treatment of DMD. However, it remains unclear the long term benefits of these ASO therapies in treating the skeletal muscle dysfunction, the diaphragmatic weakness, and the cardiomyopathy that plague all DMD patients.

Genome editing utilizing clustered regularly interspaced short palindromic repeats (CRISPR) with CRISPR-associated protein 9 (Cas9) has emerged as another novel and exciting genetic approach to permanently treating DMD patients [83–90]. The clear advantages of CRISPR-Cas9 technology over antisense-mediated exon skipping are two-fold. First, using CRISPR-Cas9 mediated genome editing offers a one time permanent treatment for DMD. Second, CRISPR-Cas9 technology provides highly sensitive and specific gene editing. This novel therapeutic method proposes delivery of the CRISPR-Cas9 machinery via adenoviral virus vectors (AVV). As such, this treatment also has the potential to trigger an undesired immune response [89, 90]. The pre-clinical data demonstrates CRISPR-Cas9 mediated genome editing remains a very promising and permanent correction to dystrophin deficiency in DMD patients [89–91].

Although all three of the above mentioned novel genetic therapeutic modalities have generated significant enthusiasm by scientists, clinicians, and patients, there remains a fundamental flaw of these proposed therapies in relation to DMD-associated cardiomyopathy. This flaw relates to the fact that they serve to functionally convert a DMD patient into a phenotype more closely resembling that of a BMD patient, rather than completely correcting or curing the DMD patient entirely of the disease process. While it is true that patients with BMD suffer less debilitating disease, approximately 70% of BMD patients over their lifespan still eventually develop advanced cardiomyopathy. Thus, while these novel genetic therapeutic modalities will surely improve the lives of DMD patients with improved skeletal muscle strength and mobility, challenges related to treating disease-related cardiomyopathy will persist [4].

Several other promising molecular therapies are also currently under investigation. Ataluren, an aminoglycoside-derived compound that functions as a stop-codon readthrough, is an investigational drug that has recently been approved by the European Medicine Agency, and is still being reviewed by the FDA [4, 92]. This therapy works to continue translation of the gene past a premature stop codon. While results in preclinical trials have shown modest improvements in cardiac dystrophin levels, there has been little evidence so far of any actual cardiac benefit derived from this therapy in clinical trials [92, 93]. Stem-cell therapy holds significant potential as a therapeutic modality in treating DMD patients. In particular, induced pluripotent stem cells have shown promise, though there are barriers in terms of successful engraftment of these cells into DMD muscle as well as the process of differentiation *in-vivo* [94]. Many potential future therapies such as these have focused on restoring dystrophin levels in skeletal muscle and while this may improve skeletal muscle weakness and ambulation, it is essential to consider whether these therapies will also improve the accompanying cardiomyopathy.

Along with emerging therapies, new diagnostic measures have also been studied. One such diagnostic tool includes newborn screening (NBS), which involves measuring the creatine kinase (CK) levels among neonates [95, 96]. The CK levels are often markedly elevated in newborns with DMD. The utilization of a two-tier system for testing, a cost-effective and accurate application of NBS, has been shown to have promising potential as a diagnostic tool to identify patients with DMD at an even earlier age [95].

In addition to these emerging therapies, there are many questions that have yet to be answered about existing treatments and therapies. Exact timing of initiation and dosage of first and second-line medications is still uncertain and remains disputed, though there is a broad consensus that earlier, anticipatory treatment is recommended for DMD patients [25, 43]. There is also a lack of supporting literature on beta-adrenergic receptor blockers, and more studies are needed to determine their exact benefits with and without the concurrent use of ACE-inhibitors or ARBs as well as MRAs [23].

Finally, DMD carriers are a relatively understudied and underappreciated group within this unique population of patients. DMD carriers are at significant risk for developing advanced cardiomyopathy, but the mechanisms underlying this phenomenon are unclear. The primary hypothesis is that skewed X chromosome inactivation occurs selectively within the cardiomyocytes of these patients, and one of the two X-chromosomes in the DMD female carrier becomes transcriptionally inactive [1, 34]. DMD carriers have an estimated 50% lifetime risk for developing cardiomyopathy [34, 97]. Researchers believe that the degree of X inactivation is correlated with the severity of cardiac manifestations in these patients, but better designed studies are required to understand the various mechanisms involved in the development of DMD-associated cardiomyopathy in DMD carriers [1].

7. Conclusion

Over the past two decades, tremendous progress has been made in understanding the pathophysiology and treatment of DMD-associated cardiomyopathy. Due to advances in neurologic, pulmonary, and orthopedic care provided to DMD patients, there has been a significant increase in the life expectancy in these patients. Therefore, more DMD patients are living into adulthood resulting in cardiomyopathy as the primary mode of death in the majority of DMD patients in 2021. Current cardiovascular guidelines directed specifically towards DMD patients are now available and provide a more solid foundation for evaluating and treating affected patients. Importantly, earlier recognition and management of the disease and its cardiac manifestations has great potential in slowing the progression of DMD-associated cardiomyopathy. Part of this success is due to the incorporation of heart failure cardiologists into the multidisciplinary team approach to DMD care and the aggressive application of guideline directed medical therapy at an early age. Though there is much progress to be made, advancements in potential novel therapies and the growing body of research in this field have created a promising future for cardiac care in DMD.

Conflict of interest

Dr. Pradeep Mammen declares the following conflicts of interests: American Heart Association (member of the AHA Career Development Research Grant

Committee), AveXis Inc. (member of the Data Monitoring and Safety Committee), California Institute of Regenerative Medicine (member of the Grants Working Group), CareDx Inc. (Site PI for the SHORE Registry), Catabasis Inc. (research grant), Dyne Therapeutics (consultant and member of the DMD Advisory Board), National Institute of Health (research grants and ad hoc grant reviewer for the NIH SMEP and MOSS Study Sections), and PhaseBio Inc. (research grant and member of the Scientific Advisory Board). The other authors have declared that no conflicts of interest exist as it pertains to the subject of the current study.

Notes/thanks/other declarations

Sources of Funding: This work was supported by the National Institute of Health (NIH) and the NIH funded UT Southwestern Senator Paul D. Wellstone Muscular Dystrophy Specialized Research Center Grant (NIH R01HL102478, U54HD087351, and P50HD087351 awarded to PPAM), Wellstone Trainee Research Awards (awarded to HL and RS), and the UT Southwestern Alfred W. Harris, M.D. Professorship in Cardiology (awarded to PPAM).

Author details

Theo Lee-Gannon[1,2], Hannah Lehrenbaum[1], Rahul Sheth[1] and Pradeep P.A. Mammen[1,2,3,4,5*]

1 Department of Internal Medicine, University of Texas Southwestern Medical Center, Dallas, TX, United States

2 Division of Cardiology, University of Texas Southwestern Medical Center, Dallas, TX, United States

3 Heart Failure, Ventricular Assist Device and Heart Transplant Program, University of Texas Southwestern Medical Center, Dallas, TX, United States

4 Hamon Center for Regenerative Science and Medicine, University of Texas Southwestern Medical Center, Dallas, TX, United States

5 Senator Paul D. Wellstone Muscular Dystrophy Specialized Research Center, University of Texas Southwestern Medical Center, Dallas, TX, United States

*Address all correspondence to: pradeep.mammen@utsouthwestern.edu

References

[1] Kamdar F, Garry DJ. Dystrophin-Deficient Cardiomyopathy. J Am Coll Cardiol. 2016;67(21):2533-46.

[2] Emery AE. The muscular dystrophies. BMJ. 1998;317(7164):991-5.

[3] Mah JK, Korngut L, Dykeman J, Day L, Pringsheim T, Jette N. A systematic review and meta-analysis on the epidemiology of Duchenne and Becker muscular dystrophy. Neuromuscular Disord. 2014;24(6):482-91.

[4] Meyers TA, Townsend D. Cardiac Pathophysiology and the Future of Cardiac Therapies in Duchenne Muscular Dystrophy. Int J Mol Sci. 2019;20(17).

[5] Hoffman EP, Brown RH, Jr., Kunkel LM. Dystrophin: the protein product of the Duchenne muscular dystrophy locus. Cell. 1987;51(6):919-28.

[6] Eagle M, Baudouin SV, Chandler C, Giddings DR, Bullock R, Bushby K. Survival in Duchenne muscular dystrophy: improvements in life expectancy since 1967 and the impact of home nocturnal ventilation. Neuromuscular Disord. 2002;12(10):926-9.

[7] Cheeran D, Khan S, Khera R, Bhatt A, Garg S, Grodin JL, et al. Predictors of Death in Adults With Duchenne Muscular Dystrophy-Associated Cardiomyopathy. J Am Heart Assoc. 2017;6(10).

[8] Koenig M, Hoffman EP, Bertelson CJ, Monaco AP, Feener C, Kunkel LM. Complete cloning of the Duchenne muscular dystrophy (DMD) cDNA and preliminary genomic organization of the DMD gene in normal and affected individuals. Cell. 1987;50(3):509-17.

[9] D'Amario D, Amodeo A, Adorisio R, Tiziano FD, Leone AM, Perri G, et al. A current approach to heart failure in Duchenne muscular dystrophy. Heart. 2017;103(22):1770-9.

[10] Laing NG, Davis MR, Bayley K, Fletcher S, Wilton SD. Molecular diagnosis of duchenne muscular dystrophy: past, present and future in relation to implementing therapies. Clin Biochem Rev. 2011;32(3):129-34.

[11] Dent KM, Dunn DM, von Niederhausern AC, Aoyagi AT, Kerr L, Bromberg MB, et al. Improved molecular diagnosis of dystrophinopathies in an unselected clinical cohort. Am J Med Genet A. 2005;134(3):295-8.

[12] Rybakova IN, Patel JR, Ervasti JM. The dystrophin complex forms a mechanically strong link between the sarcolemma and costameric actin. J Cell Biol. 2000;150(5):1209-14.

[13] Ervasti JM, Campbell KP. A role for the dystrophin-glycoprotein complex as a transmembrane linker between laminin and actin. J Cell Biol. 1993;122(4):809-23.

[14] Sharpe KM, Premsukh MD, Townsend D. Alterations of dystrophin-associated glycoproteins in the heart lacking dystrophin or dystrophin and utrophin. Journal of Muscle Research and Cell Motility. 2013;34(5-6):395-405.

[15] Johnstone VPA, Viola HM, Hool LC. Dystrophic Cardiomyopathy-Potential Role of Calcium in Pathogenesis, Treatment and Novel Therapies. Genes. 2017;8(4).

[16] Williams IA, Allen DG. Intracellular calcium handling in ventricular myocytes from mdx mice. Am J Physiol-Heart C. 2007;292(2):H846-H55.

[17] Viola HM, Davies SMK, Filipovska A, Hool LC. L-type Ca2+

channel contributes to alterations in mitochondrial calcium handling in the mdx ventricular myocyte. Am J Physiol-Heart C. 2013;304(6):H767-H75.

[18] Lorin C, Vogeli I, Niggli E. Dystrophic cardiomyopathy: role of TRPV2 channels in stretch-induced cell damage. Cardiovasc Res. 2015;106(1):153-62.

[19] Gonzalez DR, Treuer AV, Lamirault G, Mayo V, Cao Y, Dulce RA, et al. NADPH oxidase-2 inhibition restores contractility and intracellular calcium handling and reduces arrhythmogenicity in dystrophic cardiomyopathy. Am J Physiol Heart Circ Physiol. 2014;307(5):H710-21.

[20] Allen DG, Whitehead NP, Froehner SC. Absence of Dystrophin Disrupts Skeletal Muscle Signaling: Roles of Ca2+, Reactive Oxygen Species, and Nitric Oxide in the Development of Muscular Dystrophy. Physiol Rev. 2016;96(1):253-305.

[21] Dikalov SI, Nazarewicz RR. Angiotensin II-Induced Production of Mitochondrial Reactive Oxygen Species: Potential Mechanisms and Relevance for Cardiovascular Disease. Antioxid Redox Sign. 2013;19(10):1085-94.

[22] Bia BL, Cassidy PJ, Young ME, Rafael JA, Leighton B, Davies KE, et al. Decreased myocardial nNOS, increased iNOS and abnormal ECGs in mouse models of Duchenne muscular dystrophy. J Mol Cell Cardiol. 1999;31(10):1857-62.

[23] Finsterer J, Cripe L. Treatment of dystrophin cardiomyopathies. Nat Rev Cardiol. 2014;11(3):168-79.

[24] Heras-Bautista CO, Mikhael N, Lam J, Shinde V, Katsen-Globa A, Dieluweit S, et al. Cardiomyocytes facing fibrotic conditions re-express extracellular matrix transcripts. Acta Biomater. 2019;89:180-92.

[25] Buddhe S, Cripe L, Friedland-Little J, Kertesz N, Eghtesady P, Finder J, et al. Cardiac Management of the Patient With Duchenne Muscular Dystrophy. Pediatrics. 2018;142:S72-S81.

[26] Bushby K, Finkel R, Birnkrant DJ, Case LE, Clemens PR, Cripe L, et al. Diagnosis and management of Duchenne muscular dystrophy, part 1: diagnosis, and pharmacological and psychosocial management. Lancet Neurology. 2010;9(1):77-93.

[27] Aartsma-Rus A, Ginjaar IB, Bushby K. The importance of genetic diagnosis for Duchenne muscular dystrophy. J Med Genet. 2016;53(3):145-51.

[28] Birnkrant DJ, Bushby K, Bann CM, Alman BA, Apkon SD, Blackwell A, et al. Diagnosis and management of Duchenne muscular dystrophy, part 2: respiratory, cardiac, bone health, and orthopaedic management. The Lancet Neurology. 2018;17(4):347-61.

[29] van Westering T, Betts C, Wood M. Current Understanding of Molecular Pathology and Treatment of Cardiomyopathy in Duchenne Muscular Dystrophy. Molecules. 2015;20(5):8823-55.

[30] Nigro G, Comi LI, Politano L, Bain RJI. The Incidence and Evolution of Cardiomyopathy in Duchenne Muscular-Dystrophy. International Journal of Cardiology. 1990;26(3):271-7.

[31] Birnkrant DJ, Bushby K, Bann CM, Alman BA, Apkon SD, Blackwell A, et al. Diagnosis and management of Duchenne muscular dystrophy, part 2: respiratory, cardiac, bone health, and orthopaedic management. Lancet Neurology. 2018;17(4):347-61.

[32] McNally EM, Kaltman JR, Benson DW, Canter CE, Cripe LH, Duan D, et al. Contemporary cardiac

issues in Duchenne muscular dystrophy. Working Group of the National Heart, Lung, and Blood Institute in collaboration with Parent Project Muscular Dystrophy. Circulation. 2015;131(18):1590-8.

[33] Hor KN, Wansapura J, Markham LW, Mazur W, Cripe LH, Fleck R, et al. Circumferential Strain Analysis Identifies Strata of Cardiomyopathy in Duchenne Muscular Dystrophy A Cardiac Magnetic Resonance Tagging Study. Journal of the American College of Cardiology. 2009;53(14):1204-10.

[34] Politano L, Nigro V, Nigro G, Petretta VR, Passamano L, Papparella S, et al. Development of cardiomyopathy in female carriers of Duchenne and Becker muscular dystrophies. JAMA. 1996;275(17):1335-8.

[35] Viggiano E, Picillo E, Cirillo A, Politano L. Comparison of X-chromosome inactivation in Duchenne muscle/myocardium-manifesting carriers, non-manifesting carriers and related daughters. Clin Genet. 2013;84(3):265-70.

[36] Nigro G, Comi LI, Politano L, Bain RJ. The incidence and evolution of cardiomyopathy in Duchenne muscular dystrophy. Int J Cardiol. 1990;26(3):271-7.

[37] Verhaert D, Richards K, Rafael-Fortney JA, Raman SV. Cardiac involvement in patients with muscular dystrophies: magnetic resonance imaging phenotype and genotypic considerations. Circulation Cardiovascular imaging. 2011;4(1):67-76.

[38] Mann DL, Bristow MR. Mechanisms and models in heart failure: the biomechanical model and beyond. Circulation. 2005;111(21):2837-49.

[39] Khan S, Cheeran D, Garg S, Grodin J, Morlend R, Araj F, et al. Cardiac Atrophy: A Novel Mechanism for Duchenne Muscular Dystrophy (Dmd)Associated Cardiomyopathy. Journal of the American College of Cardiology. 2017;69(11):946-.

[40] Tassin T, Huang J, Gemmelli T, Kanchwala M, Punnen LM, Chung E, et al. Mechanistic Insights into Duchenne Muscular Dystrophy-Associated Cardiomyopathy. Circulation Research. 2019;123:A310.

[41] Feingold B, Mahle WT, Auerbach S, Clemens P, Domenighetti AA, Jefferies JL, et al. Management of Cardiac Involvement Associated With Neuromuscular Diseases: A Scientific Statement From the American Heart Association. Circulation. 2017;136(13):e200-e31.

[42] Birnkrant DJ, Bushby K, Bann CM, Alman BA, Apkon SD, Blackwell A, et al. Diagnosis and management of Duchenne muscular dystrophy, part 2: respiratory, cardiac, bone health, and orthopaedic management. Lancet Neurol. 2018;17(4):347-61.

[43] Duboc D, Meune C, Lerebours G, Devaux JY, Vaksmann G, Becane HM. Effect of perindopril on the onset and progression of left ventricular dysfunction in Duchenne muscular dystrophy. J Am Coll Cardiol. 2005;45(6):855-7.

[44] Ramaciotti C, Heistein LC, Coursey M, Lemler MS, Eapen RS, Iannaccone ST, et al. Left ventricular function and response to enalapril in patients with duchenne muscular dystrophy during the second decade of life. Am J Cardiol. 2006;98(6):825-7.

[45] Raman SV, Hor KN, Mazur W, Halnon NJ, Kissel JT, He X, et al. Eplerenone for early cardiomyopathy in Duchenne muscular dystrophy: a randomised, double-blind, placebo-controlled trial. Lancet Neurol. 2015;14(2):153-61.

[46] Silva MC, Magalhaes TA, Meira ZM, Rassi CH, Andrade AC, Gutierrez PS, et al. Myocardial Fibrosis Progression in Duchenne and Becker Muscular Dystrophy: A Randomized Clinical Trial. JAMA Cardiol. 2017;2(2):190-9.

[47] Spurney CF, Sali A, Guerron AD, Iantorno M, Yu Q, Gordish-Dressman H, et al. Losartan decreases cardiac muscle fibrosis and improves cardiac function in dystrophin-deficient mdx mice. J Cardiovasc Pharmacol Ther. 2011;16(1):87-95.

[48] Bish LT, Yarchoan M, Sleeper MM, Gazzara JA, Morine KJ, Acosta P, et al. Chronic losartan administration reduces mortality and preserves cardiac but not skeletal muscle function in dystrophic mice. PLoS One. 2011;6(6):e20856.

[49] Writing Committee M, Yancy CW, Jessup M, Bozkurt B, Butler J, Casey DE, Jr., et al. 2013 ACCF/AHA guideline for the management of heart failure: a report of the American College of Cardiology Foundation/American Heart Association Task Force on practice guidelines. Circulation. 2013;128(16):e240-327.

[50] Angelini C. Prevention of cardiomyopathy in Duchenne muscular dystrophy. Lancet Neurol. 2015;14(2):127-8.

[51] Rhodes J, Margossian R, Darras BT, Colan SD, Jenkins KJ, Geva T, et al. Safety and efficacy of carvedilol therapy for patients with dilated cardiomyopathy secondary to muscular dystrophy. Pediatr Cardiol. 2008;29(2):343-51.

[52] Ogata H, Ishikawa Y, Ishikawa Y, Minami R. Beneficial effects of beta-blockers and angiotensin-converting enzyme inhibitors in Duchenne muscular dystrophy. J Cardiol. 2009;53(1):72-8.

[53] Matsumura T, Tamura T, Kuru S, Kikuchi Y, Kawai M. Carvedilol can prevent cardiac events in Duchenne muscular dystrophy. Intern Med. 2010;49(14):1357-63.

[54] Viollet L, Thrush PT, Flanigan KM, Mendell JR, Allen HD. Effects of angiotensin-converting enzyme inhibitors and/or beta blockers on the cardiomyopathy in Duchenne muscular dystrophy. Am J Cardiol. 2012;110(1):98-102.

[55] Matsumura T, Tamura T, Kuru S, Kikuchi Y, Kawai M. Carvedilol can Prevent Cardiac Events in Duchenne Muscular Dystrophy. Internal Med. 2010;49(14):1357-63.

[56] Mendell JR, Moxley RT, Griggs RC, Brooke MH, Fenichel GM, Miller JP, et al. Randomized, double-blind six-month trial of prednisone in Duchenne's muscular dystrophy. N Engl J Med. 1989;320(24):1592-7.

[57] Angelini C. The role of corticosteroids in muscular dystrophy: a critical appraisal. Muscle Nerve. 2007;36(4):424-35.

[58] Finsterer J, Cripe L. Treatment of dystrophin cardiomyopathies. Nat Rev Cardiol. 2014;11(3):168-79.

[59] Yasir MG, A; Bansal, P; Sonthalia, S. Corticosteroid Adverse Effects. StatPearls. 2020.

[60] Birnkrant DJ, Bushby K, Bann CM, Apkon SD, Blackwell A, Brumbaugh D, et al. Diagnosis and management of Duchenne muscular dystrophy, part 1: diagnosis, and neuromuscular, rehabilitation, endocrine, and gastrointestinal and nutritional management. Lancet Neurol. 2018;17(3):251-67.

[61] Birnkrant DJ, Bushby K, Bann CM, Apkon SD, Blackwell A, Colvin MK, et al. Diagnosis and management of Duchenne muscular dystrophy, part 3: primary care, emergency management,

psychosocial care, and transitions of care across the lifespan. Lancet Neurol. 2018;17(5):445-55.

[62] Schram G, Fournier A, Leduc H, Dahdah N, Therien J, Vanasse M, et al. All-Cause Mortality and Cardiovascular Outcomes With Prophylactic Steroid Therapy in Duchenne Muscular Dystrophy. Journal of the American College of Cardiology. 2013;61(9):948-54.

[63] Campbell TJ, MacDonald PS. Digoxin in heart failure and cardiac arrhythmias. Med J Australia. 2003;179(2):98-102.

[64] Yancy CW, Jessup M, Bozkurt B, Butler J, Casey DE, Jr., Colvin MM, et al. 2017 ACC/AHA/HFSA Focused Update of the 2013 ACCF/AHA Guideline for the Management of Heart Failure: A Report of the American College of Cardiology/American Heart Association Task Force on Clinical Practice Guidelines and the Heart Failure Society of America. Circulation. 2017;136(6):e137-e61.

[65] Lytvyn Y, Bjornstad P, Udell JA, Lovshin JA, Cherney DZI. Sodium Glucose Cotransporter-2 Inhibition in Heart Failure: Potential Mechanisms, Clinical Applications, and Summary of Clinical Trials. Circulation. 2017;136(17):1643-58.

[66] Moss AJ, Hall WJ, Cannom DS, Klein H, Brown MW, Daubert JP, et al. Cardiac-resynchronization therapy for the prevention of heart-failure events. N Engl J Med. 2009;361(14):1329-38.

[67] Cleland JG, Daubert JC, Erdmann E, Freemantle N, Gras D, Kappenberger L, et al. The effect of cardiac resynchronization on morbidity and mortality in heart failure. N Engl J Med. 2005;352(15):1539-49.

[68] Bristow MR, Saxon LA, Boehmer J, Krueger S, Kass DA, De Marco T, et al. Cardiac-resynchronization therapy with or without an implantable defibrillator in advanced chronic heart failure. N Engl J Med. 2004;350(21):2140-50.

[69] Epstein AE, DiMarco JP, Ellenbogen KA, Estes NA, 3rd, Freedman RA, Gettes LS, et al. 2012 ACCF/AHA/HRS focused update incorporated into the ACCF/AHA/HRS 2008 guidelines for device-based therapy of cardiac rhythm abnormalities: a report of the American College of Cardiology Foundation/ American Heart Association Task Force on Practice Guidelines and the Heart Rhythm Society. J Am Coll Cardiol. 2013;61(3):e6-75.

[70] Palladino AP, A; Morra, S; Russo, V; Ergoli, M; Rago, A; Orsini, C; Nigro, G; and Politano, L. Are there real benefits to implanting cardiac devices in patients with end-stage dilated dystrophinopathic cardiomyopathy? Review of literature and personal results. Acta Myologica. 2019;38.

[71] Slaughter MS, Rogers JG, Milano CA, Russell SD, Conte JV, Feldman D, et al. Advanced heart failure treated with continuous-flow left ventricular assist device. N Engl J Med. 2009;361(23):2241-51.

[72] Akhter SA, Badami A, Murray M, Kohmoto T, Lozonschi L, Osaki S, et al. Hospital Readmissions After Continuous-Flow Left Ventricular Assist Device Implantation: Incidence, Causes, and Cost Analysis. Ann Thorac Surg. 2015;100(3):884-9.

[73] Stulak JM, Davis ME, Haglund N, Dunlay S, Cowger J, Shah P, et al. Adverse events in contemporary continuous-flow left ventricular assist devices: A multi-institutional comparison shows significant differences. J Thorac Cardiovasc Surg. 2016;151(1):177-89.

[74] Amodeo A, Adorisio R. Left ventricular assist device in Duchenne

cardiomyopathy: can we change the natural history of cardiac disease? Int J Cardiol. 2012;161(3):e43.

[75] Iodice F, Testa G, Averardi M, Brancaccio G, Amodeo A, Cogo P. Implantation of a left ventricular assist device as a destination therapy in Duchenne muscular dystrophy patients with end stage cardiac failure: management and lessons learned. Neuromuscul Disord. 2015;25(1):19-23.

[76] Stoller D, Araj F, Amin A, Fitzsimmons C, Morlend R, Thibodeau JT, et al. Implantation of a left ventricular assist device to provide long-term support for end-stage Duchenne muscular dystrophy-associated cardiomyopathy. ESC Heart Fail. 2017;4(3):379-83.

[77] Wells D, Rizwan R, Jefferies JL, Bryant R, 3rd, Ryan TD, Lorts A, et al. Heart Transplantation in Muscular Dystrophy Patients: Is it a Viable Option? Circ Heart Fail. 2020;13(4):e005447.

[78] Wu RS, Gupta S, Brown RN, Yancy CW, Wald JW, Kaiser P, et al. Clinical outcomes after cardiac transplantation in muscular dystrophy patients. J Heart Lung Transplant. 2010;29(4):432-8.

[79] Chamberlain JR, Chamberlain JS. Progress toward Gene Therapy for Duchenne Muscular Dystrophy. Mol Ther. 2017;25(5):1125-31.

[80] Yang Y, Haecker SE, Su Q, Wilson JM. Immunology of gene therapy with adenoviral vectors in mouse skeletal muscle. Hum Mol Genet. 1996;5(11):1703-12.

[81] Lu QL, Rabinowitz A, Chen YC, Yokota T, Yin H, Alter J, et al. Systemic delivery of antisense oligoribonucleotide restores dystrophin expression in body-wide skeletal muscles. Proc Natl Acad Sci U S A. 2005;102(1):198-203.

[82] Nguyen Q, Yokota T. Antisense oligonucleotides for the treatment of cardiomyopathy in Duchenne muscular dystrophy. Am J Transl Res. 2019;11(3):1202-18.

[83] Cathomen T, Ehl S. Translating the genomic revolution - targeted genome editing in primates. N Engl J Med. 2014;370(24):2342-5.

[84] Calos MP. The CRISPR Way to Think about Duchenne's. N Engl J Med. 2016;374(17):1684-6.

[85] Munshi NV. CRISPR (Clustered Regularly Interspaced Palindromic Repeat)/Cas9 System: A Revolutionary Disease-Modifying Technology. Circulation. 2016;134(11):777-9.

[86] Mendell JR, Rodino-Klapac LR. Duchenne muscular dystrophy: CRISPR/Cas9 treatment. Cell Res. 2016;26(5):513-4.

[87] Fellmann C, Gowen BG, Lin PC, Doudna JA, Corn JE. Cornerstones of CRISPR-Cas in drug discovery and therapy. Nat Rev Drug Discov. 2017;16(2):89-100.

[88] Zhang Y, Long C, Bassel-Duby R, Olson EN. Myoediting: Toward Prevention of Muscular Dystrophy by Therapeutic Genome Editing. Physiol Rev. 2018;98(3):1205-40.

[89] Min YL, Bassel-Duby R, Olson EN. CRISPR Correction of Duchenne Muscular Dystrophy. Annu Rev Med. 2019;70:239-55.

[90] Chemello F, Bassel-Duby R, Olson EN. Correction of muscular dystrophies by CRISPR gene editing. J Clin Invest. 2020;130(6):2766-76.

[91] Lim KRQ, Yoon C, Yokota T. Applications of CRISPR/Cas9 for the Treatment of Duchenne Muscular Dystrophy. J Pers Med. 2018;8(4).

[92] Namgoong JH, Bertoni C. Clinical potential of ataluren in the treatment of Duchenne muscular dystrophy. Degener Neurol Neuromuscul Dis. 2016;6:37-48.

[93] Welch EM, Barton ER, Zhuo J, Tomizawa Y, Friesen WJ, Trifillis P, et al. PTC124 targets genetic disorders caused by nonsense mutations. Nature. 2007;447(7140):87-91.

[94] Danisovic L, Culenova M, Csobonyeiova M. Induced Pluripotent Stem Cells for Duchenne Muscular Dystrophy Modeling and Therapy. Cells. 2018;7(12).

[95] Mendell JR, Shilling C, Leslie ND, Flanigan KM, al-Dahhak R, Gastier-Foster J, et al. Evidence-based path to newborn screening for Duchenne muscular dystrophy. Ann Neurol. 2012;71(3):304-13.

[96] Zellweger H, Antonik A. Newborn screening for Duchenne muscular dystrophy. Pediatrics. 1975;55(1):30-4.

[97] Lehrenbaum MH, Cheeran D, Bae Y, Ayers C, Araj F, Amin A, de Lemos JA, Drazner MH, Peshock RM, Zaha VG, Levine BD, Mammen PPA. Left ventricular structural remodeling and cardiomyopathy in Duchenne muscular dystrophy carriers. Circulation. 2020;15784:142.

Chapter 15

Cardiomyopathy in Duchenne Muscular Distrophy: Clinical Insights and Therapeutic Implications

Rachele Adorisio, Erica Mencarelli, Nicoletta Cantarutti and Maria Grandinetti

Abstract

Duchenne muscular dystrophy cardiomyopathy (DMD-DCM) is characterized by progressive ventricular dilation and dysfunction that can begin at any age and worsens over time. Thanks to the lengthening of life expectancy due to better management of respiratory involvement, end-stage heart failure (HF) is becoming the main cause of death for DMD patients. Therefore, from the time of DMD diagnosis, every effort should be focused to early detect the onset and the worsening of the DMD-DCM, with the aim of starting and modulating the therapy to slow the progression of cardiac dysfunction. In cardiac evaluation, biomarkers, electrocardiograms, and echocardiograms must be considered, but cardiac magnetic resonance (CMR) is now acquiring a leading role due to its sensitivity in the earlier identification of cardiac involvement. The management of DMD-DCM at end stage is a difficult challenge that requires a multidisciplinary team composed of clinical cardiologists, electrophysiologists, cardiac surgeons, neuromuscular specialists, and psychologists. Because of the lack of specific drugs for DMD, we will review the actual cardiovascular armamentarium including drugs used for HF.

Keywords: duchenne muscular dystrophy, DMD, dilated cardiomyopathy, neuromuscular disease, dystrophin, heart failure

1. Introduction

Duchenne muscular dystrophy (DMD) is an X-linked degenerative neuromuscular disease that affects the skeletal muscles and the heart and over time leads to loss of walking, severe respiratory complications and progressive cardiac dilation and dysfunction.

It is caused by a mutation of the DMD gene, the largest gene in the human genome, mapped on the X-chromosome that codes for dystrophin, an essential protein for the stability of the myocyte membranes. The type of mutation and the degree of reduced expression of this structural protein influences the degree of muscle and cardiac impairment and especially the speed of myopathy progression. The milder forms are generally identified with the term Becker's muscular dystrophy (BMD) while the most severe and rapidly evolving forms, due to a severe reduction or total absence of dystrophin, are properly defined as DMD. Due to the X-linked recessive inheritance, the condition of female carriers must also be considered; they have a second normally functioning allele of dystrophin gene, thus they are generally characterized by a completely normal muscular and cardiac phenotype but may also present a mild/variable expression of the disease [1].

The incidence of DMD is approximately 1 in 5000 live male births, with 2/3 of the cases due to the transmission of the X-chromosome containing the mutated gene from a carrier female to male offspring and the remaining 1/3 of cases consequent to de novo mutations.

Generally the first manifestation of the DMD is muscle weakness that begins around the age of four and worsens quickly, leading to the loss of independent walking by the age of ten and to respiratory dysfunction around the second decade of life. The cardiac involvement begins around 6–10 years of age [2, 3] while cardiovascular symptoms are rare before the age of twenty and often appear when the degree of cardiac dysfunction is severe [4].

In last decades, the life expectancy of patients with DMD has grown considerably as a result of advances in the prevention and management of respiratory complications. As a result, there has been a significant increase in manifestations of advanced cardiomyopathy that is becoming the main cause of morbidity and mortality for these patients. This has led to a growing interest in the prevention and management of DMD-DCM [5–7].

While some aspects of DMD-DCM assessment and therapy are well defined by current guidelines [8], such as the need of routine cardiac evaluation and the indication to start prophylactic cardio-protective therapy from the age of ten in all patients, many other aspects remain under investigation, especially at end stage phase.

2. Genetic basis and pathophysiology of DMD-DCM

The DMD gene, encoded on the X chromosome, is the longest gene of our genome; it contains long introns with many "hotspots" susceptible to a high rate of mutations which can lead to the deletion (60–65% of all DMD mutations) or duplication (10%) of one or many exons. Shorter mutations such as point mutations are responsible for the remaining 25% of DMD cases. One third of DMD cases are due to de novo mutations while two third are inherited. The mutations resulting in the production of a truncated protein or of a dystrophin lacking in structural domains necessary for interaction with other proteins, are responsible for the most severe forms of the disease [9].

Dystrophin is a long intracellular protein of 3685 aminoacids and a molecular weight of 427 kDa. It is composed by four domains: an *amino-terminal domain* that interacts with actin of the myocyte cytoskeleton, a *central rod-like domain* that contains sites of interaction with anionic lipids and with neural NOS, a second actin-binding motif and four short proline-rich spacers responsible of the elasticity of the protein, *a cysteine-rich domain* that provides the protein–protein interaction and stabilizes dystroglycan binding, and a *C-terminal domain*, that interacts with several cytoplasmic, integral membrane and extracellular glycoproteins to create a protein complex called DAPC (dystrophin-associated protein complex) (**Figure 1**). The DAPC, in healthy myocytes, anchors the cytoskeleton and the plasma membrane to the extracellular matrix, ensuring stability and resistance to cells during contractions [9]. The lack of dystrophin, or the presence of an abnormal dystrophin, causes the loss of stability of this complex connection system with consequent greater

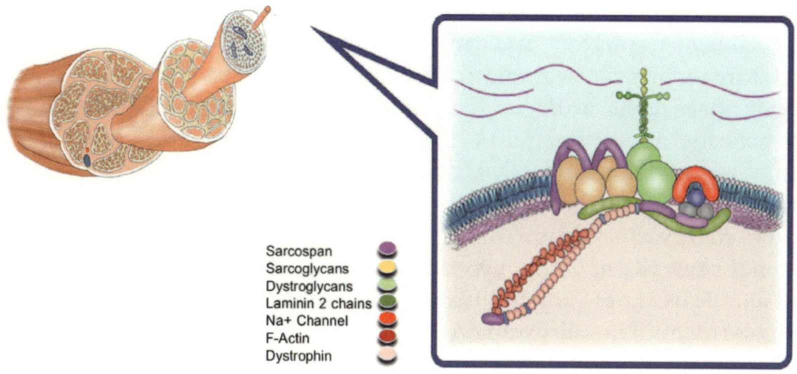

Figure 1.
The dystrophin- associated protein complex (DAPC). Dystrophin and DAPC plays an essential structural role in linking the actin of cytoskeleton to the extracellular matrix. The subunits of the DAPC, such as the sarcoglycans, have a vital role in the maintenance of muscle integrity. Dystrophin, a flexible rod-like cytoplasmic protein, directly interacts with the actin polymers of the cytoskeleton and with a complex of transmembrane glico-proteins composed by sarcoglycans, beta- and alpha-dystroglycan that creates a connection with the extracellular matrix by its linking with laminin-2.

fragility of the cell membrane of myocytes, dysregulation of cellular signaling and high susceptibility to damage and cell death. Cellular stress and cardiomyocyte death cause the release of cytokines, chemokines and cellular debris that attract neutrophils, macrophages and, later in time, fibroblasts. This process leads to the replacement of the heart muscle with fibrous tissue; it generally starts from the region behind the posterior mitral valve apparatus and proceeds toward the ventricular apex and around the heart, and from the epicardium to the endocardium, to lead, ultimately, to the dilation and the dysfunction of the ventricles [10]. In this scenario, inflammation, dysregulation of the intracellular calcium (Ca2+) signaling, alteration of synthesis of nitric oxide, inadequate anti-oxidant response, mitochondrial malfunction and deficiency of membrane repair systems are all mechanisms involved in the molecular pathogenesis of DMD-DCM and they can be addressed for the development of new disease-modifier therapies [11].

Fibrosis, abnormal Ca2+ homeostasis and elevated reactive oxygen species are also predisposing factor to the onset of ventricular arrhythmias in DMD-DCM. Recently, a predisposition to pacing induced ventricular arrhythmias was demonstrated in an animal model of DMD. In this model, the aberrant Ca2+ release through RyR2, which leads to delayed after depolarizations (DADs) and triggered ventricular arrhythmias, was related to the oxidated Ca2+/calmodulin-dependent protein kinase II, Ox-CaMKII. Genetic inhibition of Ox-CaMKII normalized intracellular Ca2+ and prevented ventricular arrhythmias in this model [12]. Another interesting study suggested that arrhythmias could also result from an alteration of the components of the cardiac gap junction; in particular it has been proposed that the dislocation and anomalous S-nitrosylation of connexin 43 (Cx43) lead to the early depolarization of the cytoplasmic membrane and the consequent generation of action potentials. Then, these channels can be therapeutic targets to prevent fatal arrhythmias in patients with DMD [13].

3. Clinical course

The diagnosis of DMD may occur around 4 yo for difficulty in gait, calf hypertrophy, delayed speech, inability to jump or stand without using the arms for assistance (Gower maneuver), toe walking and difficulty in climbing stairs.

Over the time the progressive muscle waste leads to loss of ambulatory capacity and to decline of respiratory and cardiac functions [14].

Literature reports the beginning of ongoing cardiac disease processes as around 6–10 years of age. Echocardiographic abnormalities and clinical DCM can occur at any age but often appear around 14–15 yo and are common over 18 years of age [15]. Symptoms are mild or completely absent up to the most advanced stages of cardiomyopathy, and this is mainly due to the significant reduction in oxygen consumption and in energy expenditure consequent to muscle weakness. It is remarkable that often the severity of cardiomyopathy does not correlate with the degree of skeletal muscle weakness, thus regular cardiac evaluation is very important also in patients with mild motility impairment and it is required before any invasive diagnostic procedure or surgery.

In the last decade, the increase in life expectancy, deriving from the better management of the respiratory involvement and the improved supportive cares, have resulted in a sharp increase in the number of patients with severe cardiomyopathy, and to date, end-stage HF has becoming one of the leading causes of morbidity and mortality in DMD [6].

Data from a multicentre Pediatric Cardiomyopathy Registry (PCMR) show a high prevalence of DCM also in milder forms of dystrophinopathies as in BMD (up to 90% of cases). Interestingly, in these patients, detection of cardiomyopathy often occurs at a more advanced stage and the progression of the LV dysfunction and dilation may be more rapid than in patients with DMD. Despite this, mortality rate for DMD patients with DCM is significantly worse than that of BMD patients, who can undergo heart transplant [16].

4. Noninvasive assessing of DMD-DCM

From the time of DMD diagnosis, every effort should be focused to detect early the onset and the progression of DCM. Early recognition and periodic re-evaluation are essential to guide therapy and to identify patients at increased risk of progression of cardiomyopathy and major cardiac events. Clinical evaluation remains challenging because most of these patients have often low blood pressure values and cool extremities because of reduced skeletal muscular mass even in the presence of hemodynamic compensation. Therefore, multiparametric evaluation is crucial to correctly recognize the progression of cardiac impairment [8].

4.1 Cardiovascular biomarkers

Serum biomarkers are often very useful for the diagnosis and monitoring heart disease. In particular, serum levels of cardiac troponin I/T are known to be associated to the extension of myocardial damage, but there are conflicting results about their diagnostic and prognostic implications in the DMD-DCM. Actually, only troponin I showed to be reliable in patients with neuromuscular disorder [17]. Troponin I levels seem to be significantly elevated in patients with initial myocardial fibrosis expressed by mild late gadolinium enhancement (LGE) at the cardiac magnetic resonance (CMR) compared to those without LGE. Interestingly, this positive association between troponin levels and myocardial fibrosis is lost when LGE degree becomes moderate-to-severe, probably because at advanced stage of cardiomyopathy most of myocardium is already substituted by fibro-fatty tissue, therefore the release of myocardio-necrosis enzymes is reduced [18].

Natriuretic peptides are well established markers of HF and congestion in DCM. In DMD, pulmonary hypertension caused by impairment of the respiratory muscles and restrictive physiopathology are considered to be involved in the mechanism of increased values of plasma natriuretic peptide. In addition to the more commonly used brain natriuretic peptide (BNP), a significant elevation in plasma alpha-atrial natriuretic peptide (alphaANP) levels is found as a sign of a poor prognosis and may be a useful index for the management of patients with DMD-DCM [19].

In the management of HF is very important to assess renal function. In DMD serum creatinine values are generally very low as a consequence of their reduced muscle mass and therefore creatinine cannot be considered a good marker of renal function. In these patients, serum values of cystatin C, a protein produced by all cells, not only by muscle cells, are a good parameter for assessing renal function, because they better correlate with glomerular filtration rate (GFR) and cardiac dysfunction. Furthermore, it is reported a significant correlation between Cystatin C and cardiac dysfunction, providing for the first time a novel marker to identify cardio-renal syndrome in patients with DMD [20].

4.2 Electrocardiography and cardiac imaging

Electrocardiogram and transthoracic echocardiogram are the two fundamental exams advised to establish baseline cardiac involvement and they are recommended annually in all patients since the diagnosis of DMD. After the age of ten, cardiac assessment should have been *at least* yearly because of the increased risk of DCM. Even in the absence of abnormalities on the echocardiogram, a CMR should be performed in all children without contraindications from 7 years of age, when it is possible to perform this examination without the need for anesthesia, with the aim to detect early any regional dysfunction or myocardial fibrosis. When some abnormalities are found, controls should be more frequent [8].

Electrocardiographic (EKG) changes are very common (up to 90%). Initially, myocardial dystrophy may manifest itself as mild nonspecific EKG changes such as increased R-wave voltage in right or left precordial leads, QRS fragmentation, or slight alterations in ventricular repolarization. When cardiac disease is overt, R-wave voltage decreases and abnormal Q waves may appear generally in infero-lateral leads. ECG often shows also one of the following features: right axis deviation, conduction defects or short PR intervals, polyphasic R waves in V1, right bundle branch block, flat and inverted T waves, and prolonged heart rate-corrected QT interval. Sinus tachycardia is very common in DMD and, together with the reduction of circadian index and the scarce heart rate variability, it is a sign of the autonomic dysfunction that often affect these patients. 24-hours ECG monitoring is essential to detect autonomic dysfunction and it is recommended in case of suspect of arrhythmias and for routine monitoring of advanced stage of DMD-DCM, in which the presence of atrial fibrillation, atrial or ventricular arrhythmias may affect prognosis and change the management [21].

Echocardiography allows to identify the *LV dilation*, defined in children by a LV end-diastolic diameter that exceeds the mean value expected for age and sex by two standard deviations, and *LV systolic dysfunction*, defined by a LV ejection fraction (LVEF) <55% or a fractional shortening (FS) <28% [22]. Despite the advances in 2D and 3D techniques, FS is still considered the best surrogate of LV systolic function, among the echocardiographic possibilities, for its high reproducibility and its strong correlation with CMR LVEF [23]. Furthermore, routinely recognition of diastolic dysfunction is important because it is very frequent in all stages of DCM and can precede contractile impairment.

For earlier detection of LV impairment, speckle tracking echocardiography is also very useful, as it is a technique able to evaluate subclinical LV dysfunction before development of overt LVEF reduction. Global longitudinal strain (GLS), obtained by

2D speckle tracking echocardiography is abnormal in nearly 50% of DMD patients with a normal LVEF, and a decrease of 0,34% per year of GLS in DMD patients according to age has been recently reported [24]. The lowest values of strain is often observed in the inferolateral and anterolateral mid-basal segments. However, speckle tracking analysis is often limited in DMD because echocardiographic image quality is poor in these patients and declines by 2,5% for each 1 year increase in age because of chest deformities, lung hyperinflation, and limited mobility [25].

CMR is becoming the gold standard exam in the evaluation of DMD-DCM, especially because it allows a non-invasive myocardial tissue characterization by LGE and T1 mapping techniques, using non –ionizing radiations. It also offers the possibility to better analyze the size and global and regional kinetics of the left and right ventricles, not being limited by body habitus and providing a more accurate and reproducible three-dimensional views if compared to echocardiography. LGE identifies fibrosis, it may have a subepicardial or transmural distribution, it is often initially localized in the inferolateral wall, and its extension allows to stratify the severity of cardiac involvement. LGE is an independent predictor of adverse cardiac events in DMD patients, also in those with a preserved LVEF [26]. T1 mapping technique pre- and post-contrast is able to identify diffuse fibrosis even earlier than LGE but T1 mapping value varies a lot depending on the sequence used, and it cannot discriminate diffuse myocardial fibrosis from inflammation or fat infiltration [27]. Finally, CMR can also provide myocardial strain analysis, using feature-tracking technique.

CMR can be useful also to evaluate more precisely the severity of myocardial dysfunction and fibrosis in further stages, to assess the efficacy of anti-remodeling therapy, to screen asymptomatic DMD female carriers. However, the high costs, patient's claustrophobia and the technical difficulties to obtain the exam in patients with home ventilator may limit its use in this group of patients.

5. Management of DMD-DCM from prevention to end-stage HF

In the clinical course of DMD-DCM three stages of DCM can be distinguished: a *pre-clinical stage*, a *clinical stage* and an *end-stage DCM* (**Figure 2**).

The *pre-clinical stage* is characterized by normal dimension and function of the heart. It usually limited to the early teenager years of life. In this phase, although the LV contractile function is preserved (LVEF>55%), the process of myocyte damage and fibrotic myocardial replacement has generally already begun and it can manifest itself with nonspecific EKG changes, subtle local wall motion abnormalities, diastolic dysfunction consequent to cardiomyocyte hypertrophy, reduction in ventricular strain values and LGE at CMR.

At this stage of the DMD-DCM, the aim will be to delay the onset of ventricular contractile dysfunction. Current recommendation advices to start angiotensin converting enzyme inhibitor (ACE- I) as preventive strategy. Perindopril 2–4 mg/die, [28] or an angiotensin receptor blocker (ARB) can be prescribed in all DMD patients from the age of ten. The indication to start therapy earlier, in patients with initial signs of cardiac involvement (such as the presence of mild LGE) but with preserved contractile function is still under debate and investigation [8].

At this early phase of DCM, when LV is mildly dilated, the use of mineralocorticoid receptor antagonist (MRA), such as eplerenone or spironolactone, may slow the rate of decline of LV function. Further studies are needed to determine the effect of combined cardioprotective therapy on event-free survival in these patients [29, 30].

The *clinical stage* includes a wide range of patients, with various degree of LV dilation and dysfunction, without any symptoms or with initial signs or symptoms

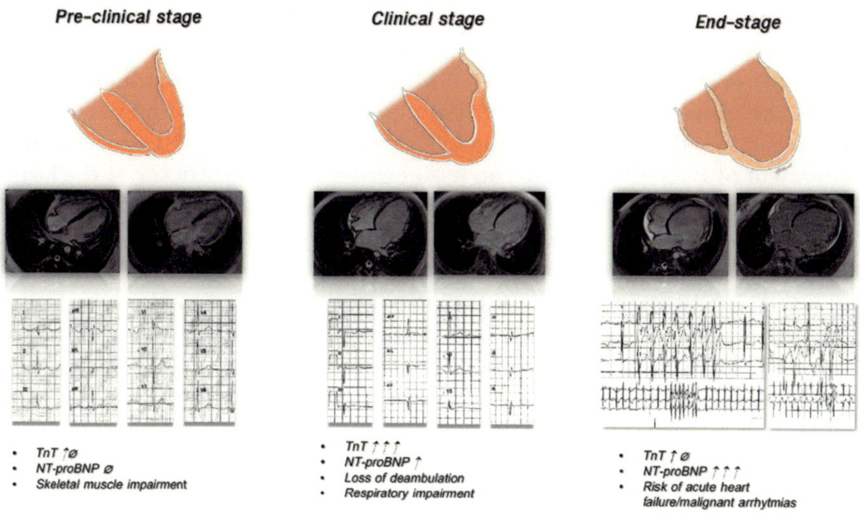

Figure 2.
Cardiac magnetic resonance (CMR), electrocardiographic (EKG) features and clinical status at different stages of the DMD-DCM progression. In the pre-clinical stage left ventricular (LV) function is still preserved, CMR may identify initial fibrosis, at the EKG some alterations such as QRS fragmentation, rsr' complexes in V1 and alterations of ventricular repolarization may appear, and blood levels of troponin T (TnT) may be slightly or moderately high while NTproBNP is normal. The clinical stage is characterized by a certain degree of LV dysfunction and dilation, inflammation and fibrotic replacement of the heart muscle are extended, as shown by the wide distribution of late gadolinium enhancement (LGE) areas at CMR imagines, abnormal Q waves appear at the ECG, and the values of TnT and NTpro BNP are usually very high and moderately high respectively. In the end-stage, LV dilation and dysfunction are severe, much of the heart muscle is replaced by fibrous tissue, filling pressure increases, and episodes of acute heart failure and ventricular arrhythmias become frequent, NTproBNP values are very high while TnT values may not be particularly high due to reduced total cardiac muscle mass.

of HF. This phase can start at any age but frequently it begins after the age of ten. Few studies have focused on treating DMD patients with mild to moderate LV systolic dysfunction (LVEF>30% <50%), and the current consensus statement supports the use of traditional treatment for HF to treat the progression of DCM. All patients with at least mild ventricular dysfunction should be treated with an ACE-I or an ARB. In particular lisinopril (ACE-I) and losartan (ARB) have shown equal effectiveness in preserving or improving ventricular function in established DCM [31]. Due to their ability to reduce the fibrotic process and stabilize LV systolic function, MRAs should be considered in this phase of DMD-DCM, even in case of mild reduction of LVEF, that is much earlier than indicated by current guidelines for the management of HF (symptomatic patients with LVEF <35%). In addition, a beta blockers (BB) such as carvedilol, is indicated when a sufficient improvement in cardiac function is not achieved with the initial therapy with ACE-I/ARB. Routine use of the BBs in DMD patients has been controversial in the past years due to conflicting results on their efficacy obtained from retrospective and non-randomized prospective studies. Nowadays, the superiority of combination therapy with an ACE-I/ARB and a BB over monotherapy with ACE-I/ARB is supported by studies that have shown more beneficial effect on LV function, on prevention of major cardiac events (death, deterioration of HF and severe arrhythmias) and on long-term survival [32–34]. Furthermore, in DMD-DCM, BBs are also useful to control sinus tachycardia caused by autonomic dysfunction and other forms of tachyarrhythmia.

The *end-stage* DCM is characterized by severe degree of LV dysfunction (LVEF <30%) and dilation, the patients might have signs and/or symptoms of HF. Also, they may have rhythm disturbances, with a higher risk of acute decompensation of HF and sudden cardiac death. Generally this phase occurs after the age of twenty but in some more aggressive forms of CMD it can manifest earlier. At this stage of disease every effort must be aimed to reduce acute events and hospitalizations and to improve symptoms and quality of life of these patients. Medical treatment includes a combination of an ACE-I/ARB, an MRA and a BB at the maximum tolerated or recommended dose, according to European and American Guidelines for the management of HF [35, 36]. Based on recent evidence of the efficacy of the heart rate reduction strategy in lowering the long term incidence of acute adverse events in DMD patients with advanced cardiac involvement, ivabradine should be considered if LVEF remains below 40% and heart rate above 70 bpm despite maximum dose of ACE-I/ARB and BB [37]. Furthermore these patients may also benefit from treatment with Sacubitril/Valsartan, the first-in-class angiotensin receptor neprilysin inhibitor (ARNI) that in last decade has become part of standard therapy for adult HF and it has shown excellent preliminary results in pediatric patients in the ongoing PANORAMA-HF trial (DMD patients included).

In end-stage CMD signs and symptoms of systemic or pulmonary congestion may be clinically evident and loop diuretics are indicated. For chronic use furosemide 1 to 6 mg/kg/die is generally effective, but in some cases the addiction of Metolazone, a thiazide-like diuretic, is required. It is important to underline that there is no evidence of the effectiveness of loop diuretics in improving survival, so they are to be considered only for relieving symptoms [38].

In patients with severe LV dysfunction an antithrombotic therapy should be considered in the primary prevention of thromboembolic events, although not routinely recommended [39].

As mentioned above, DMD patients are at risk of arrhythmias such as atrial fibrillation, atrial flutter and ventricular tachycardia and this risk increases as cardiomyopathy progresses. To date, the management of arrhythmias, with drugs and devices, in DMD-DCM is based on general international guidelines, as there are no specific recommendations for DMD. Implantable cardioverter defibrillator (ICD) has gained acceptance in selected patients [40]. The effectiveness of cardiac resynchronization therapy (CRT) in these patients seems to be poor probably due to the presence of the extensive postero-lateral fibrosis and poorly explored.

Patients with DMD are generally not considered suitable for cardiac transplant candidacy due to early walking impairment, predisposition to respiratory complications, and their short life expectancy. Heart transplant (HTx) has been considered in few highly selected cases in which respiratory compromise was not relevant and reported [40]. In BMD, HTx is considered in end stage phase of CMP.

Few cases of patients with end-stage DMD-DCM and preserved or only mild reduced respiratory function, left ventricle assist device (LVAD) has been considered as a destination therapy [41, 42]. To date, the international literature about LVAD in DMD patients is poor and proper selection of patient and ethical aspect should be accurately evaluated case by case. Share decision making process is also crucial and exploratory dialog with patients and caregivers should be routinely carried out during follow up, not only in urgent situation [43].

Recently, a retrospective study on DMD patients evaluated the effects of advanced cardiac therapies (i.e. ICD, LVAD, HTx) on large DMD population. Out of 436 DMD patients, 9 had ICD placed, 4 had LVAD and 1 HTx. The authors concluded that advanced HF therapies may be used effectively in select subjects with DMD but further studies are needed to stratify the risk and select patients [40].

In the process of choosing about advanced cardiac therapies for end-stage DMD-DCM an in-depth personalized assessment is crucial, and involves the collaboration of the patient and his family with a team of experts composed of cardiologists, cardiac surgeons, neuromuscular specialists, anesthetists, pneumologists, bioethics experts and psychologists.

6. DMD-specific drugs: corticosteroids and new target therapies

Given their effectiveness in slowing the progression of muscle damage and in prolonging the ability to walk and the life-expectancy, corticosteroids such as prednisone and deflazacort have become the standard basic treatment of patients with DMD from the moment of diagnosis or, in any case, by the age of five [44]. While some preclinical studies have suggested that corticosteroids can accelerate cardiomyopathy, subsequent clinical studies have supported their beneficial role in preserving ventricular function and delaying the progression of heart disease, especially by slowing down the inflammation and the fibrotic process and by increasing myogenic repair and myoblast proliferation [45].

Schram et al. [46] showed that steroid therapy was associated with a significantly lower all-cause mortality rate, due to a substantial reduction in HF–related deaths. In this observational study, patients treated with combination of steroid and ACE-I, experienced a much lower incidence of new-onset cardiomyopathy than those treated without steroid.

In recent years a new MRA, called Vamorolone, has been discovered. This new MRA is able to mimic the anti-inflammatory effects of glucocorticoids and it could represent, in the near future, an alternative to the others. It has been reported it seems to have less side effects and greater antifibrotic effect thanks to the inhibition of the aldosterone pathway [47].

Moreover, several other new therapeutic strategies are under investigation, focused to mitigate inflammation and fibrosis or to restore the dystrophin expression. These last strategy includes:

- *the read-through therapies*, such as Ataluren (Translarna™, PTC Therap), the first molecule approved in Europe for DMD, that enables the transcription of mRNA containing premature stop codons;

- *the antisense oligonucleotides (AONs)* that can bind pre-mRNA in specific splicing sites allowing to skip the exons containing mutations and restoring the reading frame of the dystrophin;

- *the viral gene therapies,* that exploit viral vectors to transfer truncated versions of dystrophin gene into myocytes;

- *the upregulation of Utrophin*, a protein similar to dystrophin, that can supply its structural function;

- *the cell based therapies* that consist on the administration of healthy myocytes precursors that can colonize skeletal and cardiac muscle of the recipient.

Most of these gene-targeted therapies are still under study and the evaluation of their efficacy is mainly based on the increased expression of dystrophin in skeletal myocytes and on the slowing of the myopathy progression. Whether these therapies are able to increase dystrophin expression equally in skeletal muscle cells and in cardiomyocytes is still unclear since the heart cannot be routinely biopsied. This is a crucial point as isolated improvement in muscle function would lead to increased demand on a weak heart, accelerating the progression of cardiomyopathy. In particular, Ataluren has shown a modest increase in dystrophin expression in mouse heart, while in a small cohort of humans neither measurable improvement nor deterioration in heart function were observed during 24 months of treatment. Instead, there are strong evidences regarding the benefit on heart function from gene therapies that use micro-dystrophin genes. In preclinical studies a robust expression of micro-dystrophin in cardiomyocytes has been proved, but the high dose required may be burdened significant side effects and the presence of micro-dystrophin instead of wild-type dystrophin can still lead to the development of a BMD-like cardiomyopathy. Further studies are needed to better understand the long-term effects of these therapies on the heart [48].

6.1 Cardiomyopathy in DMD female carriers

Most women carrying the DMD mutation in one of the two X chromosomes are asymptomatic for life due to the presence of sufficient normal dystrophin produced by the unchanged allele of the gene. Some of these women, called "manifesting carriers", may have mild or moderate forms of myopathy and cardiomyopathy; this is probably due to a mosaic inactivation of the healthy allele in skeletal and heart muscles, or simply to the reduced total amount of normal dystrophin in the cells. In particular, cardiomyopathy can occur in up to 8% of cases and symptoms can appear from adolescence to late adulthood even without any correlation with musculoskeletal manifestations [49]. Therefore, current guidelines recommend to perform echocardiography every 5 years in all adult dystrophinopathy carriers [14]. The severity of disease can vary widely and can worsen during concomitant events such as pregnancy and childbirth. It is interesting to note that in 45% of DMD carriers, subepicardial LGE in the inferolateral free LV wall is detectable at CMR as well as in the initial forms of cardiomyopathy in DMD male patients and this is associated with myocardial enzyme release and with a greater probability of progression of the cardiomyopathy [50].

7. Conclusion

Given the primary role of cardiomyopathy in determining the prognosis of DMD patients, every effort should be focused on preventing or slowing the progression of their cardiac dysfunction. Many drugs commonly used for HF have proven to be quite effective, especially if used from the very early stages of the disease, before heart dysfunction becomes evident. So current recommendations underline the importance of routinely cardiac evaluation since the diagnosis of DMD to early recognize heart abnormalities and start ACE-I. In this preclinical stage of DMD-DCM, CMR plays a substantial role due to its sensitivity in identifying initial areas of fibrotic replacement of the heart muscle. Because of the lack of specific DMD-DCM therapies, current drugs used for HF might be used and further studies are required to address their efficacy, especially at end-stage DCM. To date some new target therapies are available and many others are under evaluation, so that in the near future we will be able to count on a much wider range of specific therapeutic possibilities than now. Moreover, in the end-of- life management, ethical issues are still a matter of intense debate in order to identify potential advanced cardiac therapies candidates. Surely, in this challenging course of treatment, sharing decisions with the patient and his caregivers and the support of a multidisciplinary team are crucial cornerstones for obtaining the best possible results.

Conflict of interest

The authors declare no conflict of interest.

Author details

Rachele Adorisio[1*], Erica Mencarelli[1], Nicoletta Cantarutti[1] and Maria Grandinetti[1,2]

1 Department of Cardiac Surgery, Cardiology and Heart Lung Transplant, Bambino Gesù Children Hospital and Research Institute, Rome, Italy

2 Department of Cardiovascular and Thoracic Sciences, Fondazione Policlinico Universitario A. Gemelli IRCCS, Rome, Italy

*Address all correspondence to: rachele.adorisio@opbg.net

References

[1] Lim KRQ, Sheri N, Nguyen Q, Yokota T. Cardiac Involvement in Dystrophin-Deficient Females: Current Understanding and Implications for the Treatment of Dystrophinopathies. Genes (Basel). 2020 Jul 8;11(7):765. doi: 10.3390/genes11070765.

[2] Tandon A, Villa CR, Hor KN, Jefferies JL, Gao Z, Towbin JA, Wong BL, Mazur W, Fleck RJ, Sticka JJ, Benson DW, Taylor MD. Myocardial fibrosis burden predicts left ventricular ejection fraction and is associated with age and steroid treatment duration in duchenne muscular dystrophy. J Am Heart Assoc. 2015 Mar 26;4(4):e001338. doi: 10.1161/JAHA.114.001338.

[3] Hor KN, Taylor MD, Al-Khalidi HR, Cripe LH, Raman SV, Jefferies JL, O'Donnell R, Benson DW, Mazur W. Prevalence and distribution of late gadolinium enhancement in a large population of patients with Duchenne muscular dystrophy: effect of age and left ventricular systolic function. J Cardiovasc Magn Reson. 2013 Dec 21;15(1):107. doi: 10.1186/1532-429X-15-107.

[4] D'Amario D, Amodeo A, Adorisio R, Tiziano FD, Leone AM, Perri G, Bruno P, Massetti M, Ferlini A, Pane M, Niccoli G, Porto I, D'Angelo GA, Borovac JA, Mercuri E, Crea F. A current approach to heart failure in Duchenne muscular dystrophy. Heart. 2017 Nov;103(22):1770-1779. doi: 10.1136/heartjnl-2017-311269. Epub 2017 Jul 1.

[5] Fayssoil A, Yaou RB, Ogna A, Leturcq F, Nardi O, Clair B, Wahbi K, Lofaso F, Laforet P, Duboc D, Orlikowski D, Annane D. Clinical profiles and prognosis of acute heart failure in adult patients with dystrophinopathies on home mechanical ventilation. ESC Heart Fail. 2017 Nov;4(4):527-534. doi: 10.1002/ehf2.12165. Epub 2017 May 18.

[6] Buddhe S, Cripe L, Friedland-Little J, Kertesz N, Eghtesady P, Finder J, Hor K, Judge DP, Kinnett K, McNally EM, Raman S, Thompson WR, Wagner KR, Olson AK. Cardiac Management of the Patient With Duchenne Muscular Dystrophy. Pediatrics. 2018 Oct;142(Suppl 2):S72-S81. doi: 10.1542/peds.2018-0333I.

[7] Eagle M, Baudouin SV, Chandler C, Giddings DR, Bullock R, Bushby K. Survival in Duchenne muscular dystrophy: improvements in life expectancy since 1967 and the impact of home nocturnal ventilation. Neuromuscul Disord. 2002 Dec;12(10):926-9. doi: 10.1016/s0960-8966(02)00140-2

[8] Birnkrant DJ, Bushby K, Bann CM, Alman BA, Apkon SD, Blackwell A, Case LE, Cripe L, Hadjiyannakis S, Olson AK, Sheehan DW, Bolen J, Weber DR, Ward LM; DMD Care Considerations Working Group. Diagnosis and management of Duchenne muscular dystrophy, part 2: respiratory, cardiac, bone health, and orthopaedic management. Lancet Neurol. 2018 Apr;17(4):347-361. doi: 10.1016/S1474-4422(18)30025-5. Epub 2018 Feb 3.

[9] D'Amario D, Gowran A, Canonico F, Castiglioni E, Rovina D, Santoro R, Spinelli P, Adorisio R, Amodeo A, Perrucci GL, Borovac JA, Pompilio G, Crea F. Dystrophin Cardiomyopathies: Clinical Management, Molecular Pathogenesis and Evolution towards Precision Medicine. J Clin Med. 2018 Sep 19;7(9):291. doi: 10.3390/jcm7090291.

[10] Frankel KA, Rosser RJ. The pathology of the heart in progressive muscular dystrophy: epimyocardial

fibrosis. Hum Pathol. 1976 Jul;7(4):375-86. doi: 10.1016/s0046-8177(76)80053-6.

[11] van Westering TL, Betts CA, Wood MJ. Current understanding of molecular pathology and treatment of cardiomyopathy in duchenne muscular dystrophy. Molecules. 2015 May 15;20(5):8823-55. doi: 10.3390/molecules20058823.

[12] Wang Q, Quick AP, Cao S, Reynolds J, Chiang DY, Beavers D, Li N, Wang G, Rodney GG, Anderson ME, Wehrens XHT. Oxidized CaMKII (Ca2+/Calmodulin-Dependent Protein Kinase II) Is Essential for Ventricular Arrhythmia in a Mouse Model of Duchenne Muscular Dystrophy. Circ Arrhythm Electrophysiol. 2018 Apr;11(4):e005682. doi: 10.1161/CIRCEP.117.005682.

[13] Lillo MA, Himelman E, Shirokova N, Xie LH, Fraidenraich D, ContrerasJE.S-nitrosylationofconnexin43 hemichannels elicits cardiac stress-induced arrhythmias in Duchenne muscular dystrophy mice. JCI Insight. 2019 Dec 19;4(24). pii: 130091.

[14] Bushby K, Finkel R, Birnkrant DJ, Case LE, Clemens PR, Cripe L, Kaul A, Kinnett K, McDonald C, Pandya S, Poysky J, Shapiro F, Tomezsko J, Constantin C; DMD Care Considerations Working Group. Diagnosis and management of Duchenne muscular dystrophy, part 2: implementation of multidisciplinary care. Lancet Neurol. 2010 Feb;9(2):177-89. doi: 10.1016/S1474-4422(09)70272-8.

[15] Nigro G, Comi LI, Politano L, Bain RJ. The incidence and evolution of cardiomyopathy in Duchenne muscular dystrophy. Int J Cardiol. 1990 Mar;26(3):271-7. doi: 10.1016/0167-5273(90)90082-g.

[16] Connuck DM, Sleeper LA, Colan SD, Cox GF, Towbin JA, Lowe AM, Wilkinson JD, Orav EJ, Cuniberti L, Salbert BA, Lipshultz SE; Pediatric Cardiomyopathy Registry Study Group. Characteristics and outcomes of cardiomyopathy in children with Duchenne or Becker muscular dystrophy: a comparative study from the Pediatric Cardiomyopathy Registry. Am Heart J. 2008 Jun;155(6):998-1005. doi: 10.1016/j.ahj.2008.01.018. Epub 2008 Mar 19.

[17] Schmid J, Birner Gruenberger R, Liesinger L, Stojakovic T, Scharnagl H, Dieplinger B, Asslaber M, Radl R, Polacin M, Beer M, Szolar D, Quasthoff S, Binder J.S., Rainer P. Elevated cardiac troponin T but not troponin I in patients with skeletal muscle disease. European Heart Journal (2017) 38 (Supplement), 553554.

[18] Voleti S, Olivieri L, Hamann K, Gordish-Dressman H, Spurney C. Troponin I Levels Correlate with Cardiac MR LGE and Native T1 Values in Duchenne Muscular Dystrophy Cardiomyopathy and Identify Early Disease Progression. Pediatr Cardiol . 2020 May 31. doi: 10.1007/s00246-020-02372-5.

[19] Yanagisawa A, Yokota N, Miyagawa M, Kawamura J, Ishihara T, Aoyagi T, Ishikawa K. Plasma levels of atrial natriuretic peptide in patients with Duchenne's progressive muscular dystrophy. Am Heart J. 1990 Nov;120(5):1154-8. doi: 10.1016/0002-8703(90)90130-p.

[20] Villa CR, Kaddourah A, Mathew J, Ryan TD, Wong BL, Goldstein SL, Jefferies JL. Identifying evidence of cardio-renal syndrome in patients with Duchenne muscular dystrophy using cystatin C. Neuromuscul Disord. 2016 Oct;26(10):637-642

[21] Fayssoil A, Abasse S, Silverston K. Cardiac Involvement Classification and Therapeutic Management in Patients

with Duchenne Muscular Dystrophy. J Neuromuscul Dis. 2017;4(1):17-23. doi: 10.3233/JND-160194.

[22] Soslow JH, Xu M, Slaughter JC, Stanley M, Crum K, Markham LW, Parra DA.Evaluation of Echo cardiographic Measures of Left Ventricular Function in Patients with Duchenne Muscular Dystrophy: Assessment of Reproducibility and Comparison to Cardiac Magnetic Resonance Imaging. J Am Soc Echocardiogr. 2016 Oct;29(10):983-991. doi: 10.1016/j.echo.2016.07.001.

[23] Spurney CF, McCaffrey FM, Cnaan A, Morgenroth LP, Ghelani SJ, Gordish-Dressman H, Arrieta A, Connolly AM, Lotze TE, McDonald CM, Leshner RT, Clemens PR. Feasibility and Reproducibility of Echocardiographic Measures in Children with Muscular Dystrophies. J Am Soc Echocardiogr. 2015 Aug;28(8):999-1008. doi: 10.1016/j.echo.2015.03.003.

[24] Vincenti M, De La Villeon G, Lavastre K, Barrea C, Guillaumont S, Bredy C, Gamon L, Meli AC, Cazorla O, Fauconnier J, Meyer P, Rivier F, Adda J, Mura T, Lacampagne A. Speckle-Tracking Echocardiography in Children With Duchenne Muscular Dystrophy: A Prospective Multicenter Controlled Cross-Sectional Study. J Am Soc Echocardiogr. 2019 Mar;32(3):412-422. doi: 10.1016/j.echo.2018.10.017.

[25] Power A, Poonja S, Disler D, Myers K, Patton DJ, Mah JK, Fine NM, Greenway SC. Echocardiographic Image Quality Deteriorates with Age in Children and Young Adults with Duchenne Muscular Dystrophy. Front Cardiovasc Med. 2017 Dec 20;4:82. doi: 10.3389/fcvm.2017.00082.

[26] Florian A, Ludwig A, Engelen M, Waltenberger J, Rösch S, Sechtem U, Yilmaz A. Left ventricular systolic function and the pattern of late-gadolinium-enhancement independently and additively predict adverse cardiac events in muscular dystrophy patients. J Cardiovasc Magn Reson. 2014 Sep 25;16(1):81. doi: 10.1186/s12968-014-0081-1.

[27] Olivieri LJ, Kellman P, McCarter RJ, Cross RR, Hansen MS, Spurney CF. Native T1 values identify myocardial changes and stratify disease severity in patients with Duchenne muscular dystrophy. J Cardiovasc Magn Reson. 2016 Oct 28;18(1):72. doi: 10.1186/s12968-016-0292-8.

[28] Duboc D, Meune C, Lerebours G, Devaux JY, Vaksmann G, Bécane HM. Effect of perindopril on the onset and progression of left ventricular dysfunction in Duchenne muscular dystrophy. J Am Coll Cardiol. 2005 Mar 15;45(6):855-7. doi: 10.1016/j.jacc.2004.09.078.

[29] Raman SV, Hor KN, Mazur W, Halnon NJ, Kissel JT, He X, Tran T, Smart S, McCarthy B, Taylor MD, Jefferies JL, Rafael-Fortney JA, Lowe J, Roble SL, Cripe LH. Eplerenone for early cardiomyopathy in Duchenne muscular dystrophy: a randomised, double-blind, placebo-controlled trial. Lancet Neurol. 2015 Feb;14(2):153-61. doi: 10.1016/S1474-4422(14)70318-7.

[30] Raman SV, Hor KN, Mazur W, Cardona A, He X, Halnon N, Markham L, Soslow JH, Puchalski MD, Auerbach SR, Truong U, Smart S, McCarthy B, Saeed IM, Statland JM, Kissel JT, Cripe LH. Stabilization of Early Duchenne Cardiomyopathy With Aldosterone Inhibition: Results of the Multicenter AIDMD Trial. J Am Heart Assoc 2019, 8, e013501. DOI: 10.1161/JAHA.119.013501

[31] Allen HD, Flanigan KM, Thrush PT, Dvorchik I, Yin H, Canter C, Connolly AM, Parrish M, McDonald CM, Braunlin E, Colan SD, Day J, Darras B, Mendell JR. A randomized, double-blind trial of lisinopril and losartan for

the treatment of cardiomyopathy in Duchenne muscular dystrophy. PLoS Curr 2013, 5. DOI: 10.1371/currents.md.2cc69a1dae4be7dfe2bcb420024ea865

[32] Rhodes J, Margossian R, Darras BT, Colan SD, Jenkins KJ, Geva T, Powell AJ. Safety and efficacy of carvedilol therapy for patients with dilated cardiomyopathy secondary to muscular dystrophy. Pediatr Cardiol 2008, 29, 343-351. DOI: 10.1007/s00246-007-9113-z

[33] Matsumura T, Tamura T, Kuru S, Kikuchi Y, Kawai M. Carvedilol can prevent cardiac events in Duchenne muscular dystrophy. Intern Med 2010, 49, 1357-1363. DOI: 10.2169/internalmedicine.49.3259.

[34] Ogata H, Ishikawa Y, Ishikawa Y, Minami R. Beneficial effects of beta-blockers and angiotensin-converting enzyme inhibitors in Duchenne muscular dystrophy. J Cardiol 2009, 53, 72-78. DOI: 10.1016/j.jjcc.2008.08.013.

[35] Yancy CW, Jessup M, Bozkurt B, Butler J, Casey DE Jr, Drazner MH, Fonarow GC, Geraci SA, Horwich T, Januzzi JL, Johnson MR, Kasper EK, Levy WC, Masoudi FA, McBride PE, McMurray JJ, Mitchell JE, Peterson PN, Riegel B, Sam F, Stevenson LW, Tang WH, Tsai EJ, Wilkoff BL; American College of Cardiology Foundation; American Heart Association Task Force on Practice Guidelines. 2013 ACCF/AHA guideline for the management of heart failure: a report of the American College of Cardiology Foundation/American Heart Association Task Force on Practice Guidelines. J Am Coll Cardiol 2013, 62, 147-239. DOI: 10.1016/j.jacc.2013.05.019.

[36] Ponikowski P, Voors AA, Anker SD, Bueno H, Cleland JG, Coats AJ, Falk V, González-Juanatey JR, Harjola VP, Jankowska EA, Jessup M, Linde C, Nihoyannopoulos P, Parissis JT, Pieske B, Riley JP, Rosano GM, Ruilope LM, Ruschitzka F, Rutten FH, van der Meer P; Authors/Task Force Members; Document Reviewers. 2016 ESC Guidelines for the diagnosis and treatment of acute and chronic heart failure: The Task Force for the diagnosis and treatment of acute and chronic heart failure of the European Society of Cardiology (ESC). Eur J Heart Fail 2016, 18, 891-975. DOI: 10.1002/ejhf.592.

[37] Adorisio R, Calvieri C, Cantarutti N, D'Amico A, Catteruccia M, Bertini E, Baban A, Filippelli S, Perri G, Amodeo A, Drago F. Heart rate reduction strategy using ivabradine in end-stage Duchenne cardiomyopathy. Int J Cardiol 2019, 280, 99-103. DOI: 10.1016/j.ijcard.2019.01.052.

[38] Mullens W, Damman K, Harjola VP, Mebazaa A, Brunner-La Rocca HP, Martens P, Testani JM, Tang WHW, Orso F, Rossignol P, Metra M, Filippatos G, Seferovic PM, Ruschitzka F, Coats AJ. The use of diuretics in heart failure with congestion - a position statement from the Heart Failure Association of the European Society of Cardiology. Eur J Heart Fail. 2019 Feb;21(2):137-155. doi: 10.1002/ejhf.1369.

[39] Kirk R, Dipchand AI, Rosenthal DN, Addonizio L, Burch M, Chrisant M, Dubin A, Everitt M, Gajarski R, Mertens L, Miyamoto S, Morales D, Pahl E, Shaddy R, Towbin J, Weintraub R. The International Society for Heart and Lung Transplantation Guidelines for the management of pediatric heart failure: Executive summary. J Heart Lung Transplant 2014, 33, 888-909. DOI: 10.1016/j.healun.2014.06.002

[40] Amodeo A, Adorisio R. Left ventricular assist device in Duchenne cardiomyopathy: can we change the natural history of cardiac disease? Int

J Cardiol. 2012 Nov 29;161(3):e43. doi: 10.1016/j.ijcard.2012.04.009.

[41] Perri G, Filippelli S, Adorisio R, Iacobelli R, Iodice F, Testa G, Paglietti MG, D'Amario D, Massetti M, Amodeo A. Left ventricular assist device as destination therapy in cardiac end-stage dystrophinopathies: Midterm results. J Thorac Cardiovasc Surg. 2017 Mar; 153(3):669-674. doi:10.1016/j.jtcvs.2016.08.016

[42] Wittlieb-Weber CA, Villa CR, Conway J, Bock MJ, Gambetta KE, Johnson JN, Lal AK, Schumacher KR, Law SP, Deshpande SR, West SC, Friedland-Little JM, Lytrivi ID, McCulloch MA, Butts RJ, Weber DR, Knecht KR. Use of advanced heart failure therapies in Duchenne muscular dystrophy. Prog Pediatr Cardiol. 2019 Jun;53:11-14. doi: 10.1016/j.ppedcard.2019.01.001.

[43] McNally EM, Kaltman JR, Benson DW, Canter CE, Cripe LH, Duan D, Finder JD, Groh WJ, Hoffman EP, Judge DP, Kertesz N, Kinnett K, Kirsch R, Metzger JM, Pearson GD, Rafael-Fortney JA, Raman SV, Spurney CF, Targum SL, Wagner KR, Markham LW; Working Group of the National Heart, Lung, and Blood Institute; Parent Project Muscular Dystrophy. Contemporary cardiac issues in Duchenne muscular dystrophy. Working Group of the National Heart, Lung, and Blood Institute in collaboration with Parent Project Muscular Dystrophy. Circulation. 2015 May 5;131(18):1590-8. doi: 10.1161/CIRCULATIONAHA.114.015151.

[44] Bello L, Gordish-Dressman H, Morgenroth LP, Henricson EK, Duong T, Hoffman EP, Cnaan A, McDonald CM; CINRG Investigators. Prednisone/prednisolone and deflazacort regimens in the CINRG Duchenne Natural History Study. Neurology. 2015 Sep 22;85(12):1048-55. doi: 10.1212/WNL.0000000000001950.

[45] Markham LW, Kinnett K, Wong BL, Woodrow Benson D, Cripe LH. Corticosteroid treatment retards development of ventricular dysfunction in Duchenne muscular dystrophy. Neuromuscul Disord. 2008 May;18(5):365-70. doi: 10.1016/j.nmd.2008.03.002.

[46] Schram G, Fournier A, Leduc H, Dahdah N, Therien J, Vanasse M, Khairy P. All-cause mortality and cardiovascular outcomes with prophylactic steroid therapy in Duchenne muscular dystrophy. J Am Coll Cardiol. 2013 Mar 5;61(9):948-54. doi: 10.1016/j.jacc.2012.12.008

[47] Heier CR, Yu Q, Fiorillo AA, Tully CB, Tucker A, Mazala DA, Uaesoontrachoon K, Srinivassane S, Damsker JM, Hoffman EP, Nagaraju K, Spurney CF. Life Sci Alliance. 2019 Feb 11;2(1):e201800186. doi: 10.26508/lsa.201800186. Print 2019 Feb.

[48] Meyers TA, Townsend D. Cardiac Pathophysiology and the Future of Cardiac Therapies in Duchenne Muscular Dystrophy. Int J Mol Sci. 2019 Aug 22;20(17):4098. doi: 10.3390/ijms20174098.

[49] Finsterer J, Stollberger C. Muscle, cardiac, and cerebral manifestations in female carriers of dystrophin variants. J. Neurol. Sci. 2018;388:107-108. doi: 10.1016/j.jns.2018.03.01

[50] Wexberg P, Avanzini M, Mascherbauer J, Pfaffenberger S, Freudenthaler B, Bittner R, Bernert G, Weidinger F. Myocardial late gadolinium enhancement is associated with clinical presentation in Duchenne muscular dystrophy carriers. J Cardiovasc Magn Reson. 2016 Sep 22;18(1):61. doi: 10.1186/s12968-016-0281-y.

Chapter 16

Peripartum Cardiomyopathy: The Hidden Enemy

Fatima Zahra Merzouk, Sara Oualim and Mohammed Sabry

Abstract

Peripartum cardiomyopathy (PPCM) is the most common cardiomyopathy in pregnancy. It is potentially life-threatening. It is, diagnosed in women without a history of heart disease 1 month before delivery or within 5 months. It is marked by heart failure and left ventricular dyshfunction. The evolution is favorable. LV function improves within 6 months in the majority of patients, but long-lasting mortality and morbidity are not infrequent. Recent work suggests the critical toxic role for late-gestational hormones on the maternal vasculature and the genetic underpinnings of PPCM. Complications include different types of supraventricular and ventricular arrhythmias, heart failure and ischemic stroke. The brain natriuretic peptide (BNP) can be used to risk stratify women for adverse events. Management of peripartum cardiomyopathy is based on treatment of heart failure. The addition of bromocriptine seemed to improve LVEF. Close monitoring of pregnant women with cardiomyopathy by multidisciplinary team is recommended.

Keywords: pregnancy, cardiomyopathy, heart failure

1. Introduction

In the 1800s, heart failure associated with pregnancy and the peripartum period was recognized for the first time by Virchow and others [1]. However, the term peripartum cardiomyopathy (PPCM) was not introduced until 1971 by Demakis and Rahimtoola [2]. Those authors, specifically defined the syndrome as occurring in the peripartum period.

In 2010, the European Society of Cardiology provided operational definition of PPCM as cardiomyopathy with reduced EF, usually <45%, presenting toward the end of pregnancy or in the months after delivery in a woman without previously known structural heart disease [3]. Cardiac imaging before clinical presentation is almost never available in these young women, therefore, the absence of preexisting heart disease is usually only presumed [4].

Why this interest in peripartum cardiomyopathy? It is both the most common cardiomyopathy in pregnancy and the most common non-obstetric cause of maternal death.

The timing of PPCM is not certain. Most cases occur in the first weeks after delivery [2].

However, it can also present well before and up to months after delivery.

These uncertainties make the definition of this disease imprecise and reflects our still incomplete understanding of PPCM.

IntechOpen

Many potential causes have been proposed, including autoimmunity, viral myocarditis, nutritional deficiencies, and hemodynamic stresses [5]. Most recently, a role for vascular dysfunction, hormonal insults, and underlying genetics has been suggested. But, the cause of PPCM remains unknown.

Clinical recognition is integral to the management of this disease, because there must be careful exclusion of alternative etiologies. Specific diagnostic or prognostic tests are lacking.

Management of peripartum cardiomyopathy is based on standard heart failure therapy. The addition of bromocriptine seemed to improve LVEF.

2. Epidemiology

The reported incidence of PPCM varies between 1:100 and 1:20 000 deliveries worldwide and between races within countries. Accurate data are lacking because of the paucity of population-based registries.

The Kaiser Permanente Health system, which is the USA's largest non-profit health plan including 9.9 million members, provided data that identified pregnant women with heart failure from 2003 to 2014 [6]. Among these women, PPCM occurred in 333 (68.2%). An analysis of 64 million discharge US hospital records from 1000 hospitals in 47 states identified 34 219 cases of PPCM, with an incidence of 1 in 968 births [7].

A higher incidence of disease is found among African-American woman, who are 3-to 16-fold more likely to be diagnosed with PPCM [8, 9]. The incidence of PPCM in Africa and Asia suggest an incidence of $\approx$1 in 1000 live births [6]. Women of African descent are more likely to develop PPCM.

However, there are some striking hot spots of PPCM, the cause of which remains unclear. In northern Nigeria, the incidence of PPCM may be as much as 1 in 100 live births [10]. In Haiti, the incidence of PPCM has been reported as high as 1 in 300 live births [11] possibly related to racial background, a high prevalence of preeclampsia or nutritional deficiencies.

An increasing trend of PPCM has been reported in many studies. For example, from 8.5 to 11.8 per 10 000 live births between 2004 and 2011 [7] and from 2.3 to 4.5 per 10 000 live births between 1990 and 2002 [12]. This increasing incidence is probably related to the increased recognition and diagnosis of disease, rising maternal age and multifetal pregnancies, or changing demographics [12, 13].

As the incidence of PPCM increases, the mortality increases as well. In a Californian study of maternal cardiovascular deaths between 2002 and 2006, PPCM was the leading cause (23%) [14].

3. Predisposing factors

Risk factors for PPCM are not understood. Studies have shown that increasing age, African ethnicity, pre-eclampsia, multiparity, malnutrition and traditional risk factors for cardiovascular disease, such as hypertension, diabetes and smoking, are associated with PPCM.

3.1 Age

The incidence of PPCM is associated with age. More than 50% of cases occur in women over 30 years of age [7, 8] with an odds ratio of 10 in a comparison of women less than 20 years of age [7].

Although the disease can strike women of any age, most women in the United States are diagnosed in women older than 30 years [15].

3.2 Race

PPCM affects black women more often. A study in California noted an incidence of PPCM in blacks of 1 in 1421, nearly 3 times that in whites [8].

In a population study of cases in North Carolina in 2003, the incidence of PPCM in black women was 4 times that of white women (1,1087 versus 1,4266), and the fatality rate at 5-year follow-up was also 4 times as high (24% versus 6%) [16].

3.3 Preeclampsia and eclampsia

Preeclampsia strongly predispose to PPCM. However, it is important to realize that PPCM is not simply a manifestation of severe preeclampsia.

A meta-analysis of 22 studies covering 979 cases of PPCM showed an overall prevalence of preeclampsia of 22%, >4 times the 3–5% population prevalence [17]. The prevalence of preeclampsia in many of these studies may be underestimated because preeclampsia is often underreported and because the presence of preeclampsia is often used as an exclusion criterion from the diagnosis of PPCM.

PPCM is also frequently found in association with eclampsia, with an odds ratio of 12.9 in a California population study of 1888 patients with eclampsia [18].

It is important to realize that preeclampsia can also trigger pulmonary edema in the absence of PPCM. The cardiac toxicity caused by preeclampsia can be clinically silent but can also present as pulmonary edema with preserved EF or as part of PPCM. A number of echocardiographic studies have shown that preeclampsia causes diastolic dysfunction even in the absence of clinical heart failure [19]. This diastolic dysfunction is independent from blood pressure elevations and can persist up to 1 year after delivery and resolution of preeclampsia [4].

The strong association between preeclampsia and PPCM suggests that they may share pathophysiological mechanisms. The suspicion for PPCM should never be lowered in the presence of preeclampsia.

3.4 Multiple gestations

Rate of twin births is generally higher in reports of PPCM than in the general population.

PPCM is frequently reported in cases of multigestational status. According to a meta-analysis, the average rate of twin gestations in cases of PPCM across 16 studies was 9% well above the average estimated prevalence of 3% [17, 20].

Although multiparity has traditionally been defined as a risk factor for PPCM, recent studies have shown that the majority of cases of PPCM in the US occur during the first or second pregnancy [2, 15].

3.5 Hypertension

According to a meta-analysis covering 979 cases of PPCM, hypertensive disorder was present in 37% (range, 29–45%) of cases [17]. A study of US hospital discharge records in 6 states identified 535 patients with PPCM, of whom 46.9% had hypertension (odds ratio, 13.4) [21].

We may say that hypertension strongly predispose to PPCM.

3.6 Other factors

Substance abuse, anemia, asthma, diabetes mellitus, obesity, and malnutrition are other associated conditions that have been reported but less well substantiated.

4. Hemodynamic changes during normal pregnancy

4.1 Antepartum changes

During pregnancy, several hemodynamic changes occur [22]:

- *Preload increases:* Maternal blood volume begins to increase at 6 weeks' gestation. By the second trimester, maternal blood volume increases to 50% above baseline. This effect leads to increased preload and left ventricular end-diastolic volume.

- *Afterload decreases:* As the uterine circulation increases during the first trimester, the systemic vascular resistance falls. There is further peripheral vasodilatation that occurs, likely from decreased vascular responsiveness to angiotensin and norepinephrine. These cumulative changes result in a decrease in maternal blood pressure.

- *Heart rate increases*: The heart rate increases by 15–20% by the third trimester (secondary to increased sympathetic tone).

In normal pregnancy, cardiac output increases by 30–50% through increased stroke volume during the first two trimesters. During the second part of pregnancy, cardiac output increases through an increase in heart rate. These changes are illustrated in **Figure 1**.

Cardiac output varies by maternal position. When supine, the gravid uterus can compress the inferior vena cava and impede venous return to heart and the cardiac output can decrease by 25%.

Despite these dramatic hemodynamic alterations, intrinsic left ventricular contractility does not appear to change appreciably [24]. The cardiac atria and ventricles must, however, accommodate the pregnancy-induced hypervolemia.

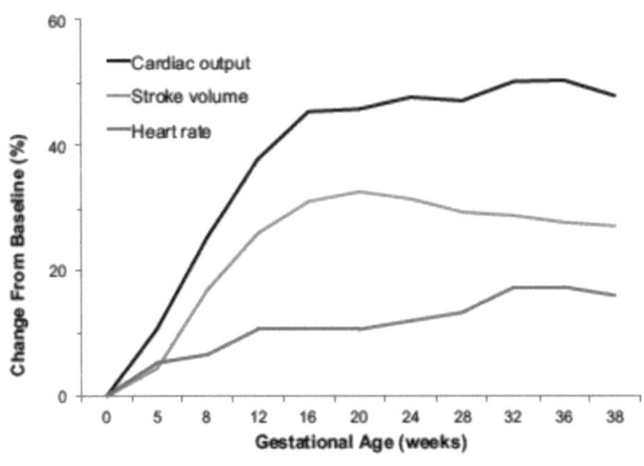

Figure 1.
Changes in hemodynamic properties throughout pregnancy. (data derived from Robson et al. [23]).

Consequently, normal pregnancy is associated with increased left ventricular mass [25, 26]. Such cardiac remodeling is a normal, physiologic response, and some, but not all, suggest these changes resolve by 3 months postpartum [27].

The increase in plasma volume during pregnancy is larger than the increase in red blood cells, which leads to physiological anemia. Systemic vascular resistance decreases at the end of the second trimester and then increases toward the end of pregnancy.

4.2 Labor and delivery

Marked fluctuations in cardiac output occur, during labor and delivery. Each uterine contraction can contribute up to 500 milliliters (ml) of maternal blood volume due to auto- transfusion of uterine blood [22].

Cardiac output can increase as much as 30% during the first stage of labor and up to 50% during the second stage due to maternal pushing [28]. Cardiac output is also augmented by the sympathetic surge induced by anxiety and pain. Immediately after delivery, the cardiac output can increase by 80% above pre-labor values due to auto-transfusion from the uterus during contractions and from the utero-placental circulation after relief of vena caval compression by the uterus. Blood loss during a normal delivery may be 500–1000 mL but is partly compensated by the increase in stroke volume.

Hemodynamic changes are fully reset after 6 months. During pregnancy and postpartum, patients remain in a hypercoagulable state.

5. Physiopathology

Until recently, the etiology and pathophysiology of peripartum cardiomyopathy have been elusive, not fully understood and likely multifactorial.

One of the oldest theories is that PPCM is simply a failed hemodynamic "stress test" of pregnancy. According to this, the cardiovascular changes during pregnancy we detailed before, ultimately lead to peripartum heart failure. We would expect then that PPCM will occur early in midpregnancy, as the maximal changes always start in this period. However, with very few exceptions, PPCM is a disease of late pregnancy and after the delivery. Thus, if peripartum cardiomyopathy were a failed stress test, it would occur much earlier and more often than it does [29].

Another old hypothesis suggested that PPCM is triggered by viral myocarditis. This observation came from findings that right-sided endomyocardial biopsies displayed evidence of inflammation. In a series of endomyocardial biopsies performed in 38 women from Niger (similar proportions of women with PPCM and controls), Inflammation was variably present in endomyocardial biopsies taken from women with the condition, however few patients met histologic criteria for myocarditis [30–32]. Cardiac magnetic resonance (CMR) imaging was performed in a cohort of 40 women in the Investigations in Pregnancy-Associated Cardiomyopathy (IPAC), only one woman had findings potentially consistent with myocarditis [33].

Other potential causes for PPCM have also been proposed. Microchimerism, with fetus-derived cells that can persist in the immune-suppressed pregnant state and can lodge in the maternal heart, has been proposed as a trigger for autoimmunity after delivery [34].

Deficiencies of iron and selenium have also been proposed. The current theory regarding the pathophysiology of peripartum cardiomyopathy suggest that it is genetically predisposed. As previously discussed, this is evidenced epidemiologically by geographic and racial variations. In a German registry, 15% of women with PPCM had a family history of cardiac disease in a first-degree relative [35]. Genetic studies have supported the notion that genetics contribute to PPCM. Mutations in the TTNC1 and TTN genes that encode cardiac myoprotein troponin C and titin have been identified in women with PPCM [36]. The titin is a critical structural component of sarcomeres in cardiac and skeletal muscle. However, over 90% of individuals with TTN truncating variants do not develop PPCM, indicating that additional environmental, genetic, or epigenetic factors are at play [37].

A landmark 2007 article first introduced that PPCM is a vascular disease triggered by the hormonal changes of late pregnancy. Although the idea was proposed in the past, experimental support for it was lacking. Recently, a 2 mice models and epidemiological data started supporting the notion that PPCM is in large part a vascular disease, triggered by the hormonal milieu of the peripartum [38, 39].

The first mouse lacked the cardioprotective STAT3 gene also accused of developing the peripartum cardiomyopathy. In this case, the oxidative stress led to cleavage of the nursing hormone, prolactin. The 16-kDa prolactin fragment had vasculotoxic and pro- apoptotic properties and vascular and myocardial dysfunction (**Figure 2**) [36].

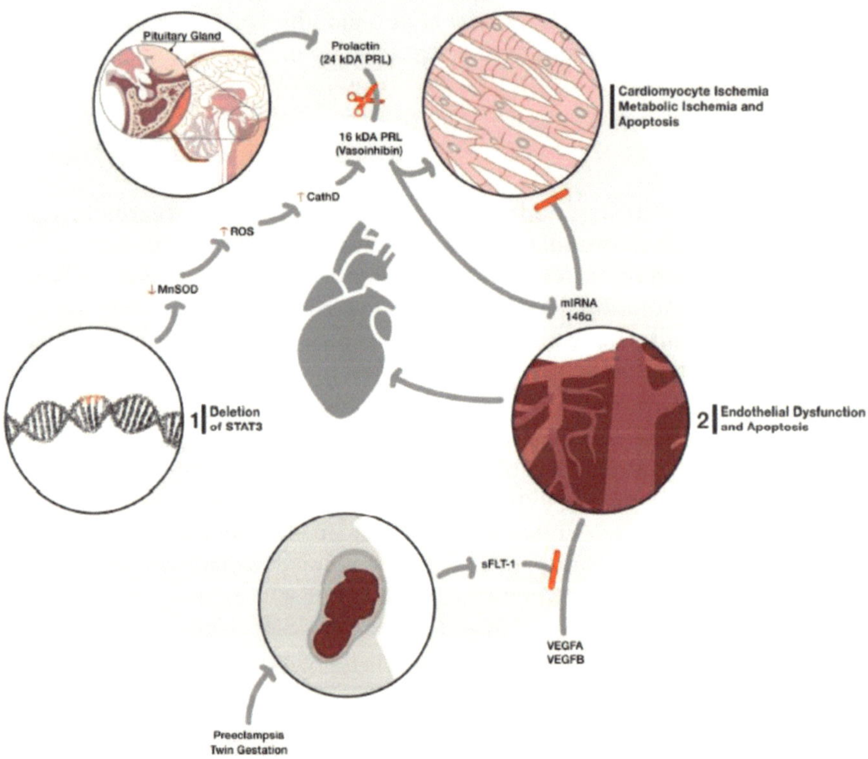

Figure 2.

Pathogenesis of peripartum cardiomyopathy: 1) genetic predisposition caused by mutations of various genes (STAT3, TTN, TTNC1) that regulate cardiomyocyte function causes secretion of cathepsin D (CathD), which cleaves pituitary prolactin (PRL) to form a 16-kDa fragment, vasoinhibin; 2) vasoinhibin acts on blood vessels to trigger apoptosis as well as microRNA-146a resulting in cardiomyocyte ischemia, metabolic insufficiency, and apoptosis. Simultaneously, the placenta, especially with the preeclampsia syndrome, secretes soluble fms-like tyrosine kinase 1 (sFlt-1), which neutralizes vascular endothelial growth factors A and B (VEGFA and VEGFB, respectively) that are critical for vascular health. MnSOD, mitochondrial antioxidant manganese superoxide dismutase; ROS, reactive oxygen species. (data from Arany and Elkayam [4]; Arany [40]. Illustrations created by Ceara Byrne, MS. Commented by Cunningham [29]).

The second mouse had another cardiac-specific genetic deletion of proliferator-activated receptor gamma coactivator-1a (PGC-1a) leading to vasculotoxicity by activation of the 16-kDa prolactin fragment and decreased expression of vascular endothelial growth factor (VEGF) [36]. VEGF is antagonized by the placental secretion of soluble Fms-like tyrosine kinase 1 (sFlt1) which is sufficient to cause profound systolic dysfunction in mice lacking cardiac PGC-1 alpha. This was incriminated in the genesis of PPCM and predicted worse outcomes [41].

6. Clinical presentation

Diagnosis of PPCM may be difficult: the symptoms of heart failure during pregnancy can mimic signs and symptoms that occur during normal pregnancy. The majority of women with PPCM are diagnosed after delivery, precisely in the first month postpartum [3]. Unfortunately, delays in diagnosis are associated with increased incidence of preventable complications and worse outcomes [16, 42, 43].

At the time of diagnosis, patients most commonly complain of signs and symptoms of congestive heart failure including dyspnea, orthopnea and paroxysmal nocturnal dyspnea. Other common symptoms include cough, palpitations, chest tightness, abdominal pain and pitting edema of the lower extremities. If chest pain is severe, the clinical picture can suggest a myocardial infarction or pulmonary embolism.

Women can have difficulty lying flat for the exam. Physical examination usually reveals signs of heart failure including tachypnea, tachycardia, elevated jugular venous pressure, third heart sound, systolic murmur of tricuspid or mitral regurgitation, pulmonary rales, and peripheral edema. Almost half women will have peripartum hypertension and, commonly, Preeclampsia [3, 18, 44]. A minority of patients will present with severe arrhythmias, cardiogenic shock and thromboembolic complications.

7. Diagnostic testing

Initial diagnostic studies will often include an electrocardiogram (ECG), chest x-ray, bloodwork, and echocardiogram. The 12-lead electrocardiogram usually shows only sinus tachycardia with non-specific ST- and T-wave changes. A normal electrocardiogram does not rule out PPCM [45]. A chest x-ray is not obligatory for diagnosis but if it is obtained, fetal shielding must be used. The chest x-ray may show an increased cardiac silhouette with varying degrees of pulmonary congestion, edema and pleural effusions.

Assessment of kidney, liver and thyroid function is recommended along with evaluation for anemia and sepsis. Proteinuria must also be quantified. Levels of brain natriuretic peptide (BNP) and N-terminal pro-BNP, are not change significantly during normal pregnancy [46], they can be mildly elevated in the setting of pre-eclampsia, but they are usually markedly elevated in PPCM [47].

Echocardiography is the gold standard for confirmation of diagnosis and must be obtained as soon as possible. It should be performed in any suspected case of PPCM as the LVEF is typically <45% [3]. It will show global reduction in LV systolic function with various degrees of LV dilatation. In addition to that, it may demonstrate right ventricular dilatation and/or dysfunction, functional mitral and/or tricuspid regurgitation, pulmonary hypertension, and left atrial or biatrial enlargement. Intracardiac thrombus may occur [48, 49], and the LV apex should be

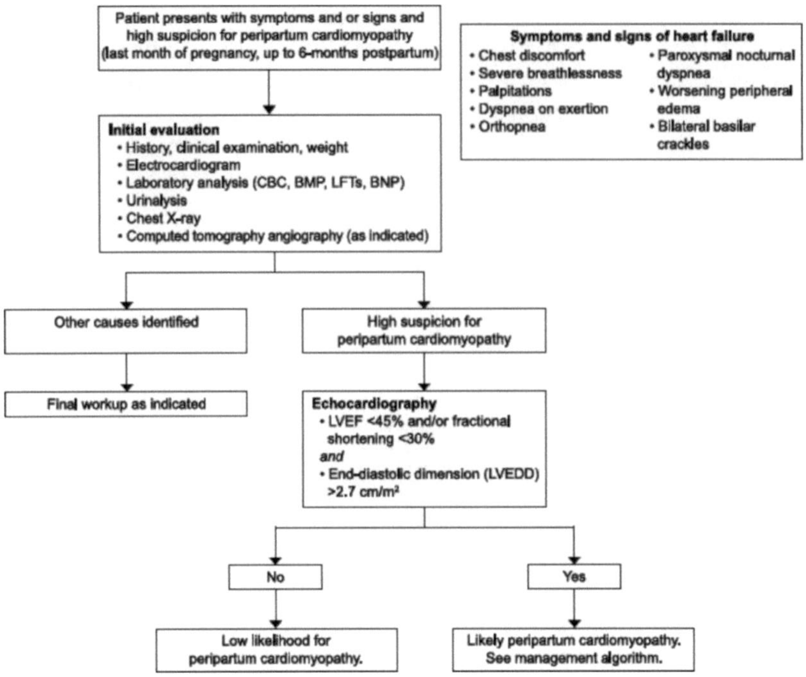

Figure 3.
Evaluation of the woman with suspected peripartum cardiomyopathy. CBC, complete blood count; BMP, basic metabolic panel; LFT, liver function test; BNP, brain natriuretic peptide; LVEF, left ventricular ejection fraction; LVEDD, left ventricular end-diastolic diameter. (Cunningham [29]).

clearly visualized. In the European worldwide registry of 411 patients, right ventricular function was severely abnormal in 10%, normal in half, mildly abnormal in approximately 35%, and [50]. Hibbard et al. proposed stringent criteria to diagnose peripartum cardiomyopathy [51].

Cardiac magnetic resonance imaging (MRI) provides accurate ejection fraction and chamber measurements when the echocardiogram is inadequate. However, the use of MRI for diagnosis of PPCM is not routine practice as gadolinium should be avoided unless it is considered absolutely essential [52].

There is no role for routine endomyocardial biopsy. The endomyocardial biopsy can only be indicated in the woman for whom there is consideration for heart transplantation.

A summary done by Cunningham of the complete evaluation recommendations are shown in **Figure 3**.

8. Differential diagnosis

PPCM is a diagnosis of exclusion. The differential diagnosis includes common causes of pulmonary edema and cardiac failure. To avoid over diagnosis, careful attention to possible pre-existing heart disease including valvular disease and cardiomyopathies is crucial.

Sepsis syndrome causes endothelial inflammation and can result in myocardial dysfunction from sepsis-induced cardiomyopathy.

Pulmonary causes such as pneumonia facilitated by the immune tolerance during pregnancy or pulmonary embolism resulting from the hypercoagulable peripartum period might mimic a PPCM as well.

Differential Diagnosis	Considerations
Takotsubo cardiomyopathy	Echocardiogram may show classic apical ballooning
Familial cardiomyopathy	Family history, genetic testing
Pre-existing cardiomyopathy	History of HF prior to pregnancy; prior echo studies with low LVEF before pregnancy
Recurrent peripartum cardiomyopathy	Ask about symptoms of HF that occurred after a prior pregnancy
Pre-eclampsia	Preserved systolic function on echocardiogram
Hypertrophic cardiomyopathy	Left ventricular hypertrophy, LVOT obstruction, preserved systolic function, genetic testing
Myocarditis	Consider if viral prodrome, histological diagnosis, fulminant presentation
Arrhythmogenic right ventricular cardiomyopathy	Consider with family history, genetic testing, echocardiographic findings
Left ventricular noncompaction	Echocardiographic and CMR findings
Chemotherapy-related cardiomyopathy	History of chemotherapy, particularly doxorubicin
Valvular heart disease	Echocardiographic findings; congenital aortic stenosis; mitral stenosis from rheumatic heart disease in endemic country. Patients with PPCM may also have valve disease, i.e., mitral regurgitation
Congenital heart disease	May be diagnosed for the first time during pregnancy by echocardiography
Tachycardia-arrhythmia mediated cardiomyopathy	Consider if specific underlying rhythm abnormality. Note that sinus tachycardia may be secondary to heart failure during pregnancy
Hypertensive heart disease	Left ventricular hypertrophy; less common in young people unless very longstanding history of hypertension
Ischemic heart disease	Cardiovascular risk factors; angina; prior CAD; consider SCAD and MINOCA diagnoses
Cardiomyopathy related to other systemic medical diseases	Consider in the appropriate context, i.e., systemic lupus erythematosus, antiphospholipid syndrome, hemochromatosis
Cardiomyopathy related to other acute conditions	May consider if patient has other conditions such as sepsis, treatment in intensive care unit, post-respiratory arrest
Pulmonary embolism	Dyspnea, tachycardia with preserved LVEF

CAD, coronary artery disease; CMR, cardiac magnetic resonance imaging; HF, heart failure; LVEF, left ventricular ejection fraction; LVOT, left ventricular outflow tract; MINOCA, myocardial infarction in non-obstructive coronary arteries; PPCM, peripartum cardiomyopathy; SCAD, spontaneous coronary artery dissection.

Table 1.
Differential diagnosis for heart failure during pregnancy.

Severe preeclampsia can cause pulmonary edema from a capillary– endothelial leak and decreased plasma oncotic pressure, and multifetal gestation and certain tocolytic agents increase this vulnerability. However, PPCM is only diagnosed in the presence of systolic dysfunction.

Other much less common causes of peripartum heart failure include thyrotoxicosis, lupus erythematosus, myocardial infarction and Takotsubo cardiomyopathy. Echocardiography is sufficient to differentiate from these causes.

Potential causes of pregnancy-related HF are listed in **Table 1** [36].

9. Treatment

9.1 Initial management

Patients with PPCM presenting with symptoms of acute severe heart failure require prompt treatment in an intensive care unit. Intravenous diuretics should be given to patients having pulmonary congestion and volume overload. The caution is required if volume control used before delivery to avoid hypotension and impaired uterine perfusion. For rapid diagnosis and decision-making, a pre-specified management algorithm and expert interdisciplinary team are crucial (**Figures 3–5**) [53, 54].

9.2 Chronic heart failure management

In postpartum, Angiotensin-converting enzyme inhibitors or angiotensin receptor blockers can be used. The Angiotensin-converting enzyme inhibitors or angiotensin receptor blockers are contraindicated before delivery, a combination of hydralazine and organic nitrates can be used instead during pregnancy.

During pregnancy, β-Blockade should be considered. to avoid promoting uterine activity, β-1–selective agents can be preferable. Digoxin may be safely used during pregnancy, but its role is currently being debated [55, 56].

9.3 Bromocriptine and cessation of breastfeeding

There's an increase of Serum levels of a fragment of prolactin, called 16 kDa prolactin during the puerperal period. In PPCM patients, the 16 kDa prolactin fragment is overexpressed and is thought to initiate and perpetrate excessive oxidative stress through reactive oxygen species, which then induces apoptosis via ischemia–reperfusion and hypoxia-reoxygenation mechanisms. This increase of 16 kDa prolactin culminates in myocardial dysfunction and symptomatic heart failure [57, 58]. Dopaminergic inhibition of prolactin secretion achieved with bromocriptine, is thought to thwart prolactin's deleterious effects on cardiac function [41].

The addition of bromocriptine to standard heart failure therapy PPCM patients appeared to result in significantly greater improvements in NYHA functional class, LV systolic and diastolic function, degree of functional mitral regurgitation, and low morbidity and mortality in PPCM patients than seen with standard therapy alone [35, 59–62].

Moreover, although bromocriptine stopped lactation in the PPCM patients, the survival and growth of those infants were normal [60].

Bromocriptine can be prescribed in women with symptoms of congestive heart failure, no other identifiable cause for heart failure finded, that developed in the last month of pregnancy or during the first month postpartum, having LVEF failure <35% by transthoracic echocardiography.

According to the guidelines of European Society of Cardiology, the use of Bromocriptine (2.5 mg once daily) for at least 1 week may be considered in uncomplicated cases, while prolonged treatment (2.5 mg twice daily for 2 weeks, then 2.5 mg once daily for 6 weeks) may be considered in patients with EF <25% and/or cardiogenic shock [63].

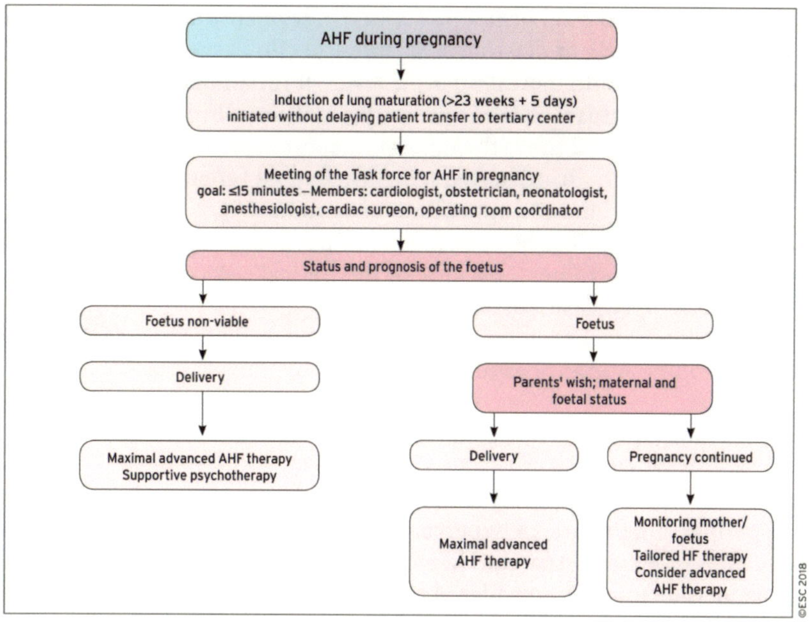

Figure 4.
Management of acute heart failure during pregnancy: Rapid interdisciplinary workup and treatment of mother and foetus (modified from Bauersachs et al. [53]). AHF, acute heart failure; HF, heart failure.

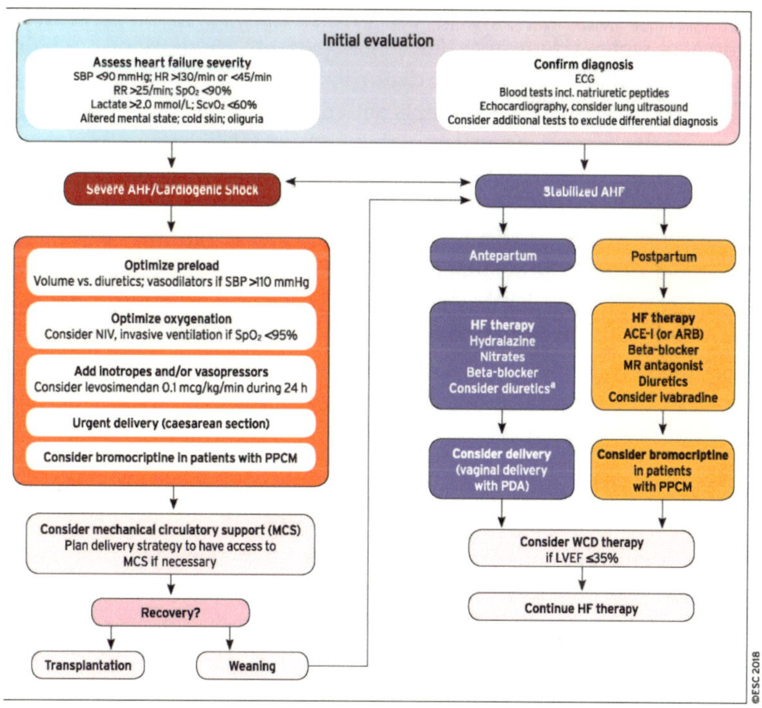

Figure 5.
Management of acute heart failure during/after pregnancy (modified from Bauersachs et al. [53]). A diuretics have to be used with caution due to potential reduction in placental blood flow. ACE-I, angiotensin-converting enzyme inhibitor; AHF, acute heart failure; ARB, angiotensin receptor blocker; ECG, electrocardiogram; HF, heart failure; HR, heart rate; LVEF, left ventricular ejection fraction; MCS, mechanical circulatory support; MR, mineralocorticoid receptor; NIV, non-invasive ventilation; PDA, Peridural analgesia; PPCM, peripartum cardiomyopathy; RR, respiratory rate; SBP, systolic blood pressure; ScvO2, central venous oxygen saturation; SpO2, peripheral oxygen saturation; WCD, wearable cardioverter-defibrillator.

The bromocriptine should be not prescribed in women with systolic blood pressure > 160 or < 95 mm Hg or diastolic >105 mm Hg; clinical conditions other than cardiomyopathy that could increase plasma levels of inflammatory markers such as sepsis, autoimmune disease, or HIV positivity; significant liver disease (defined as liver transaminase levels>2 times the upper limit of normal); history of peptic ulcer disease; history of psychiatric disorders; impaired renal function (defined as urea and/or creatinine >1.5 times the upper limit of normal [60].

Bromocriptine should not be used in the patient using triptans (for example, for the treatment of migraines), because of theoretical risks of serotoninergic syndrome or prolonged vasospastic reactions.

All patients receiving bromocriptine must receive standard heart failure therapy with at least prophylactic anticoagulation.

9.4 Thromboembolism and anticoagulation

Thromboembolic risk is higher in PPCM than other forms of cardiomyopathy [13]. The peripartum period is a hypercoagulable state [64], likely an evolutionary adaptation to minimize postpartum hemorrhaging. In patients with an LVEF <35%, the anticoagulation must be considered [65], at least during pregnancy and the first 2 months postpartum. Heparin and unfractionated heparin are safe during pregnancy, and the unfractionated heparin is preferred because of its shorter half-life.

9.5 Arrhythmias and antiarrhythmic therapies

Beta-blockers and non-vasoselective calcium-channel blockers can be used safely for rate control of tachyarrhythmias. For PPCM patients, there are no guidelines for implantation of an implantable cardiac defibrillator (ICD). However, sudden cardiac death has been reported in PPCM patients with decreased LVEF in both the acute and chronic stages of this disease, as well as in those whose LVEF has completely normalized, indicating that the risk of sudden cardiac death may persist well into recovery. It might be reasonable to consider ICD in patients with EF <30% with sustained ventricular arrhythmias or history of survival after cardiac arrest, but this decision should be carefully weighed against the evidence that LV function improves within 6 months in the majority of patients. A suitable alternative is wearable cardioverter-defibrillator devices for patients with LVEF ≤35% to prevent sudden cardiac death [66, 67].

But it would be reasonable to consider ICD implantation in patients with persistent NYHA class III or IV symptoms despite optimal medical therapy for 6 months and whose LVEF remains <30%.

9.6 Cardiac assist devices

Temporary circulatory support with inotropes, intra-aortic balloon pumps, LV and biventricular assist devices, and extracorporeal membrane oxygenation must be considered in patients who clinically deteriorate, despite optimal medical treatment, either as a bridge to recovery or transplantation [68]. As that LV function improves within 6 months in the majority of patients, the decision to refer the patient for cardiac transplantation should not be made too early. Results after transplantation in patients with PPCM are comparable to patients transplanted for other etiologies.

9.7 Obstetric management

Excessive volume depletion and angiotensin-converting enzyme inhibitors should be avoided. No published data exist to indicate that elective caesarian delivery or early delivery can ameliorate PPCM or improve fetal prognosis. Apgar scores, mean birth weight and size, are lower in neonates born to women with PPCM, likely reflecting earlier gestational age at delivery [69]. Timing and mode of delivery must therefore be made by a team of obstetricians and cardiologists. Early delivery needs should be reserved for cases of impending peril to mother or fetus [70].

9.8 Subsequent pregnancies

Several studies highlighted the higher incidence of PPCM in women with high parity [11, 71, 72]. Increased morbidity and mortality is observed during subsequent pregnancies, especially in women with persistent left ventricular dysfunction after the first pregnancy [62–73]. Early contraception should be given in PPCM women [74].

10. Prognosis

The evolution is favorable. LV function improves within 6 months in the majority of patients and will remain stable under drug treatment. The decision to refer the patient for cardiac transplantation estimated at 1–2% [12]. Prognosis of PPCM is better than the prognosis of other forms of dilated cardiomyopathy [75].

Mortality to 12 months is 4–14% [76, 77]. the addition of bromocriptine to standard heart failure therapy appeared to improve LVEF. A trial adding the prolactin blocker bromocriptine with standard therapy for heart failure reported an excellent 6-month follow-up outcome in severely diseased patients having over 60% full recovery and 0%, heart transplantation, use of assist device and mortality [60].

Mortality between 2 and 5 years, ranging from 0 to 6% in American and French women [48–79], to 15–30% in women from Brazil, [80], China, [81] South Africa, [82] Turkey, [83–85] and the Philippines [86].

In USA the mortality ranging from 7 to 16% at between 7 and 8.6 years [16, 75, 77], the mortality was 23% at 6.1 years in India [87]. In Malaysia the mortality was 8.3% at 6.4 years [88].

When myocardial recovery occurs in PPCM, There are no recommendations to determine the time of long-term treatment.

11. Conclusion

Management of peripartum cardiomyopathy is largely limited to the same neurohormonal antagonists used in other forms of cardiomyopathy, the addition of bromocriptine to standard heart failure therapy seemed to improve LVEF. LV function improves within 6 months in the majority of patients having optimal medical therapy. Whatever the evolution, long-term follow-up is essential. Early contraception should be given in PPCM women.

Author details

Fatima Zahra Merzouk*, Sara Oualim and Mohammed Sabry
Department of Cardiology, Mohammed VI University of Health Sciences Cheick Khalifa Hospital, Casablanca, Morocco

*Address all correspondence to: merzoukfatimazahra@hotmail.fr

References

[1] Porak C. *De L'influence réciproque de la grossesse et des maladies du Coeur* [thesis]. Medical Faculty of Paris, France: 1880.

[2] Demakis JG, Rahimtoola SH, Sutton GC, Meadows WR, Szanto PB, Tobin JR, Gunnar RM. Natural course of peripartum cardiomyopathy. Circulation. 1971;44:1053-1061.

[3] Sliwa K, Hilfiker-Kleiner D, Petrie MC, et al; Heart Failure Association of the European Society of Cardiology Working Group on Peripartum Cardiomyopathy. Current state of knowledge on etiology, diagnosis, management, and therapy of peripartum cardiomyopathy: a position statement from the Heart Failure Association of the European Society of Cardiology Working Group on Peripartum Cardiomyopathy. Eur J Heart Fail. 2010;12:767-778. doi: 10.1093/eurjhf/hfq120.

[4] Arany Z, Elkayam. Peripartum Cardiomyopathy. Circulation. 2016;133:1397-1409. DOI: 10.1161/ CIRCULATIONAHA.115.020491.

[5] Ntusi NB, Mayosi BM. Aetiology and risk factors of peripartum cardiomyopathy: a systematic review. Int J Cardiol. 2009;131:168-179. doi:10.1016/j.ijcard.2008.06.054.

[6] Ng AT, Duan L, Win T, et al. Maternal and fetal outcomes in pregnant women with heart failure. Heart 2018;104:1949-1954.

[7] Kolte D, Khera S, Aronow WS, et al. Temporal trends in incidence and outcomes of peripartum cardiomyopathy in the United States: a nationwide population-based study. J Am Heart Assoc. 2014;3:e001056. doi: 10.1161/JAHA.114.001056.

[8] Brar SS, Khan SS, Sandhu GK, et al. Incidence, mortality, and racial differences in peripartum cardiomyopathy. Am J Cardiol. 2007;100(2):302-304 [Epub2007/07/17].

[9] Gentry MB, Dias JK, Luis A, Pate lR, Thornton J, Reed GL. African-American women have a higher risk for developing peripartum cardiomyopathy. J Am Coll Cardiol. 2010;55(7): 654-659 [Epub2010/02/23].

[10] Isezuo SA, Abubakar SA. Epidemiologic profile of peripartum cardiomyopathy in a tertiary care hospital. Ethn Dis. 2007;17:228-233.

[11] Fett JD, Christie LG, Carraway RD, Murphy JG. Five-year prospective study of the incidence and prognosis of peripartum cardiomyopathy at a single institution. Mayo Clin Proc. 2005;80:1602-1606. doi: 10.4065/80.12.1602.

[12] Mielniczuk LM, Williams K, Davis DR, Tang AS, Lemery R, Green MS, Gollob MH, Haddad H, Birnie DH. Frequency of peripartum cardiomyopathy. Am J Cardiol. 2006;97:1765-1768. doi: 10.1016/j.

[13] Elkayam U. Clinical characteristics of peripartum cardiomyopathy in the United States: diagnosis, prognosis, and management. J Am Coll Cardiol. 2011;58(7):659 670 [Epub2011/08/06].

[14] Main EK, McCain CL, Morton CH, Holtby S, Lawton ES. Pregnancy related mortality in California: causes, characteristics, and improvement opportunities. Obstet Gynecol. 2015;125:938-947. doi: 10.1097/ AOG.0000000000000746.

[15] Elkayam U, Akhter MW, Singh H, et al. Pregnancy-associated cardiomyopathy: clinical characteristics and a comparison between early and late presentation. Circulation. 2005;111 (16):2050-2055 [Epub2005/04/27].

[16] Harper MA, Meyer RE, Berg CJ. Peripartum cardiomyopathy: population-based birth prevalence and 7-year mortality. Obstet Gynecol. 2012;120:1013-1019.

[17] Bello N, Rendon IS, Arany Z. The relationship between pre-eclampsia and peripartum cardiomyopathy: a systematic review and meta-analysis. J Am Coll Cardiol. 2013;62:1715-1723. doi: 10.1016/j.jacc.2013.08.717

[18] Fong A, Chau CT, Pan D, Ogunyemi DA. Clinical morbidities, trends, and demographics of eclampsia: a population-based study. *Am J Obstet Gynecol*. 2013;209:229.e1-229.e7. doi: 10.1016/j.ajog.2013.05.050.

[19] Melchiorre K, Sutherland GR, Baltabaeva A, Liberati M, Thilaganathan B. Maternal cardiac dysfunction and remodeling in women with preeclampsia at term. Hypertension. 2011;57:85-93. doi: 10.1161/HYPERTENSIONAHA.110.162321.

[20] Russell RB, Petrini JR, Damus K, Mattison DR, Schwarz RH. The changing epidemiology of multiple births in the United States. Obstet Gynecol. 2003;101:129-135.

[21] Kao DP, Hsich E, Lindenfeld J. Characteristics, adverse events, and racial differences among delivering mothers with peripartum cardiomyopathy. JACC Heart Fail. 2013;1:409-416. doi: 10.1016/j.jchf.2013.04.011

[22] Jennifer Lewey, Jennifer Haythe, Cardiomyopathy in pregnancy. S E M I N ARS IN PERINATOLOGY (2014) http://dx.doi.org/10.1053/j.semperi.2014.04.0210146-0005/& 2014 Elsevier.

[23] Robson SC, Hunter S, Boys RJ, Dunlop W. Serial study of factors influencing changes in cardiac output during human pregnancy. Am J Physiol. 1989;256(4Pt2):[H1060-5. Epub1989/04/01].

[24] Hibbard JU, Shroff SG, Cunningham FG. Cardiovascular alterations in normal and preeclamptic pregnancies. In: Taylor RN, Roberts JM, Cunningham FG, editors. Chesley's hypertensive disorders in pregnancy. 4th ed. Amsterdam (the Netherlands): Academic Press; 2014.

[25] Ducas RA, Elliott JE, Melnyk SF, Premecz S, DaSilva M, Cleverly K, et al. Cardiovascular magnetic resonance in pregnancy: insights from the cardiac hemodynamic imaging and remodeling in pregnancy (CHIRP) study. J Cardiovasc Magn Reson 2014;16:1.

[26] Stewart RD, Nelson DB, Matulevicius SA, Morgan JL, McIntire DD, Drazner MH, et al. Cardiac magnetic resonance imaging to assess the impact of maternal habitus on cardiac remodeling during pregnancy. Am J Obstet Gynecol 2016;214:640.e1-6.

[27] Clapp JF 3rd, Capeless E. Cardiovascular function before, during, and after the first and subsequent pregnancies. Am J Cardiol 1997;80:1469-1473.

[28] Ouzounian JG,ElkayamU. Physiologic changes during normal pregnancy and delivery. Cardiol Clin. 2012;30(3):317-329 [Epub 2012/07/21].

[29] Gary Cunningham, John J. Byrne, David B. Nelson, MD. Peripartum Cardiomyopathy. (Obstet Gynecol 2019;133:167-79). DOI: 10.1097/AOG.0000000000003011

[30] Bültmann BD, Klingel K, Näbauer M, Wallwiener D, Kandolf R. High prevalence of viral genomes and inflammation in peripartum cardiomyopathy. *Am J Obstet Gynecol* 2005;193:363-5. 10.1016/j.ajog.2005.01.022 pmid:16098856.

[31] Sanderson JE, Olsen EG, Gatei D. Peripartum heart disease: an endomyocardial biopsy study. *Br Heart J* 1986;56:285-91. 10.1136/hrt.56.3.285 pmid:3756045.

[32] Rizeq MN, Rickenbacher PR, Fowler MB, Billingham ME. Incidence of myocarditis in peripartum cardiomyopathy. *Am J Cardiol* 1994;74:474-7. 10.1016/0002-9149(94)90906-7 pmid:8059728.

[33] Schelbert EB, Elkayam U, Cooper LT, et al. Investigations of Pregnancy Associated Cardiomyopathy (IPAC) Investigators. Myocardial damage detected by late gadolinium enhancement cardiac magnetic resonance is uncommon in peripartum cardiomyopathy. J Am Heart Assoc 2017;6:e005472. 10.1161/JAHA.117.005472 pmid:28373243.

[34] Pearson GD, Veille JC, Rahimtoola SH, Hsia J, Oakley CM, Hosenpud JD, et al. Peripartum cardiomyopathy: National Heart, Lung, and Blood Institute and Office of Rare Diseases (National Institutes of Health) workshop recommendations and review. JAMA 2000;283:1183-1188.

[35] Haghikia A, Podewski E, Libhaber E, et al. Phenotyping and outcome on contemporary management in a German cohort of patients with peripartum cardiomyopathy. Basic Res Cardiol 2013;108:366.

[36] Melinda B. Davis, MD,a Zolt Arany, MD, PHD,b Dennis M. McNamara, MD, MS,c Sorel Goland, MD,d Uri Elkayam, MD. Peripartum Cardiomyopathy. JACC State-of-the-Art Review. J Am Coll Cardiol 2020;75:207-221

[37] Haggerty CM, Damrauer SM, Levin MG, et al. Genomics-first evaluation of heart disease associated with titin-truncating variants. Circulation 2019;140:42-54

[38] Hilfiker-Kleiner D, Kaminski K, Podewski E, et al. A cathepsin D-cleaved 16 kDa form of prolactin mediates postpartum cardiomyopathy. Cell 2007;128:589-600.

[39] Bello NA, Arany Z. Molecular mechanisms of peripartum cardiomyopathy: a vascular/hormonal hypothesis. Trends Cardiovasc Med 2015;25: 499-504

[40] Arany Z. Understanding peripartum cardiomyopathy. Annu Rev. Med 2018;69:165-166.

[41] Damp J, Givertz MM, Semigran M, et al. Relaxin-2 and Soluble Flt1 Levels in Peripartum Cardiomyopathy: Results of the Multicenter IPAC Study. J Am Coll Cardiol HF 2016;4:380-388

[42] Fett JD. Earlier detection can help avoid many serious complications of peripartum cardiomyopathy. Future Cardiol 2013;9:809-816.

[43] Goland S, Modi K, Bitar F, et al. Clinical profile and predictors of complications in peripartum cardiomyopathy. J Card Fail 2009;15:645-650.

[44] Hilfiker-Kleiner D, Haghikia A, Masuko D, Nonhoff J, Held D, Libhaber E, et al. Outcome of subsequent pregnancies in patients with a history of peripartum cardiomyopathy. Eur J Heart Fail 2017;19:1723-1728.

[45] Honigberg MC, Elkayam U, Rajagopalan N, et al. Electrocardiographic findings in peripartum cardiomyopathy. Clin Cardiol 2019;42:524-529.

[46] Resnik JL, Hong C, Resnik R, Kazanegra R, Beede J, Bhalla V, et al. Evaluation of B-type natriuretic peptide (BNP) levels in normal and preeclamptic women. Am J Obstet Gynecol 2005; 193:450-454.

[47] Tanous D, Siu SC, Mason J, et al. B-type natriuretic peptide in pregnant women with heart disease. J Am Coll Cardiol 2010;56:1247-1253.

[48] Amos AM, Jaber WA, Russell SD. Improved outcomes in peripartum cardiomyopathy with contemporary. Am Heart J 2006;152:509-513.

[49] Sliwa K, Forster O, Libhaber E, et al. Peripartum cardiomyopathy: inflammatory markers as predictors of outcome in 100 prospectively studied patients. Eur Heart J 2006;27:441-446.

[50] Sliwa K, Mebazza A, Hilfiker-Kleiner D, Petrie MC, Maggioni AP, Laroche C, et al. Clinical characteristics of patients from the worldwide registry on peripartum cardiomyopathy (PPCM): EURObservational Research Programme in conjunction with the Heart Failure Association of the European Society of Cardiology Study Group on PPCM. Eur J Heart Fail 2017; 19:1131-1141.

[51] Hibbard JU, Lindheimer M, Lang RM. A modified definition for peripartum cardiomyopathy and prognosis based on echocardiography. Obstet Gynecol 1999;94:311-316.

[52] Kanal E, Barkovich AJ, Bell C, et al. ACR guidance document on MR safe practices:2013. J Magn Reson Imaging. 2013;37(3): 501-530 [Epub2013/01/25].

[53] Bauersachs J, Arrigo M, Hilfiker-Kleiner D, Veltmann C, Coats AJ, Crespo-Leiro MG, De Boer RA, van der Meer P, Maack C, Mouquet F, Petrie MC, Piepoli MF, Regitz-Zagrosek V, Schaufelberger M, Seferovic P, Tavazzi L, Ruschitzka F, Mebazaa A, Sliwa K. Current management of patients with severe acute peripartum cardiomyopathy: Practical guidance from the Heart Failure Association of the European Society of Cardiology Study Group on peripartum cardiomyopathy. Eur J Heart Fail 2016;18:1096-1105.

[54] Hilfiker-Kleiner D, Westhoff-Bleck M, Gunter HH, von Kaisenberg CS, Bohnhorst B, Hoeltje M, Kuehn C. A management algorithm for acute heart failure in pregnancy. The Hannover experience. Eur Heart J 2015;36:769-770.

[55] Cleland JG, Cullington D. Digoxin: quo vadis? Circ Heart Fail. 2009;2:81-85. doi: 10.1161/CIRCHEARTFAILURE. 109.859322.

[56] Chaggar PS, Shaw SM, Williams SG. Is foxglove effective in heart failure? Cardiovasc Ther. 2015;33:236-241. doi: 10.1111/1755-5922.12130.

[57] Negoro S, Kunisada K, Fujio Y, et al. Activation of signal transducer and activator of transcription 3 protects cardiomyocytes from hypoxia/ reoxygenation-induced oxidative stress through the upregulation of manganese superoxide dismutase. Circulation 2001;104:979-981.

[58] Singh N, Dhalla AK, Seneviratne C, Singal PK. Oxidative stress and heart failure. Mol Cell Biochem 1995;147:77-81.

[59] Sliwa K, Blauwet L, Tibazarwa K, Libhaber E, Smedema JP, Becker A, McMurray J, Yamac H, Labidi S, Struman I, Hilfiker-Kleiner D. Evaluation of bromocriptine in the treatment of acute severe peripartum cardiomyopathy: A proof-of-concept pilot study. Circulation 2010;121:1465-1473.

[60] Hilfiker-Kleiner D, Haghikia A, Berliner D, Vogel-Claussen J, Schwab J, Franke A, Schwarzkopf M, Ehlermann P, Pfister R, Michels G, Westenfeld R, Stangl V, Kindermann I, Kuhl U, Angermann CE, Schlitt A, Fischer D, Podewski E, Bohm M, Sliwa K, Bauersachs J. Bromocriptine for the treatment of peripartum cardiomyopathy: A multicentre

randomized study. Eur Heart J 2017;38:2671-2679.

[61] McNamara DM, Elkayam U, Alharethi R, Damp J, Hsich E, Ewald G, Modi K, Alexis JD, Ramani GV, Semigran MJ, Haythe J, Markham DW, Marek J, Gorcsan J III, Wu WC, Lin Y, Halder I, Pisarcik J, Cooper LT, Fett JD. Clinical outcomes for peripartum cardiomyopathy in North America: Results of the IPAC study (Investigations of Pregnancy-Associated Cardiomyopathy). J Am Coll Cardiol 2015;66:905-914.

[62] Haghikia A, Podewski E, Berliner D, Sonnenschein K, Fischer D, Angermann CE, Bohm M, Rontgen P, Bauersachs J, Hilfiker-Kleiner D. Rationale and design of a randomized, controlled multicentre clinical trial to evaluate the effect of bromocriptine on left ventricular function in women with peripartum cardiomyopathy. Clin Res Cardiol 2015;104:911-917.

[63] Vera Regitz-Zagrosek, Jolien W Roos-Hesselink, Johann Bauersachs, Carina Blomström-Lundqvist, Renata Cífková, Michele De Bonis, Bernard Iung, Mark Richard Johnson, Ulrich Kintscher, Peter Kranke, Irene Marthe Lang, Joao Morais, Petronella G Pieper, Patrizia Presbitero, Susanna Price, Giuseppe M C Rosano, Ute Seeland, Tommaso Simoncini, Lorna Swan, Carole A Warnes, ESC Scientific Document Group, 2018 ESC Guidelines for the management of cardiovascular diseases during pregnancy: The Task Force for the Management of Cardiovascular Diseases during Pregnancy of the European Society of Cardiology (ESC), European Heart Journal, Volume 39, Issue 34, 07 September 2018, Pages 3165-3241, https://doi.org/10.1093/eurheartj/ehy340

[64] Greer IA. Clinical practice: pregnancy complicated by venous thrombosis. N Engl J Med. 2015;373:540-547. doi: 10.1056/NEJMcp140743

[65] Box LC, Hanak V, Arciniegas JG. Dual coronary emboli in peripartum cardiomyopathy. Tex Heart Inst J 2004;31:442-444.

[66] Duncker D, Haghikia A, Konig T, Hohmann S, Gutleben KJ, Westenfeld R, et al. Risk for ventricular fibrillation in peripartum cardiomyopathy with severely reduced left ventricular functionvalue of the wearable cardioverter/defibrillator. Eur J Heart Fail. 2014;16(12):1331-1336. https://doi.org/10.1002/ejhf.188.

[67] Duncker D, Konig T, Hohmann S, Bauersachs J, Veltmann C. Avoiding untimely implantable cardioverter/defibrillator implantation by intensified heart failure therapy optimization supported by the wearable cardioverter/defibrillator—the prolong study. J Am Heart Assoc. 2017;6(1). doi:https://doi.org/10.1161/JAHA.116.004512.

[68] Hilfiker-Kleiner D, Haghikia A, Nonhoff J, Bauersachs J. Peripartum cardiomyopathy: current management and future perspectives. Eur Heart J. 2015;36(18):1090-1097. https://doi.org/10

[69] Gunderson EP, Croen LA, Chiang V, Yoshida CK, Walton D, Go AS. Epidemiology of peripartum cardiomyopathy: incidence, predictors, and outcomes. Obstet Gynecol. 2011;118:583-591. doi: 10.1097/AOG.0b013e318229e6de.

[70] Elkayam U. Risk of subsequent pregnancy in women with a history of peripartum cardiomyopathy. J Am Coll Cardiol. 2014;64(15): 1629-1636. https://doi.org/10.1016/j.jacc.2014.07.961.

[71] Sliwa K, Skudicky D, Bergemann A, Candy G, Puren A, Sareli P. Peripartum

cardiomyopathy: analysis of clinical outcome, left ventricular function, plasma levels of cytokines and Fas/APO-1. J Am Coll Cardiol. 2000;35(3):701-705.

[72] Sliwa K, Mebazaa A, Hilfiker-Kleiner D, Petrie MC, Maggioni AP, Laroche C, et al. Clinical characteristics of patients from the worldwide registry on peripartum cardiomyopathy (PPCM): EURObservational Research Programme in conjunction with the Heart Failure Association of the European Society of Cardiology Study Group on PPCM. Eur J Heart Fail. 2017;19(9):1131-1141. https://doi.org/10.1002/ejhf.780.

[73] Sliwa K, Petrie MC, Hilfiker-Kleiner D, Mebazaa A, Jackson A, Johnson MR, et al. Long-term prognosis, subsequent pregnancy, contraception and overall management of peripartum cardiomyopathy: practical guidance paper from the Heart Failure Association of the European Society of Cardiology Study Group on Peripartum Cardiomyopathy. Eur J Heart Fail. 2018;20:951-962. https://doi.org/10.1002/ejhf.1178.

[74] Roos-Hesselink JW, Cornette J, Sliwa K, Pieper PG, Veldtman GR, Johnson MR. Contraception and cardiovascular disease. Eur Heart J. 2015;36(27):1728-34, 34a-34b. https://doi.org/10.1093/eurheartj/ehv141.

[75] Felker GM, Thompson RE, Hare JM, Hruban RH, Clemetson DE, Howard DL, et al. Underlying causes and long-term survival in patients with initially unexplained cardiomyopathy. N Engl J Med 2000;342:1077-1084.

[76] Ravikishore AG, Kaul UA, Sethi KK, Khalilullah M. Peripartum cardiomyopathy: prognostic variables at initial evaluation. Int J Cardiol 1991;32:377-380.

[77] Pillarisetti J, Kondur A, Alani A, Reddy M, Reddy M, Vacek J, Weiner CP, Ellerbeck E, Schreiber T, Lakkireddy D. Peripartum cardiomyopathy: predictors of recoveryand current state of implantable cardioverter-defibrillator use. J Am Coll Cardiol 2014;63: 2831 – 2839

[78] Habli M, O'Brien T, Nowack E, Khoury S, Barton JR, Sibai B. Peripartum cardiomyopathy: prognostic factors for long-term maternal outcome. Am J Obstet Gynecol 2008;199:415.e1 –5.

[79] Mouquet F, Mostefa Kara M, Lamblin N, Coulon C, Langlois S, Marquie C, de Groote P. Unexpected and rapid recovery of left ventricular function in patients with peripartum cardiomyopathy: impact of cardiac resynchronization therapy. Eur J Heart Fail 2012;14:526-529.

[80] de Souza JL Jr, de Carvalho Frimm C, Nastari L, Mady C. Left ventricular function after a new pregnancy in patients with peripartum cardiomyopathy. J Card Fail 2001;7:30– 35.

[81] Li W, Li H, Long Y. Clinical characteristics and long-term predictors of persistent left ventricular systolic dysfunction in peripartum cardiomyopathy. Can J Cardiol 2016;32:362– 368.

[82] Ntusi NB, Badri M, Gumedze F, Wonkam A, Mayosi BM. Clinical characteristics and outcomes of familial and idiopathic dilated cardiomyopathy in Cape Town: a comparative study of 120 cases followed up over 14 years. S Afr Med J 2011;101:399– 404

[83] Duran N, Gunes H, Duran I, Biteker M, Ozkan M. Predictors of prognosis in patients with peripartum cardiomyopathy. Int J Gynaecol Obstet 2008;101:137– 140.

[84] Biteker M, Ilhan E, Biteker G, Duman D, Bozkurt B. Delayed recovery in peripartum cardiomyopathy: an indication for long-term follow-up and sustained therapy. Eur J Heart Fail 2012;14:895-901.

[85] Akil MA, Bilik MZ, Yildiz A, Acet H, Ertas F, Simsek H, Polat N, Zengin H, Akilli R, Agacayak E, Kayan F, Ozdemir M, Alan S. Peripartum cardiomyopathy in Turkey: experience of three tertiary centres. J Obstet Gynaecol 2016;36:574– 580.

[86] Cuenza LR, Manapat N, Jalique JR. Clinical profile and predictors of outcomes of patients with peripartum cardiomyopathy: the Philippine Heart Center experience. ASEAN Heart J 2016;24:9.

[87] Mishra TK, Swain S, Routray SN. Peripartum cardiomyopathy. Int J Gynaecol Obstet 2006;95:104– 109.

[88] Chee KH. Favourable outcome after peripartum cardiomyopathy: a ten-year study on peripartum cardiomyopathy in a university hospital. Singapore Med J 2013;54:28– 31.

Section 6

Miscellaneous Cardiomyopathies

Chapter 17

Myocarditis and Inflammatory Cardiomyopathy

Emanuele Bobbio and Kristjan Karason

Abstract

Activation of the inflammatory system occurs in most patients with advanced heart failure, regardless of etiology, and contributes to the pathophysiological milieu and the progression of the disease. The term *inflammatory cardiomyopathy* (ICM) refers to a group of disorders for which an acute or chronic myocardial inflammation is the central cause of abnormal cardiac structure or impaired cardiac function. The most common cause of inflammatory cardiomyopathy is *lymphocytic myocarditis*, which is most usually triggered by a viral infection, and occasionally by other infectious agents. Rare causes of specific inflammatory cardiomyopathies include *cardiac sarcoidosis*, *giant cell myocarditis* and *eosinophilic myocarditis*. Inflammatory cardiomyopathy can also occur in connection with autoimmune inflammatory diseases. Typical manifestations of inflammatory cardiomyopathy include chest pain, heart failure, and arrhythmias, but these symptoms and signs are unspecific. Although non-invasive diagnostic methods are emerging, the gold standard of diagnosis is the histological examination of an endomyocardial biopsy. Owing to the invasive nature of this technique and a modest diagnostic sensitivity, its use is limited. Therefore, the identification of inflammatory cardiomyopathy is elusive and the true incidence of the condition remains unknown. In most cases of lymphocytic myocarditis, recovery occurs within a few weeks following supportive treatment. In patients with cardiac sarcoidosis, giant cell myocarditis or eosinophilic myocarditis the use of immunosuppressive treatment is recommended, as is the case in myocarditis associated with autoimmune disorders. Such interventions may also have beneficial effects in chronic viral myocarditis once the virus has been cleared. In severe cases, treatment with mechanical circulatory support and/ or heart transplantation may be required. Randomized intervention trials including antiviral, immunomodulating, or immunosuppressive agents are lacking. Similarly, new molecular-based methods and therapies tailored to specific pathogeneses have a potential to improve diagnosis and outcomes in patients with inflammatory cardiomyopathy. Still, such techniques and interventions are to be evaluated in adequate randomized controlled studies.

Keywords: myocarditis, inflammatory cardiomyopathy, lymphocytic myocarditis, cardiac sarcoidosis, giant cell myocarditis, eosinophilic myocarditis, heart failure, endomyocardial biopsy

1. Introduction

Myocarditis implies the presence of diffuse or focal inflammation in the cardiac muscle [1]. Although inflammation of the myocardium can be induced by

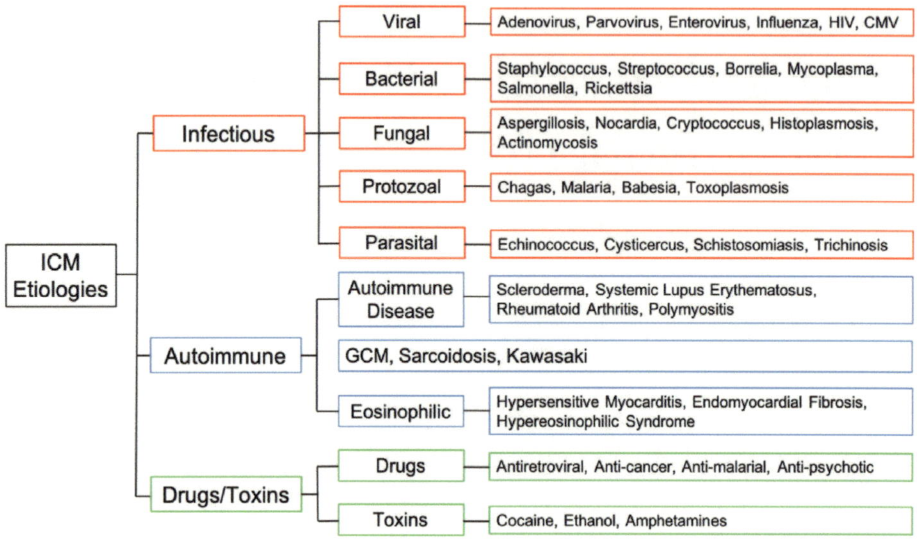

Figure 1.
Inflammatory cardiomyopathy (ICM) refers to a broad group of disorders for which inflammation of the myocardium represents the principal cause of ventricular remodeling and cardiac dysfunction.

a wide variety of autoimmune disorders, hypersensitivity reactions and toxins, the predominant etiopathogenetic factor is infectious agents; these are mostly viral, but can also include bacterial and protozoal microbes [1, 2]. Still, in the individual case the etiology can be difficult to identify. Inflammatory cardiomyopathy refers to a broad group of disorders for which inflammation of the myocardium represents the principal cause of ventricular remodeling and cardiac dysfunction (**Figure 1**) [3, 4]. This term is rather unspecific since as several cardiomyopathies a low degree of inflammation is present and an infectious agent can seldom be identified [1]. In contrast to hereditary cardiomyopathies, no monogenetic diseases cause inflammatory cardiomyopathy, although a genetic predisposition towards cardiotropic viruses and/or autoimmune reactions may occur in certain individuals [2, 5].

Myocarditis and inflammatory cardiomyopathy can be acute, subacute, or chronic [1]. The incidence and prevalence of these conditions are difficult to estimate as many cases are asymptomatic [2, 6] and the diagnosis is seldom verified with an endomyocardial biopsy (EMB) [7]. Nevertheless, myocarditis and inflammatory cardiomyopathy are noteworthy conditions related to poor outcomes, especially when complicated by heart failure and ventricular arrhythmias [5, 8]. This chapter will focus on cardiomyopathies associated with impaired cardiac structure and function for which inflammation is the primary cause.

2. Myocarditis and inflammatory cardiomyopathy

The previous histopathological diagnosis of myocarditis has traditionally been defined according to the Dallas criteria of 1986, which requires the presence of inflammatory cell infiltrates in the myocardial tissue and advocate classification into active forms with myocytolysis and borderline forms without cell necrosis [1, 5]. A histological diagnosis requires an endomyocardial biopsy, which is not only resource-intensive, but also invasive with attendant potential for complications [9]. The Dallas criteria represented the first attempt to develop standardized diagnostic guidelines for the histopathological classification of myocarditis [10]. However, the practical use of these criteria is limited by their low sensitivity owing to variation in collection of the samples and inter-observer variability between different pathologists [7, 11].

In addition to histological examination, an endomyocardial biopsy can be examined with polymerase chain reaction (PCR) techniques to screen for cardiotropic viruses and with immunohistochemical methods to detect low-grade inflammation [1]. The value of these analyses is still unclear, however, as the results do not provide a clear guide with respect to the management and prognosis of inflammatory cardiomyopathy. For these reasons, many practitioners refrain from obtaining endomyocardial biopsies, with the result that myocarditis often becomes an exclusion diagnosis based on clinical features and other clinical examinations [1].

Cardiac magnetic resonance (MR) has been used more extensively in recent years to diagnose and exclude myocarditis and inflammatory cardiomyopathy (**Figure 2A**) [12]. The 'Lake Louise criteria', a consensus guide to cardiac MR in myocardial inflammation were published in 2009 [13]. These criteria focused on three diagnostic targets in the myocardial tissue derived from a signal intensity assessment in T2-weighted images with early and late gadolinium enhancement: 1) edema; 2) hyperemia; and 3) necrosis or scar. A high likelihood of myocarditis is assumed to occur if two out of these three criteria are positive [13]. The Lake Louise Criteria have subsequently been widely used in both clinical and research settings.

^{18}Ffluoro-deoxy-glucose (FDG) positron emission tomography/computed tomography (PET/CT) is emerging as a diagnostic tool for the assessment of myocarditis and inflammatory cardiomyopathy (**Figure 2B**) [14]. As the activation of inflammatory cells is associated with increased glucose utilization, [15] myocarditis can be detected by PET after intravenous administration of FDG. The CT is added to identify the localization of myocardial inflammation, which correlates anatomically with increased glucose turnover. As compared with cardiac MR,

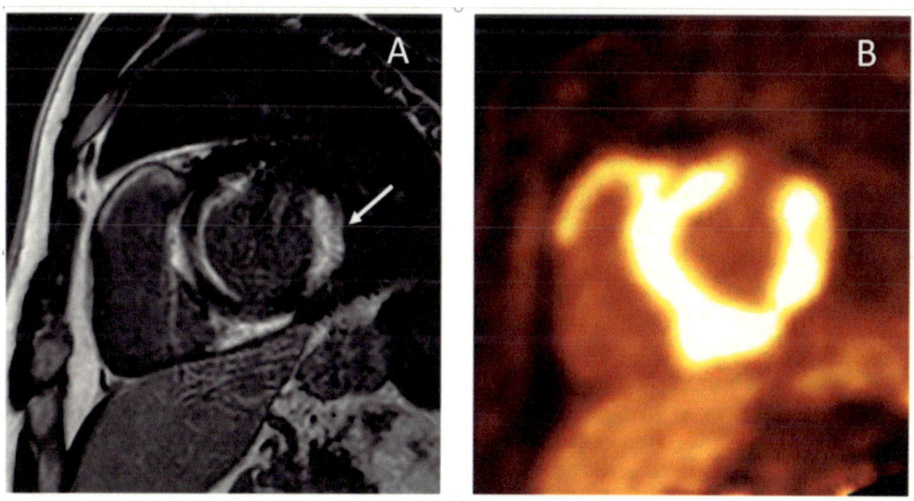

Figure 2.
Images from a patient with cardiac sarcoidosis: A) cardiac MR (T2-weighted image) showing delayed enhancement (arrow) indicating inflammation and B) PET/CT displaying a general increase in glucose uptake in the cardiac muscle also indicating inflammation. Figure courtesy of Dr. Christian Polte.

PET/CT is associated with reduced radiation exposure, and demonstrates higher sensitivity of for mild or borderline myocarditis, and increased specificity for chronic myocarditis [14].

3. Etiology

Cardiotropic viruses are the commonest causes of myocarditis in Europe and North America [2]. The most frequently-encountered etiological agents include enterovirus (Coxsackie B virus), adenovirus and parvovirus. Other viruses that are sometimes detected include influenza virus, hepatitis C virus, and HIV. The spirochete bacterium, *Borrelia burgdorferi*, may in rare cases cause myocarditis, which mainly affects the cardiac electrical system resulting in atrioventricular (AV) block [2, 5].

Chagas' disease (American trypanosomiasis) is prevalent various countries of Central-and South America. The infection is caused by Trypanosoma cruzi, which is a protozoan parasite transmitted to humans by various species of triatomine bugs [16]. Trypanosoma cruzi can cause both acute myocarditis and a chronic inflammation leading to severe cardiomyopathy and advanced heart failure [16].

Myocarditis can also occur in connection with autoimmune diseases, mainly systemic lupus erythematosus, systemic sclerosis, and rheumatoid arthritis. Various pharmaceuticals and chemicals can cause myocarditis via a toxic or allergic reaction affecting the heart. Radiation, heat stroke and hypothermia are examples of physical injuries that have been associated with cardiac inflammation [1, 2].

4. Pathophysiology

The pathophysiological mechanisms of lymphocytic myocarditis have been studied in animal models for Coxsackie B virus and other cardiotropic viruses [17]. Coxsackie B virus, which is an RNA virus, is incorporated into the myocyte via a receptor and mediated endocytosis, after which virus replication occurs in the cytoplasm [2, 18]. Following toxic cell necrosis, the virus particles come into contact with the myocardial interstitial tissue and trigger an innate immune response. The myocardial tissue becomes infiltrated by macrophages and natural killer (NK) cells, which eliminate infected myocytes and produce several cytokines, including virus-inhibiting interferon and tumor necrosis factor-α (TNF-α), a cardio-depressant [2]. Over time, the adaptive immune system is also stimulated, leading to recruitment of cytotoxic T-cells and neutralizing antibodies that contribute to viral clearance. An experimental form of viral myocarditis has been proposed to cause cardiomyopathy through three different mechanisms (**Figure 3**) [2].

1. Adequate immune activation leads to healing of the myocarditis within two to three weeks, but the damage is so extensive that a clinical phenotype of dilated cardiomyopathy arises [18].

2. An upregulated and overactive immune response may cause tissue damage through infiltrations of T-cells and autoantibodies (autoimmune cardiomyopathy).

3. A downregulated and ineffective immune response can lead to continuous apoptosis through a persistence virus infection (viral cardiomyopathy) [1].

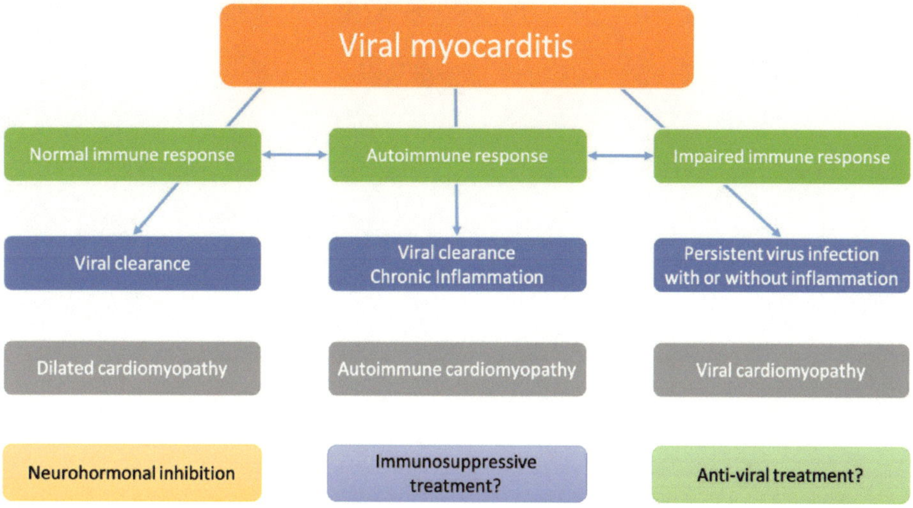

Figure 3.
An experimental form of viral myocarditis has been proposed to cause cardiomyopathy through three different mechanisms.

Findings that support the relationship between cardiotropic viruses and the development of cardiomyopathy in human studies include disturbances of T-cell regulation, inadequate expression of human leucocyte antigens (HLA) expressed and the presence of autoantibodies against cardiac epitopes [2].

5. Clinical features

Patients with myocarditis or inflammatory cardiomyopathy may present with a wide variety of symptoms and signs. The spectrum ranges from asymptomatic patients with minor changes on the electrocardiogram (ECG), or echocardiogram, to patients with fatigue, breathlessness, and palpitations and syncope due to impaired cardiac function or arrhythmias, and finally to patients with circulatory shock as a consequence of fulminant heart failure [19]. In some cases, the clinical presentation is preceded by influenza symptoms, upper respiratory tract infection or gastrointestinal discomfort, but in many cases, there are no prodromal symptoms [8].

Despite a large heterogeneity of the clinical picture, a few distinct forms can be identified.

1. Acute lymphocytic myocarditis presents with chest symptoms, comprising discomfort, pain, or palpitations, often combined with fatigue or breathlessness [19]. Fever and signs of infection can accompany the symptoms and myocardial biomarkers are frequently elevated. The ECG shows ST-T changes or arrhythmias and an echocardiogram can show regional hypokinesia or impaired systolic function [20]. The most usual differential diagnosis is acute coronary syndrome, which in most cases requires an exclusionary coronary angiogram. The treatment is mainly supportive (**Figure 4A**).

2. Fulminant myocarditis is an unusual but a very serious condition [6, 21]. The patient presents with cardiogenic chock including hypotension, tachycardia, and anuria without any other explanation for heart failure [22].

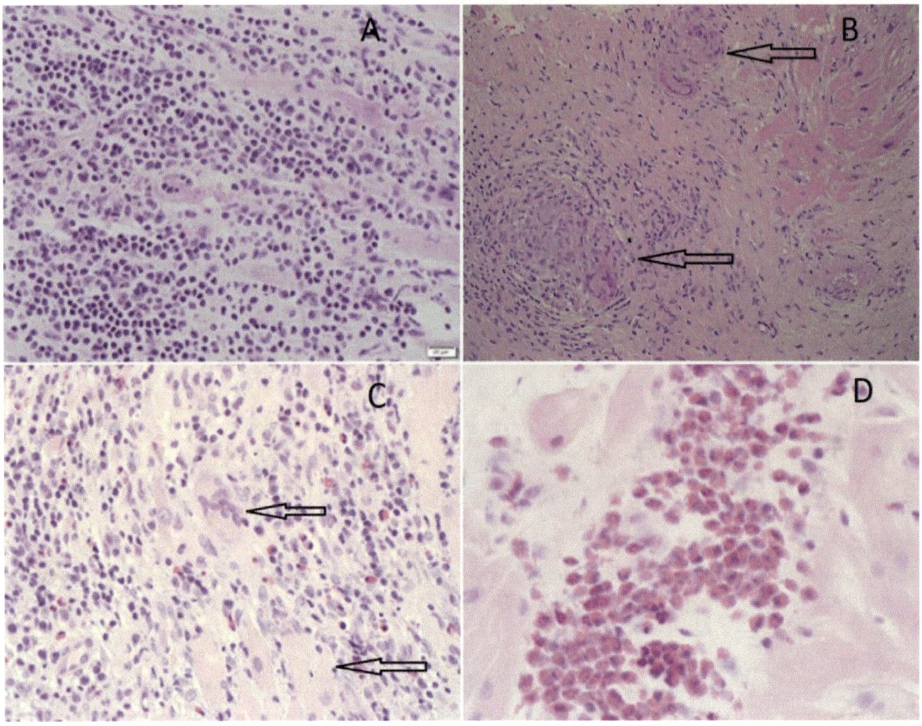

Figure 4.
Histopathological findings on endomyocardial biopsies from patients with inflammatory cardiomyopathy (tissue-staining with hematoxylin and eosin). A) Lymphocytic myocarditis. *Dense lymphocytic cell infiltration with some residual cardiomyocytes. B)* Cardiac sarcoidosis. *Non-caseating epithelioid cell granulomas (arrows) and fibrosis. C)* Giant cell myocarditis. *Widespread myocardial lesions with degenerated and necrotic cardiomyocytes and infiltration of mononuclear inflammatory cells, giant multinuclear cells (arrow) and some eosinophils. D)* Eosinophilic myocarditis. *Massive interstitial eosinophilic cell infiltration. Figure courtesy of prof. Anders Oldfors.*

The echocardiogram displays poor ventricular contractility without dilation and a myocardial biopsy can be normal or show a varying degree of inflammation [22]. Such patients often require intensive care, with administration of an inotropic and/or vasoconstrictive drug and, in some case short-term mechanical circulatory support (MCS) [4]. The pronounced ventricular failure frequently recovers within a few weeks. It has been speculated that the temporary cardio-depressive feature can be caused by an extensive storm of toxic cytokines, which would explain why the myocardial biopsy can be normal [21].

3. Cardiac sarcoidosis, giant cell myocarditis and eosinophilic myocarditis are examples of three additional clinical entities, which will be discussed separately below.

6. Diagnostics

Laboratory analysis often reveals elevation of inflammatory activity and increases in circulating markers of myocardial injury, such as creatine kinase (CK) and troponin [8]. Elevation of natriuretic peptides indicates overt heart failure.

Virus serology is seldom conclusive. An ECG can show unspecific ST-T changes, T-wave inversions, AV block or tachyarrhythmia [20]. An echocardiogram can detect regional hypokinesia, as well as ventricular dilation and reduced ejection fraction [23]. A suspicion of myocarditis most often arises after a coronary angiogram has excluded an underlying coronary artery disease.

Cardiac MR is used for the workup of suspected myocarditis. With delayed enhancement techniques, general or focal accumulation of contrast can be seen, which differs from ischemic injuries and can be of value when deciding the localization of an endomyocardial biopsy [24]. The Lake Louise criteria can be applied to evaluate the likelihood for myocardial inflammation. A PET/CT that shows increased focal or general myocardial uptake of FDG supports the diagnosis.

An endomyocardial biopsy should be considered when acute or chronic heart failure of unclear genesis presents, as well as in patients with impaired left ventricular function of unknown etiology with contemporary arrhythmias of ventricular origin or a significant AV block [9]. If myocarditis is diagnosed this will influence treatment and determine the prognosis. Even if a myocardial biopsy is limited by suboptimal sensitivity and some risk, this investigation still serves as a pivotal tool for diagnosis of myocardial inflammation [7].

7. Treatment

Treatment of myocarditis and inflammatory cardiomyopathy is mainly supportive and conforms with standard medical therapy for other dilated cardiomyopathies [6]. Patients should receive conventional, guideline-directed medical heart failure treatment including beta-blockers, inhibition of the renin-angiotensin-aldosterone system with angiotensin-converting enzyme (ACE) inhibitors or an angiotensin-receptor blocker (ARB), or as applied more recently, valsartan/sacubitril (an ARB combined with a neprilysin inhibitor [ARNI]), as well as a mineral corticoid antagonist (spironolactone or eplerenone) [25]. Sodium–glucose cotransporter-2 (SGLT-2) inhibitors are emerging as a new oral new therapy for heart failure patients who have reduced ejection fraction and are added to conventional therapy for patients both with or without diabetes [26, 27]. Loop diuretics should be added in patients who show signs of fluid retention [28]. If necessary, anti-arrhythmic therapy involving a pacemaker (PM) and/or an implantable cardioverter defibrillator (ICD) is indicated [6]. With severe heart failure, inotropic support may be necessary, or alternatively a short-term MCS [22]. The role of immunosuppression in myocarditis is controversial and its use as a general strategy is not advocated [29, 30].

Persons with acute myocarditis and mild myocardial infection frequently recover without any sequelae, but should refrain from heavy physical activity or sporting for at least 3 months due to an increased risk of ventricular arrhythmias [4].

8. Cardiac sarcoidosis

Sarcoidosis is a multisystem inflammatory disease of unknown etiology characterized by the presence of mononuclear phagocytes and non-caseating granuloma in different organ systems [31]. Although clinical heart disease has been confirmed in around 5% of patients with systemic sarcoidosis, up to 25% of such patients display signs of cardiac sarcoidosis at autopsy, indicating asymptomatic cardiac disease [32, 33].

The incidence of cardiac involvement varies between different ethnic groups: for example cardiac sarcoidosis is much more common among Japanese patients and African Americans than Caucasians [31]. A pronounced myocardial fibrosis can lead to a mixed picture of restrictive and dilated cardiomyopathy. The conduction system is more often affected in cardiac sarcoidosis than in other inflammatory cardiomyopathies, possibly due to an inflammation that is located in the atrium and the antero-septal wall of the left ventricle, which frequently leads to AV block [34, 35]. Granuloma formation can occur in all parts of the heart, but the cardiac valves and coronary arteries are usually spared [31]. The pericardium may also be involved, and pericardial fluid is present in 5-15% of cases [31].

It has been suggested that the incidence of cardiac sarcoidosis is increasing [36]. In the US, the incidence of transplant patients with cardiac sarcoidosis as their underlying condition increased from 0.1% to 0.5% between 1994 and 2014 [37]. Similar trends were reported from a Finnish nationwide cohort study [36]. However, this increase in incidence may be due to a progress in imaging techniques, increasing awareness and more aggressive diagnostics involving endomyocardial biopsies [36].

8.1 Etiology

Sarcoidosis is an inflammatory disease whose pathogenesis and inciting events are not well understood. Accumulating evidence suggests that the disease is caused by an immunological response to an antigenic trigger of unknown origin in genetically susceptible individuals [38]. Supportive of this are alleles of the *HLA-DRB1* locus, which are more common in patients with sarcoidosis [39]. In addition, exposure to environmental triggers and to various micro-organisms have been linked to the development of the disease [40].

8.2 Pathophysiology

Non-caseating granulomas are the histopathological hallmark of cardiac sarcoidosis (**Figure 4B**). The granuloma consists of a tightly packed follicle made up of lymphocytes (in particular CD4+ T cells), giant cells and epithelioid cells surrounded by a rim of fibroblasts and lymphocytes [41].

Clinical features of cardiac sarcoidosis depend on the location, extent, and activity of the disease. Cardiac sarcoidosis can also occur without clinical manifestations [31], but common symptoms include palpitations, dizziness and/or fainting [36]. Symptomatic cardiac sarcoidosis is a potentially serious condition that can lead to heart failure, life-threatening arrhythmias, and sudden death [42, 43].

8.3 Diagnostics

Emergence of symptoms and signs of heart disease in patients with known extracardiac sarcoidosis, especially young individuals with electrical conduction disturbances, should raise the suspicion of cardiac sarcoidosis. A careful history should be obtained with respect to palpitations, syncope and pre-syncope [31, 44]. An ECG may reveal unspecific ST-T changes, T-inversions, conduction disturbances or ventricular arrhythmias. Long-term electrocardiography can provide valuable additional information in the form of the numbers of both supraventricular and ventricular premature extra-systoles and supraventricular and ventricular tackyarrhythmias [45]. In clinically silent cardiac sarcoidosis, the echocardiogram is often normal, but with manifest disease, structural and functional aberrations become apparent [45, 46]. Those defects are variable and usually non-specific, although interventricular thinning, especially basal, left and/or right ventricle diastolic and systolic dysfunction, and isolated wall motion abnormalities, may indicate cardiac sarcoidosis [31]. Cardiac MR, and to an increasing extent FDG-PET/CT, are today considered to be the best methods for detecting and visualizing sarcoidosis in the heart muscle [31]. Both techniques can visualize active inflammation (**Figure 2**) [47–49]. Although the pattern of late gadolinium enhancement on Cardiac MR is usually patchy and multifocal, with sparing of the endocardial border, this is neither specific nor diagnostic for cardiac sarcoidosis [50, 51]. An endomyocardial biopsy that displays non-caseating granulomas strongly supports the diagnosis, but is not pathognomonic.

In patients with extra-cardiac sarcoidosis, a lymph node or lung biopsy is typically preferred to endomyocardial biopsy because of the lesser procedural risk and higher diagnostic yield [36, 48]. However, in the case of a negative extra-cardiac biopsy, an endomyocardial biopsy may be required. Nevertheless, owing to the patchy distribution of the disease, and endomyocardial biopsy reveals non-caseating granulomas in less than 25% of patients [52].

8.4 Treatment

A strong suspicion of cardiac sarcoidosis motivates treatment with high dose corticosteroids with slow tapering. Studies have shown regression of high-grade AV block after corticosteroid treatment, as well as a reduced frequency of ventricular arrhythmias in the acute phase of the disease [53]. Most patients - but not all - benefit from this treatment. Methotrexate is also an option, but is mainly given to facilitate tapering of steroids and, thus, alleviate their side effects [31]. The optimal treatment period for corticosteroids is still debated, but should not be less than one year and, in most cases, should be longer. If a decision is made to end corticosteroid treatment, it is important to follow the patient closely for possible relapse, especially during the first year [36].

Antiarrhythmic drugs usually have only a limited effect on rhythm disturbances in patients with cardiac sarcoidosis. Beta-blockers are the first choice for both supraventricular and ventricular arrhythmias [53] and amiodarone can be tested in acute situations with ventricular tachycardia (VT). If the arrhythmia events are associated with active inflammation, corticosteroids should be added or their dose increased. If satisfactory results are not achieved, VT ablation may be considered [34, 35]. Class I anti-arrhythmic agents are not recommended in patients with cardiac sarcoidosis as most patients have structural myocardial changes in the form of myocardial fibrosis. Because of the tendency towards persistent VT attacks and a high risk of sudden death, implantation of an ICD must be considered and should be discussed with the patient at an early stage. A recent international consensus document on sarcoidosis-related arrhythmias provides guidance on which patients should be considered for ICD implantation [34]. In those with a high-grade AV block, an implantation of a permanent pacemaker is indicated [44].

Heart failure owing to cardiac sarcoidosis should always be treated with guideline-directed medical therapy, as described above. Heart transplantation is an option for patients in NYHA functional class IIIB-IV or in those with intractable arrhythmias, with satisfactory outcomes [54]. However, there is a risk of recurrence of the sarcoidosis in the transplanted heart and little is known about long-term morbidity and mortality in this group after heart transplantation [55].

9. Giant cell myocarditis

Giant cell myocarditis (GCM) is a rare inflammatory heart disease of unknown etiology, which is associated with thymoma, inflammatory bowel disease and other autoimmune disorders [1]. The myocardial inflammation is characterized by widespread infiltration of giant cells along with several other inflammatory cell types that cause myocyte destruction [43]. Giant cells themselves are abnormal cell masses generated by the fusion of several macrophages (**Figure 4C**). Evidence suggests that this phenomenon may arise in response to immune dysregulation mediated by T-lymphocytes [43]. Giant cell myocarditis has been commonly depicted as a rapidly progressive and usually fatal condition for which heart transplantation is the treatment of choice [56]. The disease caught attention in the 1990's when the International Multicenter Giant Cell Myocarditis Study Group reported that 89% of the 63 included patients with the disease either required heart transplantation or died. The median transplant-free survival rate was only 5.5 months [56]. In a later analysis, the overall transplant-free survival at 5 years in patients with giant cell myocarditis was reported to be as low as 10% [57]. However, previous epidemiological studies are confounded by the fact that most patients were diagnosed after heart transplantation or at autopsy.

The initial symptoms of giant cell myocarditis comprise chest pain, palpitations, fatigue, breathlessness and ankle swelling. Individuals with giant cell myocarditis often exhibit advanced heart failure and life-threating arrhythmias [21]. Endomyocardial biopsy is the gold standard for diagnosis [9]. Cardiac MR and PET/CT are useful for identifying targets for biopsy. The combination of cardiac MR and endomyocardial biopsy has been shown to improve detection rates. When a clinical suspicion remains high despite a negative biopsy, repeat sampling is recommended [1].

Patients who are diagnosed in the early phase of the disease may respond to immunosuppressive treatment, including calcineurin inhibitors (tacrolimus or cyclosporine), an antimetabolite (mycophenolate mofetil or azathioprine) and prednisolone, but an ongoing disease process rapidly damages the heart, which is why heart transplantation often becomes the only realistic treatment option. Owing to the severity of heart failure and the presence of treatment-resistant ventricular arrhythmias, patients with giant cell myocarditis frequently develop multiorgan failure and require durable mechanical support with either a left ventricular or a bi-ventricular assist device as a bridge-to-transplantation [55]. Patients treated with combined immunosuppression have a median survival of 12.3 months from the onset of symptoms, compared to 3.0 months without immunosuppression [58]. Early and aggressive arrhythmia management, including radiofrequency catheter ablation, has been suggested to prolong survival [59]. Early initiation of immunosuppressive therapy also seems to improve outcomes in patients with this aggressive cardiac disease [59].

10. Eosinophilic myocarditis

Eosinophilic myocarditis is a rare and potentially lethal disease characterized by eosinophilic infiltrates in the myocardial tissue (**Figure 4D**). It may occur in association with malignancy, parasite infection, hypersensitivity, and also an idiopathic hyper-eosinophilic syndrome [60, 61]. However, the relative associations between proposed triggers and myocardial eosinophilia remain elusive and, in most cases, the underlying cause remains unknown [1, 60]. The clinical presentation can range from mild symptoms to chronic restrictive cardiomyopathy (Loeffler cardiomyopathy) or acute fulminant myocarditis (also called acute necrotizing eosinophilic myocarditis) [60]. The definite diagnosis of eosinophilic myocarditis can only be achieved with an endomyocardial biopsy, although clinicians often base the diagnosis on laboratory findings and imaging examinations, mainly cardiac MR [1, 9].

In most cases, eosinophilia can be detected in peripheral blood samples and this finding together with cardiac symptoms should always raise suspicions of eosinophilic myocarditis. However, in the early stage of the disease, peripheral eosinophilia may be absent and it may not develop at all in a subgroup of patients. Circulating markers of inflammation and myocardial injury are often increased and natriuretic peptides increase in parallel with the severity of the heart failure syndrome. Normal laboratory tests do not, however, exclude the presence of the disease [60].

The ECG is often abnormal, mainly demonstrating ST-T segment abnormalities, but this is neither sensitive nor specific for eosinophilic myocarditis. The echocardiogram is of pivotal importance with respect to excluding other heart failure etiologies, evaluating left ventricular systolic and diastolic function and monitoring the presence of pericardial effusion. Cardiac MR allows for the identification of edema and diffuse foci of delayed enhancement reflecting myocardial inflammation, necrosis and fibrosis. In stable patients, it is reasonable to perform cardiac MR imaging prior to endomyocardial biopsy, as the former may help to identify focal pathology through late enhancement and guide myocardial tissue sampling. However, in unstable patients an endomyocardial biopsy should be prioritized [60, 62, 63]. Eosinophilic myocarditis, particularly in its fulminant form, is associated with high in-hospital mortality, but owing to the rarity of the disease, no reliable data on mortality rates are available. Its incidence and prevalence are probably under-estimated, as the disease is most usually discovered post-mortem [60].

The treatment and prognosis of eosinophilic myocarditis depends on its etiology. In the acute phase, restriction of physical activity is an important measure. In selected patients, particularly in those with suspected autoreactive etiology and negative virology, early treatment with corticosteroids has resulted in advantageous outcomes [64]. Nevertheless, the evidence supporting corticosteroid therapy is limited, deriving from small, non-randomized studies. Moreover, the initial dosage and treatment duration vary between different reports and, therefore, no evidence-based recommendations can be presented. It is not unreasonable, however, to adjust the steroid dose and treatment duration to the severity of the disease and the primary underlying disorder [60, 62, 64]. The monoclonal antibody benralizumab, which binds to the interleukin-5 receptor on the cell surface and causes apoptosis of eosinophils, has recently been advocated as a promising new therapeutic strategy for eosinophil myocarditis [60].

11. Conclusions

Inflammatory cardiomyopathy refers to a diverse group of disorders in which inflammation of the heart muscle is accompanied by disturbances of cardiac structure and/or function. The diagnosis of these disorders remains challenging despite recent advances in imaging and molecular biology techniques. Together with careful anamnestic enquiry, physical examination and laboratory tests, a comprehensive diagnostic work-up, including both non-invasive and invasive methods, is required to reach a conclusion with respect to identification, management and prognosis. Although cardiac MR and PET/CT represent fundamental non-invasive diagnostic methods, endomyocardial biopsy remains the gold standard. Regular treatment of inflammatory cardiomyopathies is based on the guideline-directed therapy for heart failure and arrhythmias. More targeted therapies, including immunomodulating treatment, can be indicated only when histopathological findings from the endomyocardial biopsy are known. However, owing to a lack of evidence, an individual assessment of each patient is of vital importance for the management of inflammatory cardiomyopathies. Large prospective multicenter randomized studies are needed to generate evidence-based treatment recommendations in this specific group of patients.

Acknowledgements

The authors thank Dr. Christian Polte for providing us with **Figure 2** and Professor Anders Oldfors for providing us with **Figure 4**. We also express gratitude to Hughes associates, Oxford, UK, for reviewing the English used in this book chapter.

Conflict of interest

The authors declare no conflict of interest.

Author details

Emanuele Bobbio[1,3] and Kristjan Karason[1,2,3]*

1 Department of Cardiology, Sahlgrenska University Hospital, Gotenburg, Sweden

2 Transplant Institute, Sahlgrenska University Hospital, Gotenburg, Sweden

3 Institute of Medicine at Sahlgrenska Academy, University of Gothenburg, Sweden

*Address all correspondence to: kristjan.karason@medfak.gu.se

References

[1] Trachtenberg BH, Hare JM. Inflammatory Cardiomyopathic Syndromes. Circ Res. 2017;121(7): 803-18.

[2] Tschope C, Ammirati E, Bozkurt B, Caforio ALP, Cooper LT, Felix SB, et al. Myocarditis and inflammatory cardiomyopathy: current evidence and future directions. Nat Rev Cardiol. 2021;18(3):169-93.

[3] Richardson P, McKenna W, Bristow M, Maisch B, Mautner B, O'Connell J, et al. Report of the 1995 World Health Organization/ International Society and Federation of Cardiology Task Force on the Definition and Classification of cardiomyopathies. Circulation. 1996;93(5):841-2.

[4] Caforio AL, Pankuweit S, Arbustini E, Basso C, Gimeno-Blanes J, Felix SB, et al. Current state of knowledge on aetiology, diagnosis, management, and therapy of myocarditis: a position statement of the European Society of Cardiology Working Group on Myocardial and Pericardial Diseases. Eur Heart J. 2013;34(33):2636-48, 48a-48d.

[5] Krejci J, Mlejnek D, Sochorova D, Nemec P. Inflammatory Cardiomyopathy: A Current View on the Pathophysiology, Diagnosis, and Treatment. Biomed Res Int. 2016;2016:4087632.

[6] Ammirati E, Frigerio M, Adler ED, Basso C, Birnie DH, Brambatti M, et al. Management of Acute Myocarditis and Chronic Inflammatory Cardiomyopathy: An Expert Consensus Document. Circ Heart Fail. 2020;13(11):e007405.

[7] Ammirati E, Cipriani M, Bonacina E, Garascia A, Oliva F. [Endomyocardial biopsy should be performed in selected patients with suspected myocarditis]. G Ital Cardiol (Rome). 2015;16(10):539-43.

[8] Ammirati E, Cipriani M, Moro C, Raineri C, Pini D, Sormani P, et al. Clinical Presentation and Outcome in a Contemporary Cohort of Patients With Acute Myocarditis: Multicenter Lombardy Registry. Circulation. 2018;138(11):1088-99.

[9] Elliott P, Arbustini E. The role of endomyocardial biopsy in the management of cardiovascular disease: a commentary on joint AHA/ACC/ESC guidelines. Heart. 2009;95(9):759-60.

[10] Aretz HT, Billingham ME, Edwards WD, Factor SM, Fallon JT, Fenoglio JJ, Jr., et al. Myocarditis. A histopathologic definition and classification. Am J Cardiovasc Pathol. 1987;1(1):3-14.

[11] Magnani JW, Danik HJ, Dec GW, Jr., DiSalvo TG. Survival in biopsy-proven myocarditis: a long-term retrospective analysis of the histopathologic, clinical, and hemodynamic predictors. Am Heart J. 2006;151(2):463-70.

[12] Ferreira VM, Schulz-Menger J, Holmvang G, Kramer CM, Carbone I, Sechtem U, et al. Cardiovascular Magnetic Resonance in Nonischemic Myocardial Inflammation: Expert Recommendations. J Am Coll Cardiol. 2018;72(24):3158-76.

[13] Friedrich MG, Sechtem U, Schulz-Menger J, Holmvang G, Alakija P, Cooper LT, et al. Cardiovascular magnetic resonance in myocarditis: A JACC White Paper. J Am Coll Cardiol. 2009;53(17):1475-87.

[14] Chen W, Jeudy J. Assessment of Myocarditis: Cardiac MR, PET/CT, or PET/MR? Curr Cardiol Rep. 2019;21(8):76.

[15] Calder PC, Dimitriadis G, Newsholme P. Glucose metabolism in lymphoid and inflammatory cells and

tissues. Curr Opin Clin Nutr Metab Care. 2007;10(4):531-40.

[16] Nunes MCP, Beaton A, Acquatella H, Bern C, Bolger AF, Echeverria LE, et al. Chagas Cardiomyopathy: An Update of Current Clinical Knowledge and Management: A Scientific Statement From the American Heart Association. Circulation. 2018;138(12):e169-e209.

[17] Dominguez F, Kuhl U, Pieske B, Garcia-Pavia P, Tschope C. Update on Myocarditis and Inflammatory Cardiomyopathy: Reemergence of Endomyocardial Biopsy. Rev Esp Cardiol (Engl Ed). 2016;69(2):178-87.

[18] Kuhl U, Pauschinger M, Noutsias M, Seeberg B, Bock T, Lassner D, et al. High prevalence of viral genomes and multiple viral infections in the myocardium of adults with "idiopathic" left ventricular dysfunction. Circulation. 2005;111(7):887-93.

[19] Lieberman EB, Hutchins GM, Herskowitz A, Rose NR, Baughman KL. Clinicopathologic description of myocarditis. J Am Coll Cardiol. 1991;18(7):1617-26.

[20] Butta C, Zappia L, Laterra G, Roberto M. Diagnostic and prognostic role of electrocardiogram in acute myocarditis: A comprehensive review. Ann Noninvasive Electrocardiol. 2020;25(3).

[21] Ammirati E, Camici PG. Still poor prognosis for patients with giant cell myocarditis in the era of temporary mechanical circulatory supports. Int J Cardiol. 2018;253:122-3.

[22] Veronese G, Ammirati E, Cipriani M, Frigerio M. Fulminant myocarditis: Characteristics, treatment, and outcomes. Anatol J Cardiol. 2018;19(4):279-86.

[23] Felker GM, Boehmer JP, Hruban RH, Hutchins GM, Kasper EK, Baughman KL, et al. Echocardiographic findings in fulminant and acute myocarditis. J Am Coll Cardiol. 2000;36(1):227-32.

[24] Friedrich MG, Sechtem U, Schulz-Menger J, Holmvang G, Alakija P, Cooper LT, et al. Cardiovascular magnetic resonance in myocarditis: A JACC White Paper. J Am Coll Cardiol. 2009;53(17):1475-87.

[25] Ponikowski P, Voors AA, Anker SD, Bueno H, Cleland JG, Coats AJ, et al. 2016 ESC Guidelines for the diagnosis and treatment of acute and chronic heart failure: The Task Force for the diagnosis and treatment of acute and chronic heart failure of the European Society of Cardiology (ESC). Developed with the special contribution of the Heart Failure Association (HFA) of the ESC. Eur J Heart Fail. 2016;18(8):891-975.

[26] Zinman B, Wanner C, Lachin JM, Fitchett D, Bluhmki E, Hantel S, et al. Empagliflozin, Cardiovascular Outcomes, and Mortality in Type 2 Diabetes. N Engl J Med. 2015;373(22):2117-28.

[27] McMurray JJV, Solomon SD, Inzucchi SE, Køber L, Kosiborod MN, Martinez FA, et al. Dapagliflozin in Patients with Heart Failure and Reduced Ejection Fraction. N Engl J Med. 2019;381(21):1995-2008.

[28] Metra M, Davison B, Bettari L, Sun H, Edwards C, Lazzarini V, et al. Is worsening renal function an ominous prognostic sign in patients with acute heart failure? The role of congestion and its interaction with renal function. Circ Heart Fail. 2012;5(1):54-62.

[29] Mason JW, O'Connell JB, Herskowitz A, Rose NR, McManus BM, Billingham ME, et al. A clinical trial of immunosuppressive therapy for myocarditis. The Myocarditis Treatment Trial Investigators. N Engl J Med. 1995;333(5):269-75.

[30] Frustaci A, Chimenti C, Calabrese F, Pieroni M, Thiene G, Maseri A. Immunosuppressive therapy for active lymphocytic myocarditis: virological and immunologic profile of responders versus nonresponders. Circulation. 2003;107(6):857-63.

[31] Birnie DH. Cardiac Sarcoidosis. Semin Respir Crit Care Med. 2020;41(5):626-40.

[32] Birnie DH, Nery PB. Debating the Definition and Incidence of Isolated Cardiac Sarcoidosis. JACC Clin Electrophysiol. 2020;6(9):1190-1.

[33] Trivieri MG, Spagnolo P, Birnie D, Liu P, Drake W, Kovacic JC, et al. Challenges in Cardiac and Pulmonary Sarcoidosis: JACC State-of-the-Art Review. J Am Coll Cardiol. 2020;76(16):1878-901.

[34] Birnie DH, Sauer WH, Bogun F, Cooper JM, Culver DA, Duvernoy CS, et al. HRS expert consensus statement on the diagnosis and management of arrhythmias associated with cardiac sarcoidosis. Heart Rhythm. 2014;11(7):1305-23.

[35] Birnie DH, Sauer WH, Judson MA. Consensus statement on the diagnosis and management of arrhythmias associated with cardiac sarcoidosis. Heart. 2016;102(6):411-4.

[36] Kandolin R, Lehtonen J, Airaksinen J, Vihinen T, Miettinen H, Ylitalo K, et al. Cardiac sarcoidosis: epidemiology, characteristics, and outcome over 25 years in a nationwide study. Circulation. 2015;131(7):624-32.

[37] Al-Kindi SG, Oliveira GH. Letter by Al-Kindi and Oliveira regarding article "cardiac sarcoidosis: epidemiology, characteristics, and outcome over 25 years in a nationwide study". Circulation. 2015;132(17):e211.

[38] Muchtar E, Blauwet LA, Gertz MA. Restrictive Cardiomyopathy: Genetics, Pathogenesis, Clinical Manifestations, Diagnosis, and Therapy. Circ Res. 2017;121(7):819-37.

[39] Rossman MD, Thompson B, Frederick M, Maliarik M, Iannuzzi MC, Rybicki BA, et al. HLA-DRB1*1101: a significant risk factor for sarcoidosis in blacks and whites. Am J Hum Genet. 2003;73(4):720-35.

[40] Rossman MD, Thompson B, Frederick M, Iannuzzi MC, Rybicki BA, Pander JP, et al. HLA and environmental interactions in sarcoidosis. Sarcoidosis Vasc Diffuse Lung Dis. 2008;25(2):125-32.

[41] Agostini C, Adami F, Semenzato G. New pathogenetic insights into the sarcoid granuloma. Curr Opin Rheumatol. 2000;12(1):71-6.

[42] Ekstrom K, Lehtonen J, Nordenswan HK, Mayranpaa MI, Raisanen-Sokolowski A, Kandolin R, et al. Sudden death in cardiac sarcoidosis: an analysis of nationwide clinical and cause-of-death registries. Eur Heart J. 2019;40(37):3121-8.

[43] Kandolin R, Lehtonen J, Kupari M. Cardiac sarcoidosis and giant cell myocarditis as causes of atrioventricular block in young and middle-aged adults. Circ Arrhythm Electrophysiol. 2011;4(3):303-9.

[44] Nordenswan HK, Lehtonen J, Ekstrom K, Kandolin R, Simonen P, Mayranpaa M, et al. Outcome of Cardiac Sarcoidosis Presenting With High-Grade Atrioventricular Block. Circ Arrhythm Electrophysiol. 2018;11(8):e006145.

[45] Mehta D, Lubitz SA, Frankel Z, Wisnivesky JP, Einstein AJ, Goldman M, et al. Cardiac involvement in patients with sarcoidosis: diagnostic and prognostic value of outpatient testing. Chest. 2008;133(6):1426-35.

[46] Skold CM, Larsen FF, Rasmussen E, Pehrsson SK, Eklund AG. Determination of cardiac involvement in sarcoidosis by magnetic resonance imaging and Doppler echocardiography. J Intern Med. 2002;252(5):465-71.

[47] Ekstrom K, Lehtonen J, Hanninen H, Kandolin R, Kivisto S, Kupari M. Magnetic Resonance Imaging as a Predictor of Survival Free of Life-Threatening Arrhythmias and Transplantation in Cardiac Sarcoidosis. J Am Heart Assoc. 2016;5(5).

[48] Kandolin R, Lehtonen J, Graner M, Schildt J, Salmenkivi K, Kivisto SM, et al. Diagnosing isolated cardiac sarcoidosis. J Intern Med. 2011;270(5):461-8.

[49] Ohira H, Birnie DH, Pena E, Bernick J, Mc Ardle B, Leung E, et al. Comparison of (18) F-fluorodeoxyglucose positron emission tomography (FDG PET) and cardiac magnetic resonance (CMR) in corticosteroid-naive patients with conduction system disease due to cardiac sarcoidosis. Eur J Nucl Med Mol Imaging. 2016;43(2):259-69.

[50] Ichinose A, Otani H, Oikawa M, Takase K, Saito H, Shimokawa H, et al. MRI of cardiac sarcoidosis: basal and subepicardial localization of myocardial lesions and their effect on left ventricular function. AJR Am J Roentgenol. 2008;191(3):862-9.

[51] Erthal F, Juneau D, Lim SP, Dwivedi G, Nery PB, Birnie D, et al. Imaging of cardiac sarcoidosis. Q J Nucl Med Mol Imaging. 2016;60(3):252-63.

[52] Bennett MK, Gilotra NA, Harrington C, Rao S, Dunn JM, Freitag TB, et al. Evaluation of the role of endomyocardial biopsy in 851 patients with unexplained heart failure from 2000-2009. Circ Heart Fail. 2013;6(4):676-84.

[53] Ekstrom K, Lehtonen J, Kandolin R, Raisanen-Sokolowski A, Salmenkivi K, Kupari M. Incidence, Risk Factors, and Outcome of Life-Threatening Ventricular Arrhythmias in Giant Cell Myocarditis. Circ Arrhythm Electrophysiol. 2016;9(12).

[54] Toma M, Birnie D. Heart Transplantation for End-Stage Cardiac Sarcoidosis: Increasingly Used With Excellent Results. Can J Cardiol. 2018;34(8):956-8.

[55] Bobbio E, Lingbrant M, Nwaru BI, Hessman E, Lehtonen J, Karason K, et al. Inflammatory cardiomyopathies: short- and long-term outcomes after heart transplantation-a protocol for a systematic review and meta-analysis. Heart Fail Rev. 2020;25(3):481-5.

[56] Cooper LT, Jr., Berry GJ, Shabetai R. Idiopathic giant-cell myocarditis--natural history and treatment. Multicenter Giant Cell Myocarditis Study Group Investigators. The New England journal of medicine. 1997;336(26):1860-6.

[57] Okura Y, Dec GW, Hare JM, Kodama M, Berry GJ, Tazelaar HD, et al. A clinical and histopathologic comparison of cardiac sarcoidosis and idiopathic giant cell myocarditis. Journal of the American College of Cardiology. 2003;41(2):322-9.

[58] Frustaci A, Russo MA, Chimenti C. Randomized study on the efficacy of immunosuppressive therapy in patients with virus-negative inflammatory cardiomyopathy: the TIMIC study. Eur Heart J. 2009;30(16):1995-2002.

[59] Ekstrom K, Lehtonen J, Kandolin R, Raisanen-Sokolowski A, Salmenkivi K, Kupari M. Long-term outcome and its predictors in giant cell myocarditis. Eur J Heart Fail. 2016;18(12):1452-8.

[60] Brambatti M, Matassini MV, Adler ED, Klingel K, Camici PG,

Ammirati E. Eosinophilic Myocarditis: Characteristics, Treatment, and Outcomes. J Am Coll Cardiol. 2017;70(19):2363-75.

[61] Ammirati E, Stucchi M, Brambatti M, Spano F, Bonacina E, Recalcati F, et al. Eosinophilic myocarditis: a paraneoplastic event. Lancet. 2015;385(9986):2546.

[62] Kuchynka P, Palecek T, Masek M, Cerny V, Lambert L, Vitkova I, et al. Current Diagnostic and Therapeutic Aspects of Eosinophilic Myocarditis. BioMed Research International. 2016;2016:2829583.

[63] Li H, Dai Z, Wang B, Huang W. A case report of eosinophilic myocarditis and a review of the relevant literature. BMC Cardiovascular Disorders. 2015;15(1):15.

[64] Yanagisawa T, Inomata T, Watanabe I, Maekawa E, Mizutani T, Shinagawa H, et al. Clinical significance of corticosteroid therapy for eosinophilic myocarditis. Int Heart J. 2011;52(2):110-3.

Chapter 18

Cardiac Amyloidosis

Csilla Andrea Eötvös, Giorgia Pastiu, Iulia Zehan, Cerasela Goidescu, Roxana Chiorescu, Roxana Lazar, Florina Frîngu, Raluca Tomoaia, Monica Pop, Adrian Molnar, Sorin Pop and Dan Blendea

Abstract

Amyloidosis represents a heterogeneous group of disorders caused by amyloid fibril deposition in the extracellular space in different organs. Among the many types of amyloidosis cardiac involvement occurs almost exclusively with immunoglobulin light chain amyloidosis (AL amyloidosis) or transthyretin amyloidosis (ATTR amyloidosis). When present cardiac amyloidosis (CA) has a significant impact on disease prognosis. The typical clinical presentation in CA is that of a restrictive cardiomyopathy. Clinical suspicion of CA is based on clinical, laboratory and electrocardiographic findings. The diagnosis is confirmed using echocardiography, cardiac magnetic resonance imaging, biopsy, and/or bone scintigraphy. A precise definition of amyloidosis type is essential for choosing the specific treatment for this condition. Treatment of CA has two components: general treatment of congestive HF, and specific treatment of the underlying protein misfolding disorder.

Keywords: cardiomyopathy, amyloidosis, restrictive cardiomyopathy

1. Introduction

All types of amyloidosis involve deposition of amyloidogenic protein, composed of low molecular weight subunits, most of which circulate as plasma components. The amyloid deposits are formed by subunit proteins which originate from soluble precursors. These proteins have undergone conformational changes that generated an antiparallel beta-pleated sheet.

There are more than 30 precursor proteins that can form deposits in the extracellular space and can generate progressive organ dysfunction.

The majority of cases of amyloidosis are caused by 3 subtypes: the most common form, which accounts for approximately 70% of all cases is AL amyloidosis, due to the deposition of misfolded immunoglobulin light chains. The other two forms with increased prevalence are ATTR amyloidosis caused by deposition of transthyretin either as wild-type (ATTRwt) form, or mutated/variant (ATTRv) [1].

CA is a myocardial infiltrative disease due to amyloid fibril deposition in the extracellular space of the heart. The infiltrative process results in increased thickness of the left ventricular wall, diastolic dysfunction and HF.

Until about a decade ago amyloidosis used to be considered a rare condition, managed primarily by hematologists, neurologists and nephrologists. CA used to be diagnosed late in the evolution of the disease, with negative impact on prognosis of these patients. In the last few years there has been and increased emphasis on early diagnosis on optimization of screening and diagnosis of CA. The reason for this is the advent of targeted therapies, which showed increased efficacy in treating CA if they are applied early in the course of the disease [2].

Systemic forms of amyloidosis affecting the heart, are mainly AL, ATTRwt, and some forms of ATTRv amyloidosis [1].

2. Pathophysiology and epidemiology of CA

The pathophysiology of CA is complex. Amyloid infiltration of the heart leads to a decrease in ventricular compliance. This in turn creates the premises for diastolic dysfunction. The decrease in ventricular compliance is associated with an elevation in ventricular filling pressures. Backward transmission of high filling pressures results in bi-atrial dilatation and stasis.

AL amyloidosis is usually caused by a small clonal B cell or plasma cell population, with about 10% of patients having multiple myeloma [3]. From a pathophysiological standpoint there is interstitial deposition of immunoglobulin light chains, as well as direct toxicity on the myocytes caused by the free light chains. These chains can induce lysosomal dysfunction, oxidative stress, apoptosis, and dysregulation of MAP kinase signaling transduction pathways as well as autophagy [4]. The amount of cardiac involvement independently predicts mortality [4].

Transthyretin (TTR), which is a transport protein for retinol and thyroid hormone synthesized by the liver, can form amyloid fibrils when it dissociates from tetramers into monomers. The destabilization tetramers with accumulation of TTR monomers can result from gene mutations in the TTR gene (ATTRv) or are the result of age-related processes (ATTRwt) [4].

The pathophysiology of CA is complex. Amyloid infiltration of the heart leads to a decrease in ventricular compliance. This in turn creates the premises for diastolic dysfunction. The decrease in ventricular compliance is associated with an elevation in ventricular filling pressures. Backward transmission of high filling pressures results in bi-atrial dilatation and stasis.

Detailed information regarding the epidemiology of CA is lacking. Gilstrap et al., in a study published in 2019, found a prevalence rate of CA among Medicare beneficiaries of 8–17 per 100,000 person-years. The incidence rate in the same study was 18–55 per 100,000 person-years [5]. The prevalence of AL amyloidosis has increased 2.6-fold in the United States between from 15.5 cases per million in 2007 to 40.5 in 2015 [6].

Cardiac involvement in AL amyloidosis is a major determinant of prognosis, with mean survival time is only about 6 months without treatment in cases with advanced cardiac disease and HF [7]. The median overall survival is extended to >5 years if modern treatment strategies are used [1].

3. Clinical manifestations

The clinical presentation of patients with amyloidosis is heterogeneous and nonspecific and, varies depending on the degree of organ involvement. The onset of symptoms depends on the type of amyloidosis.

Amyloid infiltration of the heart can generate symptoms and signs that are common in restrictive cardiomyopathy.

Lower extremity edema is a nonspecific clinical manifestation, which is common in different conditions associated with heart failure (HF). It can be associated with the elevation of jugular venous pressure, pleural effusion, ascites, pain in the right hypochondriac region caused by liver congestion, dyspnea at exertion or at rest and orthopnea. These symptoms are related predominantly to right ventricular failure and restrictive cardiomyopathy, which is one of the most common forms of presentation in CA [8].

Another symptom that can occur in CA is presyncope or syncope consequent to bradyarrhythmias or high-degree/complete atrioventricular block. Loss of consciousness is often present in AL amyloidosis and in some cases can have combined etiology [9]. Furthermore, hypotension induced by autonomic neuropathy may lead to syncope in patients with amyloidosis.

Sometimes, patients complain of palpitations which occur in the setting of atrial fibrillation (AF) due to the infiltration of the atrium with amyloid deposits or by the dilated atrium secondary to restrictive cardiomyopathy. This is the most common described arrhythmia, found in 10–15% of the patients [10]. Ventricular tachyarrhythmias can occur in advanced stages of the cardiomyopathy, however sudden cardiac death often due to electromechanical dissociation [9].

In advanced forms of CA with systolic dysfunction, the patient can exhibit signs and symptoms of low cardiac output such as fatigue, dizziness, weakness, hypotension, delayed capillary refill and decreased pressure of pulse wave.

Angina or myocardial infarction, rare manifestations of CA, may develop as a cause of microvascular dysfunction or amyloid deposits in the coronary arteries [8]. However, an in vitro experiment performed by Liao R. et al. showed that amyloidogenic light chains may have a direct toxic effect on cardiac myocytes [11] and it can explain why patients with AL amyloidosis have poorer quality of life than patients with ATTR amyloidosis with the same degree of cardiac involvement.

Extracardiac organ involvement leads to a plethora of other signs and symptoms in amyloidosis. Because of the variety of the manifestations such as nephrotic syndrome, gastrointestinal symptoms, pulmonary disease, bleeding diathesis, macroglossia, purpura, musculoskeletal abnormalities, carpal tunnel syndrome, the diagnosis is often delayed [12].

Due to the multisystemic involvement of this pathology, it is worth to mention that pulmonary disease is seen in about 50% of cases. Pulmonary amyloidosis has different patterns such as diffuse alveolar septal involvement, tracheobronchial and nodular parenchymal amyloidosis. Clinical manifestations of pulmonary amyloidosis could be misinterpreted because of the nonspecific signs and symptoms such as dyspnea at exertion, weight loss or productive cough. Because of the poor prognosis of these patients, as we can see in CA too, pulmonary involvement must be searched during the work-up and specific treatment should be initiated.

Given these clinical considerations, CA should be considered in the differential diagnosis in a patient with HF, unexplained left ventricular hypertrophy and preserved ejection fraction.

4. Laboratory and electrocardiographic findings in CA

There is no specific serum biomarker for the ATTR subtype. In the case of AL amyloidosis however, blood screening tests are available and these include electrophoresis and immunofixation of serum and urine proteins, as well as quantification of immunoglobulin free light chain levels with evaluation of the kappa - lambda ratio [13]. Due to the possible presence of a monoclonal gammopathy of undetermined significance (MGUS) in up to 5% of the general population aged >65 years, positive laboratory findings need to be carefully evaluated [13]. In the meantime, the cardiac amyloidosis' ATTR subtype may coexist with MGUS and needs to be differentiated from the AL subtype by seeking evidence of amyloid infiltration in affected organs with identification of the precursor protein [13].

Amyloid fibrils deposition in the myocardium is often correlated with the onset of arrhythmias and conduction abnormalities, consequently highlighting the key role of the electrocardiogram (ECG) in the diagnostic assessment [14]. One of the ECG findings is the presence of diffuse low voltage in the limb and/or precordial leads [15]. Even if this ECG finding is not very sensitive and it generally occurs only in late the stages of the disease, it is common, specific and has prognostic signficance in patients with CA [16]. In order to increase the diagnostic sensitivity, a low-voltage-to-mass ratio assessment was suggested (given the discordance between the low voltage on the ECG and the left ventricular hypertrophy on cardiac imaging) (**Figure 1**) [16].

Another important finding on the ECG, which is present in up to 70% of these patients, is the pseudoinfarction pattern which consists of pathologic Q or QS waves in any two consecutive leads, but without any history of infarction and without wall motion abnormalities [16]. As previously mentioned, patients with CA also tend to develop, as the disease progresses, arrhythmias which range from brady- and tachyarrhythmias or sudden cardiac death [17]. The most common arrhythmia noted in CA is AF (up to 70% of patients), but ventricular arrhythmias such as premature ventricular beats or ventricular tachycardia can also occur [18]. Conduction disease is also common and appears to be more frequent in the wtATTR subtype. This last condition can require implant of a pacemaker [18].

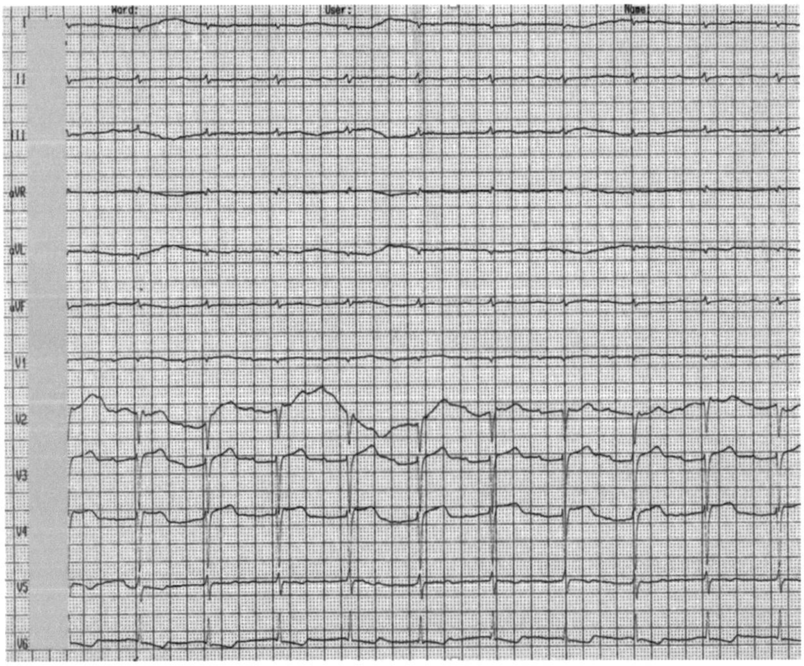

Figure 1.
ECG with low voltage seen in the frontal plane leads in a patient with AL type cardiac amyloidosis.

5. Diagnostic suspicion of CA

In the past CA used to be underdiagnosed, given its nonspecific symptoms and because it was thought to be a rare condition. In order to improve diagnostic specificity and sensitivity different "red flag" signs can be used to raise the clinical suspicion and allow an early diagnosis [16].

ATTR amyloidosis which consequentially determines cardiac amyloid infiltration is usually preceded years before onset by various clinical entities such as: carpal tunnel syndrome, lumbar spinal stenosis, and biceps tendon rupture [16]. Moreover, ATTR is also often associated with sensoriomotor polyneuropathy, autonomic dysfunction as orthostatic hypotension, erectile dysfunction, gastrointestinal motility disorders or urinary retention [16].

Even if not sensitive, macroglossia and periorbital purpura are specific signs for the AL amyloidosis and are rare seen in ATTR subtype. Other "red flags" for AL subtype include hepatomegaly and peripheral neuropathy, but these are neither sensitive, nor specific for this condition. Also, when facing patients with undifferentiated cardiac hypertrophy and nephrotic proteinuria, AL amyloidosis should be considered as a possible diagnosis [16].

6. Echocardiography in CA

Transthoracic echocardiogram is the most common non-invasive imaging tool used in patients with suspected or confirmed amyloidosis. In 1975 Chew et al. described for the first time the echocardiographic appearance of CA, based on M-mode tracings. The features seen were: normal diastolic size of the left ventricle, increased systolic dimension and pericardial effusion; given these findings, the term" stiff heart" was chosen in these patients [19, 20].

Later on more echocardiographic features were added to the amyloid phenotype: symmetric thickness of the left ventricular wall in patients with no history of hypertension or aortic valvular abnormalities, hypokinetic interventricular septum and posterior left ventricular wall with decreased systolic thickening, normal or small left ventricle cavity, increased thickness of the right ventricular anterior wall, dilated left atrium, a decrease of the E-F slope (given reduced ventricular compliance) [19, 21–23].

6.1 Two-dimensional echocardiography

The development of two-dimensional echocardiography offered the posibility to describe further the amyloid phenotype [20]. Some defining features of CA are represented by left ventricular hypertrophy with a normal/reduced cavity volume, increased thickness of the right ventricular wall and the valves (especially aortic and mitral valves), and bi-atrial enlargement (**Figures 2** and **3**) [24, 25].

Concerning the left ventricular wall thickness, it has a different pattern depending on the amyloidosis type: symmetrical in AL and asymmetrical in ATTR [26]. The presence of extracellular amyloid deposits gives the myocardium a, "granular sparkling" appearance, better visualized at the interventricular septum [27]. A small pericardial effusion or dilated inferior vena cava are often observed as signs of a restrictive filling pattern [28].

6.2 Doppler

In the 80s, Doppler ultrasound offered new possibilities to characterize the heart's function and structure, providing a more accurate diagnosis, and the

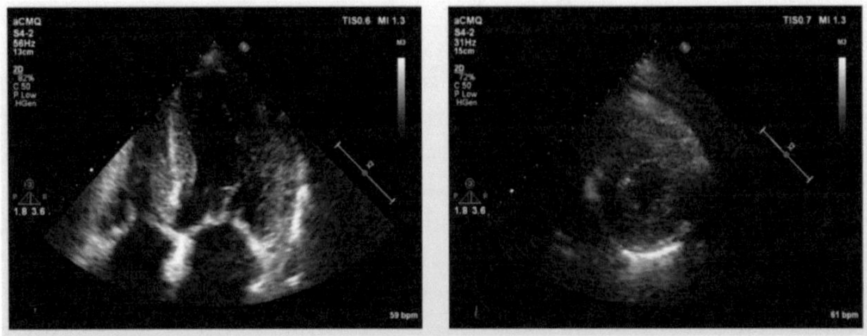

Figure 2.
2D echocardiogram (apical 4 chamber view and parasternal short axis view) in a patient with AL type cardiac amyloidosis revealing increased thickness of the left ventricular walls.

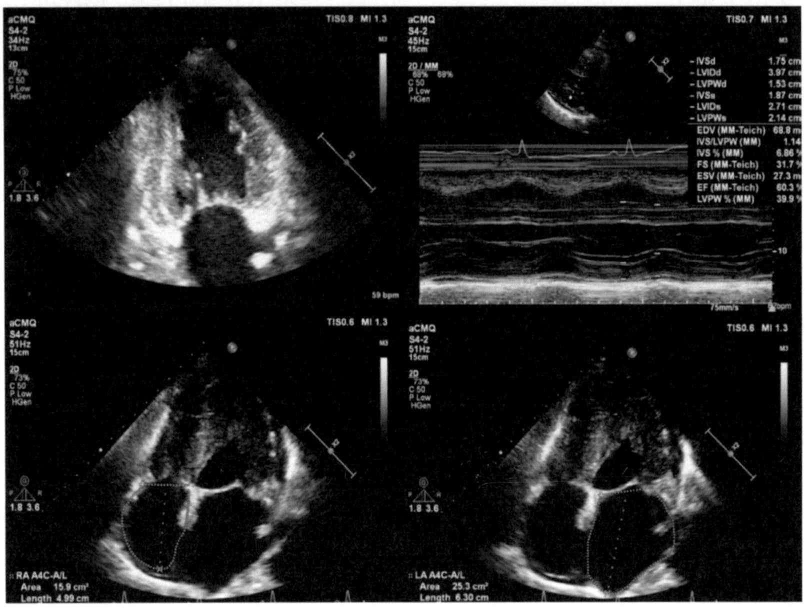

Figure 3.
2D echocardiogram (apical 2 chamber view, M-mode in parasternal long axis view and apical 4 chamber view) in a patient with AL type cardiac amyloidosis revealing increased thickness of the left ventricular walls, biatrial dilatation and hypertrophic interatrial septum.

diastolic dysfunction became a main feature of CA. First studies, performed by Klein et al. revealed that in early stages, when the parietal thickness of the left ventricle is 12-15 mm, there is an abnormal relaxation with a reduced early filling velocity, elevated late velocity, reduced early to late velocitsy ratio and longer isovolumic relaxation time. Contrary to this, in late-stage CA associated with significant ventricular wall thickening (parietal thickness equal to or more than 15 mm) an elevated E/A ratio was observed, suggesting a restrictive cardiomyopathy [19, 27]. In late-stage disease the deceleration time is markedly reduced (restrictive pattern).

The diastolic function is usually severely impaired, with a restrictive pattern defined by a decrease deceleration time on the transmitral pulsed Doppler and low tissue Doppler velocities in the left ventricular wall; E/e' is often higher than 15, which suggests elevated filling pressures (**Figure 4**) [29].

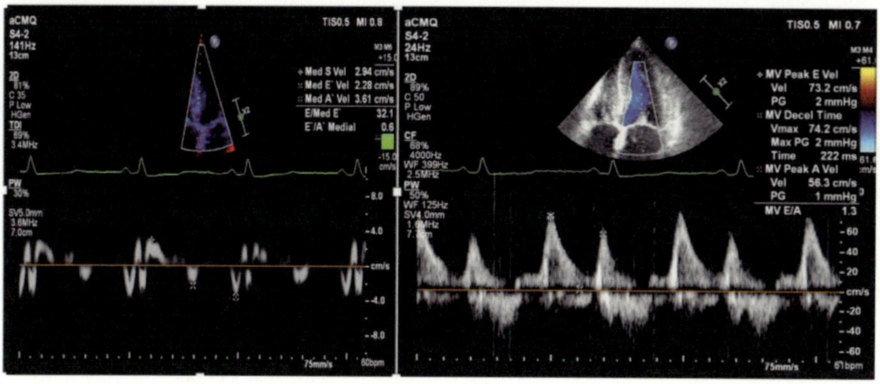

Figure 4.
2D echocardiogram with tissue Doppler sample at base of the interventricular septum and pulsed-wave Doppler at mitral valve inflow in a patient with AL type cardiac amyloidosis revealing impaired relaxation, septal e' of the LV decreased and a pseudonormal pattern.

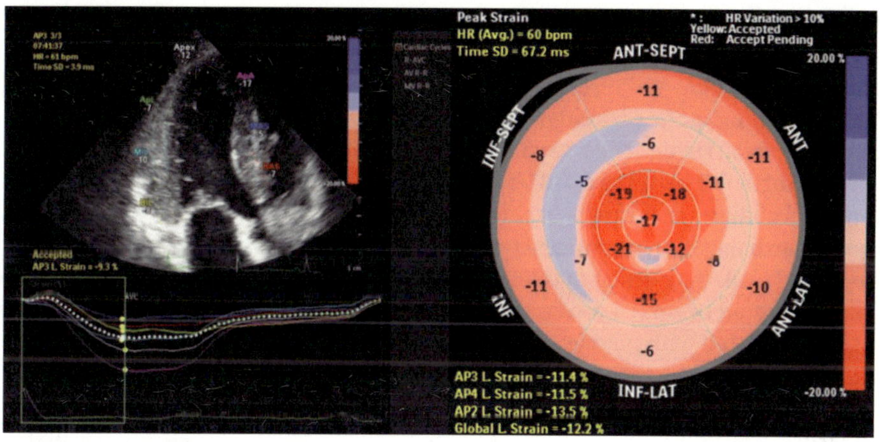

Figure 5.
Left ventricular strain image with impaired longitudinal shortening at basal and mid-ventricular level with preserved longitudinal function at the apex (relative apical sparing) as seen in the bull's eye plot on the right.

6.3 Speckle-tracking echocardiography

The speckle-tracking echocardiography (STE) plays a major role in evaluation of patients with CA, being a sensitive echocardiographic technique which detects cardiac damage due to amyloid infiltration from early stages, even when other classic parameters are still in range [30]. In patients with CA, a reduced global longitudinal strain can be observed when the left ventricular ejection fraction is still preserved [31].

Speckle tracking imagining in CA reveals reduced longitudinal shortening at the basal and mid-ventricular level with preserved longitudinal function at the apex [31]. This pattern, described by Phelan et al. as 'relative apical sparing' is a helpful tool, both sensitive and specific, to make a diagnosis of CA [32]. Longitudinal strain bull's eye plot has a typical pattern that is easy to recognize. The mechanism that determines this pattern is not yet clearly understood. Proposed mechanisms include: 1. a reduced infiltration with amyloid fibrils at the apex, compared to basal segments; 2. an increased tendency towards apoptosis at basal level, as a result of the higher parietal stress [25, 28, 33]. This typical appearance was first described in late-stage CA, but there are studies that suggest its presence in less affected hearts [31, 34].

2D STE is helpful in differentiating the thickness of myocardium caused by amyloidosis from a real left ventricular hypertrophy. In CA a systolic septal longitudinal base-to-apex strain ratio more than 2.1 in association with a low deceleration time is useful to differentiate it from patterns encountered in other types of ventricular thickening, such as true hypertrophy (**Figure 5**) [19, 31].

7. Magnetic resonance imaging in CA

The use of cardiac magnetic resonance (CMR) in patients with CA allows a good definition of cardiac morphology, ventricular and valvular function, and the possibility to analyze the structure of the ventricular wall [35]. However, the main benefit of CMR imaging in this disease remains the evaluation of the ventricular diastolic function and the structure of the ventricular wall.

The gadolinium contrast agents are very useful in characterizing the myocardial wall structure due to the differences in clearance of gadolinium between normal myocardium, edematous or scarred myocardium, and myocardium with amyloid deposits.

The gadolinium contrast agents accumulate in extracellular spaces of both normal myocardium and diseased one, but it is rapidly washed out from the normal areas, remaining in the pathological areas, late after the contrast has washed out from the normal tissue. The late gadolinium enhancement (LGE) of the myocardium has different patterns in different diseases, which, together with the other functional changes that can be evaluated by MRI. The ischemic scars appear as subendocardial LGE in a coronary territory, usually associating the thinning of the myocardial wall. In contrast to this, the amyloid deposits appear as subendocardial LGE that extend beyond a coronary artery territory (the "arch" shaped LGE) and is usually associated with increased wall thickness. In more severe stages the subendocardial LGE can be diffuse (the "annular" shaped LGE) or it can even become a transmural LGE [36]. These aspects can combine in the same patient, as they represent a continuum from no amyloid deposits and no LGE to subendocardial LGE and then to diffuse and transmural, intense LGE [37].

The expansion of the extracellular space due to amyloid deposition can also be measured by the T1 mapping technique allowing monitoring of the treatment response [38]. The extracellular volume (ECV) is below 28% in normal situations and can increase significantly with edema and fibrosis, but also with amyloid deposition. An increase above 40% of ECV is a highly suggestive sign for amyloidosis in patients with high pretest probability; this sign appears early, before LGE

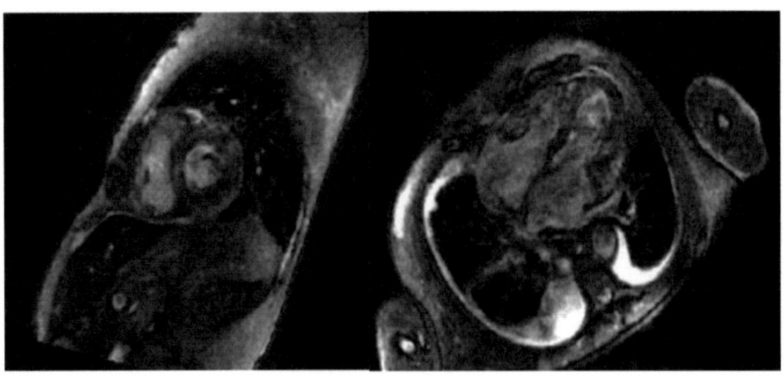

Figure 6.
MRI images: short axis 2D myocardial delayed enhancement (left) and four-chamber 2D myocardial delayed enhancement (right): diffuse, inhomogeneous late gadolinium enhancement, suggestive of cardiac amyloidosis.

appearance [39]. Given the T1 mapping technique which allows objective measurement of the extracellular volume, the response to treatment can be monitored (**Figure 6**) [40].

8. Nuclear medicine: radionuclide scintigraphy

Bone affinity isotope scintigraphy plays an important part in the early diagnosis of ATTR-type CA and in its differentiation from AL amyloidosis and other types of hypertrophic heart disease [41].

The radiotracers recommended in diagnosing ATTR amyloidosis are: 99 mTc - PYP (pyrophosphate), 99mTc - DPD (3,3-diphosphono-1,2-propanodiacarboxylic acid) and 99mTc-labeled hydroxymethylene diphosphonate (HMDP) [42]. They have an increased affinity for calcium. In ATTR-type amyloidosis, the extracellularly deposited amyloid, at the cardiac level, contains a protein that binds amyloid fibers through a calcium-dependent mechanism, which explains the affinity of these radiotracers for this type of amyloid [43]. There are comparative studies on endomyocardial biopsies, which show that patients with ATTR amyloidosis present more frequent microcalcifications in comparison to those with AL amyloidosis. In very few cases, however, patients with AL amyloidosis may have microcalcifications and in these situations scintigraphy with bone affinity radiotracers may be slightly positive [44].

Other radiotracers that can be used to highlight CA and differentiate it from other hypertrophic cardiomyopathies are as follows: 11C-Pittsburgh compound B (11C-GDP), 18F-florbetaben, and 18F-florbetapir. They have affinity for both the AL-type amyloid and ATTR and require further clinical trials for validation [41, 43].

The scintigraphy using the 123I-metaiodobenzylguanidine tracer can also detect the sympathetic denervation of the heart and thus patients at risk of cardiac arrhythmias can be identified [41, 45].

High levels of light serum and urinary chains or of medullary plasma cells are suggestive of AL-type amyloidosis, and biopsy is required to confirm amyloid deposits. In this case, myocardial scintigraphy is performed only to obtain additional information [41].

When monoclonal gammopathy is not present, myocardial scintigraphy with bone avidity radiotracers is required. If it reveals abnormal uptake of the radiotracer at the myocardial level, the diagnosis of ATTR amyloidosis is made with a sensitivity of 100%. Biopsy is not required for detecting amyloid deposits [41].

The myocardial scintigraphy protocol with bone affinity radiotracers involves monoplane imaging (anterior and posterior), 3 hours after the intravenous administration of the isotope, which allows the identification of radioactive tracer uptake and its quantification by visual evaluation of the Perugini score (0- no uptake, 1 - low uptake, of subcostal intensity, 2 - significant uptake, of intensity equal to that of the ribs, 3 - important uptake, of supracostal intensity) [43, 46].

Another way of assessing the uptake of radiotracer at the level of the heart involves performing the ratio between the values measured in a certain region at the level of the heart (H) and at the contralateral level (CL), one hour after the administration of the radiotracer [25, 47].

When the value of the Perugini score is higher than or equal to 2 and/or if the value of the H/CL ratio is higher than or equal to 1.5, the diagnosis of ATTR amyloidosis is made [47].

The H/CL ratio also has a prognostic value. Thus, values higher than 1.5 are associated with the survival reduction to 5 years (together with the echocardiographic characteristics of a more advanced stage of the disease) [43].

9. Diagnostic strategy in CA

Diagnosis of CA can be difficult given the polymorphic and nonspecific clinical manifestations [41] of this systemic disease. CA must be considered in the differential diagnosis in HF with left ventricular hypertrophy and preserved ejection fraction. By the time of the onset of signs and symptoms, it is essential not to delay the diagnosis because it has a negative influence on evolution and prognosis of the patient. Below is an algorithm for an easier approach to the diagnosis CA [41, 48, 49]. Two important steps in this algorithm in patients with clinical suspicion of CA are screening for monoclonal protein (for identification of kappa or lambda free light chains) and, in case this is positive, biopsy, most of the time from fat pad, which has a sensitivity and specificity of 79% and 80% respectively for diagnosing amyloidosis (**Figure** 7) [50].

10. General treatment of heart failure in CA

Therapy of HF along with the treatment of the underlying disease stand for different sides of the same coin in CA. There are several dissimilarities regarding medications used in CA with HF, compared to those used in patients with non-CA HF with reduced ejection fraction (HFrEF). The median survival after the onset of HF is less than 6 months in untreated patients [51].

10.1 Medical treatment of heart failure in CA

General treatment management in patients with CA and HF is challenging due to lack of randomized clinical trials on which to fundament treatment strategies [52]. Therapy should first focus on a sodium restriction diet and daily weight monitoring in conjunction with diuretics, in order to improve congestion and relieve symptoms. Neurohormonal blockade is recommended by current HF guidelines [53, 54] for patients with HFrEF regardless of its etiology, but various concerns have been raised in patients with CA-HF due to potential harmful effects [55].

Thus, diuretics and especially loop diuretics in combined with a mineralocorticoid receptor antagonist, represent the cornerstone of therapeutic strategies in this group of patients [52, 55, 56]. Clinical benefit of other usual HF therapies including beta-blockers (BB), calcium channel blockers (CCB) and angiotensin-converting enzyme inhibitors (ACEI) has not yet been proven, moreover these therapies may even be harmful in CA patients [55, 57, 58].

In amyloid cardiomyopathy, CCB and digitalis are contraindicated because they can bind to amyloid fibrils and determine severe adverse effects such as serious hypotension and syncope [58, 59]. Moreover, BB and ACEI can cause marked hypotension due to low cardiac output and fatigue, leading to a limited tolerability among these patients. Orthostatic hypotension caused by autonomic dysfunction can be exacerbated by ACEI or angiotensin receptor blockers, and the coexistence of renal dysfunction can limit their usage [52, 58]. Still, these medications should be cautiously considered in selected cases of severe nephrotic syndrome with marked proteinuria [58].

Beta-blockers with their negative chronotropic and inotropic effects, interfere with contractility and heart rate which help maintain cardiac output, resulting in significant hypotension, extreme bradycardia and even heart block since amyloid patients are already predisposed to electrical conduction anomalies [52, 55, 58]. However, in case of atrial tachyarrhythmias, BB (particularly in low doses) might present real benefits for rate control [52, 55, 58].

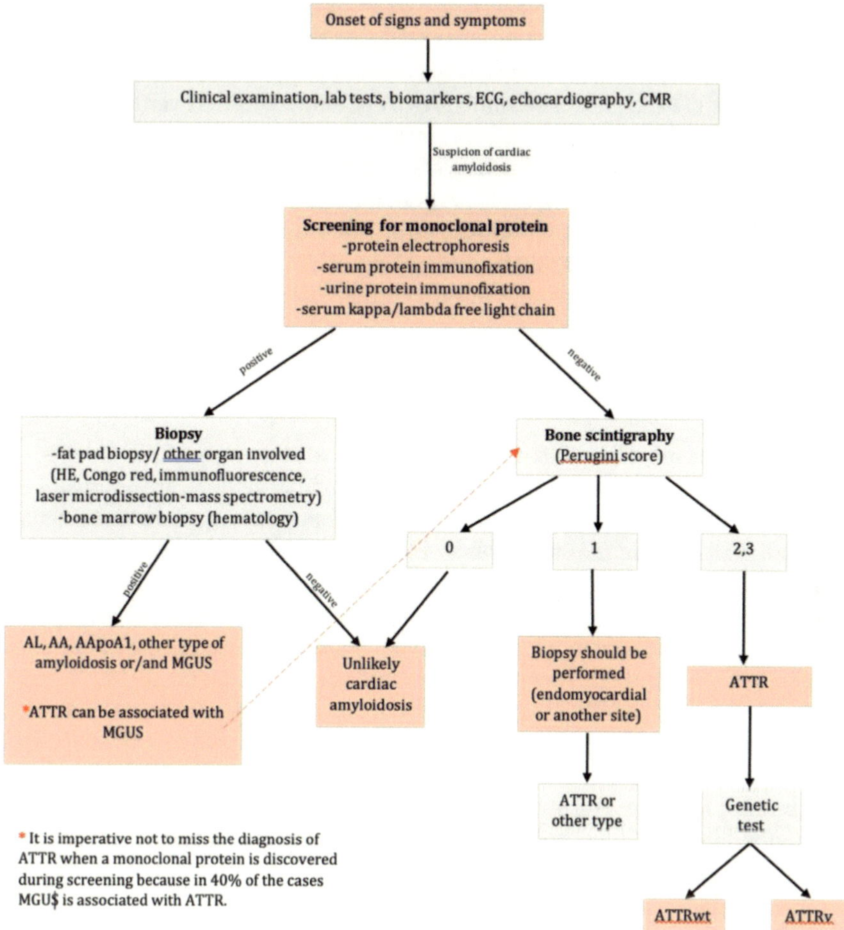

Figure 7.
Diagnostic strategy in CA. (ECG, electrocardiography; CMR, cardiovascular magnetic resonance imaging; HE, hematoxylin eosin staining; AL, amyloid light-chain amyloidosis; AA, amyloid A protein amyloidosis, AApoA1, apolipoprotein AI-derived amyloidosis; MGUS, monoclonal gammopathy of undetermined significance; ATTR, transthyretin amyloidosis; ATTRwt, wild-type transthyretin amyloidosis; ATTRv, mutant transthyretin amyloidosis).

Overall, authors agree that common medications for subjects with non-amyloid-HFrEF, should be carefully considered in those with CA-HFrEF [52, 55, 58]. Furthermore, these therapies should be discouraged in HF with preserved ejection fraction (HFpEF) and CA [56].

10.2 Heart transplantation and ventricular assist devices

Previously, overall heart transplantation in CA was thought to be contraindicated since amyloidosis represents a systemic disease and there is an increased risk of relapse [55, 58, 60]. In transplanted amyloid patients compared to standard heart transplant patients, there was no difference in survival rate, and those with end stage disease continue to have an extremely poor prognosis (50% death on the waiting list) [61, 62].

Many authors focused their attention in the last decade on mechanical circulatory support (MCS) for end-stage CA. Left ventricular assist device (LVAD), biventricular assist device (BiVAD) and total artificial heart (TAH) nowadays represent either bridge to transplantation (BTT) or destination therapies [63–68]. Some studies reveal that TAH is a feasible bridging therapy, with 82% survival, and should be preferred over LVAD therapy for durable support in selected patients [64]. Accordingly, LVAD is not suitable for CA patients with left ventricular end-diastolic diameter under 46 mm and was even associated with higher mortality post-implantation [64, 66]. Other studies found no significant difference in wait-list and up-to 5-years survival after heart transplantation in subjects sustained by BiVAD or TAH as bridging therapies [65, 66]. Outcomes become acceptable with advances in specific therapies for the underlying disease and heart transplant or heart/liver transplant could even be curative in selected cases, but there is still need for additional studies [57, 60].

10.3 Atrial fibrillation and anticoagulation

While AF is the most frequent arrhythmia in HF patients, in amyloid patients, traditional therapies could lead to severe side effects and in general, are poorly tolerated [18, 53]. Rate and rhythm management among this population continue to be challenging. For rate management the usage of beta-blockers in low doses may be attempted, but their clinical benefit remains unproven in CA. Nondihydropyridine CCB and digoxin are not recommended and may even be toxic for these patients [18, 52, 55]. Options for pharmacologic rhythm control are restricted, but studies support the use of amiodarone as first choice antiarrhythmic therapy, since it tends to be well tolerated [18, 52].

Some experts advise following a rhythm control strategy over a rate control strategy in amyloid patients, but there are no studies to support this strategy until present days.

Last but not least, several studies concluded that chronic oral anticoagulation is recommended in all patients with CA and AF irrespective of CHADS-VASC score due to an increased risk of thromboembolic events [55, 57, 69].

10.4 Cardiac implantable electronic devices

Implantable electronic devices such as pacemaker and/or implantable cardioverter-defibrillator (ICD) have not been shown to prevent sudden cardiac death or improve survival in CA patients [18, 52, 55, 57, 70]. Moreover, since overall mortality after implantation outweighs its benefits, cardiac implantable electronic devices should be used mainly for secondary prevention (hemodynamic instability due to ventricular arrhythmias) in patients with more than a year survival rate [52, 54, 55, 57]. However, permanent pacemakers, especially biventricular pacing, were shown to improve symptoms and should be considered in patients with CA and severe conduction disease [18, 57].

11. Specific treatment of AL amyloidosis cardiomyopathy

The last two decades have brought in a decrease in mortality rates and improved survival in patients with AL amyloidosis, mainly due to early diagnosis and better treatment implementation [71]. During the same period, new treatment options have become available for these complex patients, among which the most notable are new chemotherapy regimens, autologous stem cell transplantation, proteasome inhibitors and monoclonal antibodies [72].

Treatment should be adapted according to the patient's comorbidities and severity of organ involvement in order to achieve the most efficient and safe therapeutic regimen [73].

Apart from patients with monoclonal gammopathies of undetermined significance (MGUS) or smoldering myeloma, in whom initiation of specific therapy could be delayed until the first sign of organ involvement, all patients diagnosed with AL amyloidosis should be initiated on specific therapy as soon as possible [74, 75].

The treatment of these subjects should be decided by a multidisciplinary team, coordinated by a hematologist and with the involvement of other relevant medical specialties: nephrology, cardiology, pneumology, neurology and gastroenterology [76].

In addition to specific HF therapy, which has several peculiarities compared to that of the general population, patients with AL amyloidosis and cardiac involvement require treatment of the underlying disease [77].

The purpose of therapy in cardiac AL amyloidosis is to reduce the serum free light-chain levels and to obtain organ response. This should be done promptly and for as long as possible, in order to obtain a reduction of more than 90 percent in free light-chain levels, therefore preventing further amyloid deposition and fibrillogenesis [75, 78].

The standard treatment includes high-dose chemotherapy in combination with autologous stem cell transplantation (ASCT), alkylating agents, steroids, proteasome inhibitors, and immunomodulatory drugs [76]. An adequate level of response may not be obtainable in all patients. Because of this, treatment efficacy should be assessed at 3 months after ASCT (autologous stem cell transplantation) and 1–2 months after nontransplantation therapies. A decision to shift to other regimens depends on the hematologic response [76]. Patients with important cardiac involvement have a higher mortality despite good initial hematologic response, while a rapid improvement of cardiac biomarkers and left ventricular ejection fraction can be seen in those with mild CA when free light chain can be significantly reduced [73, 75].

Risk stratification is essential when choosing the treatment strategy. Only 20% of the patients newly diagnosed with AL amyloidosis are eligible for ASCT, these being considered low risk patients. Effective up-front therapy may increase this percentage, making certain other patients eligible [78]. Generally, in order to be eligible for ASCT, patients should meet the following criteria: age ≤ 70 years, cTnT <0.06 ng/mL, NT-proBNP <5000 ng/L, systolic blood pressure ≥ 100 mmHg, LVEF >45%, New York Heart Association (NYHA) functional class I or II, creatinine clearance ≥50 mL/min (unless on chronic stable dialysis), Eastern Cooperative Oncology Group (ECOG) performance status ≤2, DLCO >50%, less than 3 organs significantly involved (heart, liver, kidney, or autonomic nervous system) [76, 77].

Treatment with bortezomib, a proteasome inhibitor, should be considered in low-risk patients prior to ASCT if there are no contraindications, in order to achieve high rates of deep and durable hematologic response. This should be followed by high dose melphalan, an alkylating agent, combined with autologous stem cell transplantion, rather than chemotherapy alone [78]. ASCT allows the administration of high doses of melphalan, with myeloablative effect, thus contributing to the suppression the underlying plasma cell dyscrasia [79].

As mentioned above, the majority of AL amyloidosis patients are not eligible for ASCT, being staged in a class of intermediate or high risk [76]. For these patients, the most common initial chemotherapy regimens used nowadays are bortezomib-based, such as combinations with cyclophosphamide and dexamethasone (CyBorD) or melphalan and dexamethasone (BMDex). These regimens have a significantly higher hematological response rate, a longer progression-free period and increased overall survival compared to the older regimen of dexamethasone and prednisone, which has been the standard of care for many years in these subjects [79, 80].

Daratumumab is an anti-CD38 monoclonal antibody, which has a direct on-tumor and immunomodulatory mechanism of action, with proven activity in AL amyloidosis, which is particularly attractive in case of severe cardiac involvement. High risk patients with important cardiac involvement and NYHA class III or IV and ECOG PS = 4, need a very rapidly acting and safe regimen and supportive therapy during the chemotherapy cycles in order to sustain organ function [81]. Recently, in the phase 3 ANDROMEDA-trial, a combination of daratumumab with CyBorD in patients with newly diagnosed AL amyloidosis resulted in significantly higher hematologic, cardiac, and renal response rates typically within one cycle, and was well tolerated. Therefore, it should be considered a promising novel therapy for AL amyloidosis [82].

In patients in whom a rapid and significant reduction in the serum free light-chain levels is not achieved, a second-line treatment should be considered after hematological response assessment. In responders, maintenance therapy is not indicated [76, 83].

Organ response criteria are essential during treatment follow-up. Cardiac biomarkers, especially NT-pro BNP, have a particular importance for the cardiac response, although they are influenced by therapy related complications, fluid status and supraventricular tachyarrhythmias, very common in CA [84]. A decrease with more than 30% and > 300 ng/l, in NT-pro BNP levels and an improvement of NYHA functional class has been demonstrated to be associated with increased overall survival [83].

In patients resistant to alkylating agents and proteasome inhibitors, immunosuppressive therapy is the only remaining option. Treatment regimens that include immunosuppressant agents (lenalidomide, thalidomide) have demonstrated efficacy among patients with relapsed or resistant AL amyloidosis. These are generally avoided due to significant cardiac and renal toxicity, and are especially useful in patients with contraindications to bortezomib or in subjects with refractory disease.

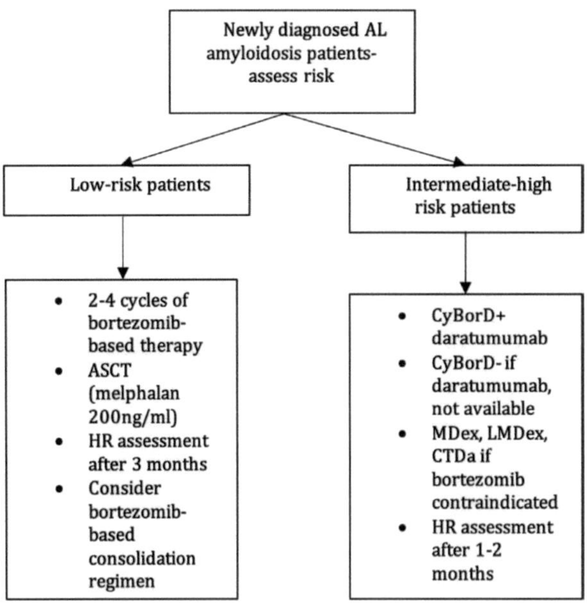

Figure 8.
Treatment algorithm of AL Amyloidosis. CyBorD = cyclophosphamide and dexamethasone; ASCT = autologous stem cell transplantation; MDex = melphalan and dexamethasone; LMDex = lenalidomide, melphalan, and dexamethasone; CTDa = cyclophosphamide and dexamethasone; HR = heart rate.

Treatment with these agents is associated with increased NT-pro BNP levels and affects the assessment of cardiac response, Also, worsening of renal failure and increased proteinuria can be detected [85, 86].

Low dose thalidomide in addition to cyclophosphamide and dexamethasone (CTDa) was demonstrated to have the highest response rates, with acceptable toxicity, but it is not recommended as a routine maintenance therapy due to cumulative neurotoxicity [87]. Lenalidomide in combination with low dose dexamethasone, with or without cyclophosphamide, could be taken into consideration in patients with relapsed AL amyloidosis, but with an increased risk of thrombotic complications (**Figure 8**) [88].

12. Specific treatment of ATTR amyloid cardiomyopathy

Recent findings in the research of molecular pathogenic mechanisms revolutionized the treatment of ATTR amyloidosis. New agents have recently been developed to suppress the production of amyloid in both wild-type and hereditary CA. Current treatment strategies include management of underlying disease process in association with symptomatic relief.

12.1 Disease modifying therapies

1. TTR synthesis inhibitors target by inhibiting the hepatic synthesis of TTR.

   - Patisiran (0.3 mg/kg iv., once daily, every three weeks for 18 months) is a second-generation small interfering RNA (siRNA), which blocks the expression of TTR, leading to reduction in TTR levels [89].

   - Inotersen (200 mg sc., once a week) is a second-generation antisense oligonucleotide, which lowers hepatic production of TTR by bonding to the mRNA [89].

   Both these drugs lead to a reduction of >85% in the concentration of circulating TTR. Two recent randomized trials have demonstrated reduction in the progression of polyneuropathy in patients with ATTRv: the APOLLO trial [90]. (The Study of an Investigational Drug, Patisiran, for the Treatment of TTR Amyloidosis) and the NEURO-TTR [91]. trial (Efficacy and Safety of Inotersen in Familial Amyloid Polyneuropathy). Even though not explicitly tested, TTR synthesis inhibitors may have beneficial cardiac effects [91, 92]. In order to demonstrate cardiac benefits, two clinical trials assessing the efficacy of TTR synthesis inhibitors in patients with cardiomyopathy are currently ongoing: 24 Month Open Label Study in the Tolerability and Efficacy of Inotersen in TTR Amyloid Cardiomyopathy Patients and the APOLLO-B trial (A Study to Evaluate Patisiran in Participants With TTR Amyloidosis With Cardiomyopathy).

2. TTR stabilizers prevent the misfolding of TTR by binding to TTR tetramer.

   - Tafamidis slows the dissociation of TTR tetramers into monomers by binding to the thyroxine-binding site of the TTR. In the ATTR-ACR randomized trial (Safety and Efficacy of Tafamidis in Patients with TTR Cardiomyopathy), which recruited both patients with ATTRv cardiomyopathy and ATTRwt cardiomyopathy, there was a significant lower all-cause mortality and cardiovascular-related hospitalization after 30 months after receiving Tafamidis when compared to placebo. Moreover, there was a lower rate of decline in the 6-minute walk test and in the quality of life under both Tafamidis doses (20 and 80 mg orally) [93]. Tafamidis was approved for the use in TTR cardiomyopathy in May 2019.

- Diflunisal is a non-steroidal anti-inflammatory drug, which significantly reduced the progression of polyneuropathy by stabilizing TTR tertramers in a randomized trial [94]. Although no controlled trials evaluated the effect of Diflunisal on TTR cardiomyopathy, two single center studies demonstrated some benefits (250 mg orally twice daily) [95, 96]. However, side effects are not rare (thrombocytopenia and renal dysfunction), administration should be avoided in patients with eGFR<45 mL/min/1.73m^2, thrombocytopenia or signs of hemodynamic or renal instability [97]. Diflunisal is not approved for TTR amyloidosis and can be used off-label.

- AG10 is a synthetic TTR ligand, which acts by binding to the TTR tetramer and therefore prevents amyloid fibril formation and deposition. A phase II randomized multicenter study demonstrated that AG10 (400 mg or 800 mg twice daily for 28 days) induced almost complete stabilization of TTR and patients treated with AG10 showed reduced mortality and cardiovascular hospitalization at 15 months [97].

- Tolcapone is approved for the treatment of Parkinson disease and acts by inhibiting TTR aggregation. It is currently under investigation in patients with TTR amyloidosis [55].

3. TTR disruptors target the clearance of amyloid fibrils from tissue.

- The combination of Doxycycline and TUDCA (tauroursodeoxycholic acid) removed amyloid deposits in preclinical studies, but there was a high incidence of side effects [98, 99]. The role of these therapies is therefore uncertain.

12.2 Symptomatic relief

The control of peripheral and autonomic neuropathy leads to significant improvement in the quality of life. Implantation of a cardiac pacemaker might be beneficial in patients with TTRv and conduction disorders [100]. Implantable cardioverter-defibrillators (ICD) are recommended in patients with significant arrhythmias or aborted sudden cardiac death with expected survival of more than one year. Although reduction in cardiac filling pressures is also necessary, it must be performed with caution, as these patients are dependent of the cardiac output. On the same principle, many drugs used in the treatment of HF might not be beneficial in patients with CA and some agents might have an abnormal distribution by binding to amyloid fibrils (eg. digoxin) [100].

12.3 Management of TTR amyloidosis in patients with aortic stenosis

Recent data demonstrated that the association between CA and aortic stenosis (AS) is more common than previously known and TTR cardiac amyloidosis is the most prevalent type to coexist with AS [101]. Since there are no randomized trials to evaluate the best therapeutic management in patients with TTR cardiac amyloidosis and AS, the treatment of CA follows the general principles and should be instituted immediately after the diagnosis is confirmed. Regarding the management of AS, the majority of the studies reported a high risk of mortality after surgical aortic valve replacement (SAVR) [101–106].

One study performed on a limited number of patients demonstrated that in patients with CA and AS outcomes might be better with trans-aortic valve replacement (TAVR) than SAVR [102]. Two ongoing prospective trials, ATTRact-AS (The Role of Occult Cardiac Amyloid in the Elderly With Aortic Stenosis) and Amylo-CARTESIAN (Prevalence and Post-surgical Outcomes of CARdiac Wild-type TransthyrEtin amyloidoSIs in Elderly Patients With Aortic stenosis Referred for Valvular Replacement) might lead to better understanding of the prevalence and management of patients who present both pathologies. One recently published sub-study of the ATTRact-AS trial showed that there was no difference in mortality after TAVR between patients with CA and AS or AS alone [107]. Thus, TAVR might be a better option for patients with intermediate to high surgical risk. However, since some patients might be prone to complications during TAVR because of the fragility of the infiltrated myocardium [108]. A multidisciplinary heart team should discuss the optimal therapy.

13. Summary

Amyloidosis represents a heterogeneous group of disorders that present as a multi-organ disease presenting with unspecific symptoms. The diagnosis of amyloidosis often is difficult and can be delayed, and therefore the number of unreported cases is likely quite significant.

Amyloid can infiltrate all structures of the heart including ventricular and atrial walls, the conduction system, the heart valves, and the coronaries. The typical clinical presentation in CA is that of a restrictive cardiomyopathy. When present, cardiac amyloidosis has a significant impact on disease prognosis.

Cardiac biomarkers, echocardiography, and other imaging techniques such as CMR or 99mTc-phosphate scintigraphy are available for the diagnosis of CA as well as determination of the extent of this disease. Endomyocardial biopsy remains the main method used for histopathological confirmation and subtyping of CA.

The main goal of the diagnostic strategy is to detect CA early, to define the extent of CA, and to enable targeted therapy.

14. Conclusion

Until recently, amyloidosis was still considered a rare multi-organ disease. The diagnosis of CA was often missed or only documented at a late stage with negative impact on the prognosis of the patients.

Meanwhile, it has become evident that CA is more prevalent than once thought and can be the only manifestation of amyloidosis so that early diagnosis and subsequent therapy are becoming increasingly important.

Conflict of interest

The authors declare no conflict of interest.

Notes/thanks/other declarations

All authors contributed equally to this chapter.

Author details

Csilla Andrea Eötvös[1,2], Giorgia Pastiu[1,2], Iulia Zehan[1,2], Cerasela Goidescu[1,3], Roxana Chiorescu[2,5], Roxana Lazar[1,2], Florina Frîngu[2,4], Raluca Tomoaia[2,4], Monica Pop[2,6], Adrian Molnar[1,2], Sorin Pop[2,5] and Dan Blendea[2,5]*

1 "Niculae Stancioiu" Heart Institute, Cluj-Napoca, Romania

2 University of Medicine and Pharmacy "Iuliu Hatieganu", Cluj-Napoca, Romania

3 Emergency Military Clinical Hospital "Dr. Constantin Papilian", Cluj-Napoca, Romania

4 Rehabilitation Hospital, Cluj-Napoca, Romania

5 Cluj County Emergency Hospital, Cluj-Napoca, Romania

6 "Leon Daniello" Pneumophtisiology Hospital, Cluj-Napoca, Romania

*Address all correspondence to: dblendea1@gmail.com

References

[1] Yilmaz A, Bauersachs J, Bengel F, Buchel R, Kindermann I, Klingel K, et al. Diagnosis and treatment of cardiac amyloidosis: position statement of the German Cardiac Society (DGK). Clin Res Cardiol. 2021.

[2] Canepa M, Tini G, Montecucco F. The impossible quest to make cardiac amyloidosis diagnosis easy. Eur J Clin Invest. 2021:e13512.

[3] Ashmun RA, Look AT. Metalloprotease activity of CD13/aminopeptidase N on the surface of human myeloid cells. Blood. 1990;75(2):462-9.

[4] Ablasser K, Verheyen N, Glantschnig T, Agnetti G, Rainer PP. Unfolding Cardiac Amyloidosis-From Pathophysiology to Cure. Curr Med Chem. 2019;26(16):2865-78.

[5] Gilstrap LG, Dominici F, Wang Y, El-Sady MS, Singh A, Di Carli MF, et al. Epidemiology of Cardiac Amyloidosis-Associated Heart Failure Hospitalizations Among Fee-for-Service Medicare Beneficiaries in the United States. Circ Heart Fail. 2019;12(6):e005407.

[6] Quock TP, Yan T, Chang E, Guthrie S, Broder MS. Epidemiology of AL amyloidosis: a real-world study using US claims data. Blood Adv. 2018;2(10):1046-53.

[7] Kyle RA, Linos A, Beard CM, Linke RP, Gertz MA, O'Fallon WM, et al. Incidence and natural history of primary systemic amyloidosis in Olmsted County, Minnesota, 1950 through 1989. Blood. 1992;79(7):1817-22.

[8] Bhogal S, Ladia V, Sitwala P, Cook E, Bajaj K, Ramu V, et al. Cardiac Amyloidosis: An Updated Review With Emphasis on Diagnosis and Future Directions. Curr Probl Cardiol. 2018;43(1):10-34.

[9] Chamarthi B, Dubrey SW, Cha K, Skinner M, Falk RH. Features and prognosis of exertional syncope in light-chain associated AL cardiac amyloidosis. Am J Cardiol. 1997;80(9):1242-5.

[10] Falk RH. Diagnosis and management of the cardiac amyloidoses. Circulation. 2005;112(13):2047-60.

[11] Liao R, Jain M, Teller P, Connors LH, Ngoy S, Skinner M, et al. Infusion of light chains from patients with cardiac amyloidosis causes diastolic dysfunction in isolated mouse hearts. Circulation. 2001;104(14):1594-7.

[12] Bishop E, Brown EE, Fajardo J, Barouch LA, Judge DP, Halushka MK. Seven factors predict a delayed diagnosis of cardiac amyloidosis. Amyloid. 2018;25(3):174-9.

[13] Papathanasiou M, Carpinteiro A, Rischpler C, Hagenacker T, Rassaf T, Luedike P. Diagnosing cardiac amyloidosis in every-day practice: A practical guide for the cardiologist. Int J Cardiol Heart Vasc. 2020;28:100519.

[14] Rahman JE, Helou EF, Gelzer-Bell R, Thompson RE, Kuo C, Rodriguez ER, et al. Noninvasive diagnosis of biopsy-proven cardiac amyloidosis. J Am Coll Cardiol. 2004;43(3):410-5.

[15] Cyrille NB, Goldsmith J, Alvarez J, Maurer MS. Prevalence and prognostic significance of low QRS voltage among the three main types of cardiac amyloidosis. Am J Cardiol. 2014;114(7):1089-93.

[16] Rubin J, Maurer MS. Cardiac Amyloidosis: Overlooked, Underappreciated, and Treatable. Annu Rev Med. 2020;71:203-19.

[17] Cheung CC, Roston TM, Andrade JG, Bennett MT, Davis MK. Arrhythmias in Cardiac Amyloidosis: Challenges in Risk Stratification and Treatment. Can J Cardiol. 2020;36(3):416-23.

[18] Giancaterino S, Urey MA, Darden D, Hsu JC. Management of Arrhythmias in Cardiac Amyloidosis. JACC Clin Electrophysiol. 2020;6(4):351-61.

[19] Koyama J, Ikeda S, Ikeda U. Echocardiographic assessment of the cardiac amyloidoses. Circ J. 2015;79(4):721-34.

[20] Quintana-Quezada RA, Yusuf SW, Banchs J. Use of Noninvasive Imaging in Cardiac Amyloidosis. Curr Treat Options Cardiovasc Med. 2016;18(7):46.

[21] Chew C, Ziady GM, Raphael MJ, Oakley CM. The functional defect in amyloid heart disease. The "stiff heart" syndrome. Am J Cardiol. 1975;36(4):438-44.

[22] Child JS, Levisman JA, Abbasi AS, MacAlpin RN. Echocardiographic manifestations of infiltrative cardiomyopathy. A report of seven cases due to amyloid. Chest. 1976;70(6):726-31.

[23] Borer JS, Henry WL, Epstein SE. Echocardiographic observations in patients with systemic infiltrative disease involving the heart. Am J Cardiol. 1977;39(2):184-8.

[24] Habib G, Bucciarelli-Ducci C, Caforio ALP, Cardim N, Charron P, Cosyns B, et al. Multimodality Imaging in Restrictive Cardiomyopathies: An EACVI expert consensus document In collaboration with the "Working Group on myocardial and pericardial diseases" of the European Society of Cardiology Endorsed by The Indian Academy of Echocardiography. Eur Heart J Cardiovasc Imaging. 2017;18(10):1090-121.

[25] Jurcut R, Onciul S, Adam R, Stan C, Coriu D, Rapezzi C, et al. Multimodality imaging in cardiac amyloidosis: a primer for cardiologists. Eur Heart J Cardiovasc Imaging. 2020;21(8):833-44.

[26] Chacko L, Martone R, Cappelli F, Fontana M. Cardiac Amyloidosis: Updates in Imaging. Curr Cardiol Rep. 2019;21(9):108.

[27] Di Nunzio D, Recupero A, de Gregorio C, Zito C, Carerj S, Di Bella G. Echocardiographic Findings in Cardiac Amyloidosis: Inside Two-Dimensional, Doppler, and Strain Imaging. Curr Cardiol Rep. 2019;21(2):7.

[28] Martinez-Naharro A, Baksi AJ, Hawkins PN, Fontana M. Diagnostic imaging of cardiac amyloidosis. Nat Rev Cardiol. 2020;17(7):413-26.

[29] Falk RH, Alexander KM, Liao R, Dorbala S. AL (Light-Chain) Cardiac Amyloidosis: A Review of Diagnosis and Therapy. J Am Coll Cardiol. 2016;68(12):1323-41.

[30] Koyama J, Ray-Sequin PA, Falk RH. Longitudinal myocardial function assessed by tissue velocity, strain, and strain rate tissue Doppler echocardiography in patients with AL (primary) cardiac amyloidosis. Circulation. 2003;107(19):2446-52.

[31] Stricagnoli M, Cameli M, Incampo E, Lunghetti S, Mondillo S. Speckle tracking echocardiography in cardiac amyloidosis. Heart Fail Rev. 2019;24(5):701-7.

[32] Phelan D, Collier P, Thavendiranathan P, Popovic ZB, Hanna M, Plana JC, et al. Relative apical sparing of longitudinal strain using two-dimensional speckle-tracking echocardiography is both sensitive and specific for the diagnosis of cardiac amyloidosis. Heart. 2012;98(19):1442-8.

[33] Rapezzi C, Fontana M. Relative Left Ventricular Apical Sparing of Longitudinal Strain in Cardiac Amyloidosis: Is it Just Amyloid Infiltration? JACC Cardiovasc Imaging. 2019;12(7 Pt 1):1174-6.

[34] Ono K, Ishimaru G, Hayashi M, Bae Y, Ito T, Izumo T, et al. The Imaging Diagnosis of Less Advanced Cases of Cardiac Amyloidosis: The Relative Apical Sparing Pattern. Intern Med. 2017;56(3):315-9.

[35] Mann DL, Zipes DP, Libby P, Bonow RO, Braunwald E. Braunwald's heart disease: a textbook of cardiovascular medicine. 10th edition. ed. Philadelphia, PA: Elsevier/ Saunders; 2015.

[36] Dungu JN, Valencia O, Pinney JH, Gibbs SD, Rowczenio D, Gilbertson JA, et al. CMR-based differentiation of AL and ATTR cardiac amyloidosis. JACC Cardiovasc Imaging. 2014;7(2):133-42.

[37] Tang CX, Petersen SE, Sanghvi MM, Lu GM, Zhang LJ. Cardiovascular magnetic resonance imaging for amyloidosis: The state-of-the-art. Trends Cardiovasc Med. 2019;29(2):83-94.

[38] Martinez-Naharro A, Hawkins PN, Fontana M. Cardiac amyloidosis. Clin Med (Lond). 2018;18(Suppl 2): s30-s5.

[39] Banypersad SM, Sado DM, Flett AS, Gibbs SD, Pinney JH, Maestrini V, et al. Quantification of myocardial extracellular volume fraction in systemic AL amyloidosis: an equilibrium contrast cardiovascular magnetic resonance study. Circ Cardiovasc Imaging. 2013;6(1):34-9.

[40] Fontana M, Corovic A, Scully P, Moon JC. Myocardial Amyloidosis: The Exemplar Interstitial Disease. JACC Cardiovasc Imaging. 2019;12(11 Pt 2):2345-56.

[41] Maurer MS, Bokhari S, Damy T, Dorbala S, Drachman BM, Fontana M, et al. Expert Consensus Recommendations for the Suspicion and Diagnosis of Transthyretin Cardiac Amyloidosis. Circ Heart Fail. 2019;12(9):e006075.

[42] Benson MD, Dasgupta NR, Rao R. Diagnosis and Screening of Patients with Hereditary Transthyretin Amyloidosis (hATTR): Current Strategies and Guidelines. Ther Clin Risk Manag. 2020;16:749-58.

[43] Singh V, Falk R, Di Carli MF, Kijewski M, Rapezzi C, Dorbala S. State-of-the-art radionuclide imaging in cardiac transthyretin amyloidosis. J Nucl Cardiol. 2019;26(1):158-73.

[44] Stats MA, Stone JR. Varying levels of small microcalcifications and macrophages in ATTR and AL cardiac amyloidosis: implications for utilizing nuclear medicine studies to subtype amyloidosis. Cardiovasc Pathol. 2016;25(5):413-7.

[45] Kyriakou P, Mouselimis D, Tsarouchas A, Rigopoulos A, Bakogiannis C, Noutsias M, et al. Diagnosis of cardiac amyloidosis: a systematic review on the role of imaging and biomarkers. BMC Cardiovasc Disord. 2018;18(1):221.

[46] Glaudemans AW, van Rheenen RW, van den Berg MP, Noordzij W, Koole M, Blokzijl H, et al. Bone scintigraphy with (99m)technetium-hydroxymethylene diphosphonate allows early diagnosis of cardiac involvement in patients with transthyretin-derived systemic amyloidosis. Amyloid. 2014;21(1): 35-44.

[47] Small GR, Ruddy TD. Straightening out the wrinkles in technetium-99m-labeled bone scintigraphy tracer assessment of cardiac amyloidosis. J Nucl Cardiol. 2019.

[48] Ruberg FL, Berk JL. Transthyretin (TTR) cardiac amyloidosis. Circulation. 2012;126(10):1286-300.

[49] Nativi-Nicolau J, Maurer MS. Amyloidosis cardiomyopathy: update in the diagnosis and treatment of the most common types. Curr Opin Cardiol. 2018;33(5):571-9.

[50] Fernandez de Larrea C, Verga L, Morbini P, Klersy C, Lavatelli F, Foli A, et al. A practical approach to the diagnosis of systemic amyloidoses. Blood. 2015;125(14):2239-44.

[51] Perlini S, Mussinelli R, Salinaro F. New and Evolving Concepts Regarding the Prognosis and Treatment of Cardiac Amyloidosis. Curr Heart Fail Rep. 2016;13(6):267-72.

[52] Siddiqi OK, Ruberg FL. Cardiac amyloidosis: An update on pathophysiology, diagnosis, and treatment. Trends Cardiovasc Med. 2018;28(1):10-21.

[53] Yancy CW, Jessup M, Bozkurt B, Butler J, Casey DE, Jr., Drazner MH, et al. 2013 ACCF/AHA guideline for the management of heart failure: a report of the American College of Cardiology Foundation/American Heart Association Task Force on Practice Guidelines. J Am Coll Cardiol. 2013;62(16):e147-239.

[54] Ponikowski P, Voors AA, Anker SD, Bueno H, Cleland JG, Coats AJ, et al. 2016 ESC Guidelines for the diagnosis and treatment of acute and chronic heart failure: The Task Force for the diagnosis and treatment of acute and chronic heart failure of the European Society of Cardiology (ESC). Developed with the special contribution of the Heart Failure Association (HFA) of the ESC. Eur J Heart Fail. 2016;18(8):891-975.

[55] Macedo AVS, Schwartzmann PV, de Gusmao BM, Melo MDT, Coelho-Filho OR. Advances in the Treatment of Cardiac Amyloidosis. Curr Treat Options Oncol. 2020;21(5):36.

[56] Bonderman D, Polzl G, Ablasser K, Agis H, Aschauer S, Auer-Grumbach M, et al. Diagnosis and treatment of cardiac amyloidosis: an interdisciplinary consensus statement. Wien Klin Wochenschr. 2020;132(23-24):742-61.

[57] Fine NM, Davis MK, Anderson K, Delgado DH, Giraldeau G, Kitchlu A, et al. Canadian Cardiovascular Society/Canadian Heart Failure Society Joint Position Statement on the Evaluation and Management of Patients With Cardiac Amyloidosis. Can J Cardiol. 2020;36(3):322-34.

[58] Itzhaki Ben Zadok O, Kornowski R. Cardiac Care of Patients with Cardiac Amyloidosis. Acta Haematol. 2020;143(4):343-51.

[59] Kristen AV. Amyloid cardiomyopathy. Herz. 2020;45(3):267-71.

[60] Sousa M, Monohan G, Rajagopalan N, Grigorian A, Guglin M. Heart transplantation in cardiac amyloidosis. Heart Fail Rev. 2017;22(3):317-27.

[61] Maurer MS, Raina A, Hesdorffer C, Bijou R, Colombo P, Deng M, et al. Cardiac transplantation using extended-donor criteria organs for systemic amyloidosis complicated by heart failure. Transplantation. 2007;83(5):539-45.

[62] Estep JD, Bhimaraj A, Cordero-Reyes AM, Bruckner B, Loebe M, Torre-Amione G. Heart transplantation and end-stage cardiac amyloidosis: a review and approach to evaluation and management. Methodist Debakey Cardiovasc J. 2012;8(3):8-16.

[63] Caldeira CCB, Machado RC, Caldeira DCB. Implantation of Short-Term and Long-Term Right Ventricular

Assist Devices. Braz J Cardiovasc Surg. 2017;32(5):435-7.

[64] Kittleson MM, Cole RM, Patel J, Ramzy D, Passano E, Chang DH, et al. Mechanical circulatory support for cardiac amyloidosis. Clin Transplant. 2019;33(10):e13663.

[65] Cheng A, Trivedi JR, Van Berkel VH, Massey HT, Slaughter MS. Comparison of total artificial heart and biventricular assist device support as bridge-to-transplantation. J Card Surg. 2016;31(10):648-53.

[66] Nguyen A, Pozzi M, Mastroianni C, Leger P, Loisance D, Pavie A, et al. Bridge to transplantation using paracorporeal biventricular assist devices or the syncardia temporary total artificial heart: is there a difference? J Cardiovasc Surg (Torino). 2015;56(3):493-502.

[67] Grupper A, Park SJ, Pereira NL, Schettle SD, Gerber Y, Topilsky Y, et al. Role of ventricular assist therapy for patients with heart failure and restrictive physiology: Improving outcomes for a lethal disease. J Heart Lung Transplant. 2015;34(8):1042-9.

[68] Chen Q, Moriguchi J, Levine R, Chan J, Dimbil S, Patel J, et al. Outcomes of Heart Transplantation in Cardiac Amyloidosis Patients: A Single Center Experience. Transplant Proc. 2021;53(1):329-34.

[69] Longhi S, Quarta CC, Milandri A, Lorenzini M, Gagliardi C, Manuzzi L, et al. Atrial fibrillation in amyloidotic cardiomyopathy: prevalence, incidence, risk factors and prognostic role. Amyloid. 2015;22(3):147-55.

[70] Kim EJ, Holmes BB, Huang S, Lugo R, Al Aboud A, Goodman S, et al. Outcomes in patients with cardiac amyloidosis and implantable cardioverter-defibrillator. Europace. 2020;22(8):1216-23.

[71] Muchtar E, Gertz MA, Kumar SK, Lacy MQ, Dingli D, Buadi FK, et al. Improved outcomes for newly diagnosed AL amyloidosis between 2000 and 2014: cracking the glass ceiling of early death. Blood. 2017;129(15):2111-9.

[72] Ozga M, Zhao Q, Benson D, Elder P, Williams N, Bumma N, et al. AL Amyloidosis: The Effect of Maintenance Therapy on Autologous Stem Cell Transplantation Outcomes. J Clin Med. 2020;9(11).

[73] Muchtar E, Gertz MA, Lacy MQ, Leung N, Buadi FK, Dingli D, et al. Refining amyloid complete hematological response: Quantitative serum free light chains superior to ratio. Am J Hematol. 2020;95(11):1280-7.

[74] Kourelis TV, Kyle RA, Dingli D, Buadi FK, Kumar SK, Gertz MA, et al. Presentation and Outcomes of Localized Immunoglobulin Light Chain Amyloidosis: The Mayo Clinic Experience. Mayo Clin Proc. 2017;92(6):908-17.

[75] Kumar SK, Callander NS, Hillengass J, Liedtke M, Baljevic M, Campagnaro E, et al. NCCN Guidelines Insights: Multiple Myeloma, Version 1.2020. J Natl Compr Canc Netw. 2019;17(10):1154-65.

[76] Palladini G, Milani P, Merlini G. Management of AL amyloidosis in 2020. Hematology Am Soc Hematol Educ Program. 2020;2020(1):363-71.

[77] Maurer MS, Elliott P, Comenzo R, Semigran M, Rapezzi C. Addressing Common Questions Encountered in the Diagnosis and Management of Cardiac Amyloidosis. Circulation. 2017;135(14):1357-77.

[78] Sidiqi MH, Aljama MA, Buadi FK, Warsame RM, Lacy MQ, Dispenzieri A, et al. Stem Cell Transplantation for Light Chain Amyloidosis: Decreased

Early Mortality Over Time. J Clin Oncol. 2018;36(13):1323-9.

[79] Comenzo RL, Vosburgh E, Falk RH, Sanchorawala V, Reisinger J, Dubrey S, et al. Dose-intensive melphalan with blood stem-cell support for the treatment of AL (amyloid light-chain) amyloidosis: survival and responses in 25 patients. Blood. 1998;91(10):3662-70.

[80] Kastritis E, Leleu X, Arnulf B, Zamagni E, Cibeira MT, Kwok F, et al. Bortezomib, Melphalan, and Dexamethasone for Light-Chain Amyloidosis. J Clin Oncol. 2020;38(28):3252-60.

[81] Dimopoulos MA, Oriol A, Nahi H, San-Miguel J, Bahlis NJ, Usmani SZ, et al. Daratumumab, Lenalidomide, and Dexamethasone for Multiple Myeloma. N Engl J Med. 2016;375(14):1319-31.

[82] Palladini G, Kastritis E, Maurer MS, Zonder J, Minnema MC, Wechalekar AD, et al. Daratumumab plus CyBorD for patients with newly diagnosed AL amyloidosis: safety run-in results of ANDROMEDA. Blood. 2020;136(1):71-80.

[83] Palladini G, Dispenzieri A, Gertz MA, Kumar S, Wechalekar A, Hawkins PN, et al. New criteria for response to treatment in immunoglobulin light chain amyloidosis based on free light chain measurement and cardiac biomarkers: impact on survival outcomes. J Clin Oncol. 2012;30(36):4541-9.

[84] Sandri MT, Salvatici M, Cardinale D, Zorzino L, Passerini R, Lentati P, et al. N-terminal pro-B-type natriuretic peptide after high-dose chemotherapy: a marker predictive of cardiac dysfunction? Clin Chem. 2005;51(8):1405-10.

[85] Kumar SK, Hayman SR, Buadi FK, Roy V, Lacy MQ, Gertz MA, et al. Lenalidomide, cyclophosphamide, and dexamethasone (CRd) for light-chain amyloidosis: long-term results from a phase 2 trial. Blood. 2012;119(21):4860-7.

[86] Dispenzieri A, Lacy MQ, Zeldenrust SR, Hayman SR, Kumar SK, Geyer SM, et al. The activity of lenalidomide with or without dexamethasone in patients with primary systemic amyloidosis. Blood. 2007;109(2):465-70.

[87] Wechalekar AD, Goodman HJ, Lachmann HJ, Offer M, Hawkins PN, Gillmore JD. Safety and efficacy of risk-adapted cyclophosphamide, thalidomide, and dexamethasone in systemic AL amyloidosis. Blood. 2007;109(2):457-64.

[88] Sanchorawala V, Wright DG, Rosenzweig M, Finn KT, Fennessey S, Zeldis JB, et al. Lenalidomide and dexamethasone in the treatment of AL amyloidosis: results of a phase 2 trial. Blood. 2007;109(2):492-6.

[89] Kittleson MM, Maurer MS, Ambardekar AV, Bullock-Palmer RP, Chang PP, Eisen HJ, et al. Cardiac Amyloidosis: Evolving Diagnosis and Management: A Scientific Statement From the American Heart Association. Circulation. 2020;142(1):e7-e22.

[90] Adams D, Gonzalez-Duarte A, O'Riordan WD, Yang CC, Ueda M, Kristen AV, et al. Patisiran, an RNAi Therapeutic, for Hereditary Transthyretin Amyloidosis. N Engl J Med. 2018;379(1):11-21.

[91] Benson MD, Waddington-Cruz M, Berk JL, Polydefkis M, Dyck PJ, Wang AK, et al. Inotersen Treatment for Patients with Hereditary Transthyretin Amyloidosis. N Engl J Med. 2018;379(1):22-31.

[92] Solomon SD, Adams D, Kristen A, Grogan M, Gonzalez-Duarte A, Maurer MS, et al. Effects

of Patisiran, an RNA Interference Therapeutic, on Cardiac Parameters in Patients With Hereditary Transthyretin-Mediated Amyloidosis. Circulation. 2019;139(4):431-43.

[93] Maurer MS, Schwartz JH, Gundapaneni B, Elliott PM, Merlini G, Waddington-Cruz M, et al. Tafamidis Treatment for Patients with Transthyretin Amyloid Cardiomyopathy. N Engl J Med. 2018;379(11):1007-16.

[94] Berk JL, Suhr OB, Obici L, Sekijima Y, Zeldenrust SR, Yamashita T, et al. Repurposing diflunisal for familial amyloid polyneuropathy: a randomized clinical trial. JAMA. 2013;310(24):2658-67.

[95] Rosenblum H, Castano A, Alvarez J, Goldsmith J, Helmke S, Maurer MS. TTR (Transthyretin) Stabilizers Are Associated With Improved Survival in Patients With TTR Cardiac Amyloidosis. Circ Heart Fail. 2018;11(4):e004769.

[96] Ikram A, Donnelly JP, Sperry BW, Samaras C, Valent J, Hanna M. Diflunisal tolerability in transthyretin cardiac amyloidosis: a single center's experience. Amyloid. 2018;25(3):197-202.

[97] Judge DP, Heitner SB, Falk RH, Maurer MS, Shah SJ, Witteles RM, et al. Transthyretin Stabilization by AG10 in Symptomatic Transthyretin Amyloid Cardiomyopathy. J Am Coll Cardiol. 2019;74(3):285-95.

[98] Obici L, Cortese A, Lozza A, Lucchetti J, Gobbi M, Palladini G, et al. Doxycycline plus tauroursodeoxycholic acid for transthyretin amyloidosis: a phase II study. Amyloid. 2012;19 Suppl 1:34-6.

[99] Wixner J, Pilebro B, Lundgren HE, Olsson M, Anan I. Effect of doxycycline and ursodeoxycholic acid on transthyretin amyloidosis. Amyloid. 2017;24(sup1):78-9.

[100] Hawkins PN, Ando Y, Dispenzeri A, Gonzalez-Duarte A, Adams D, Suhr OB. Evolving landscape in the management of transthyretin amyloidosis. Ann Med. 2015;47(8):625-38.

[101] Ternacle J, Krapf L, Mohty D, Magne J, Nguyen A, Galat A, et al. Aortic Stenosis and Cardiac Amyloidosis: JACC Review Topic of the Week. J Am Coll Cardiol. 2019;74(21):2638-51.

[102] Galat A, Guellich A, Bodez D, Slama M, Dijos M, Zeitoun DM, et al. Aortic stenosis and transthyretin cardiac amyloidosis: the chicken or the egg? Eur Heart J. 2016;37(47):3525-31.

[103] Treibel TA, Fontana M, Gilbertson JA, Castelletti S, White SK, Scully PR, et al. Occult Transthyretin Cardiac Amyloid in Severe Calcific Aortic Stenosis: Prevalence and Prognosis in Patients Undergoing Surgical Aortic Valve Replacement. Circ Cardiovasc Imaging. 2016;9(8).

[104] Cavalcante JL, Rijal S, Abdelkarim I, Althouse AD, Sharbaugh MS, Fridman Y, et al. Cardiac amyloidosis is prevalent in older patients with aortic stenosis and carries worse prognosis. J Cardiovasc Magn Reson. 2017;19(1):98.

[105] Sperry BW, Jones BM, Vranian MN, Hanna M, Jaber WA. Recognizing Transthyretin Cardiac Amyloidosis in Patients With Aortic Stenosis: Impact on Prognosis. JACC Cardiovasc Imaging. 2016;9(7):904-6.

[106] Java AP, Greason KL, Dispenzieri A, Grogan M, King KS, Maleszewski JJ, et al. Aortic valve replacement in patients with amyloidosis. J Thorac Cardiovasc Surg. 2018;156(1):98-103.

[107] Scully PR, Patel KP, Treibel TA, Thornton GD, Hughes RK, Chadalavada S, et al. Prevalence and

outcome of dual aortic stenosis and cardiac amyloid pathology in patients referred for transcatheter aortic valve implantation. Eur Heart J. 2020;41(29):2759-67.

[108] Monticelli FC, Kunz SN, Keller T, Bleiziffer S. Cardiac amyloidosis as a potential risk factor for transapical transcatheter aortic valve implantation. J Card Surg. 2014;29(5):623-4.

Chapter 19

Reversible Cardiomyopathies

Niel Shah, Miguel Rodriguez-Guerra, Muhammad Saad, Anthony Kang and Timothy J. Vittorio

Abstract

Cardiomyopathy includes a diverse and heterogeneous group of disorders affecting the myocardium and eventually leading to cardiac dysfunction. Cardiomyopathy is the leading cause of hospitalization in patients older than 65 years of age and it is an important cause for enormous healthcare expenditure. All reversible cardiomyopathies can be associated with cardiomegaly, systolic heart failure, structural changes, and an increase in mortality, but when the offensive agent is identified and stopped, these conditions tend to stop their progression and reverse. The prognosis of reversible nonischemic cardiomyopathies is better than ischemic or other nonreversible cardiomyopathies. Additionally, it is important to diagnose etiology of HF early and precisely to determine prognosis and effective treatment. Most patients with reversible cardiomyopathy present with clinical picture similar to that of systolic heart failure. Here in this book chapter, we discuss about different types of reversible cardiomyopathy including pathogenesis, clinical picture, diagnosis and treatment.

Keywords: arrhythmogenic, cirrhotic, uremic, nutritional, metabolic, inflammatory

1. Introduction

The heart is composed of a special tissue and a unique electrical system. Though there are some hypotheses about the possibility of regeneration, the cardiac tissue is composed of non-regenerative muscle cells called myocytes which have the capacity to revert acute damages before necrosis and subsequent fibrosis are present. It is thought that this reversion could be related to multiple factors. A decrease in inflammatory markers, perfusion recovery, and possible RNA reactions reduce the fiber tension and inflammation that cause the shortening of the dilated fibers, and then the transient condition will improve. All reversible cardiomyopathies can be associated with cardiomegaly, systolic heart failure, structural changes, and an increase in mortality, but when the offensive agent is identified and stopped, these conditions tend to stop their progression and reverse. In a period of 6 weeks, we are usually able to evaluate positive results after the stunning myocardial cells recover. Most patients with reversible cardiomyopathy present with clinical picture similar to that of systolic heart failure (HF) as follows:

- Dyspnea
- Chest discomfort/pain
- Lower extremity edema or peripheral edema

- Weight gain
- Orthopnea or paroxysmal nocturnal dyspnea (PND)
- Decrease in exercise tolerance etc.

In this chapter, we have focused on important types of reversible cardiomyopathy (**Figure 1**).

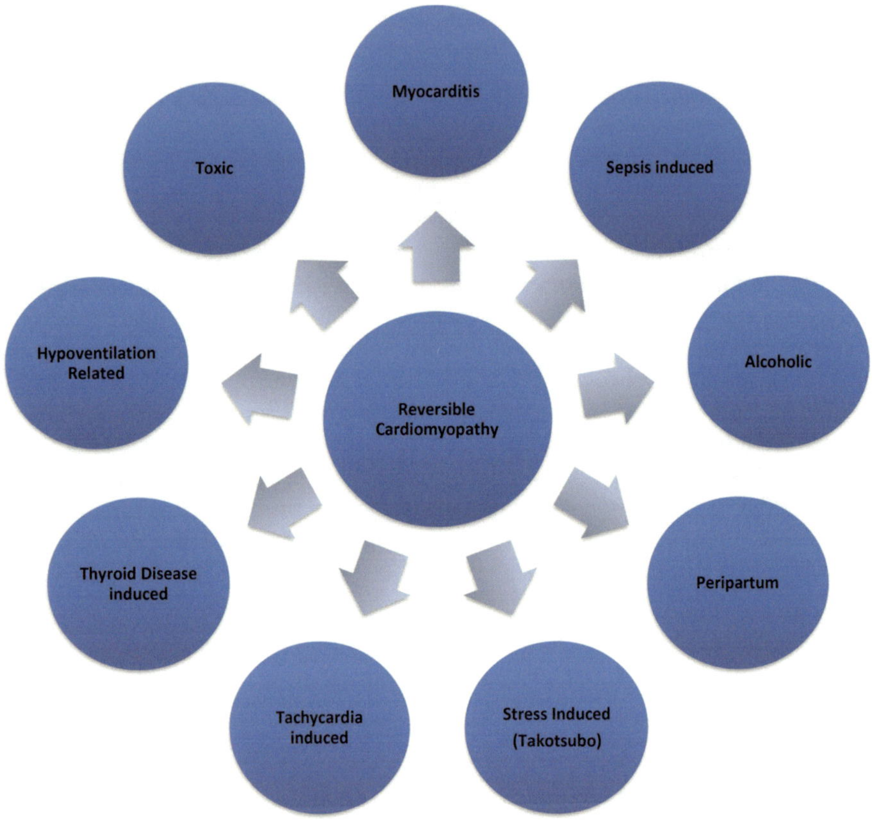

Figure 1.
Different types of reversible cardiomyopathy.

2. Epidemiology

Cardiomyopathy includes a diverse and heterogeneous group of disorders affecting the myocardium and eventually leading to cardiac dysfunction [1]. The HF is a widely prevalent syndrome today and affects 5.1 million adult Americans over the age of 20 [1]. Cardiomyopathy is the leading cause of hospitalization in patients older than 65 years of age and it is an important cause for enormous healthcare expenditure. Interestingly, ischemic cardiomyopathy is responsible for about half of these patients. On the other hand, the prevalence of reversible nonischemic cardiomyopathy is also significant, as per several large clinical trials, and ranges from 20–50% [1]. The prognosis of reversible nonischemic cardiomyopathies is better than ischemic or other nonreversible cardiomyopathies which were suggested by the epidemiological evidence [1]. Additionally, it is important to diagnose etiology of HF early and precisely to determine prognosis and effective treatment.

3. Tachycardia-induced cardiomyopathy

Arrhythmia-induced cardiomyopathy (also known as tachycardia-induced cardiomyopathy, tachycardia-mediated cardiomyopathy, or tachymyopathy) is one of the reversible causes of dilated cardiomyopathy. Arrhythmia-induced cardiomyopathy is defined by the presence of a sustained tachycardia (or frequent episodes of tachycardia or very frequent ectopy) which results in left ventricular (LV) systolic dysfunction. It is a relatively rare, but well-recognized entity caused by long-standing tachycardia, which can be treated readily in most instances and have a good prognosis. A common clinical problem is differentiating whether tachycardia is the primary cause of the patient's cardiomyopathy, or if the tachycardia is secondary to another cardiomyopathy of a different etiology. Arrhythmia-induced cardiomyopathy has been reported with nearly all types of tachyarrhythmia and frequent ectopy, both supraventricular and ventricular [2]. Different types of tachyarrhythmias associated with arrhythmia-induced cardiomyopathy include atrial fibrillation (AF), atrial flutter, atrial tachycardia, reentrant supraventricular tachycardias, and ventricular tachycardia. Regardless of the type of arrhythmia, therapy to restore normal sinus rhythm or to slow the ventricular rate (or eliminate ectopy) usually result in an improvement in left ventricular function.

The incidence of arrhythmia-induced cardiomyopathy is unclear, but an association between tachycardia and cardiomyopathy is well known. An insight into the prevalence of arrhythmia-induced cardiomyopathy can be derived from cohort studies. In one study of 1269 patients undergoing ablation for atrial flutter, 184 had reduced ejection fractions (<40 percent) at baseline [3]. In another study with a cohort of 625 patients undergoing catheter ablation for a variety of tachyarrhythmias, tachycardia-induced cardiomyopathy was present in 2.7 percent (17 of 625 patients) [4]. Similarly, in one cohort of 331 patients who had catheter ablation of incessant atrial tachycardia (AT), myocardial dysfunction was present in 9 percent of patients [5]. Additionally, the patients in the cohort with arrhythmia-induced cardiomyopathy were younger, predominantly male, and had continuous or very frequent paroxysmal tachycardia.

In general, chronic tachycardia eventually causes significant structural changes in the heart, including left ventricular dilatation and cellular morphologic changes. However, the exact mechanism by which tachycardia produces such changes is not well explained. Additionally, the morphologic and biochemical changes that result from arrhythmia-induced cardiomyopathy may produce electrophysiological abnormalities. Chronic tachycardia was associated with ventricular arrhythmias (including polymorphic ventricular tachycardia and sudden death) in a canine model which result from a prolongation in repolarization [6]. Many alterations in neurohumoral and cellular activation have been described in arrhythmia-induced cardiomyopathy patients, and several factors may contribute to the development of rate-related myocardial dysfunction. However, data supporting certain potential mechanisms are lacking, and it remains unclear whether such changes play an etiologic role or if they arise because of tachycardia.

The clinical presentation of arrhythmia-induced cardiomyopathy can vary and usually involves signs and/or symptoms related to HF (dyspnea, fatigue, orthopnea, PND, chest pain or discomfort, lower extremities edema), cardiac tachyarrhythmias (palpitations, lightheadedness, dizziness, anxiety, etc) or both. The approach to the patient with suspected arrhythmia-induced cardiomyopathy includes a thorough history and physical examination with appropriately selected tests to establish the diagnosis and assess acuity, severity, and etiology. All patients should have an electrocardiogram (ECG) to determine the cardiac rhythm and ventricular heart rate (**Figure 2**). There are no specific ECG findings that distinguish patients with

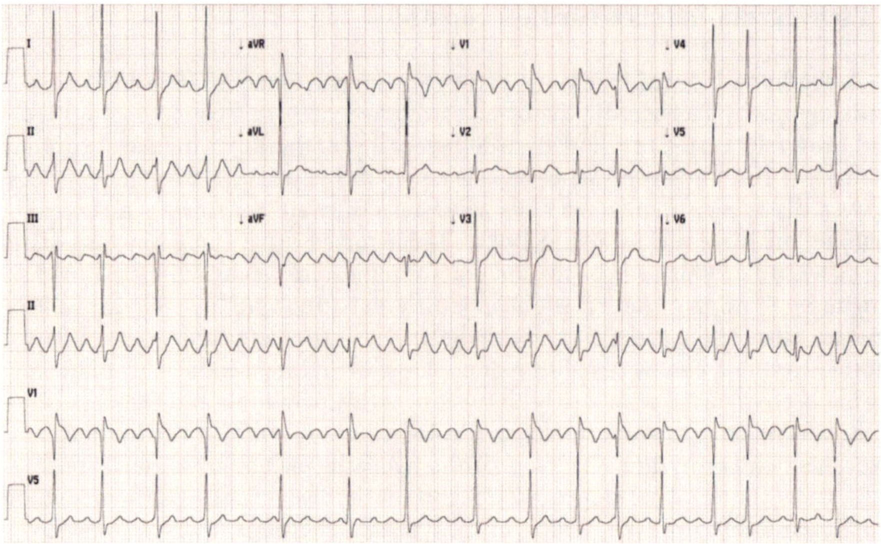

Figure 2.
ECG showing Atrial flutter that can lead to tachycardia-induced cardiomyopathy.

and without arrhythmia-induced cardiomyopathy, and the ECG findings will vary depending upon the underlying tachyarrhythmia. It is important to determine which is the primary pathology, the arrhythmia, or the cardiomyopathy. Usually, the diagnosis of arrhythmia-induced cardiomyopathy can only be made after a successful trial of therapy to slow down the ventricular rate or to restore sinus rhythm after excluding the other potential causes of cardiomyopathy. Patients with suspected arrhythmia-induced cardiomyopathy should have continuous cardiac monitoring for 24 to 48 hours and have non-invasive imaging to assess cardiac structure and function. A transthoracic echocardiogram (TTE) is the preferred modality for assessing cardiac structure and function for most patients due to its widespread availability and ease of performance. However, cardiac magnetic resonance (CMR) imaging is also a reasonable alternative approach in centers with expertise in this modality.

The initial treatments for a patient with HF and suspected arrhythmia-induced cardiomyopathy are similar to those of HF with reduced ejection fraction (HFrEF) and tachyarrhythmias. Treatment of HFrEF generally includes the use of angiotensin-converting enzyme (ACE) inhibitors, angiotensin receptor blockers (ARBs), angiotensin receptor-neprilysin inhibitor (ARNI), beta-blockers, or diuretics. On the other hand, treatment of tachyarrhythmia includes rate-control medications, consideration of antiarrhythmic drugs, and/or cardioversion. Aggressive efforts should be made to achieve good ventricular heart rate control or to restore sinus rhythm due to the potentially reversible nature of arrhythmia-induced cardiomyopathy [2]. Additionally, an adequate trial of medical therapy is required before evaluating the patient for the need for cardiac resynchronization therapy (CRT) or an implantable cardioverter-defibrillator (ICD).

Following the restoration of sinus rhythm or appropriate ventricular rate control, most patients show significant improvement and/or normalization of left ventricular ejection fraction (LVEF) over a period of months. Generally, patients who have not experienced sudden cardiac arrest or sustained ventricular arrhythmia and whose LVEF has improved to 40% or greater, do not require implantation of an ICD. If arrhythmia-induced cardiomyopathy recurs, then these patients are at substantial risk for sudden death and ICD implantation should be considered.

In some patients, the LV chamber may remain somewhat enlarged even after LVEF has normalized. Patients will also have ultrastructural abnormalities of the myocardium, despite improvement in cardiac function when a tachycardia has been terminated or rate controlled [7].

4. Alcoholic cardiomyopathy

Long-term excess alcohol consumption is a leading cause of secondary dilated cardiomyopathy and is associated with up to 40% of dilated cardiomyopathy. Alcohol use can cause atrial enlargement, global chamber dilation, cardiomegaly, and heart failure. Once the structural changes are present, patients with alcoholic cardiomyopathy are at high risk for arrhythmias, especially atrial fibrillation (AF). The prevalence of alcoholic cardiomyopathy is similar in men and women; however, there is a higher disease burden in men. It is more common in the age group of 45–59 years old. Most patients who develop alcoholic cardiomyopathy have been drinking more than 80 to 90 g of ethanol per day for more than five years. This corresponds to approximately eight bottles of beer, one liter of wine, or one-half pint of hard liquor every day. The pathogenesis of alcoholic cardiomyopathy is not well understood, but experimental data have suggested that alcohol consumption may directly or indirectly cause oxidative stress, apoptosis, impaired mitochondrial bioenergetics, altered fatty acid metabolism, and increased myocardial protein catabolism via its metabolites. The pathophysiology of alcoholic cardiomyopathy can also be explained by myocardial toxicity due to adenosine accumulation caused by the impairment of ATP production secondary to thiamine deficiency (Thiamine serves as a co-factor for ATP production).

Common clinical features include classic symptoms of HF (dyspnea, fatigue, orthopnea, PND, chest pain or discomfort, lower extremities edema) and cardiac arrhythmias (palpitations, lightheadedness, dizziness, anxiety, etc). Patients may have a normal physical exam but can also have findings of heart failure such as the decreased intensity of the heart sounds, new S3 or S4 gallop, new murmurs due to valvular insufficiency, increased jugular venous pressure, hepatojugular reflux, and peripheral edema. An EKG usually does not show any specific findings, but may show atrial fibrillation, atrial enlargement, or left ventricular hypertrophy as the most common findings. The mainstay of treatment is abstinence from alcohol which can help in reversing the disease and management of HF. Thus, prognosis in such patients is usually good if they continue to avoid alcohol. If the patient does not stop drinking alcohol, the alcoholic cardiomyopathy may cause severe HF and could advance to severe valvular insufficiency, fatal arrhythmias, and sudden cardiac death.

5. Cardiomyopathy due to acute myocarditis

Myocarditis is a global cardiomyopathy that leads to acute chamber dilation. It is a major cause of death in young adults, reaching up to 20% of deaths. The incidence of myocarditis, according to the International Classification of Diseases' diagnosis codes, was 22 patients per 100,000 patients in the 2013 world population. Myocarditis is an inflammatory disease of the heart that may occur because of infections, immune system activation, or exposure to drugs. The common causes include coxsackievirus (most common), Lyme disease, Chagas disease [8], rheumatic fever, toxic (monoxide, diphtheria, doxorubicin, daunorubicin, cocaine) [9, 10], autoimmune or systemic diseases (SLE, sclerosis, sarcoidosis) [11]. Most patients diagnosed with acute myocarditis recover without clinically relevant residual damage. Patients usually present with viral illness (Fever, malaise, fatigue, etc.) [12]. Patients can also present with symptoms of acute heart failure and conduction abnormalities (Premature atrial complex, supraventricular tachycardia, ventricular ectopies, bradyarrhythmia) including fatal arrhythmia (Ventricular tachycardia, fibrillation) leading to sudden cardiac death [13].

Common physical examination findings may include chest pain, new gallop, friction rub, or new valvular insufficiency on auscultation; hepatomegaly, cardiogenic shock, tachypnea with or without respiratory distress [14]. The ECG in some patients with myocarditis is similar to the ECG pattern of acute isolated pericarditis (which is suggestive of myopericarditis) or acute MI, myocarditis may be associated with regional ST elevations and Q waves like acute MI [15]. Laboratory tests can reveal elevated levels of troponin, pro-BNP, and CK-MB [16]. Echocardiography can be useful by showing wall motion abnormalities and acute valvular insufficiency [17].

Coronary angiography should be considered in patients when acute coronary syndrome (ACS) cannot be distinguished from the myocarditis clinically [18]. CMR is indicated in patients with suspected myocarditis with elevated troponin level and/or ventricular dysfunction, without a clear cause such as ischemic heart disease [19]. The definitive diagnosis of myocarditis can be made by endomyocardial biopsy (EMB). The need for an EMB should be based upon the likelihood that the results will change management. Histologic examination of EMB in myocarditis reveals cellular infiltrates, which are usually histiocytic and mononuclear with or without associated myocyte damage; specific histological forms of myocarditis include eosinophilic, granulomatous, and giant cell myocarditis. Possible late complications include severe valvulopathies, biventricular failure, and conduction abnormalities [20]. The mainstay treatment is to treat the underlying cause. Most patients with acute myocarditis have partial or full clinical recovery. In some cases, the process may continue subclinically which eventually causes DCM [21]. The likelihood of these late complications is increased in patients who present with greatly diminished left ventricular function.

6. Sepsis-induced cardiomyopathy

Sepsis-induced cardiomyopathy is a reversible condition causing left ventricular dilation that could lead to low filling pressures and low ejection fraction. It usually starts to normalize within 10 days of treatment of underlying sepsis [22]. Sepsis-induced myocardial dysfunction is one of the major predictors of morbidity and mortality in sepsis [23]. It is usually present in more than 40% of cases of sepsis and its presence can increase the mortality rate up to 70% [24, 25]. The exact physiopathology is not completely understood but the role of cytokines and endotoxins is thought to have an important role in the myocardial depression found in this condition. Other factors that are also related are metabolic disturbances, hypoxia, coagulopathies, and oxygen deprivation leading to myocardial injury [26]. Another theory is the high consumption of oxygen by the mitochondria creating an energy imbalance. Pro-inflammatory factors from infectious agents cause a release of cytokines and endotoxins that accelerate the oxygen consumption in a low oxygen environment eventually leading to the production of e metabolites such as free radicals and nitrogen species [27]. These metabolites then create a toxic environment and a transient myocardial injury [28, 29]. Sepsis can also cause Takotsubo cardiomyopathy which is described separately.

The clinical features include fever, elevated WBCs, weakness, and malaise along with clinical features of HF. Physical exam findings may include rash, conjunctivitis, wounds, or evident infection. Patients may also present with hypotension, chest pain, or altered mental status. EKG usually does not show any specific findings, but may show findings suggestive of ACS due to underlying myocardial inflammation [30]. Laboratory tests may show elevated inflammatory markers, such as elevated C-reactive protein (CRP), erythrocyte sedimentation rate (ESR), ferritin due to systemic inflammation [31]. Additionally, cardiac markers may be also elevated due to underlying myocardial injury [32, 33]. Furthermore, cultures should be obtained to identify the causative agent before starting a patient on antibiotics. The treatment mainly includes treatment of underlying sepsis and stabilization of the patient when they are hemodynamically unstable to avoid myocardial injury secondary to profound hypotension or arrhythmia. The prognosis of the patient usually varies depending on the severity of sepsis, but generally, the prognosis is reserved.

7. Stress cardiomyopathy or Takotsubo cardiomyopathy

Stress cardiomyopathy is also known as Takotsubo cardiomyopathy or broken heart syndrome, and the clinical presentation mimics acute myocardial infarction [34]. This condition is most common in post-menopausal women. The possible reason for involvement in such a patient group could be explained by hypotheses demonstrating a potential protective effect of estrogen in stress CM [35–37]. The patient with such type of cardiomyopathy should be treated as ACS until the obstructive coronary disease is ruled out by coronary angiography. The pathophysiology behind stress cardiomyopathy is not well understood [38], but the possible mechanism can be explained by the sudden release of catecholamine (Norepinephrine, epinephrine, and dopamine) [39, 40] that causes cardiac stunning by myocyte perfusion impairment and lead to myocardial tissue edema, necrosis, and fibrosis [41].

The clinical features include anxiety, tachycardia, and chest pain which can mimic chest pain of acute MI. EKG may vary from ST segment elevation (most common finding), ST segment depression (less common), QT interval prolongation, T wave inversion, abnormal Q waves, and non-specific abnormalities. Serum cardiac troponin levels are elevated in most patients with stress CM, while creatine kinase (CK) levels are generally normal or mildly elevated. Furthermore, brain natriuretic peptide (BNP) or N-terminal pro-BNP (NT-proBNP) levels are elevated in most patients with stress CM. Radionuclide myocardial perfusion imaging is generally not indicated in patients presenting with suspected stress cardiomyopathy since most have high-risk features for ACS and will require coronary angiography. Patients with suspected non-ST elevation ACS with low to intermediate-risk features may undergo radionuclide myocardial perfusion imaging. An echocardiogram can show a decrease in LVEF and LV wall motion abnormalities (**Figure 3**). Patterns of LV wall motion abnormality in patients with stress-induced cardiomyopathy include the apical type (most common), and atypical variants including mid-ventricular, basal, focal (limited to an isolated segment), and global types. CMR may be helpful in the diagnosis and evaluation of stress cardiomyopathy when the echocardiogram is technically suboptimal and/or there is coexistent coronary artery disease. Late gadolinium enhancement (LGE) on CMR is usually absent in stress cardiomyopathy in contrast to MI in which intense subendocardial or transmural LGE is seen.

Stress-induced cardiomyopathy is generally a reversible disorder that is managed with supportive therapy [42]. Rapid resolution of symptoms can be usually seen with conservative treatment and resolution of the physical or emotional stress. However, some patients may develop acute complications such as shock and acute HF that require intensive therapy. Appropriate management of shock varies and depends on whether significant left ventricular outflow tract (LVOT) obstruction is present [43]. HF management during an acute presentation and following stabilization is generally performed according to standard guidelines. However, caution should be performed to avoid volume depletion and with use of vasodilator therapy in patients with LVOT obstruction. Recommendations for anticoagulation to prevent thromboembolism in patients with stress cardiomyopathy with LV thrombus or severe LV systolic dysfunction are similar to those for post-MI patients [44, 45].

8. Peripartum cardiomyopathy

Peripartum cardiomyopathy is an important cause of dilated cardiomyopathy and HF. It is also known as pregnancy-associated cardiomyopathy [46]. The diagnosis can be missed due to the lack of regular screening and overlap between clinical signs or symptoms of HF signs or symptoms of the pregnancy [47]. Peripartum cardiomyopathy usually occurs during the last trimester or within the 6 months of the postpartum period. Several risk factors have been identified which include greater age, multiple gestations, African descent, and a history of preeclampsia, eclampsia, or postpartum hypertension. The pathophysiology is not clearly understood but Honigberg and Givertz suggested the possible role of oxidative stress on myocardium caused by elevated prolactin levels [48].

The clinical features of peripartum cardiomyopathy are usually masked by signs and symptoms of pregnancy and are difficult to diagnose solely based on clinical findings. Patients usually present with similar clinical presentation as HF patients (shortness of breath, fatigue, orthopnea, lower extremities pitting edema). An echocardiogram is the modality of choice for definitive diagnosis of peripartum cardiomyopathy and usually shows dilated cardiomyopathy with an impairment of the ejection fraction [49]. Echocardiogram generally reveals a global reduction in LV systolic function with LVEF nearly always <45 percent. Management is similar to the treatment of HF with reduced EF, such as ACE inhibitors or ARBs or ARNI, beta-blockers, and diuretics. In addition to this treatment, use of bromocriptine should also be considered [50]. However, prophylactic anticoagulation should always be considered along with bromocriptine treatment as thromboembolic events have been noticed during the use of bromocriptine [50]. Patients should get a repeat echocardiogram six weeks after diagnosis has been made for prognostication [51].

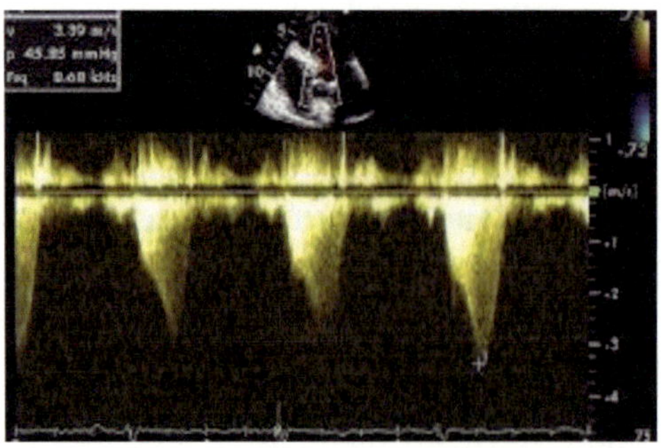

Figure 3.
Doppler image showing LVOT obstruction in a patient with Takotsubo Cardiomyopathy.

9. Thyroid disease induced cardiomyopathy

Metabolic cardiomyopathy is a secondary cardiomyopathy that results from disturbed energy production leading to impaired cardiac function. It may be caused by a myriad of endocrine disorders, nutritional deficiencies, and familial storage diseases [52]. Thyroid hormones have been shown to affect myocytes by acting on various thyroid hormone receptors in the myocardium, including a-myosin heavy chain fusion, sarcoplasmic reticulum calcium-activated ATPase (SERCA), the cellular membrane Na+/K+ pump (Na+/K+ ATPase), β-adrenergic receptors, cardiac troponin I, and atrial natriuretic peptide (ANP) [53]. These interactions help upregulate α-chains but downregulate β-chains in myocytes, which ultimately leads to faster myocardial fibril shortening [54]. Thyroid hormones have also been shown to affect the ion channels, including Na+/K+ ATPase, Na+/Ca + 2 exchanger, and various K+ channels by inducing positive inotropic effects, thereby prolonging activation of Na + channels and shortening action potential durations [55]. Additionally, thyroid hormones have been known to have a vasodilatory effect on peripheral arteries [56]. The combined effort of these mechanisms can cause systemic changes in cardiac function by reducing peripheral vascular resistance, activating the renin-angiotensin mechanism, increasing LV end-diastolic volume (LVEDV), and increasing preload [57]. The increased preload and decreased peripheral vascular resistance lead to a high cardiac output, even at rest, resulting in cardiomyopathy. In contrast to hyperthyroidism, hypothyroidism causes a low cardiac output cardiomyopathy via the same pathways mentioned above, however, by downregulating the previously mentioned receptors/channels causing decreased myocardial excitation and contractility leading to a low-output cardiomyopathy [58]. The clinical features are similar to those seen in patients with HF.

Management of thyroid disease-induced cardiomyopathy follows a similar algorithm to the cardiomyopathies mentioned above, which includes the typical HF treatment regimen. Management also includes addressing the root etiology, whether it be excess or deficiency of thyroid hormones. However, there is promising data showing that the use of β-adrenergic blockade may be beneficial in these patients. Biondi et al. conducted a small study which demonstrated that hyperthyroid patients treated with the selective β1-adrenoceptor antagonist bisoprolol experienced normalization of the LV mass index and LV systolic function after 6 months of treatment [59]. Similar results were established in a case study published a year later in which the use of β-adrenoceptor blockers showed clinical improvement in a patient with dilated cardiomyopathy caused by hyperthyroidism [60]. It is also worth mentioning the association between hyperthyroidism and AF. The prevalence of AF in thyrotoxicosis is estimated to be 13% according to one study. This is especially important as uncontrolled AF is associated with tachycardia-induced cardiomyopathy as discussed above [61, 62].

10. Cardiomyopathy related to obstructive sleep apnea or hypoventilation

Obstructive sleep apnea (OSA) is a potentially life-threatening condition that is characterized by repeated cessation of breathing while sleeping mostly due to complete or partial pharyngeal obstruction [63]. There has been evidence supporting the associations between obstructive sleep apnea and cardiovascular morbidity and mortality. The National Commission on sleep disorders research estimated that sleep apnea is probably responsible for 38,000 cardiovascular deaths per year [64]. Also, obstructive sleep apnea increases the risk of coronary artery disease by 30%, heart failure by 140%, and stroke by 60% [65]. OSA can be identified by a combination of symptoms and laboratory results, such as repetitive apneas and hypopneas accompanied by hypoxia, sleep arousals, and hemodynamic changes [66–69]. Furthermore, activation of the sympathetic nervous system during respiratory events potentiates vasoconstriction and often triggers increases in blood pressure and heart rate [67, 70]. OSA is also associated with several cardiorespiratory problems such as loud snoring, loud gasps, and daytime breathlessness [71, 72].

The underlying mechanisms showing the associations between OSA and cardiovascular disease are not completely understood, but several intermediate mechanisms have been proposed. They include sustained sympathetic activation, changes in intrathoracic pressure and oxidative stress, and later vascular inflammation caused by nocturnal hypoxia and reoxygenation cycles [73, 74]. These mechanisms then results in increases in systolic blood pressure that might eventually lead to hypertension or worsening of this condition. A similar mechanism might explain the link between OSA and tachyarrhythmia [75]; whereas bradyarrhythmia, which is more common than tachyarrhythmia, might be the effect of an increase in vagal tone due to stimulation of receptor sites in the upper airway [76]. Other abnormalities observed among patients with OSA such as disorders in coagulation factors, endothelial damage, platelet activation, and an increase in inflammatory mediators might also be involved in the pathogenesis of cardiovascular disease [74, 76–79]. Patients with OSA have characteristically higher levels of endothelin and lower levels of nitric oxide than healthy sleepers [74, 77]. This increased endothelin level is known to impair blood pressure regulation as well. Thus, patients with OSA often experience greater blood vessel constriction. Interestingly, with continuous positive airway pressure (CPAP) treatment, levels of endothelin and circulating nitric oxide invariably return to normal [77].

Recently, research interests have centered on the relative contribution of oxidative stress in explaining the associations between sleep apnea and cardiovascular morbidity [74, 79, 80]. Investigators have proposed that hypoxia, which is commonly observed in sleep apnea, promotes the formation of reactive oxygen species (ROS), which could activate the transcriptional activator hypoxia-inducible factor 1 (HIF-1), particularly during the reoxygenation period [81, 82]. ROS regulates the activation of critical transcription factors that are redox-sensitive, resulting in increased expression of genes, which encode proteins promoting adaptation to hypoxia [81]. It has been suggested that redox-sensitive transcription factors, which elicit inflammatory pathways are also activated, thereby affecting inflammatory and immune responses by promoting activation of endothelial cells, leukocytes, and platelets [74]. These cells once activated can express adhesion molecules and proinflammatory cytokines that may lead to endothelial injury and dysfunction, which inevitably lead to the development of cardiovascular morbidity [74]. Observing this chain of events, investigators surmise that atherogenesis apparently starts soon after the onset of sleep apnea [74]. Substantial atherosclerotic insults are likely incurred by the time a diagnosis is rendered since symptoms often become apparent around the age of 45 years [74, 80]. It is unclear whether such atherogenic damages can be reversed, but treatment can retard their progress [83].

Using CPAP therapy, investigators have shown significant reductions in levels of C-reactive protein and interleukin-6 [83], and atherogenic plaque regression has been observed among patients with dyslipidemia [84]. Therefore, sleep apnea diagnosis and treatment should be made as early as possible in order to prevent cardiovascular morbidity. The use of CPAP or bilevel PAP therapy have showed positive benefits in clinical trials. This therapeutic modality is highly effective in improving left ventricular ejection fraction and quality of life by decreasing blood pressure and sympathetic activity and reducing mortality among patients with congestive heart failure [85, 86]. Additionally, CPAP treatment significantly reduces risks of ACS, cardiovascular death, and hospitalization for heart failure among patients with coronary artery disease [87]. Furthermore, CPAP therapy has significant effects on lipid levels. CPAP studies show significant improvement in insulin sensitivity and left ventricular function with a corresponding decrease in blood pressure [88].

11. Toxic cardiomyopathy

Dilated cardiomyopathy can result from direct exposure to toxins, such as cocaine, alcohol, medications, particularly chemotherapeutic drugs, and radiation in the absence of abnormal underlying cardiovascular conditions such as hypertension, valvular disease, or coronary artery disease. The true prevalence of toxic cardiomyopathy in the general population is not known. The mechanism of toxic cardiomyopathy caused by some common toxic substances has been mentioned here. Alcoholic cardiomyopathy has been discussed separately. Patients with toxic cardiomyopathy usually present with clinical features similar to patients with systolic HF and the treatment involves the avoidance of toxic substances along with treatment for systolic HF.

11.1 Cocaine

Cocaine use is associated with the development of cardiomyopathy. However, the relationship is not well understood as compared to the relationship between cocaine use and coronary ischemia. Multiple mechanisms have been explained including the excessive sympathetic stimulation with increased myocardial oxygen consumption, direct toxic effect, and infectious cardiomyopathy in a parenteral cocaine user. In young persons, cardiomegaly with otherwise unexplained HF should raise the suspicion of cocaine abuse. Abstinence from cocaine usually leads to complete reversal of the myocardial dysfunction.

11.2 Medications

A number of medications such as anticancer drugs, anti-diabetic drugs, or antiretroviral drugs are associated with cardiomyopathy, and discontinuation of such drugs may result in significant improvement in cardiac function.

Anticancer drugs, such as anthracycline, trastuzumab, and cyclophosphamide are known to cause CM. Anthracycline-induced cardiomyopathy has been the most extensively studied. The mechanisms of anthracycline-induced cardiotoxicity are primarily due to its mechanisms of action as anticancer drugs which is inhibition of topoisomerase II β and DNA cleavage. Additionally, metabolic or oxidative stress factors may play a part, together with interference with iron metabolism. On the other hand, trastuzumab is a monoclonal antibody directed against the c-erbB-2 (HER2/neu) receptor that is used in the treatment of breast cancer. Since the HER2 signaling pathway plays an important role in cardiac development and protection, there is biological plausibility for cardiac toxicity with the use of trastuzumab [89, 90]. cardiomyopathy is also known to develop when a loss of function mutation occurs in HER2 in ventricular myocytes [91].

Antidiabetic medications such as thiazolidinedione class drugs are known to cause cardiotoxicity. The possible mechanisms of cardiotoxicity caused by these drugs include oxidative stress and interference with mitochondrial respiration. On the other hand, antiretroviral medications like azidothymidine are also cardiotoxic as a result of mitochondrial toxicity. Azidothymidine also increases the production of mitochondrial reactive oxygen species (ROS) in addition to energy depletion.

11.3 Methamphetamine

Methamphetamine and related compounds are the second most widely used illicit drug in the United States after cannabis [92]. Methamphetamine-associated cardiomyopathy (MACM) may be seen in chronic methamphetamine users. The primary mechanism of action of methamphetamine is the increased release and decreased uptake of catecholamines at the neuronal synapse producing a marked effect on the cardiovascular system [92]. The increased levels of catecholamines can stimulate alpha and beta-adrenergic receptors leading to hypertension and tachycardia. Methamphetamine can lead to irreversible structural and functional changes in the heart which eventually lead to decompensated heart failure and ultimately requiring heart transplantation.

11.4 Carbon monoxide

Carbon monoxide (CO) exposure is known to cause cardiomyopathy by causing hypoxic injury. CO causes direct toxic damage to the mitochondria leading to an impairment of the mitochondrial respiratory chain at the cytochrome c oxidase level and a decrease of glutathione concentrations and ATP production. In survivors of an acute exposure, there is no evidence for a delayed dilated cardiomyopathy. In one retrospective study of 626 patients with CO exposure, only 3.04% (n = 19) patients had CO induced CM [93].

11.5 Trace elements

Trace elements are known to play an important role in myocardial metabolism and their accumulation (cobalt, arsenic) or deficiency (selenium) can be responsible for a form of dilated cardiomyopathy that is indistinguishable from an idiopathic CM. The role of trace elements was assessed in one study in which myocardial and skeletal muscle biopsies were obtained from 13 patients with an idiopathic DCM, 35 patients with valvular or ischemic heart disease, and 4 normal subjects [94]. Patients with a dilated cardiomyopathy had a significant increase in the myocardial concentration of mercury (22,000 times normal), antimony (12,000-fold higher), gold (11-fold higher), chromium (13-fold higher), and cobalt (4 times higher). On the other hand, patients with valvular or ischemic heart disease had myocardial concentrations of trace elements that were ≤ 5 times greater than normal. Concentrations of trace elements in skeletal muscle were normal in all groups of patients.

Cobalt-associated cardiomyopathy probably results from interference with energy production and contractile mechanisms. Cobalt associated cardiomyopathy has been reported in drinkers of beer containing cobalt sulfate for foam stabilization (known as Quebec beer-drinkers' cardiomyopathy) [95], individuals with work-related cobalt exposure, and in some individuals exposed to cobalt from metal hip prostheses [96]. There have been some reported cases where degeneration of metallic hip implants can lead to cobalt cardiomyopathy [97, 98]. Antimony may cause lethal oxidative stress and cell death mediated by elevation in intracellular calcium. Proposed mechanisms for mercury toxicity include depletion of glutathione, ROS production and interruption in selenium-dependent endogenous enzymatic reactions. The existence of lithium-induced cardiomyopathy is still debated.

12. Uremic cardiomyopathy

Cardiovascular diseases are the leading cause of morbidity and mortality in chronic kidney disease (CKD) patients [99]. These adverse cardiovascular consequences are due to CKD related cardiomyopathy, which is termed uremic cardiomyopathy [100]. Uremic cardiomyopathy in patients with CKD or end-stage renal disease (ESRD) is the result of pressure overload, volume overload, and the uremic state itself. Epidemiological studies and studies using cardiac MRI have suggested that the primary manifestation of uremic cardiomyopathy is LV hypertrophy (LVH). It is present even in patients with very early stages of CKD. The prevalence of LVH in pre-dialysis patients is up to 65%. The pathogenesis of uremic cardiomyopathy is poorly understood and is generally multifactorial. Patients with CKD usually continue to have abnormal myocardial remodeling despite improvements made to dialysis and advancements in the treatment of CKD, hypertension, hypervolemia, anemia. Two factors play an important role in the pathophysiology of patients with CKD and mineral and bone disease (CKD-MBD) which include the hormone FGF23, and its cofactor, αKlotho. FGF23 is deleterious to the myocardium, while αKlotho is protective. Although αKlotho is an obligatory cofactor for FGF23 action as the primary phosphaturic hormone in phosphorus homeostasis, both factors are seen to have independent and antagonistic effects on the myocardium. Briefly, the main pathophysiology of uremic cardiomyopathy includes a triad of hyperphosphatemia, αKlotho deficiency, and elevated FGF23 levels [100].

The cause for very high cardiovascular risk in CKD patients can be explained by effects of traditional and non-traditional cardiovascular risk factors which are augmented by sequelae of CKD, such as uremia, anemia, hypervolemia, oxidative stress, inflammation, and insulin resistance eventually leading to faster progression of cardiovascular disease and increasing the number of cardiovascular events and mortality [101]. About 40% of deaths in dialysis patients are due to sudden cardiac death (SCD) which outweighs deaths due to HF, acute myocardial infarction (MI), and stroke in such population [102]. The major reason for sudden cardiac death in patients with uremic cardiomyopathy is fatal arrhythmia which is in contrast to the general population where the most common reason for SCD is acute MI. The risk factors for adverse cardiovascular events in dialysis patients include anemia, high parathyroid hormone levels, hypo or hypercalcemia, hyperphosphatemia, fast electrolyte shift, chronic volume overload, inflammation, coronary artery disease, autonomic dysfunction, atrial fibrillation, heart failure with systolic dysfunction, and left ventricular hypertrophy (LVH) [103].

The clinical features in uremic cardiomyopathy patients are similar to that of HF patients such as dyspnea, orthopnea, fatigue, weakness, elevated jugular venous pressure, an S3 gallop, rales, and peripheral edema. ECG can show findings suggestive of LVH and may show nonspecific ischemic changes. Echocardiography may reveal LV systolic dysfunction, LV diastolic dysfunction, or valve dysfunction. Laboratory tests may show elevated natriuretic peptides and cardiac enzymes like other cardiomyopathies, but the interpretation of those tests is difficult in a patient with CKD or ESRD as these patients usually have elevated levels of cardiac biomarkers at baseline due to poor renal clearance. Thus, an entire clinical picture with lab tests, ECG findings, and echocardiogram findings should be taken to make a diagnosis of uremic cardiomyopathy.

Conventional hemodialysis is the main treatment for uremic cardiomyopathy, and it may cause regression of LVH. Hemodialysis is also known to reverse the systolic dysfunction and thus improve LVEF in some patients with ESRD. However, patients tend to continue to have cardiac dysfunction or uremic cardiomyopathy even while on hemodialysis treatment, thus conventional hemodialysis may not be adequate treatment despite being the treatment of choice. Renal transplantation has been shown to reverse uremic cardiomyopathy and to confer a significant survival advantage over hemodialysis [104]. Future therapies targeting the underlying cellular mechanisms of uremic cardiomyopathy may help to reduce the burden of uremic cardiomyopathy in the CKD and ESRD population. In a study on uremic mice, Rapamycin has been shown to reduce cardiac hypertrophy and fibrosis [105]. Thus, rapamycin has the potential to be an effective therapy for uremic cardiomyopathy. LVH is the early and pertinent manifestation of uremic cardiomyopathy as well as a powerful independent predictor of survival in CKD. The regression of LVH can reduce cardiovascular risk and improve survival.

13. Cirrhotic cardiomyopathy

Cirrhotic cardiomyopathy (CCM) is defined as a cardiac dysfunction in patients with cirrhosis, which is characterized by impaired contractile responsiveness to stress and/or altered diastolic relaxation, with electrophysiological abnormalities, in the absence of other known cardiac disorder [106–108]. For years CCM was confused with alcoholic cardiomyopathy, but in 1953, Kowalski and Abelmann demonstrated the existence of a circulatory dysfunction specific to liver cirrhosis [109]. Since then many experimental and clinical studies have established the existence of CCM different than alcoholic cardiomyopathy. Cirrhosis of the liver leads to a hyperdynamic circulatory state, which induces cardiac dysfunctions that characterize the CCM syndrome which includes a combination of systolic and diastolic dysfunctions, prolonged ventricular repolarization, and the inability of the sinus node to increase heart rate during exercise [108].

CCM is a condition in which patients usually remain asymptomatic for months to years as they have a near-normal cardiac function at rest and develop symptoms only under conditions of physical or pharmacological stress [110]. Thus, the diagnosis of CCM is challenging and the actual prevalence of this condition remains unknown. Pathogenesis of CCM includes mechanisms such as the increased activity of the vasodilator pathway through the actions of NO, cytokines, cannabinoids, carbon monoxide, and cytokines, decreased beta-adrenergic function, and sodium and calcium transport kinetics downregulation in the cardiac muscle which can lead to an impaired contractile function of the cardiomyocyte. CCM is generally a silent condition as patients at rest do not develop any signs or symptoms of heart failure as peripheral vasodilatation protects the heart by reducing afterload [108]. However, CCM should be suspected in patients with cirrhosis presenting with a decrease in exercise tolerance and HF symptoms in the absence of any other underlying heart disease.

Echocardiogram and ECG are the most important tests to diagnose CCM. ECG can reveal prolongation of QT interval in such patients. The most common echocardiography finding in such patients is first-degree diastolic dysfunction which is characterized by reduced early diastolic ventricular filling and increased atrial filling ($E/A < 1.0$), deceleration time > 200 ms, and prolonged isovolumetric relaxation time (ITVR >80 ms) representing increased resistance to ventricular inflow [111]. Stress echocardiography is also a useful method that should be used in patients with advanced liver disease as it can detect subtle systolic and diastolic dysfunctions before the ventricular ejection fraction is decreased [112]. Laboratory tests usually show elevated levels of troponin, atrial natriuretic peptide (ANP), and NT-proBNP. Additionally, CMR can also serve as a useful tool in the diagnosis of CCM. In patients with CCM, late gadolinium enhancement has a diffuse myocardial distribution in MR images with the appearance of myocarditis [113].

The treatment of CCM is similar to the treatment of HF in non-cirrhotic patients. However, reduction in afterload is not recommended in patients with advanced cirrhosis as these patients are already significantly dilated. However, in patients with final-stage liver disease and associated with CCM, liver transplantation is the only effective established treatment. Liver transplantation has been shown to reverse the systolic and diastolic dysfunction and prolonged QT interval [114, 115]. However, the unavailability of organ donors and cost concerns should be considered. The candidates must be well evaluated, as patients are at risk of death by HF, coronary artery disease, tachyarrhythmias, and other cardiac deaths in the post-operative term of liver transplantation. There is no accurate data on the prognosis for liver transplantation in patients with CCM. Patients with CCM should avoid physical effort and other forms of stress and should be provided with oxygen in some situations.

14. Conclusion

Reversible cardiomyopathies have been considered as one of the under diagnosed etiologies of non-ischemic cardiomyopathy that require careful clinical insight. Although reversible in nature but if remain undiagnosed, it can lead to catastrophic effects. It is hypothesized to have better prognosis compared to ischemic cardiomyopathy. Early diagnosis is warranted to guide efficient treatment. Further research regarding diagnostic and therapeutic algorithm for this subset of cardiomyopathy is needed to improve long term outcomes (**Table 1**).

Etiology of cardiomyopathy	Pathophysiology	Management
Myocarditis	Inflammation due to infectious agent, most commonly viral.	Natural course with recovery, no definitive treatment. Steroid may be used in Giant cell myocarditis
Sepsis-induced	Not well understood. Probably reaction due to cytokines release.	Treatment of underlying infection.
Alcoholic	High incidence of cardiomegaly. Toxicity mediated due to adenosine accumulation.	Alcohol cessation
Peripartum	Most commonly in the last trimester. Could be misdiagnosed. Not clear mechanism.	Standard CHF treatment. Bromocriptine may be helpful
Stress Induced	Known as Takotsubo Cardiomyopathy. Caused by sudden release of catecholamine due to stress.	Spontaneous recovery
Tachycardia induced	Arrythmia such as atrial tachycardia and PVC induced	Arrythmia ablation
Thyroid disease-induced	It is a part of Metabolic Cardiomyopathy. Caused by hyper or hypothyroidism. Could lead to arrhythmias especially atrial fibrillation.	Treatment of underlying condition
Hypoventilation Related	Most commonly due to OSA. Could cause structure and hemodynamic changes.	Better prognosis if early intervention of the OSA before severe changes in the intracardiac pressures.
Toxic	Could be cause by licit or ilicit agents that results cardiotoxic	Most of the times reversible once the agent is stopped.

Table 1.
Summary of Reversible Cardiomyopathies.

Author details

Niel Shah[1], Miguel Rodriguez-Guerra[1], Muhammad Saad[2], Anthony Kang[3] and Timothy J. Vittorio[2*]

1 Division of Medicine, BronxCare Hospital Center, Bronx, NY, USA

2 Division of Cardiology, BronxCare Hospital Center, Bronx, NY, USA

3 Division of Pharmacy, BronxCare Hospital Center, Bronx, NY, USA

*Address all correspondence to: tjvittorio@gmail.com

References

[1] Nagarakanti R, Whellan D, Rubin S, Mather PJ. Reversible cardiomyopathies. Cardiol Rev. 2007 Jul-Aug;15(4):178-83. doi: 10.1097/CRD.0b013e31804c98b1. PMID: 17575481

[2] Gopinathannair R, Etheridge SP, Marchlinski FE, et al. Arrhythmia-Induced Cardiomyopathies: Mechanisms, Recognition, and Management. J Am Coll Cardiol 2015; 66:1714.

[3] Brembilla-Perrot B, Ferreira JP, Manenti V, et al. Predictors and prognostic significance of tachy cardiomyopathy: insights from a cohort of 1269 patients undergoing atrial flutter ablation. Eur J Heart Fail 2016; 18:394.

[4] Donghua Z, Jian P, Zhongbo X, et al. Reversal of cardiomyopathy in patients with congestive heart failure secondary to tachycardia. J Interv Card Electrophysiol 2013; 36:27.

[5] Medi C, Kalman JM, Haqqani H, et al. Tachycardia-mediated cardiomyopathy secondary to focal atrial tachycardia: long-term outcome after catheter ablation. J Am Coll Cardiol 2009; 53:1791.

[6] Pak PH, Nuss HB, Tunin RS, et al. Repolarization abnormalities, arrhythmia and sudden death in canine tachycardia-induced cardiomyopathy. J Am Coll Cardiol 1997; 30:576.

[7] Nerheim P, Birger-Botkin S, Piracha L, Olshansky B. Heart failure and sudden death in patients with tachycardia-induced cardiomyopathy and recurrent tachycardia. Circulation 2004; 110:247.

[8] Khan FY. Imported *Plasmodium vivax* malaria complicated by reversible myocarditis. J Fam Community Med 2019;26:232-4.

[9] Freeman R. Reversible Myocarditis Due to Chronic Lead Poisoning in Childhood. Archives of Disease in Childhood. 1965;40(212):389-393. doi:10.1136/adc.40.212.389

[10] Çetin M, Mis MD, Karaman K, et al. Carbamazepine-induced DRESS syndrome leading to reversible myocarditis in a child. Central European Journal of Immunology. 2019;44(1): 102-105. doi:10.5114/ceji.2019.83700

[11] Chen M-X, Yu B-L, Peng D-Q, Zhou S-H. Eosinophilic myocarditis due to Churg–Strauss syndrome mimicking reversible dilated cardiomyopathy. Heart & Lung. 2014;43(1):45-47. doi:10.1016/j.hrtlng.2013.09.006

[12] Becher PM, Gotzhein F, Klingel K, et al. Cardiac Function Remains Impaired Despite Reversible Cardiac Remodeling after Acute Experimental Viral Myocarditis. Journal of Immunology Research. 2017;2017:1-17. doi:10.1155/2017/6590609

[13] Fabre, A., & Sheppard, M. N. (2006). Sudden adult death syndrome and other non-ischaemic causes of sudden cardiac death. Heart (British Cardiac Society), 92(3), 316-320. https://doi.org/10.1136/hrt.2004.045518

[14] Hufnagel, G., Pankuweit, S., Richter, A., Schönian, U., & Maisch, B. (2000). The European Study of Epidemiology and Treatment of Cardiac Inflammatory Diseases (ESETCID). First epidemiological results. Herz, 25(3), 279-285. https://doi.org/10.1007/s000590050021

[15] Morgera, T., Di Lenarda, A., Dreas, L., Pinamonti, B., Humar, F., Bussani, R., Silvestri, F., Chersevani, D., & Camerini, F. (1992). Electro cardiography of myocarditis revisited: clinical and prognostic significance of electrocardiographic changes. American

heart journal, 124(2), 455-467. https://doi.org/10.1016/0002-8703(92)90613-z

[16] Lauer, B., Niederau, C., Kühl, U., Schannwell, M., Pauschinger, M., Strauer, B. E., & Schultheiss, H. P. (1997). Cardiac troponin T in patients with clinically suspected myocarditis. Journal of the American College of Cardiology, 30(5), 1354-1359. https://doi.org/10.1016/s0735-1097(97)00317-3

[17] Felker, G. M., Boehmer, J. P., Hruban, R. H., Hutchins, G. M., Kasper, E. K., Baughman, K. L., & Hare, J. M. (2000). Echocardiographic findings in fulminant and acute myocarditis. Journal of the American College of Cardiology, 36(1), 227-232. https://doi.org/10.1016/s0735-1097(00)00690-2

[18] J.P. Laissy, F. Hyafil, L.J. Feldman, et al. Differentiating acute myocardial infarction from myocarditis: diagnostic value of early- and delayed-perfusion cardiac MR imaging Radiology, 237 (2005), pp. 75-82. https://doi.org/10.1148/radiol.2371041322

[19] Mahrholdt, H., Goedecke, C., Wagner, A., Meinhardt, G., Athanasiadis, A., Vogelsberg, H., Fritz, P., Klingel, K., Kandolf, R., & Sechtem, U. (2004). Cardiovascular magnetic resonance assessment of human myocarditis: a comparison to histology and molecular pathology. Circulation, 109(10), 1250-1258. https://doi.org/10.1161/01.CIR.0000118493.13323.81

[20] Baughman K. L. (2006). Diagnosis of myocarditis: death of Dallas criteria. Circulation, 113(4), 593-595. https://doi.org/10.1161/CIRCULATIONAHA.105.589663

[21] Talmon, G., Fink, D. L., Horowitz, Y., & Miron, D. (2015). Harefuah, 154(10), 641-675.

[22] Romero-Bermejo, F. J., Ruiz-Bailen, M., Gil-Cebrian, J., & Huertos-Ranchal, M. J. (2011). Sepsis-induced cardiomyopathy. Current cardiology reviews, 7(3), 163-183. https://doi.org/10.2174/157340311798220494

[23] Annane, D., Bellissant, E., & Cavaillon, J. M. (2005). Septic shock. Lancet (London, England), 365(9453), 63-78. https://doi.org/10.1016/S0140-6736(04)17667-

[24] Dombrovskiy, V. Y., Martin, A. A., Sunderram, J., & Paz, H. L. (2007). Rapid increase in hospitalization and mortality rates for severe sepsis in the United States: a trend analysis from 1993 to 2003. Critical care medicine, 35(5), 1244-1250. https://doi.org/10.1097/01.CCM.0000261890.41311.E9

[25] Martin, G. S., Mannino, D. M., Eaton, S., & Moss, M. (2003). The epidemiology of sepsis in the United States from 1979 through 2000. The New England journal of medicine, 348(16), 1546-1554. https://doi.org/10.1056/NEJMoa022139

[26] Angus, D. C., Linde-Zwirble, W. T., Lidicker, J., Clermont, G., Carcillo, J., & Pinsky, M. R. (2001). Epidemiology of severe sepsis in the United States: analysis of incidence, outcome, and associated costs of care. Critical care medicine, 29(7), 1303-1310. https://doi.org/10.1097/00003246-200107000-00002

[27] Fernandes, C. J., Jr, Akamine, N., & Knobel, E. (2008). Myocardial depression in sepsis. Shock (Augusta, Ga.), 30 Suppl 1, 14-17. https://doi.org/10.1097/SHK.0b013e3181818617

[28] Parker, M. M., Shelhamer, J. H., Bacharach, S. L., Green, M. V., Natanson, C., Frederick, T. M., Damske, B. A., & Parrillo, J. E. (1984). Profound but reversible myocardial depression in patients with septic shock. Annals of internal medicine, 100(4), 483-490. https://doi.org/10.7326/0003-4819-100-4-483

[29] Jardin, F., Fourme, T., Page, B., Loubières, Y., Vieillard-Baron, A., Beauchet, A., & Bourdarias, J. P. (1999). Persistent preload defect in severe sepsis despite fluid loading: A longitudinal echocardiographic study in patients with septic shock. Chest, 116(5), 1354-1359. https://doi.org/10.1378/chest.116.5.1354

[30] Sharkey, S. W., Shear, W., Hodges, M., & Herzog, C. A. (1998). Reversible myocardial contraction abnormalities in patients with an acute noncardiac illness. Chest, 114(1), 98-105. https://doi.org/10.1378/chest.114.1.98

[31] Pereira, J., Ribeiro, A., Ferreira-Coimbra, J. et al. Is there a C-reactive protein value beyond which one should consider infection as the cause of acute heart failure?. BMC Cardiovasc Disord 18, 40 (2018). https://doi.org/10.1186/s12872-018-0778-4

[32] Ammann, P., Maggiorini, M., Bertel, O., Haenseler, E., Joller-Jemelka, H. I., Oechslin, E., Minder, E. I., Rickli, H., & Fehr, T. (2003). Troponin as a risk factor for mortality in critically ill patients without acute coronary syndromes. Journal of the American College of Cardiology, 41(11), 2004-2009. https://doi.org/10.1016/s0735-1097(03)00421-2

[33] Arlati, S., Brenna, S., Prencipe, L., Marocchi, A., Casella, G. P., Lanzani, M., & Gandini, C. (2000). Myocardial necrosis in ICU patients with acute non-cardiac disease: a prospective study. Intensive care medicine, 26(1), 31-37. https://doi.org/10.1007/s001340050008

[34] Chan WL, Firdaus MA-BM, Said MRM, Abidin IZ. Atypical Presentation of Takotsubo Cardiomyopathy: Stroke as a Predisposing Factor. Medeniyet Medical Journal. 2020. doi:10.5222/mmj.2020.47374

[35] Chmielecki M, Strozyk A, Jaguszewski M, Gruchala M, Rynkiewicz A. Takotsubo cardiomyopathy related to compound electrolyte aberration and anemia in Crohn's disease. International Journal of Cardiology. 2012;157(3). doi:10.1016/j.ijcard.2011.10.143

[36] Simsek, E. C., Emren, S. V., & Ozdogan, O. (2018). Unusual combined cause of Takotsubo cardiomyopathy: Hyponatremia and seizure. Northern clinics of Istanbul, 6(3), 304-307. https://doi.org/10.14744/nci.2018.65148

[37] Nakamura M, Nagamine T. Severe Lamotrigine-induced Hyponatremia Associated with Takotsubo Cardiomyopathy. INNOVATIONS IN CLINICAL NEUROSCIENCE. 2019;16(7-8).

[38] Andreozzi F, Cominetti G, Karmali R, Kamgang P. Electrolyte Disorders as Triggers for Takotsubo Cardiomyopathy. European Journal of Case Reports in Internal Medicine. 2018;(LATEST ONLINE):1. doi:10.12890/2018_000760

[39] Alexandre J, Benouda L, Champ-Rigot L, Labombarda F. Takotsubo cardiomyopathy triggered by alcohol withdrawal. Drug and Alcohol Review. 2011;30(4):434-437. doi:10.1111/j.1465-3362.2011.00289.x

[40] Matsuoka R, Muneuchi J, Yusaku Nagatomo. Takotsubo cardiomyopathy associated with Paragonimiasis westermani. Paediatrics and international child health. 2018;38(4). doi:10.1080/20469047.2017.1371482

[41] Guglin, M., & Novotorova, I. (2011). Neurogenic stunned myocardium and takotsubo cardiomyopathy are the same syndrome: a pooled analysis. Congestive heart failure (Greenwich, Conn.), 17(3), 127-132. https://doi.org/10.1111/j.1751-7133.2011.00210.x

[42] Middlemost, S., & Mabin, T. (2008). Takotsubo cardiomyopathy: an acute and reversible cardiomyopathy mimicking acute myocardial infarction. Cardiovascular journal of Africa, 19(1), 33-38.

[43] Izumo, M., & Akashi, Y. J. (2018). Role of echocardiography for takotsubo cardiomyopathy: clinical and prognostic implications. Cardiovascular diagnosis and therapy, 8(1), 90-100. https://doi.org/10.21037/cdt.2017.07.03

[44] Kurisu, S., Inoue, I., Kawagoe, T., Ishihara, M., Shimatani, Y., Nakama, Y., Maruhashi, T., Kagawa, E., & Dai, K. (2011). Incidence and treatment of left ventricular apical thrombosis in Tako-tsubo cardiomyopathy. International journal of cardiology, 146(3), e58–e60. https://doi.org/10.1016/j.ijcard.2008.12.208

[45] Schneider, B., Athanasiadis, A., Schwab, J., Pistner, W., Gottwald, U., Schoeller, R., Toepel, W., Winter, K. D., Stellbrink, C., Müller-Honold, T., Wegner, C., & Sechtem, U. (2014). Complications in the clinical course of tako-tsubo cardiomyopathy. International journal of cardiology, 176(1), 199-205. https://doi.org/10.1016/j.ijcard.2014.07.002

[46] Kim, M. J., & Shin, M. S. (2017). Practical management of peripartum cardiomyopathy. The Korean journal of internal medicine, 32(3), 393-403. https://doi.org/10.3904/kjim.2016.360

[47] Sliwa, K., Hilfiker-Kleiner, D., Petrie, M. C., Mebazaa, A., Pieske, B., Buchmann, E., Regitz-Zagrosek, V., Schaufelberger, M., Tavazzi, L., van Veldhuisen, D. J., Watkins, H., Shah, A. J., Seferovic, P. M., Elkayam, U., Pankuweit, S., Papp, Z., Mouquet, F., McMurray, J. J., & Heart Failure Association of the European Society of Cardiology Working Group on Peripartum Cardiomyopathy (2010). Current state of knowledge on aetiology, diagnosis, management, and therapy of peripartum cardiomyopathy: a position statement from the Heart Failure Association of the European Society of Cardiology Working Group on peripartum cardiomyopathy. European journal of heart failure, 12(8), 767-778. https://doi.org/10.1093/eurjhf/hfq120

[48] M. C. Honigberg and M. M. Givertz, "Peripartum cardiomyopathy," BMJ, vol. 364, p. k5287, 2019.. doi: https://doi.org/10.1136/bmj.k5287

[49] Pearson, G. D., Veille, J. C., Rahimtoola, S., Hsia, J., Oakley, C. M., Hosenpud, J. D., Ansari, A., & Baughman, K. L. (2000). Peripartum cardiomyopathy: National Heart, Lung, and Blood Institute and Office of Rare Diseases (National Institutes of Health) workshop recommendations and review. JAMA, 283(9), 1183-1188. https://doi.org/10.1001/jama.283.9.1183

[50] Bauersachs J, König T, van der Meer P, Petrie MC, et al. Pathophysiology, diagnosis and management of peripartum cardiomyopathy: a position statement from the Heart Failure Association of the European Society of Cardiology Study Group on peripartum cardiomyopathy. Eur J Heart Fail. 2019 Jul;21(7):827-843. doi: 10.1002/ejhf.1493. Epub 2019 Jun 27. PMID: 31243866

[51] Hibbard, J. U., Lindheimer, M., & Lang, R. M. (1999). A modified definition for peripartum cardiomyopathy and prognosis based on echocardiography. Obstetrics and gynecology, 94(2), 311-316. https://doi.org/10.1016/s0029-7844(99)00293-8

[52] Patel H, Madanieh R, Kosmas CE, Vatti SK, Vittorio TJ. Reversible Cardiomyopathies. Clin Med Insights Cardiol. 2015;9(Suppl 2):7-14. Published 2015 May 21. doi:10.4137/CMC.S19703

[53] Ertek S, Cicero AF. Hyperthyroidism and cardiovascular complications: a

narrative review on the basis of pathophysiology. Archives of medical science: AMS. 2013;9(5):944-52.

[54] Ojamaa K, Klemperer JD, MacGilvray SS, Klein I, Samarel A. Thyroid hormone and hemodynamic regulation of beta-myosin heavy chain promoter in the heart. Endocrinology. 1996;137(3):802-8.

[55] Walker JD, Crawford FA Jr, Mukherjee R, Spinale FG. The direct effects of 3,5,3′-triiodo-L-thyronine (T3) on myocyte contractile processes: Insights into mechanisms of action. The Journal of thoracic and cardiovascular surgery. 1995;110(5):1369-80.

[56] Park KW, Dai HB, Ojamaa K, Lowenstein E, Klein I, Sellke FW. The direct vasomotor effect of thyroid hormones on rat skeletal muscle resistance arteries. Anesthesia & Analgesia. 1997;85(4):734-8.

[57] Fadel BM, Ellahham S, Ringel MD, Lindsay J Jr, Wartofsky L, Burman KD. Hyperthyroid heart disease. Clinical cardiology. 2000;23(6):402-8.

[58] Klein I, Danzi S. Thyroid disease and the heart. Circulation. October 9, 2007;116(15):1725-35.

[59] Biondi B, Fazio S, Carella C et al. Control of adrenergic overactivity by betablockade improves the quality of life in patients receiving long term suppressive therapy with levothyroxine. The Journal of Clinical Endocrinology & Metabolism. 1994;78(5):1028-33.

[60] Watanabe E, Ohsawa H, Noike H et al. Dilated cardiomyopathy associated with hyperthyroidism. Internal medicine (Tokyo, Japan). 1995;34(8):762-7.

[61] Grogan M, Smith HC, Gersh BJ, Wood DL. Left ventricular dysfunction due to atrial fibrillation in patients initially believed to have idiopathic dilated cardiomyopathy. The American journal of cardiology. 1992;69(19):1570-3.

[62] Sairaku A, Nakano Y, Oda N, Uchimura Y et al. Incomplete Cure of Tachycardia-Induced Cardiomyopathy Secondary to Rapid Atrial Fibrillation by Heart Rate Control Without Sinus Conversion. J Cardiovasc Electrophysiol. 2014;25(10):1037-43.

[63] Jean-Louis G, Zizi F, Clark LT, Brown CD, McFarlane SI. Obstructive sleep apnea and cardiovascular disease: role of the metabolic syndrome and its components. J Clin Sleep Med. 2008;4(3):261-272.

[64] The National Commission on Sleep Disorders Research. Wake up America: a national sleep alert. Washington DC: US Government Printing Office 2002

[65] Shahar E, Whitney CW, Redline S, et al. Sleep-disordered breathing and cardiovascular disease: cross-sectional results of the Sleep Heart Health Study. Am J Respir Crit Care Med 2001;163:19-25.

[66] Pinto JM, Garpestad E, Weiss JW, et al. Hemodynamic changes associated with obstructive sleep apnea followed by arousal in a porcine model. J Appl Physiol 1993;75:1439-43.

[67] Somers VK, Dyken ME, Clary MP, et al. Sympathetic neural mechanisms in obstructive sleep apnea. J Clin Invest 1995;96:1897-904.

[68] Patil SP, Schneider H, Schwartz AR, et al. Adult obstructive sleep apnea: pathophysiology and diagnosis. Chest 2007;132:325-37.

[69] Hudgel DW. Mechanisms of obstructive sleep apnea. Chest 1992;101(2):541-549.

[70] Narkiewicz K, Montano N, Cogliati C, et al. Altered cardiovascular

variability in obstructive sleep apnea. Circulation 1998;98:1071-7.

[71] Netzer NC, Hoegel JJ, Loube D, et al. Prevalence of symptoms and risk of sleep apnea in primary care. Chest 2003;124:1406-14.

[72] Teculescu D, Benamghar L, Hannhart B, et al. [Habitual snoring. Prevalence and risk factors in a sample of the French male population]. Rev Mal Respir 2007;24(3, Pt 1):281-7.

[73] Fletcher EC. Cardiovascular disease associated with obstructive sleep apnea. Monaldi Arch Chest Dis 2003;59:254-61.

[74] Lavie L. Obstructive sleep apnoea syndrome--an oxidative stress disorder. Sleep Med Rev 2003;7:35-51.

[75] Gami AS, Pressman G, Caples SM. Association of atrial fibrillation and obstructive sleep apnea. Circulation 2004;27:367

[76] Zwillich C, Devlin T, White D, et al. Bradycardia during sleep apnea. Characteristics and mechanism. J Clin Invest 1982;69:1292

[77] Ip MS, Lam B, Chan LY, et al. Circulating nitric oxide is suppressed in obstructive sleep apnea and is reversed by nasal continuous positive airway pressure. Am J Respir Crit Care Med 2000;162:2166-71.

[78] Budhiraja R, Parthasarathy S, Quan SF. Endothelial dysfunction in obstructive sleep apnea. J Clin Sleep Med 2007;3:409-15.

[79] Kasasbeh E, Chi DS, Krishnaswamy G. Inflammatory aspects of sleep apnea and their cardiovascular consequences. South Med J 2006;99:58-67.

[80] Lavie L. Sleep-disordered breathing and cerebrovascular disease: a mechanistic approach. Neurol Clin 2005;23:1059-75.

[81] Semenza GL, Prabhakar NR. HIF-1-dependent respiratory, cardiovascular, and redox responses to chronic intermittent hypoxia. Antioxid Redox Signal 2007;9:1391-6.

[82] Nanduri J, Nanduri RP. Cellular mechanisms associated with intermittent hypoxia. Essays Biochem 2007;43:91-104.

[83] Yokoe T, Minoguchi K, Matsuo H, et al. Elevated levels of Creactive protein and interleukin-6, in patients with obstructive sleep apnea syndrome are decreased by nasal continuous positive airway pressure. Circulation 2003;107:1129-34.

[84] Brown G, Albers JJ, Fisher LD, et al. Regression of coronary artery disease as a result of intensive lipid-lowering therapy in men with high levels of apolipoprotein B. N Engl J Med 1990;323:1289-98

[85] Kaneko Y, Floras JS, Usui K, et al. Cardiovascular effects of continuous positive airway pressure in patients with heart failure and obstructive sleep apnea. N Engl J Med 2003;348:1233-41.

[86] Bradley TD, Logan AG, Kimoff RJ, et al. Continuous positive airway pressure for central sleep apnea and heart failure. N Engl J Med 2005;353:2025-33.

[87] Milleron O, Pilliere R, Foucher A, et al. Benefits of obstructive sleep apnoea treatment in coronary artery disease: a long-term follow-up study. Eur Heart J 2004;25:728-34.

[88] Harsch IA, Hahn EG, Konturek PC. Insulin resistance and other metabolic aspects of the obstructive sleep apnea syndrome. Med Sci Monit 2005;11:RA70-5.

[89] Lee KF, Simon H, Chen H, et al. Requirement for neuregulin receptor erbB2 in neural and cardiac development. Nature 1995; 378:394.

[90] Crone SA, Zhao YY, Fan L, et al. ErbB2 is essential in the prevention of dilated cardiomyopathy. Nat Med 2002; 8:459.

[91] Ozcelik C, Erdmann B, Pilz B, et al. Conditional mutation of the ErbB2 (HER2) receptor in cardiomyocytes leads to dilated cardiomyopat

[92] Qutrio Baloch Z, Hussain M, Agha Abbas S, Perez JL, Ayyaz M. Methamphetamine-Induced Cardiomyopathy (MACM) in a Middle-Aged Man; a Case Report. Emerg (Tehran). 2018;6(1):e9.

[93] Jung YS, Lee JS, Min YG, Park JS, Jeon WC, Park EJ, Shin JH, Oh S, Choi SC. Carbon monoxide-induced cardiomyopathy. Circ J. 2014;78(6): 1437-44. doi: 10.1253/circj.cj-13-1282. Epub 2014 Apr 4. PMID: 24705389.hy. Proc Natl Acad Sci U S A 2002; 99:8880.

[94] Frustaci A, Magnavita N, Chimenti C, et al. Marked elevation of myocardial trace elements in idiopathic dilated cardiomyopathy compared with secondary cardiac dysfunction. J Am Coll Cardiol 1999; 33:1578.

[95] Morin Y, Daniel P. Quebec beer-drinkers' cardiomyopathy: etiological considerations. Can Med Assoc J 1967; 97:926.

[96] Simonsen LO, Harbak H, Bennekou P. Cobalt metabolism and toxicology--a brief update. Sci Total Environ 2012; 432:210.

[97] Allen LA, Ambardekar AV, Devaraj KM, et al. Clinical problem-solving. Missing elements of the history. N Engl J Med 2014; 370:559.

[98] Dahms K, Sharkova Y, Heitland P, et al. Cobalt intoxication diagnosed with the help of Dr House. Lancet 2014; 383:574.

[99] Go AS. Cardiovascular disease consequences of CKD. Semin Nephrol. (2016) 36:293-304. 10.1016/j.semnephrol.2016.05.006

[100] de Albuquerque Suassuna PG, Sanders-Pinheiro H, de Paula RB. Uremic Cardiomyopathy: A New Piece in the Chronic Kidney Disease-Mineral and Bone Disorder Puzzle. Front Med (Lausanne). 2018;5:206. Published 2018 Jul 24. doi:10.3389/fmed.2018.00206

[101] Liu M, Li XC, Lu L, Cao Y, Sun RR, Chen S, et al. . Cardiovascular disease and its relationship with chronic kidney disease. Eur Rev Med Pharmacol. Sci. (2014) 18:2918-26. Available online at: https://www.europeanreview.org/wp/wp-content/uploads/2918-2926.pdf

[102] Saran R, Robinson B, Abbott KC, Agodoa LYC, Bhave N, Bragg-Gresham J, et al.., US Renal Data System 2017 Annual Data Report: epidemiology of kidney disease in the United States. Am J Kidney Dis. (2018) 71:A7. 10.1053/j.ajkd.2018.01.002

[103] Alpert MA. Sudden cardiac arrest and sudden cardiac death on dialysis: epidemiology, evaluation, treatment, and prevention. Hemodial Int. (2011) 15(Suppl 1):S22-9. 10.1111/j.1542-4758.2011.00598.x

[104] Zolty R, Hynes PJ, Vittorio TJ. Severe left ventricular systolic dysfunction may reverse with renal transplantation: uremic cardiomyopathy and cardiorenal syndrome. Am J Transplant. 2008 Nov;8(11):2219-24. doi: 10.1111/j.1600-6143.2008.02407.x. Epub 2008 Sep 19. PMID: 18808406.

[105] Siedlecki AM, Jin X, Muslin AJ. Uremic cardiac hypertrophy is reversed

by rapamycin but not by lowering of blood pressure. Kidney Int. 2009 Apr;75(8):800-8. doi: 10.1038/ki.2008.690. Epub 2009 Jan 21. PMID: 19165175; PMCID: PMC2764402.

[106] Wiese S, Hove JD, Bendtsen F, Moller S. Cirrhotic cardiomyopathy: pathogenesis and clinical relevance. Nat Rev Gastroenterol Hepatol. 2014;11:177-186. doi: 10.1038/nrgastro.2013.210.

[107] Moller S, Hove JD, Dixen U, Bendtsen F. New insights into cirrhotic cardiomyopathy. Int J Cardiol. 2013;167:1101-1108. doi: 10.1016/j.ijcard.2012.09.089.

[108] Carvalho MVH, Kroll PC, Kroll RTM, Carvalho VN. Cirrhotic cardiomyopathy: the liver affects the heart. Braz J Med Biol Res. 2019;52(2):e7809. Published 2019 Feb 14. doi:10.1590/1414-431X20187809

[109] Kowalski HJ, Abelmann WH. The cardiac output at rest in Laennec's cirrhosis. J Clin Invest. 1953;32:1025-1033. doi: 10.1172/JCI102813.

[110] Huffman C, Wagman G, Fudim M, Zolty R, Vittorio T. Reversible cardiomyopathies--a review. Transplant Proc. 2010 Nov;42(9):3673-8. doi: 10.1016/j.transproceed.2010.08.034. PMID: 21094837.

[111] Licata A, Novo G, Colomba D, Tuttolomondo A, Galia M, Camma C. Cardiac involvement in patients with cirrhosis: a focus on clinical features and diagnosis. J Cardiovasc Med. 2016;17:26-36. doi: 10.2459/JCM.000000 0000000288.

[112] Barbosa M, Guardado J, Marinho C, Rosa B, Quelhas I, Lourenço A, et al. Cirrhotic cardiomyopathy: isn't stress evaluation always required for diagnosis? World J Hepatol. 2016;28:200-206. doi: 10.4254/wjh.v8.i3.200.

[113] Lossnitzer D, Steen H, Zahn A, Lehrke S, Weiss C, Weiss KH, et al. Myocardial late gadolinium enhancement cardiovascular magnetic resonance in patients with cirrhosis. J Cardiovasc Magn Reson. 2010;12:47. doi: 10.1186/1532-429X-12-47.

[114] Torregrosa M, Aguadé S, Dos L, Segura R, Gónzalez A, Evangelista A, et al. Cardiac alterations in cirrhosis: reversibily after liver transplantation. J Hepatol. 2005;42:68-74. doi: 10.1016/j.jhep.2004.09.008.

[115] Timoh T, Protano MA, Wagman G, Bloom M, Vittorio TJ. A perspective on cirrhotic cardiomyopathy. Transplant Proc. 2011 Jun;43(5):1649-53. doi: 10.1016/j.transproceed.2011.01.188. PMID: 21693251.

Chapter 20

Ischemic Heart Disease

Saraí López De Lucio and Marco Antonio López Hernández

Abstract

All over the world ischemic heart disease remains as the leading cause of death, followed by stroke. Ischemic heart disease, also called coronary artery disease has a broad spectrum of clinical manifestations from the acute coronary syndromes which include, unstable angina pectoris and acute myocardial infarction with and without elevation of the ST segment and chronic coronary disease. In patients with diabetes mellitus the cardiovascular complications mainly ischemic heart disease, are the main cause of morbidity and mortality. However, in population-based studies, the risk of heart failure in patients with diabetes mellitus is significantly increased following adjustment for well-established heart failure risk factors such as hypertension or ischemic heart disease. Ischemic heart failure angiographically diagnosed is associated with a shorter survival than non-ischemic heart failure. Coronary artery disease is independently associated with higher mortality.

Keywords: myocardial infarction, coronary artery disease, heart failure, Ischemic heart disease

1. Introduction

Ischemic disorders, such as peripheral vascular disease, stroke and myocardial infarction, are the most common causes death in the world. Cardiovascular diseases are the main cause of death globally, with an estimated 17.9 million deaths each year, representing 31% of all global deaths. Of these deaths, 85% are a consequence of myocardial infarction and stroke. Over 75% of cardiovascular disease deaths take place in low- and middle-income countries [1]. The main cause of myocardial infarction is coronary artery disease, and in turn the main cause of coronary artery disease is atherosclerosis. The rupture of atheroma plaque is the event that lead to the thrombus formation with the subsequent occlusion of the blood supply distal to the affected vessel segment. The magnitude of the tissue injury is directly related to the extent of the territory affected by the reduction in blood flow and the length of the ischemic period, which influences the levels at which intracellular pH and ATP are reduced. Follow-up of groups of patients with characteristics that favor the appearance of atherosclerosis over time, has allowed the identification of risk factors for cardiovascular disease, as well as the development of various predictive models, such as the Framingham score.

The main cause of ischemic heart disease is coronary artery disease caused by atherosclerosis. There are secondary causes of ischemia, these can cause ischemic heart disease and non-obstructive myocardial infarction of the coronary arteries (INOCA and MINOCA), these secondary causes are classified in coronary, myocardial and non-cardiac causes.

IntechOpen

2. Atherosclerotic artery disease

The term atherosclerosis is rooted in the Greek word αθερα ("athero", which means crushed food in the form of a mass) for the aspect of the necrotic core area and the word σκλεροζ ("scleros" which means hard) for hardening or induration, referring to the fibrous layer of the luminal edge. Atherosclerosis is an inflammatory process that begins from childhood and develops over the years, is asymptomatic most of the time; is distinguished by retention, oxidation and modification of lipids in the form of fatty streaks on the walls of the arteries that later evolve to fibrous plaques causing wall thickening in the affected artery, decreasing its internal diameter over time. Rupture of this plaque cause thrombosis and occlusion of the blood supply to the myocardial tissue irrigated by the affected artery [2].

The main cause of Ischemic heart disease is atherosclerosis. Coronary atherosclerotic disease can be classified into three types: obstructive coronary artery disease, non-obstructive coronary artery disease, and microvascular coronary artery disease. In addition to arteriosclerosis and thrombosis of the coronary arteries, other causes of acute myocardial infarction are extremely rare. Cases have been described of infarction caused by embolization within the coronary arteries from clot fragments from elsewhere, or septic embolization due to endocarditis of the aortic valve.

3. Definition of myocardial infarction

The introduction of more sensitive cardiac biomarkers has led the American College of Cardiology (ACC) and the European Society of Cardiology (ESC) to collaborate for the redefinition of myocardial infarction using a clinical and biochemical approach. These societies reported that myocardial injury detected by abnormal biomarkers in the context of acute myocardial ischemia should be labeled as in the fourth universal definition of myocardial infarction. In other words, myocardial infarction is defined as the presence of acute myocardial damage detected by the elevation of cardiac biomarkers in the context of evidence of acute myocardial ischemia [3].

Myocardial infarction can be defined from the point of view of pathological anatomy as myocardial cell death due to prolonged ischemia. The first ultrastructural changes are diminished cellular glycogen, sarcolemmal disruption, and relaxed myofibrils and they are seen as early as 10–15 min after the onset of ischemia. Mitochondrial abnormalities are observed as early as 10 minutes after coronary occlusion by electron microscopy [4, 5].

Cardiac troponins are regulatory proteins that mediate interaction between actin and myiosin, there are two types of cardiuacx troponins; troponin T (cTnT) and troponin I (cTnI), The cTnI has not been identified outside the myocardium. Cardiac troponin T is expressed to a small extent in skeletal muscle; however, the current cTnT assay does not identify skeletal troponins Myocardial injury is defined by detection of an elevated cardiac troponin (cTn) value above the 99th percentile URL. The injury is considered acute if there is a rise and/or fall of cTn values. The biomarkers of choice for the evaluation of myocardial damage are cTnI and cTnT; the use of high-sensitivity cTn (hs-cTn) is recommended in routine clinical practice [6]. Other biomarkers, such as the MB fraction of creatine kinase (CK-MB), are less sensitive and specific (**Table 1**).

Of patients with acute coronary syndrome, 1 to 14% do not have identifiable obstructive coronary lesions on coronary angiography.

DOI: http://dx.doi.org/10.5772/intechopen.97515

Classification of myocardial infarction	
Myocardial infarction type I	Usually precipitated by atherosclerotic plaque disruption in atherothrombotic coronary artery disease.
Myocardial infarction type 2	Caused by mismatch between oxygen supply and demand, the pathophysiological mechanism lead to ischaemic myocardial injury.
Myocardial infarction type 3	Patients that manifest with a typical presentation of myocardial ischemia/ infarction, including presumed new ischaemic ECG changes or ventricular fibrillation, and die before it is possible to obtain blood for cardiac biomarker determination; or the patient may succumb soon after the onset of symptoms before an elevation of biomarker values has occurred.
Myocardial infarction type 4	Type 4a. Associated with percutaneous coronary intervention.
	Type 4b. Stent/scaffold thrombosis associated with percutaneous coronary intervention.
	Type 4c. Restenosis associated with percutaneous coronary intervention.
Myocardial infarction type 5	Associated with coronary artery bypass grafting.

Table 1.
Classification of myocardial infarction according the fourth universal definition of myocardial infarction.

Patients with myocardial infarction and non-obstructive coronary arteries (MINOCA), represent a conundrum given the many potential underlying etiologies. MINOCA is defined as angiographic stenosis <50% and myocardial infarction Possible causes of MINOCA can be subdivided into coronary, myocardial, and non-cardiac disorders (**Figure 1**).

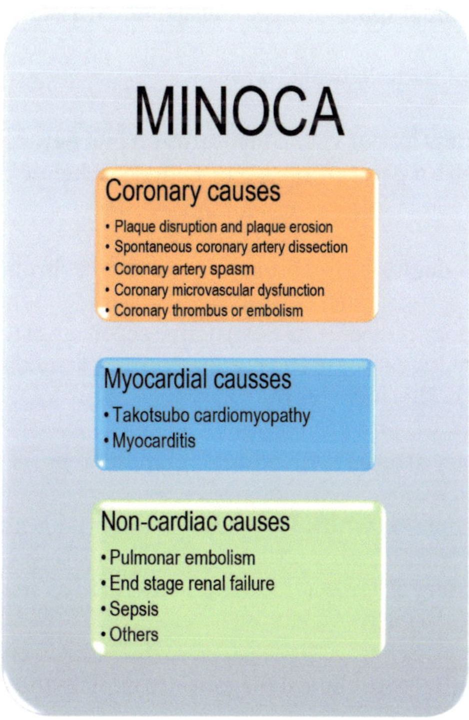

Figure 1.
Etiologies of MINOCA.

MINOCA is found in up to 14% of patients presenting with an acute coronary syndrome. Many terms have been used to describe patients with acute myocardial infarction or acute coronary syndrome with normal or near-normal coronary arteries, such as MINOCA, MINCA (MI with normal coronary arteries) and INOCA (ischemia and no obstructive coronary artery disease) The most common pathologies associated with an acute coronary syndromes are plaque rupture, erosion and calcified nodules which are present in 44%, 31% and 8% respectively.

Plaque formation starts with the formation of fatty streaks and intimal thickening, leading to fibrous cap atheroma and eventually to fibrous cap thinning. This so-called thin-cap fibroatheroma can rupture. In plaque erosion, there is an abundance of smooth muscle cells without an extensive necrotic core, hemorrhage or calcification. It differs from plaque rupture, as there is an absence of fibrous cap disruption. Identification of vulnerable plaques on coronary angiography can be challenging. Intravascular coronary imaging and computed tomography angiography could play an important role in finding these plaques in the future.

An elevated troponin beyond the 99th percentile of the upper reference level is a hallmark of myocardial injury in the same way that it is for myocardial infarction. However, myocardial injury is attributable to non-ischemic mechanisms of myocyte injury and in this way these entities differ conceptually from ischemic heart disease.

The diagnosis of MINOCA requires the fulfillment of the following criteria:

1. Acute myocardial infarction. Detection of a rise or fall of cTn value with at least one value above the 99th percentile upper reference limit and corroborative clinical evidence of infarction evidenced by at least one of the following criteria:

    - Symptoms consistent with myocardial ischemia.
    - New electrocardiographic changes consistent with ischemia.
    - Development of pathological Q waves.
    - Evidence of a new loss of viable myocardium or a new regional wall motion abnormality with a pattern consistent with an ischemic cause on imaging studies.
    - Evidence by angiography or autopsy of a coronary thrombus.

2. Evidence on angiography of non-obstructive coronary arteries, defined as the absence of obstructive disease (no coronary artery stenosis ≥50% in any major epicardial vessel). This includes the following cases:

    - Normal coronary arteries with no angiographic stenosis.
    - Angiographic stenosis with <30% stenosis and mild luminal irregularities.
    - Moderate coronary atherosclerotic lesions defined as stenosis >30% but <50%.

3. Absence of an alternate clinical diagnosis to explain the presentation

    - Alternate diagnoses include but are not limited to non-ischemic causes such as pulmonary embolism, sepsis, and myocarditis.

Among MINOCA patients coronary plaque disruption is common. The terms plaque rupture, plaque erosion, and calcific nodules are included in the term plaque disruption. Plaque rupture is an event that can trigger the formation of a thrombus that leads to myocardial infarction due to superimposed coronary spasm, distal embolization, or in some cases, transient complete thrombosis that resolves with spontaneous thrombolysis.

Coronary artery spasm is an intense vasoconstriction with more than 90% lumen occlusion of an epicardial coronary artery that compromises myocardial blood flow. Hyperresponsiveness to toxins or drugs of vascular smooth muscle cells can lead to vasospasm of the coronary arteries, or it can occur spontaneously due to disorders in coronary vasomotor tone.

In 30–50% of patients with non-obstructive coronary artery disease documented by invasive coronary angiography and presenting with chest pain or discomfort, coronary microvascular dysfunction can be detected. Microvascular dysfunction is seen more frequently in women and patients with classic cardiovascular risk factors. Microvascular dysfunction can be a cause of ischemia, but it can also be a consequence of myocardial injury.

Coronary embolism or thrombosis can cause MINOCA if it involves the microcirculation or if there is partial lysis of the epicardial coronary thrombus it can result in coronary disease that is not obstructive by coronary angiography. This can occur with or without a hypercoagulable state. Disorders with increased coagulability that cause coronary thrombosis can be classified as inherited or acquired. Among these disorders is the antiphospholipid syndrome, which is a heterogeneous disorder characterized by the presence of autoantibodies against protein-phospholipid complexes. Hereditary thrombophilia is prevalent in the general population, with a variable prevalence depending on race/ethnicity. Acquired hypercoagulable states include thrombotic thrombocytopenic purpura, antiphospholipid syndrome, heparin-induced thrombocytopenia, and myeloproliferative neoplasms.

Spontaneous coronary artery dissection is a relatively rare non atherosclerotic mechanism of myocardial infarction. The separation of the medial and adventitial vascular walls associated with intramural hematoma protrusion into the lumen cause obstruction to coronary blood flow. The primary source of the dissection is still controversial and the exact mechanism is not entirely known.

4. Myocardial ischemia-reperfusion injury

Occlusion of a coronary artery causes sudden cessation of regional perfusion, rapidly leading to the cessation of aerobic metabolism, creatine phosphate depletion, and the onset of anaerobic glycolysis; this continues to build up of lactate and catabolites and progressively reduces ATP levels. If ischemia continues, tissue acidosis develops and cellular ion exchange is impaired, the function of the cell membrane is impaired, triggering the onset of myocyte death. Irreversible myocardial damage begins in the subendocardium 20 minutes after coronary occlusion and extends as a wave front towards the subepicardial layers; after one hour of coronary occlusion, the dependent subendocardium and part of the myocardium are irreversibly damaged; transmural extension is completed with 4–6 h of ischemia.

Reperfusion entails a replenishment of substrates, mainly oxygen, which will intervene in the oxidation of fatty acids at the mitochondrial level. Complete restoration of contractile function is achieved when adenosine triphosphate (ATP) levels normalize and excess adenosine diphosphate (ADP, platelet aggregation agonist) disappears. There are other factors, such as changes in calcium flux due to membrane alterations or alterations in the metabolism of free fatty acids, which are responsible for the prolonged abnormality of contraction after ischemia [7–9]. Endothelial damage activates the coagulation cascade with platelet and red cell aggregation that contribute to microvascular dysfunction [10]; the inflammatory response with complement activation also influences myocardial perfusion dysfunction [11] and other changes such as glycogen and ATP depletion, mitochondrial edema and nuclear chromatin clumping correlate with worsening myocardial function after ischemia (stunned myocardium) [12–14].

Reperfusion of the affected vessel during an acute myocardial infarction is crucial to save the ischemic myocardium, but it also causes a metabolic injury that can be reversible, as in the case of myocardial stunning [15–17], but it can also be irreversible and manifest as microvascular dysfunction and an increase in the size of the infarcted myocardium. This phenomenon is known as myocardial ischemia–reperfusion injury.

Several molecular mechanisms have been shown to be involved in the etiology of myocardial ischemia–reperfusion injury including defects in calcium handling, mitochondrial damage, reactive oxygen species production, and inflammation.

5. Apoptosis

Both calcium overload and oxidative stress can induce on the mitochondrial permeability transition pores abrupt opening. This abrupt opening of these pores causes uncoupling of oxidative phosphorylation and mitochondrial swelling, thereby inducing apoptosis and cell necrosis [18–19]. The apoptosis process is energy-dependent. It gets activated during ischemia, but it is not effected until the oxygen supply is reinitiated during reperfusion. Caspase activation is a primordial event in apoptosis. Caspase inhibition during early reperfusion has been demonstrated to protect the myocardium against reperfusion injury in a murine model [20].

6. Defects in calcium handling

For the maintenance of the excitation-contraction coupling in cardiomyocytes, calcium homeostasis plays an essential role. During the cardiac action potential, extracellular calcium enters the cell through L-type calcium channels, the ryanodine receptor 2 (RyR2) is activated by intracellular calcium leading to increased release of calcium from the sarcoplasmic reticulum. Intracellular calcium present at a certain level cause myocardial contraction, by binding to the myofilament of the contractile protein troponin C. On the one hand, the sarcoplasmic reticulum calcium-ATPase (SERCA) recaptures intracellular calcium, bringing it back to the sarcoplasmic reticulum. On the other hand, the sodium-calcium exchanger (NCX) expels calcium from the cells and the dissociation of calcium from the myofilament protein leads to cardiomyocite relaxation. SERCA, NCX, RyR2, and mitochondria regulate the calcium levels in myocardial cells, and also participate in calcium overload during ischemic injury. The common clinical characteristics of the myocardial induced reperfusion injury are myocardial reperfusion arrhythmias, stunning, intramyocardial hemorrhage, microvascular obstruction, and enlargement of the myocardial infarction [21–24].

After a period of hypoxia and ischemia, myocardial cells have an increase in anaerobic metabolism, this leads to the intracellular aggregation of hydrogen ions, which causes a low intracellular pH and an increase in intracellular sodium through hydrogen-sodium exchange (HNX). Excess intracellular sodium leads to sodium excretion and calcium uptake by the sodium calcium exchanger ultimately resulting in calcium overload.

Calcium plays a fundamental role in the coupling of cardiac excitation-contraction. Thus, the calcium overload will increase the reperfusion injury and the size of the infarcted myocardium. Excess intracellular calcium will enter the mitochondria and this excess mitochondrial calcium inhibits ATP production, exacerbates energy metabolism disorders, and ultimately leads to apoptosis of myocardial cells. Mitochondrial damage is known to be a marker of irreversible damage in cardiomyocytes [25–26].

Disturbances of calcium homeostasis play a key role in the development of reperfusion arrhythmias, including idioventricular rhythm, ventricular tachycardia, and ventricular fibrillation [27]. Inhibition of intracellular calcium overload improves recovery of cardiac function [28].

7. Autophagy and mitophagy

The phenomenon called "mitophagy" consists of the activation of cellular autophagy and degradation of damaged mitochondria by lysosomes and is generally beneficial because they reduce the reperfusion injury [29].

Ischemia is known to stimulate autophagy. This occurs through a mechanism dependent on adenosine monophosphate activated protein kinase (AMPK), while ischemia–reperfusion causes left ventricular dysfunction and autophagic myocardial cell death through a Beclin-1 dependent mechanism, but independent of AMPK. The increase in autophagosomes containing damaged mitochondria is associated with the latter event [30, 31].

8. Inflammation

A sequence of cellular events leading to collagen-based scar formation leads to healing of the infarcted myocardium. This is a consequence of the fact that the heart of adult mammals has little regenerative capacity. Three overlapping phases describe the repair of the infarcted myocardium: the inflammatory, the proliferative and the maturation phases. Inflammation exerts a key role in cardiovascular diseases, as extensively reported in the literature. Inflammatory responses exert a different effect in the acute and chronic phase. Activation of inflammatory responses acutely contributes to the healing process including release of cytokines and infiltration of inflammatory cells into the myocardium, while prolonged activation of inflammation triggers pro-apoptotic pathways [32–34].

Reperfusion of the infarcted area of the myocardium triggers a complex inflammatory reaction accompanied by infiltration of inflammatory leukocytes into the compromised myocardial region and the release of cytokines. This release of cytokines and the inflammatory response after myocardial infarction are an integral part of the healing process and contribute to the remodeling of cardiac tissue, however, excessive inflammatory responses are detrimental to the integrity of the extracellular matrix and to cell survival. This occurs through enhanced activation of pro-apoptotic signaling pathways, with a subsequent poor clinical outcome [35–37].

Tissue injury generates endogenous signals that activate the innate immune system; these molecules belong to a large group of mediators that warn the body of injury and are known as damage-associated molecular patterns (DAMPs). A group of structurally diverse endogenous signals are released after tissue necrosis occurs, promoting cell activation of innate immune systems through binding to recognition pattern receptors, these are known by the term alarmins. High mobility group B1 (HMGB1) is the best characterized alarmin and is a key initiator of inflammatory injury following myocardial ischemia through actions that might involve the receptor for advanced glycation end products (RAGE) and toll-like receptors (TLRs). The fact that both harmful and beneficial effects of HMGB1 have been reported in the infarcted myocardium is not surprising given the critical role of alarmin-mediated signaling in inflammation and repair of myocardial tissue. The identification of danger signals by innate immune cells occurs through participation of TLRs, a family of transmembrane receptors that activate subsequent pro-inflammatory cascades. Studies of loss of genetic function indicate that TLR2 and TLR4, both located on the cell surface, are important mediators of the post-infarction inflammatory reaction.

A molecular program that leads to the recruitment of inflammatory cells in the healing infarct is activated by alarmin-mediated signaling. The pro-inflammatory chemokines induced in the infarcted heart generate chemotactic gradients that lead to the recruitment of subpopulations of leukocytes through interactions with the corresponding chemokine receptors. Upregulation of pro-inflammatory cytokines (such as IL-1β, members of the IL-6 family and tumor necrosis factor [TNF]) induce molecule synthesis, endothelial cell adhesion, and activate leukocyte integrins, mediating strong adhesive interactions that ultimately lead to extravasation of inflammatory cells into the infarct.

In the infarcted myocardium the expression of the two main chemokine sub families (C-C y C-X-C) mediate the inflammatory leukocyte recruitment, The neutrophyl recruitment is mediated by the chemokines CX-C with amminoacid secuence Glu-Leu-Arg which are quickly induced by the infarcted myocardium.

9. Oxidative stress

Oxidative stress can be produced from enzymatic sources and non-enzymatic sources. Common enzymatic sources include the xanthine oxidase system, mitochondrial electron transport chain, NADPH oxidase system, and uncoupled nitric oxide synthase (NOS) system. Non-enzymatic sources are a minor source of oxidative stress, and include hemoglobin and myoglobin. The xanthine oxidase system, NADPH oxidase system, and mitochondrial electron transport chain are broadly implicated in oxidative stress in several organs, including the heart, lung, brain, muscle, intestine, liver, pancreas, stomach, and kidney. NOS is a major oxidative stress factor in the liver, heart, and aortic endothelial cells [38–40].

The onset of acute myocardial ischemia during an acute myocardial infarction induces cell damage and the death of different constituents of the myocardium. This, in turn, initiates an acute pro-inflammatory response through the concerted action of several processes including the production of reactive oxygen species, the activation of the complement cascade, and the damage-associated molecular patterns that serve as ligands for pattern recognition receptors (PRRs) a family of cytosolic nucleotide-binding oligomerization domain receptors (NLRP3, also known as Nod-like receptors) and toll like receptors This result in the release of a variety of pro-inflammatory mediators such as cytokines and chemokines, which induce the recruitment of inflammatory cells into the infarcted zone, and augment the pro-inflammatory response following acute myocardial infarction.

Infiltrating leukocytes can induce cardiomyocyte death by targeting the viable borderline area of the infarct, thus extending the ischemic lesion beyond the area of the original infarction.

10. Heart failure

Heart failure is a complex syndrome responsible for high rates of death and hospitalization among the general population worldwide. One of the most frequent causes of HF is ischemic heart disease.

Heart failure is a clinical syndrome characterized by typical symptoms (breathlessness, ankle swelling, and fatigue) that may be accompanied by signs (e.g. elevated jugular venous pressure, pulmonary crackles, and peripheral oedema) caused by a structural and/or functional cardiac abnormality, resulting in a reduced cardiac output and/or elevated intracardiac pressures at rest or during stress. Demonstration of an underlying cardiac cause is central to the diagnosis. This is usually a myocardial abnormality causing systolic and/or diastolic ventricular dysfunction (**Figure 2**).

The two main types of heart failure are the acute and chronic forms. In chronic heart failure which is the most common type, symptoms appear slowly over time and gradually worsen with various underlying mechanisms such as mechanical stress, ischemia, infections, autoimmune diseases, and genetic diseases [41–45].

The regeneration process in ischemic heart disease after myocardial infarction begins with the infiltration of leukocytes. This is triggered by ischemia and the presence of necrotic cardiomyocytes to eliminate irreparably damaged or dead cells and allows repair of the infarcted area through the formation of scars to maintain cardiac integrity [46, 47].

A significant number of inflammatory cells, including monocytes/macrophages and neutrophils that infiltrate the infarct area, are considered to be an essential component of very early wound healing processes. It is through the polarization of macrophages towards a reparative phenotype that neutrophils orchestrate post-infarction healing. The polarization of neutrophils is mediated by DAMPs and the neutrophils themselves can polarize towards different phenotypes, for example, neutrophils N1 and N2 in the infarct region [48–51]. The cellular immune response and the subsequent inflammatory response are considered a key factor in adverse left ventricular remodeling after an acute myocardial infarction. The New York Heart Association (NYHA) functional classification has been used to describe the

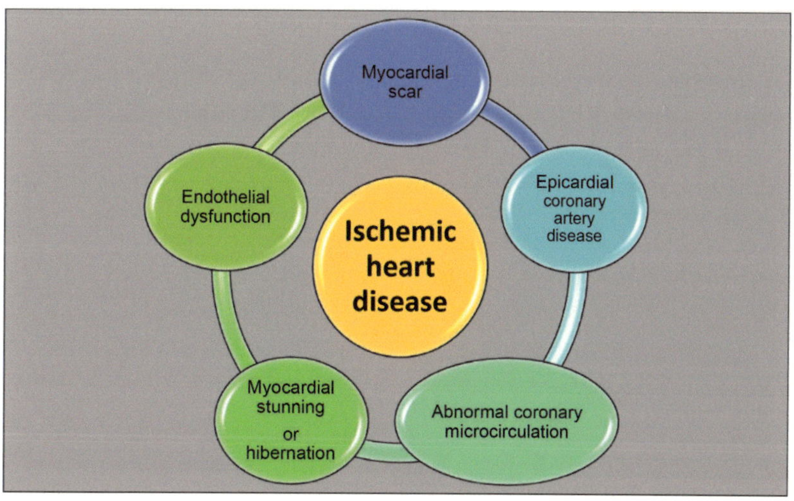

Figure 2.
Ischemic heart disease features in the etiology of heart failure.

severity of symptoms and exercise intolerance in heart failure. Although there is a clear relationship between the severity of symptoms and survival, the severity of symptoms is poorly correlated with many measures of left ventricular function, and patients with mild symptoms may be at high risk of hospitalization and death (**Figure 3**) [52–54].

Estimation of prognosis for morbidity, disability and death helps patients, their families and clinicians decide on the appropriate type and timing of therapies (in particular, decisions about a rapid transition to advanced therapies) and assists with planning of health and social services and resources (**Figure 3**) [55].

Virtually any measurement that can be performed in a biological system is included in the definition of a biomarker, this term in the context of heart failure is limited to substances measured in the blood other than electrolytes and commonly used markers of kidney or liver function. The plasma concentration of natriuretic peptides (NPs) can be used as an initial diagnostic test, especially in the non-acute setting when echocardiography is not immediately available. Elevated NPs help establish an initial working diagnosis, identifying those who require further cardiac investigation; patients with values below the cut-point for the exclusion of important cardiac dysfunction do not require echocardiography [55].

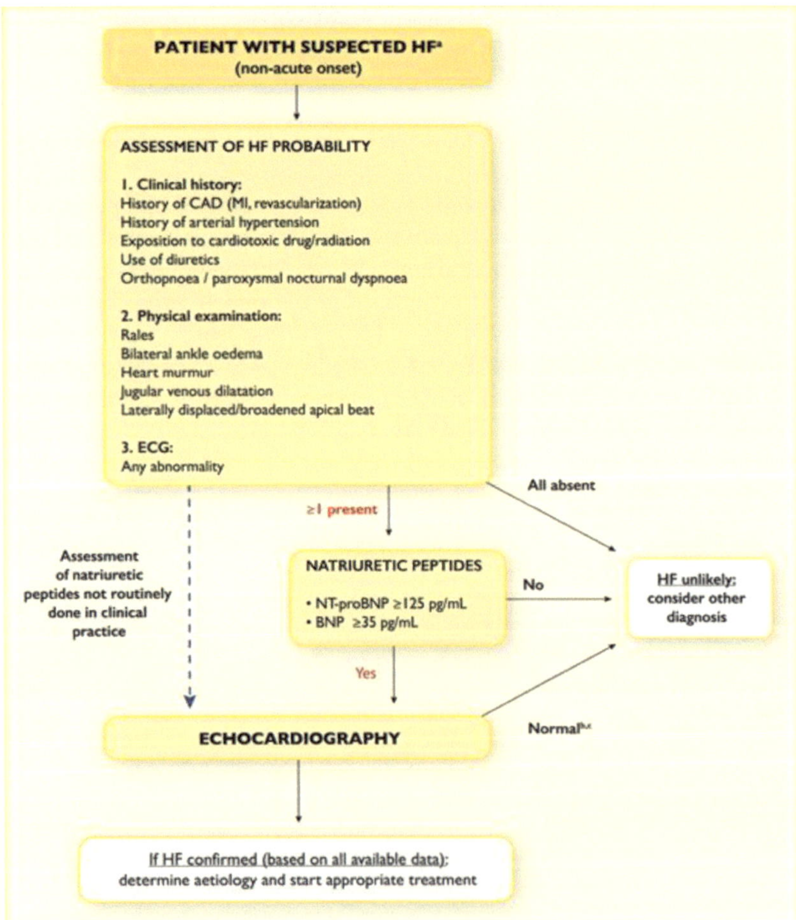

Figure 3.
Diagnostic algorithm from the ESC guidelines for the diagnosis and treatment of acute and chronic heart failure for the diagnosis of heart failure of non-acute onset [55]. BNP = B-type natriuretic peptide; CAD = coronary artery disease; HF = heart failure; MI = myocardial infarction; NT-proBNP = N-terminal pro-B type natriuretic peptide.

The fact that several drugs for HF have shown detrimental effects on long-term outcomes, despite showing beneficial effects on shorter-term surrogate markers, has led regulatory bodies and clinical practice guidelines to seek mortality/morbidity data for approving/recommending therapeutic interventions for HF. However, it is now recognized that preventing HF hospitalization and improving functional capacity are important benefits to be considered if a mortality excess is ruled out.

After of myocardial infarction the presence of ischemic heart failure mortality is a frequent complication. Several factors, such as infarct size, recurrent myocardial ischemia, ventricular remodeling, mechanical complications, stunned myocardium, and hibernating myocardium influence the appearance of left ventricular systolic dysfunction with or without clinical heart failure [56–58].

In 30–40% patients, the etiology of heart failure is nonischemic, the ischemic etiology is a significant independent predictor of mortality in patients with heart failure [59]. In the VALIANT registry were included 5573 consecutive MI patients at 84 hospitals in nine countries from 1999 to 2001. A multivariable logistic survival model was constructed using baseline variables to determine the adjusted mortality risk for those with in-hospital heart failure and/or left ventricular systolic disfunction. The presence of heart failure precedes 80.3% of all in-hospital deaths after myocardial infarction, and the survivors. Heart failure post high risk myocardial infarction occurs in a time-dependent fashion and is usually not directly related to re-infarction [60, 61].

11. Conclusions

Ischemic heart disease remains as the leading cause of death in the world. Coronary atherosclerosis and related ischemic heart failure is a leading cause of heart failure with reduced ejection fraction, the heart failure of ischemic ethiology is associated with a shorter survival and more complications than non-ischemic heart failure. The heart failure and systolic left ventricle dysfunction are present in more than the 80% of in-hospital deaths after myocardial infarction. Substantial improvements in the prevention and management of heart failure present formidable challenges, but these challenges may be met because much of the necessary ground work has already been carried out.

It is important to highlight that for the clinician who faces the challenge of treating patients with ischemic heart disease, it is important to know its mechanisms and the therapies aimed at both the management of patients with acute myocardial infarction and heart failure. The goals of treatment in patients with HF are to improve their clinical status, functional capacity, quality of life, prevent hospital admission, and reduce mortality.

Author details

Saraí López De Lucio[1*] and Marco Antonio López Hernández[2]

1 Lasalle University, USA

2 Internal Medicine Division, Ecatepec General Hospital, Mexico

*Address all correspondence to: ameliedelucio@icloud.com

References

[1] World Health Organization. https://www.who.int/en/news-room/fact-sheets/detail/cardiovascular-diseases-(cvds).

[2] Insull W. The pathology of atherosclerosis: Plaque development and plaque responses to medical treatment. Am J Med 2009;122

[3] Fourth Universal Definition of Myocardial Infarction, Thygesen K, Alpert JS, Jaffe AS, Chaitman BR, Bax JJ, Morrow DA, White HD, (2018); Executive Group on behalf of the Joint European Society of Cardiology (ESC)/ American College of Cardiology (ACC)/ American Heart Association (AHA)/ World Heart Federation (WHF) Task Force for the Universal Definition of Myocardial Infarction. Circulation. 2018 Nov 13;138(20): e618-e651.

[4] Jennings RB, Ganote CE. Structural changes in myocardium during acute ischemia. Circ Res 1974;35:156-172.

[5] Virmani R, Forman MB, Kolodgie FD. Myocardial reperfusion injury. Histopathological effects of perfluorochemical. Circulation 1990;81:IV57–IV68

[6] Thygesen K, Mair J, Giannitsis E, Mueller C, Lindahl B, Blankenberg S, Huber K, Plebani M, Biasucci LM. Tubaro M, Collinson P, Venge P, Hasin Y, Galvani M, Koenig W, Hamm C, Alpert JS, Katus H, Jaffe AS; Study Group on Biomarkers in Cardiology of the ESC Working Group on Acute Cardiac Care. How to use high-sensitivity cardiac troponins in acute cardiac care. Eur Heart J. 2012;33: 2252-2257.

[7] Kloner R.A., Jennings R.B. Consequences of brief ischemia: Stunning, preconditionig, and their clinical implications. Part 1. Circulation. 2001;104:2981-2989.

[8] Downey J.M., Cohen M.V. Reducing infarct size in the setting of acute myocardial infarction. Prog Cardiovasc Dis. 2006;48:363-371.

[9] Peng C.F., Davis J.L., Murphy M.L., et al. Straub KD. Effects of reperfusion on myocardial wall thickness, oxidative phosphorylation, and Ca + + metabolism following total and partial myocardial ischemia. Am Heart J. 1986;112:1238-1244.

[10] Piper H.M., García-Dorado D., Ovize M. A fresh look at reperfusion injury. Cardiovasc Res. 1998;38:291-300.

[11] Frink R.J., Rooney P.A., Trowbridge J.O., et al. Coronary thrombosis and platelet/fibrin microemboli in death associated with acute myocardial infarction. Br Heart J. 1988;59:196-200.

[12] Bcranck J.T. C reactive protein and complement in myocardial infarction and postinfarction heart failure. 1997;18:1834-1836.

[13] Knight C.H., Fox K. From antianginal drugs to myocardial cytoprotective agents. Am J Cardiol. 1995;76:4B-7B.

[14] Pomar F., Cosín J., Portolés M., et al. Functional and ultrastructural alterations of canine myocardium subjected to very brief coronary occlusions. Eur Heart J. 1995;16:1482-1490.

[15] Bolli R. Myocardial 'stunning' in man. Circulation. 1992;86:1671-1691

[16] Heusch G. The Coronary Circulation as a Target of Cardioprotection. Circ. Res. 2016;118:1643-1658.

[17] Heusch G. Coronary microvascular obstruction: The new frontier in cardioprotection. Basic Res. Cardiol. 2019;114:45.

[18] Shanmuganathan S., Hausenloy D.J., Duchen M.R., Yellon D.M. Mitochondrial permeability transition pore as a target for cardioprotection in the human heart. Am. J. Physiol. Heart Circ. Physiol. 2005;289:H237–H242

[19] Heusch G. Molecular basis of cardioprotection: Signal transduction in ischemic pre-, post-, and remote conditioning. Circ. Res. 2015;116:674-699

[20] Mocanu M.M., Baxter G.F., Yellon D.M. Caspase inhibition and limitation of myocardial infarct size: Protection against lethal reperfusion injury. Br. J. Pharm. 2000;130:197-200.

[21] Manning A.S., Hearse D.J. Reperfusion-induced arrhythmias: Mechanisms and prevention. J. Mol. Cell. Cardiol. 1984;16:497-518.

[22] Bolli R., Marban E. Molecular and cellular mechanisms of myocardial stunning. Physiol. Rev. 1999;79:609-634.

[23] Entman M.L., Michael L., Rossen R.D., Dreyer W.J., Anderson D.C., Taylor A.A., Smith C.W. Inflammation in the course of early myocardial ischemia. FASEB J. Off. Publ. Fed. Am. Soc. Exp. Biol. 1991;5:2529-2537.

[24] Krug A., De Rochemont W.D.M., Korb G. Blood supply of the myocardium after temporary coronary occlusion. Circ. Res. 1966;19:57-62

[25] Dorn G. W., Maack C. (2013). SR and mitochondria: Calcium cross-talk between kissing cousins. J. Mol. Cell. Cardiol. 55, 42-49.

[26] Williams G. S. B., Boyman L., Lederer W. J. (2015). Mitochondrial calcium and the regulation of metabolism in the heart. J. Mol. Cell. Cardiol. 78, 35-45.

[27] Kukreja R.C., Janin Y. Reperfusion Injury: Basic Concepts and Protection Strategies. J. Thromb. Thrombolysis. 1997;4:7-24.

[28] Chen C.C., Morishige N., Masuda M., Lin W., Wieland W., Thone F., Mubagwa K., Borgers M., Flameng W. R56865, a Na(+)- and Ca(2+)-overload inhibitor, reduces myocardial ischemia-reperfusion injury in blood-perfused rabbit hearts. J. Mol. Cell. Cardiol. 1993;25:1445-1459.

[29] Przyklenk K., Dong Y., Undyala V.V., Whittaker P. Autophagy as a therapeutic target for ischemia /reperfusion injury? Concepts, controversies, and challenges. Cardiovasc. Res. 2012;94:197-205

[30] Matsui Y., Takagi H., Qu X., Abdellatif M., Sakoda H., Asano T., Levine B., Sadoshima J. Distinct roles of autophagy in the heart during ischemia and reperfusion: Roles of AMP-activated protein kinase and Beclin 1 in mediating autophagy. Circ. Res. 2007;100:914-922.

[31] Yu P., Zhang J., Yu S., Luo Z., Hua F., Yuan L., Zhou Z., Liu Q., Du X., Chen S., et al. Protective Effect of Sevoflurane Postconditioning against Cardiac Ischemia/Reperfusion Injury via Ameliorating Mitochondrial Impairment, Oxidative Stress and Rescuing Autophagic Clearance, PLoS ONE. 2015;10:e0134666.

[32] Fiordelisi A., Iaccarino G., Morisco C., Coscioni E., Sorriento D. NFkappaB is a Key Player in the Crosstalk between Inflammation and Cardiovascular Diseases. Int. J. Mol. Sci. 2019;20:1599. doi: 10.3390/ijms20071599.

[33] Sorriento D., Iaccarino G. Inflammation and Cardiovascular Diseases: The Most Recent Findings. Int. J. Mol. Sci. 2019;20:3879.

[34] Liu J., Wang H., Li J. Inflammation and Inflammatory Cells in Myocardial Infarction and Reperfusion Injury: A

Double-Edged Sword. Clinical Medicine Insights. Cardiology. 2016;10:79-84.

[35] Yellon DM, Hausenloy DJ. Myocardial reperfusion injury. N Engl J Med. 2007;357(11):1121-1135..

[36] Nahrendorf M, Pittet MJ, Swirski FK. Monocytes: protagonists of infarct inflammation and repair after myocardial infarction. Circulation. 2010;121(22):2437-2445.

[37] Swirski FK, Nahrendorf M. Leukocyte behavior in atherosclerosis, myocardial infarction, and heart failure. Science. 2013;339(6116):161-166.

[38] De Pascali F, Hemann C, Samons K, Chen CA, Zweier JL: Hypoxia and reoxygenation induce endothelial nitric oxide synthase uncoupling in endothelial cells through tetrahydrobiopterin depletion and S-glutathionylation. Biochemistry 2014;53:3679-3688.

[39] Moens AL, Champion HC, Claeys MJ, Tavazzi B, Kaminski PM, Wolin MS, Borgonjon DJ, Van Nassauw L, Haile A, Zviman M, Bedja D, Wuyts FL, Elsaesser RS, Cos P, Gabrielson KL, Lazzarino G, Paolocci N, Timmermans J-P, Vrints CJ, Kass DA: High-Dose Folic Acid Pretreatment Blunts Cardiac Dysfunction During Ischemia Coupled to Maintenance of High-Energy Phosphates and Reduces Postreperfusion Injury. Circulation 2008;117:1810-1819.

[40] Perkins K-AA, Pershad S, Chen Q, McGraw S, Adams JS, Zambrano C, Krass S, Emrich J, Bell B, Iyamu M, Prince C, Kay H, Teng JC-W, Young LH: The effects of modulating eNOS activity and coupling in ischemia/ reperfusion (I/R). Naunyn Schmiedebergs Arch Pharmacol 2012;385:27-38.

[41] Sun Y. Myocardial repair/ remodelling following infarction: roles of local factors. Cardiovasc Res 2009; 81: 482-490.

[42] Levine RA, Hagége AA, Judge DP, Padala M, Dal-Bianco JP, Aikawa E, Beaudoin J, Bischoff J, Bouatia-Naji N, Bruneval P, Butcher JT, Carpentier A, Chaput M, Chester AH, Clusel C, Delling FN, Dietz HC, Dina C, Durst R, Fernandez-Friera L, Handschumacher MD, Jensen MO, Jeunemaitre XP, Le Marec H, Le Tourneau T, Markwald RR, Mérot J, Messas E, Milan DP, Neri T, Norris RA, Peal D, Perrocheau M, Probst V, Pucéat M, Rosenthal N, Solis J, Schott JJ, Schwammenthal E, Slaugenhaupt SA, Song JK, Yacoub MH; Leducq Mitral Transatlantic Network. Mitral valve disease—morphology and mechanisms. Nat Rev Cardiol 2015; 12: 689-710.

[43] Manning WJ. Asymptomatic aortic stenosis in the elderly: a clinical review. JAMA 2013; 310: 1490-1497.

[44] Eriksson U, Ricci R, Hunziker L, Kurrer MO, Oudit GY, Watts TH, Sonderegger I, Bachmaier K, Kopf M, Penninger JM. Dendritic cell-induced autoimmune heart failure requires cooperation between adaptive and innate immunity. Nat Med 2003; 9: 1484-1490.

[45] Cooper LT. Myocarditis. N Engl J Med 2009; 360: 1526-1538.

[46] Latet SC, Hoymans VY, Van Herck PL, Vrints CJ. The cellular immune system in the post-myocardial infarction repair process. Int J Cardiol 2015;179:240-247.

[47] van der Laan AM, Nahrendorf M, Piek JJ. Healing and adverse remodelling after acute myocardial infarction: role of the cellular immune response. Heart 2012;98:1384-1390.

[48] Swirski FK, Nahrendorf M. Leukocyte behavior in atherosclerosis, myocardial infarction, and heart failure. Science 2013;339:161-166.

[49] Yan X, Anzai A, Katsumata Y, Matsuhashi T, Ito K, Endo J,

Yamamoto T, Takeshima A, Shinmura K, Shen W, Fukuda K, Sano M. Temporal dynamics of cardiac immune cell accumulation following acute myocardial infarction. J Mol Cell Cardiol 2013;62:24-35.

[50] Horckmans M, Ring L, Duchene J, Santovito D, Schloss MJ, Drechsler M, Weber C, Soehnlein O, Steffens S. Neutrophils orchestrate post-myocardial infarction healing by polarizing macrophages towards a reparative phenotype. Eur Heart J 2017;38:187-197.

[51] Ma Y, Yabluchanskiy A, Iyer RP, Cannon PL, Flynn ER, Jung M, Henry J, Cates CA, Deleon-Pennell KY, Lindsey ML. Temporal neutrophil polarization following myocardial infarction. Cardiovasc Res 2016;110:51-61.

[52] McMurray JJ V. Clinical practice. Systolic heart failure. N Engl J Med 2010;3623:228-238.

[53] Chen J , Normand S-LT, Wang Y, Krumholz HM. National and regional trends in heart failure hospitalization and mortality rates for Medicare beneficiaries, 1998-2008. JAMA 2011;306:1669-1678.

[54] Dunlay SM , Redfield MM, Weston SA, Therneau TM, Hall Long K, Shah ND, Roger VL. Hospitalizations after heart failure diagnosis a community perspective. J Am Coll Cardiol 2009;54:1695-1702.

[55] P. Ponikowski, A.A. Voors, S.D. Anker, et al. 2016 ESC Guidelines for the diagnosis and treatment of acute and chronic heart failure: The Task Force for the diagnosis and treatment of acute and chronic heart failure of the European Society of Cardiology (ESC) Developed with the special contribution of the Heart Failure Association (HFA) of the ESC. Eur Heart J, 37 (2016), pp. 2129-2200,

[56] Pfeffer MA, Braunwald E. Ventricular remodeling after myocardial infarction: experimental observations and clinical implications. Circulation. 1990; 81: 1161-1172.

[57] Zornoff LAM, Paiva SAR, Duarte DR, et al. Ventricular remodeling after myocardial infarction: concepts and clinical implications. Arq Bras Cardiol. 2009; 92: 157-164.

[58] Cleland JGF, Torabi A, Khan NK. Epidemiology and management of heart failure and left ventricular systolic dysfunction in the aftermath of a myocardial infarction. Heart. 2005; 91: ii7– ii13.

[59] Bart BA, Shaw LK, Mc Cantis CB et al, Clinical Determinants of Mortality in Patients With Angiographically Diagnosed Ischemic or Nonischemic Cardiomyopathy. JACC, 1997, 30(4);1002-1008.

[60] Velazquez EJ, Francis GS, Amstrong PW et al. An international perspective on heart failure and left ventricular systolic dysfunction complicating myocardial infarction: the VALIANT registry. Eur Heart J 2004 Nov;25(21):1911-1919

[61] Lewis EF, Velazquez EJ, Solomon SD, et al. Predictors of the first heart failure hospitalization in patients who are stable survivors of myocardial infarction complicated by pulmonary congestion and/or left ventricular dysfunction: a VALIANT study. Eur Heart J 2008 Mar;29(6):748-756

Section 7

Treatment and Future Perspectives

Chapter 21

Gene Therapy for Heart Disease: Modified mRNA Perspectives

Lior Zangi, Ravinder K. Kaundal and Keerat Kaur

Abstract

Ischemic heart disease (IHD) presents a gigantic clinical challenge that demands effective therapeutic approaches. With increasing knowledge of the basic molecular mechanisms guiding the progress of this disease, it is now possible to target the key pathological players through gene therapy. Modified mRNA-based gene delivery presents a promising alternative to traditional gene therapy, because modRNA approaches have high potency, non-immunogenicity, greater efficiency and controlled nucleic acid transfer to the body. However, until recently the therapeutic applications of mRNA have been limited, as naturally occurring mRNA is rapidly degraded and cleared from the circulation. In this chapter, we outline the compositional changes made to mRNA to enhance its translational capacity and discuss the available carrier molecules currently being employed to deliver modRNA to the heart. We provide a detailed overview of modRNA applicability for cardiac repair and regeneration and consider future directions for novel delivery methods that can facilitate its cardiac therapeutic use.

Keywords: cardiac repair, cardiac regeneration, gene therapy, modified mRNA, non-viral gene delivery

1. Introduction

1.1 Ischemic heart disease

Ischemic heart disease (IHD), a life-threatening cardiac condition, is the most common cause of heart failure, which is the leading cause of mortality worldwide, and in developed countries its burden is rivaled only by cancer. Systolic dysfunction and reduced cardiac output are the major hallmarks of ischemic heart failure (IHF). It is hard to determine the etiology of IHF, which is often associated with multiple underlying diseases, including ischemic cardiomyopathy, coronary artery disease or previous myocardial infarction (MI), that cause an imbalance between myocardial oxygen demand and supply. Decreased or complete loss of blood supply to an area of the myocardium for a prolonged period has detrimental effects on cardiomyocytes (CM). Myocardial ischemia progressively results in either reversible, via myocardial stunning and hibernation, or irreversible loss of CM. Following myocardial ischemia, a heavy burst of cell damage or death occurs in the infarct region, mostly within the first 24 hours [1]. However, low-grade cell death continues in the peri-infarct zone for months due to a complex cascade of molecular and cellular events [2]. Because the adult heart cannot regenerate, newer therapeutic approaches are needed to halt the ongoing damage that follows myocardial ischemia. Multiple studies have consistently indicated that attenuating apoptotic cell death pathways (death receptor and mitochondrial apoptosis pathways) could be a viable therapeutic strategy for MI [3–6].

Soon after MI, a spectrum of clinical changes occurs in the heart and eventually results in heart failure. Billions of CMs die, triggering a multiphase reparative response known as cardiac remodeling that can be divided into three distinct but overlapping phases: the inflammatory phase, the proliferative phase and the maturation or healing phase [7]. The early inflammatory phase, characterized by immune cell recruitment and infiltration, clears dead cells and debris from the infarct region and prepares the injured region for the proliferative phase, during which mesenchymal reparative cells, mainly myofibroblasts and endothelial cells, proliferate and form granulation tissue. Myofibroblasts secrete excessive extracellular matrix proteins that play a critical role in preserving the structural integrity of the damaged heart. As myofibroblast and endothelial cell apoptosis ends, the maturation phase begins and heals the infarct into a collagen-rich fibrotic scar [8]. Post-ischemic myocardial remodeling replaces most of the dead necrotic infarct with fibrotic nonfunctional scar tissue, which increases the mechanical load on the adjacent myocardium and thus reduces the pumping capacity of the heart muscle. Informed by a detailed understanding of these mechanisms, gene-based therapy for IHD aims to upregulate the genes involved in (a) activating adult CM proliferation, (b) preventing cardiac cell apoptosis and necrosis, (c) reducing the innate and adaptive immune response and (d) inducing angiogenesis. Several studies utilize gene therapy strategies to investigate and treat IHD.

In the last two decades, emerging gene therapies have sought to improve heart function after MI. However, treatments involving traditional vectors have produced few meaningful results. Efforts to use DNA-based or viral gene delivery methods to induce cardiac repair processes post MI or in HF conditions have failed due to poor, uncontrolled gene delivery [9, 10]. Current pharmacological therapeutics help manage symptoms and improve quality of life, but these approaches lack organ specificity and cannot permanently remedy the disease. Synthetic modified mRNA (modRNA) is a promising gene delivery vector, and the Pfizer-BioNTech and Moderna vaccines against the novel coronavirus SARS-COV-2 have generated great optimism about its prospects in other areas. ModRNA therapeutics offer several advantages over conventional vectors, as they offer safe, non-immunogenic, efficient, transient, local, controlled delivery of an almost limitless range of nucleic acids to nearly any part of the human body. Over the last eight years, i.e. since the first time modRNA was delivered to the heart [11], various pre-clinical studies have explored using modRNA for gene introduction following IHD. In this chapter, we will focus on structural modifications that allow modRNA to escape the immune response, modRNA carrier systems in the heart and the use of modRNA for upregulating genes that support cardiovascular regeneration.

2. Exogenous mRNA translation

The process of gene expression begins with DNA transcription to messenger RNA (mRNA), which is then translated into a protein. Following the pre-mRNA transcript for synthesis, post-transcriptional or co-transcriptional modifications produce a mature, functional RNA molecule that can leave the nucleus to perform a variety of functions in the cell. These post-transcriptional modifications significantly alter the chemical structure of the RNA molecule in three major ways: (a) capping at 5′ end, (b) polyadenylation at 3′ end and (c) splicing introns in the coding region. These processes are vital to mature mRNA production and translation.

Capping is the first modification and involves adding N7-methylated guanosine to the first nucleotide at the 5′-end of growing nascent mRNA transcripts.

Synchronized with transcription, this modification takes effect immediately as the first 25–30 nucleotides of the nascent transcript are synthesized [12]. The 5′ cap not only protects nascent mRNA from 5′ to 3′ exonuclease cleavage and degradation but also facilitates mRNA splicing, polyadenylation and nuclear export. There is also evidence that 5′ untranslated region (UTR) plays a critical role in initiating protein synthesis [13]. Polyadenylation is another major post-transcriptional modification of the pre-mRNA transcript that occurs before the mature mRNA leaves the nucleus. As transcriptions terminate, polyadenylation begins when an endonuclease-protein complex releases the functional pre-mRNA by cleaving it between an AAUAAA consensus sequence and a GU-rich sequence at the 3′ end from the growing transcript. An enzyme called poly (A) polymerase (PAP), which is part of the endonuclease-protein complex, catalyzes the addition of an approximately 200-adenine-nucleotide string, also known as a polyA tail, to the 3′ end of cleaved pre-mRNA [14, 15]. Changes in these components of mRNA are discussed later the chapter.

These post-transcriptional pre-mRNA processes take place in the nucleus, and only the successfully processed mature mRNA molecules are exported out of the nucleus, whereas the faulty mRNAs and spliced-out introns are degraded by a specialized multi-subunit exosome complex. In the cytoplasm, the mature functional mRNA will be either directed to ribosomes for translation or shuttled to other compartments for sequestration and/or degradation [16].

3. Innate immune response

The innate immune system is the first line of defense against pathogens. It plays a critical role in initiating the protective immune response by detecting exogenous motifs, a process also known as recognizing pathogen-associated molecular patterns (PAMPs) via pattern recognition receptors (PRRs) present in many immune cell types, particularly sentinel APCs. Nucleic acids (DNA and RNA) have been documented as key PAMPs and are known to initiate a complex cascade of intracellular signaling pathways leading to the production of proinflammatory cytokines and chemokines. Therefore, synthetic or exogenously administered mRNA molecules are inherently immunogenic. Toll-like receptors (TLRs), the type I transmembrane proteins, are the major PRRs that contribute to RNA recognition in the endosomal compartment. TLR3 is localized in the endosomes of innate immune cells and recognizes the dsRNA. Upon binding to dsRNA, TLR3 is activated and recruits its downstream adaptor TRIF (TIR-domain containing protein inducing type 1 Interferon (IFN)-I), which facilitates the formation of TRIF signaling complex. This complex activates NF-κB and IRF3/IRF7 transcription factors that ultimately boost the transcription of proinflammatory cytokines and interferons (IFNs), respectively.

Alternatively, single-stranded RNA (ssRNA) and their degradative products in the endosomes are sensed by Toll-like receptor 7 (TLR7) and TLR8 [17], which recognize and bind to ssRNA, leading to confirmation changes in receptor dimers. These changes facilitate recruitment of downstream adaptor myeloid differentiation marker 88 (MyD88), which enables the formation of a multiprotein signaling complex, Myddosome. This complex activates downstream NF-κB and IRF7 signaling that induces the production of proinflammatory cytokines and IFNs, respectively [18], which activate antigen-presenting cells (APC). At the same time, higher INF levels activate the type I interferon (IFN-I) pathway which upregulates an array of genes including those involved in degrading cellular mRNA and ribosomal RNA-like oligoadenylate synthetase (OAS) [18] and inhibiting translation e.g. 2′-5′- and protein kinase R (PKR) [19, 20].

In the cytosol, unmodified mRNAs are detected by different sets of PRRs including retinoic acid-inducible gene-I-like receptors (RLRs), nucleotide oligomerization domain (NOD)-like receptors (NLRs), oligoadenylate synthetase (OAS) receptors and RNA-dependent protein kinase (PKR). Almost all mammalian cell types express RLRs, which are the chief family of cytosolic RNA sensors [21]. The RLR family includes retinoic acid-inducible gene 1 (RIG-I), melanoma differentiation-associated-5 (MDA-5) and laboratory of genetics and physiology 2 (LGP2). Upon binding with the RNA, RIG-I and MDA5 undergo conformational changes and interact with mitochondrial antiviral-signaling protein (MAVS). MAVS plays an essential role in RLR signal transduction by recruiting a series of kinases which in turn elevate the expression of proinflammatory cytokines and IFN genes via IRF-3/7 and NF-kB pathways [22–24].

Given its immunostimulatory properties, synthetic modRNA has undergone various design modifications to ensure adequate escape from the innate immune response, thereby averting toxic overactivation and facilitating efficient translation of the exogenous mRNA.

4. mRNA alterations to escape immune response and enhance stability

As discussed above, the major obstacles to RNA therapeutics are their instability due to high RNAses activity and the higher immunogenicity of RNA molecules. The possible feedback loop between innate immune activation and reduced mRNA translation further decreases therapeutic mRNA potency. Thus, to push cardiac mRNA therapy towards clinical use, researchers seek to optimize the chemical structure of mRNA by changing its phosphate backbone, RNA terminals or nucleosides. Synthetic modRNA construction has been discussed previously [25]. In this section, we highlight recent progress in modifying RNA to regulate RNA stability.

4.1 Nucleotide modifications

Non-immunogenic mRNA is engineered by transcribing plasmid DNA in vitro. This flexible method can substitute uridine with modified nucleosides such as pseudouridine, 2-thiouridine, 5-methyluridine, 5-methylcytidine or N6-methyladenosine [26]. These modifications have been shown to bypass TLR7 and TLR8 activation. Specifically, completely replacing uridine with 1-Methylpseudouridine-5′-Triphosphate (N1m Ψ) enables more robust translation than other changes in mRNA structure [27]. Psuedouridine (Ψ) is a naturally occurring uridine isomer generated by a C-C, instead of N-C, bond to uridine. The bonding process entails breaking the glycosidic bond, rotating the base 180° and reforming bonds but retains the normal base pairing preference for adenosine [28]. Transcriptome-wide analyses have revealed thousands of Ψ sites in human mRNAs, demonstrating it is endogenous to the human body. Although Ψ-modified mRNA binds to RIG-I with high affinity post endocytosis, it fails to trigger the canonical RIG-I conformational changes associated with robust signaling, thus escaping the immune response.

4.2 Replacing mRNA capping

The 5′-cap is a hallmark of eukaryotic mRNA and plays an essential role in cap-dependent initiation of protein synthesis, stabilization of eukaryotic mRNA splicing, nuclear export and mRNA decay. This cap interacts with the cap binding complex to trigger mRNA export from the nucleus. Once in cytoplasm, its interaction with the eukaryotic translation initiation factor 4E (eIF4E) causes 5′ to 3′ mRNA looping to recruit multiple ribosomes and enhance the protein translation rate. Chemically, the 5′-cap consists of an inverted 7-methylguanosine (m7G) linked to the first nucleotide of the RNA via a reverse 5′ to 5′ triphosphate bridge. As the abnormally capped (cap 0) or uncapped (5'ppp or 5'pp) mRNAs are recognized by PRRs, modifications like adding the 2′O methylation of +1 nucleotide (cap 1 or m7GpppNm) are central to the non-self-discrimination of the innate immune response against foreign RNA. However, Cap 1 can sometimes attach the mRNA strand in a reverse orientation, i.e., Gpppm7 instead of m7Gppp, which reduces translation efficiency. Thus, the second-generation capping system of anti-reverse cap analogs (ARCA) 3′-O- Mem7G(5′)ppp(5′)G, which cannot incorporate in the reverse orientation, is frequently used in vitro and in vivo to ensure correct capping orientation and higher translational efficiency [29, 30]. One downside of this chemical capping strategy is that the need for higher-ratio ARCA and GTP concentrations to produce a high percentage of capped mRNA significantly elevates the cost of modRNA production. Yet changing ratios of 5′ ARCA cap and N1m Ψ to favor ARCA over N1m Ψ greatly increases the yield per reaction, improves translation, reduces immunogenicity and lowers costs, making modRNA more affordable for basic and translational research [31].

4.3 Changes in untranslated regions

UTRs are important regulators of mRNA decay and translational efficiency as they serve as ribosome entry points during translation. The 5'UTR carries structural elements which are recognized by cell-specific RNA-binding proteins that may regulate translation initiation in a cap-dependent or cap-independent manner. The impact of the UTR on mRNA translation varies by species, cell type, and cell state; applying bioinformatics tools to diverse 5'UTR and 3'UTR combinatory libraries may be able to estimate mRNA translation efficiency. In vitro screening for optimized mRNA 5' UTR combinations has shown improved expression of arginase 1 (ARG1), a potential therapeutic mRNA target, with the 5'UTR for complement factor 3 (C3) and cytochrome p4502E1 (CYP2E1) [32]. Using a transcriptomic and proteomic analysis, Sultana et al. recently identified 5' UTR from the fatty acid metabolism gene carboxylesterase 1D (Ces1d) as an mRNA translation enhancer post cardiac and hepatic ischemic injuries. Ces1D belongs to the carboxylesterases family and plays vital roles in lipid metabolism. Thus, the fact that the heart switches to fatty acid metabolism under ischemic conditions may be why modRNA with Ces1D 5'UTR produces higher translation [33].

Like 5'UTR, 3'UTR located after ORF can also contribute to mRNA translation and controls multiple aspects of mRNA metabolism, including nuclear export, cytoplasmic localization, translational efficiency and mRNA stability [34]. Nevertheless, 3'UTR has proven conceptually more difficult to mechanistically regulate than 5'UTR. The 3'UTR length is a key regulator of mRNA expression: mRNAs with longer 3′ UTRs have a shorter half-life whereas mRNAs with shorter 3′ UTRs are less efficiently translated. To date, erythrocyte proteins, alpha [35] and beta [36] globin 3′UTR have primarily been used in modRNA production; their longer half-lives improve protein production and prolong modRNA expression. New cellular library screenings that explore cell-based selection processes to identify 3′ UTRs may further augment mRNA translation levels. Amino-terminal enhancer of split (AES), mRNA-mitochondrially encoded 12S rRNA (mtRNR1) and mtRNR1-AES-based 3′ UTRs can upgrade RNA translation in mRNA vaccination and mRNA-based reprogramming of human fibroblasts [37]. Apart from using stable mRNA sequences, 3'UTR also offers the binding site for miRNA, which are responsible for mRNA degradation. Thus, either limiting the number of miRNA sites or artificially incorporating miRNA-binding sites in the mRNA sequence can reduce gene expression in nontargeted tissues and promote mRNA stability.

4.4 Optimizing polyA tail length

The final approach for controlling RNA stability and regulating translation are polyA tails, which are homopolymeric sequences at the 3′ ends of RNA molecules. Post transcription, about 20 factors work cohesively to recognize the polyadenylation site at the 3'end, cleave the pre-mRNA, add a polyA tail and trigger transcription termination. Beside adenosines, full-length polyA and mRNA sequencing reported the presence of non-A nucleotides, mostly cytosines, in the polyA tail region [38]. Conventionally, polyA tails were thought to be synthesized by adding ~250 adenosines to the 3'UTR; however, recent developments using the PAL-seq and TAIL-seq have shown that most mRNAs have much shorter tails, with a median between 50 and 100 nt. Additionally, tail length correlates negatively with expression, half-life and ribosome occupancy. In the case of modRNA expression in the heart, reporter gene comparisons have demonstrated higher translation levels for modRNA containing 173 polyA compared to 120 adenosine, thus suggesting that longer polyA tail length produces higher-translating modRNA [39].

5. Modified mRNA delivery systems in the heart

An efficient delivery system is critical for achieving therapeutic effects with modRNA. The delivery vehicle must protect the mRNA from RNAses and the innate immune system. For exogenous mRNA to be translated, it must pass the lipid bilayer barrier in order to reach the cytoplasm, a rather arduous process. Successful mRNA uptake greatly depends on the targeted cell type and the physiological properties of the mRNA delivery complexes. modRNA is a larger molecule than those used in other gene delivery methods, and its size makes diffusion through the cell membrane more challenging. Furthermore, because modRNA contains a negatively charged phosphate backbone, the cell membrane creates repulsion that influences cellular delivery and organ distribution. By enhancing stability and translation, the recent chemical modifications in modRNA components have led to encouraging progress in the development of various carrier systems that can deliver large mRNA molecules to hard-to-reach organs, especially the heart (**Figure 1**).

Lipid nanoparticle (LNP) complexes are a popular choice for in vivo modRNA delivery. Compared to other complexes, LNPs can encapsulate larger modRNA volumes, offer better protection against RNAses and renal clearance and induce higher cellular uptake. These carrier molecules are primarily composed of ionizable lipids to ensure self-assembly of this large mo.ecule (~100 nm), phospholipids to support the lipid bilayer, cholesterol, a stabilizing agent and polyethylene glycol (PEG) lipids that increase the half-life and hence the stability of the formulations. To efficiently deliver modRNA in the heart, Turnbull et al. used a custom formulation consisting of an epoxide-derived lipidoid (mixed in ethanol with the stabilizers DSPC, cholesterol and PEG-DMG) in addition to modRNA to generate formulated lipid nanoparticles (FLNPs) via nanoprecipitation. The custom-made FLNPs were more stable and showed faster translation than the traditional formulations [40, 41]. Even though LNPs are the most appealing and commonly used mRNA delivery vehicles, some remaining challenges need to be addressed. First, the lipid formulations may cause some toxicity in vivo, and second, the formulations need to be

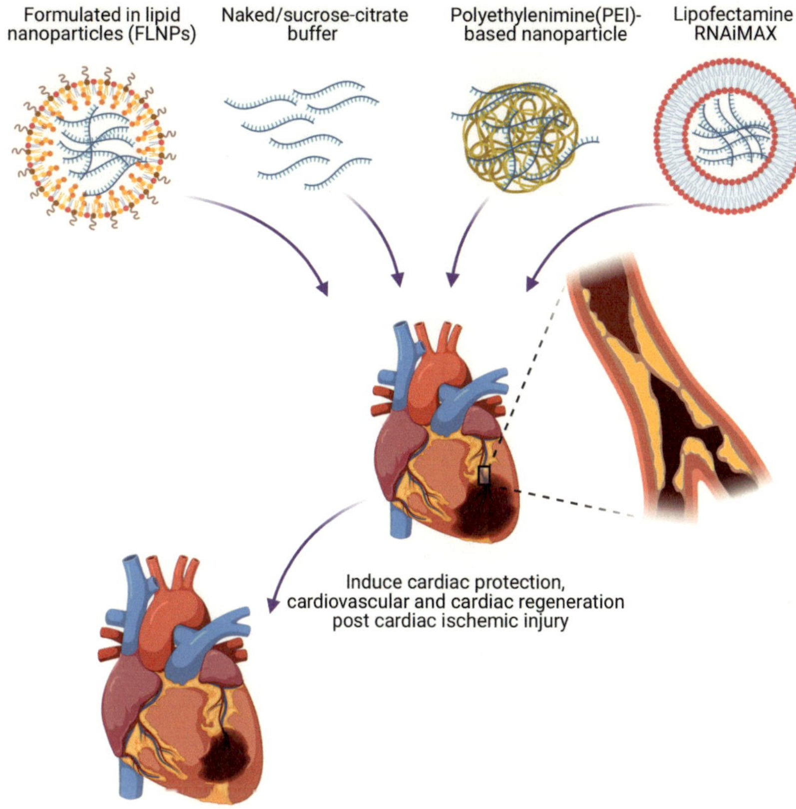

Figure 1.
Modified mRNA carrier systems for cardiac delivery.

adjusted depending on the administration route. An experimental study showed that reporter genes were expressed significantly more when delivered intradermally compared to intravenously [42]. Furthermore, the systemically delivered LNPs favor expression in the liver due to apolipoprotein E binding and subsequent receptor-mediated uptake by hepatocytes. Thus, fine-tuning LNP a component is pivotal to beneficial cardiac therapy [43].

Although developed for siRNA transfections, cationic lipid nanoparticles, commonly known as lipofectamine, also have promising outcomes for modRNA delivery in the heart. Lipofectamine particles consist of a 3:1 mixture of DOSPA (2,3-dioleoyloxy-N- [2(sperminecarboxamido)ethyl]-N,N-dimethyl-1-propaniminium trifluoroacetate) and DOPE (1,2-Dioleoyl-sn-glycero-3-phosphoethanolamine) generating a cationic molecule that readily encapsulates the negatively charged modRNA and carries it across the plasma membrane due to the neutral co-lipid mediating fusion between the liposome and the cell membrane [44]. Kondrat et al. have formulated modRNA with RNAimax for myocardial delivery [25]. For in vitro and in vivo cardiac cell delivery, lipofectamine RNAimax and modRNA can be delivered in optiMEM medium and gel-based formulations. For instance, a mixture of Cre recombinase modRNA mixed with lipofectamine and polyacrylic acid successfully expressed the protein when painted on the surface of transgenic Rosa26^{mtmg} heart [45]. Further, Singh et al. reported alginate carrying microencapsulated modRNA (M^3RNA) can cause rapid protein expression in primary CMs and targeted expression in mouse and porcine hearts. Forming alginate matrix by crosslinking alignate in the presence of Ca^{2+} provides an excellent platform for modRNA delivery in infarcted hearts [46].

Delivery Method	Species	Administration Route	Protein Target	Results	Mechanism	Publication
Formulated lipidoid nanoparticles (FLNP)	Rat and Pig	Intramyocardial/ intracoronary	eGFP	Reported highly efficient, rapid and short-term mRNA expression in the heart	Epoxide-derived lipidoid complex enhanced eGFP mRNA levels in heart tissue	Turnbull et al. [40]
	Rat	Intramyocardial	EGFP	Protocol	Protocol	Turnbull et al. [41]
Alginate, nanomaterial encapsulated	Mouse and Pig	Intramyocardial/ intracoronary	FLuc, EGFP and mCherry	M^3RNA enabled rapid and targeted protein expression in mouse and porcine hearts.	The crosslinkage of alginate gel with Ca^{2+} at the infarcted site provided an in situ alginate matrix to encapsulate therapeutic mRNA	Singh et al. [46]
Polyethylenimine-based nanoparticle	Mouse	Intracardiac	IGF-1	Reduced cell apoptosis, enhanced cell survival	IGF1 increased the levels of Akt and Erk phosphorylation	Huang et al. [47]
Lipofectamine RNAimax	Mouse	Intracardiac	VEGFA	Induced angiogenesis, improved myocardial function and mice survival	Changed the fate of heart progenitor cells and induced vascular regeneration after MI	Zangi et al. [11]
	Mouse	Intracardiac	VEGFA	Endothelial specification, engraftment, proliferation and reduced apoptosis of the human Isl1+ progenitors in vivo	Induced $Isl1^+$ cells to endothelial cell fate, proliferation and survival of Isl1+ progenitors	Lui et al. [45]
	Mouse	Intracardiac/gel application	DN-IGF-1R, IGFR	Reduced cell differentiation into adipocytes after MI	Adipogenic differentiation ceased post MI	Zangi et al. [51]

DOI: http://dx.doi.org/10.5772/intechopen.97184

Delivery Method	Species	Administration Route	Protein Target	Results	Mechanism	Publication
Sucrose-citrate buffer	Mouse	Intracardiac	mutated FSTL1	CM proliferation and limited cardiac remodeling	Replaced asparagine with glutamine in the N-glycosylation site at position 180 of FSTL1	Magadum et al. [52]
	Mouse	Intracardiac	Pkm2	CM cell cycle induction, decreased oxidative stress	PKM2 interacted with β-catenin and upregulated downstream targets Cyclin D1 and C-Myc	Magadum et al. [53]
	Mouse	Intracardiac	AC	Reduced cell apoptosis, increased cell survival, improved cardiac function	Decreased ceramide levels and lowered abundance of proinflammatory detrimental neutrophils	Hadas et al. [54]
	Mouse	Intracardiac	GFP, Luciferase	Optimized time and amount for efficient modRNA delivery in the heart	Optimized time and amount for efficient modRNA delivery in the heart	Sultana et al. [50]
	Human	Epicardial injection	VEGFA	Expected to increase blood flow in the heart	Increased angiogenesis	Moderna Therapeutics [55]
	Mouse	Intracardiac	Luciferase	Increased translation by replacing 5'UTR	Ces1D enhanced mRNA translation post cardiac and hepatic ischemic injury	Sultana et al. [33]
	Mouse	Intracardiac	Luciferase, Cre	Delivered modRNA in a MI model	Protocol	Kaur et al. [49]
	Minipig	Intracardiac	VEGFA	Promoted capillary density, improved heart function post MI, reduced fibrosis	Increased angiogenesis	Carlsson et al. [56]
	Mouse	Intracardiac injection	aYAP	Decreased CM necrosis, attenuated innate immune responses	YAP/TEAD1 suppressed toll like receptor pathway	Chen et al. [57]
	Mouse	Intracardiac injection	Cre	Specific modRNA translation system	L7Ae based modRNA delivery exclusively to CMs.	Magadum et al. [58]

Table 1.
Recent modRNA studies in the heart: Delivery system, target and findings.

To increase the efficiency of modRNA uptake in vivo, cationic polymers have occasionally been used to upregulate therapeutic genes in the heart. These chemically diverse and positively charged molecules are highly compatible with the negatively charged modRNA and thus hold great potential for functionalization. Polymers can be linear, branched or dendrimers; the latter comprise many branched repeats. One cardiac modRNA variant is polyethylenimine (PEI), which can efficiently promote gene transfection in vivo, as described by Huang et al. [47]. With a nitrogen atom at every third position along the polymer, PEI has a high charge density at reduced pH values, which may promote mRNA condensation and endosomal escape [48]. ModRNA transfection also depends on final formulations and reportedly works best at a nitrogen residue/phosphate (N/P) ratio of 6 of jetPEI/modRNA [47]. Despite PEI's initial use in modRNA delivery in mice, its molecular weight and linear versus branched form need to be optimized, as these are reportedly major determinants of transfection efficiency and cytotoxicity.

Lastly, the safest, most efficient modRNA delivery method to the heart, as presented by Kaur et al. [49], is naked delivery without conjugation of any nanoparticle. Unlike the nanoparticle formulations, naked modRNA in saline or sucrose-citrate buffer does not form any of the complexes that make its efficacy questionable in vitro. While the transfection reagent masks the negatively charged mRNA, allowing electromagnetic attachment to and endocytosis of the negatively charged cell membrane, these formulations are associated with increased cell death. While comparing various modRNA various delivery reagents, naked modRNA with sucrose-citrate buffer or saline yields higher protein translation compared to modRNA encapsulated in nanoparticles in the heart. This could be explained by the sucrose acting as a readily available energy source to enhance endocytosis of the modRNA. The composition of the sucrose-citrate buffer also provides appropriate viscosity and thus prevents clumping to ensure single-stranded mRNA enters the myocardium to achieve high translation and avoid activating the immune response. Further, encapsulating modRNA with RNAimax has proven to be detrimental in the heart and triggers apoptosis locally. Another study showed that delivering 100ug of Luciferase/Cre recombinase modRNA in sucrose-citrate buffer was sufficient to produce optimal gene translation, resulting in ~20% transfection of the left ventricle [50]. The studies using various modRNA delivery systems in the heart are compiled in **Table 1**.

6. Modified mRNA to induce cardiac repair

ModRNA holds enormous potential as a non-viral gene delivery method for cardiovascular diseases. Recent developments in the understanding of basic blood vessel formation mechanisms have shown it may be possible to use therapeutic vascular growth to treat heart disease. Traditional vectors have delivered several growth factors to achieve new vessel growth in the heart [59]. To circumvent the complications associated with recombinant protein- and gene transfer-based therapies, Zangi et al. published a landmark study using in vitro transcribed modRNA to efficiently deliver vascular endothelial growth factor A (VEGFA) into the heart with minimal induction of innate immune responses. Their work demonstrated that direct intramyocardial injection of synthetic mRNA containing pseudouridine and 5-methylcytidine, encoding VEGFA, promoted vascular growth, improved heart function and enhanced long-term survival following MI injury [11]. Furthermore, VEGFA also had a pro-survival effect on vascular and endothelial cells and enhanced endothelial proliferation of epicardial-derived progenitor cells [51].

Subsequent to this study in mice, Carlsson et al. established the efficacy of clinical-grade VEGFA modRNA, AZD8601 for heart regeneration after MI in porcine models. The group showed that the modRNA formulated in biocompatible citrate-buffered saline can transiently deliver genes into the heart. They also confirmed that intradermally or intravenously administered modRNA did not exhibit any signs of acute toxicity or inflammation in rats and cynomolgus monkeys. Epicardially injected AZD8601 administered 7 days after permanent ligation of the mid-left anterior descending coronary artery led to improved cardiac function in mini-pigs. The study demonstrated significant improvements in left ventricular ejection fraction, contractility and myocardial compliance with increased neovessel formation in the peri-infarct area and attenuated cardiac fibrosis 2 months after injection [56]. The promising results in the pig model led to the first clinical trial involving modRNA therapy for cardiac regeneration, by AstraZeneca (AZD8601) in collaboration with Moderna [55]. This phase 2a clinical trial (clinical trial number: NCT03370887) is expected to prove the safety and efficacy of epicardially injected VEGFA modRNA and authenticate improved myocardial blood flow in patients who underwent coronary artery bypass grafting surgery. Furthermore, the VEFGA modRNA, AZD8601 has progressed to a phase 1 clinical testing study in men with type 2 diabetes mellitus. The study involves delivering AZD8601 intradermally as a single dose into the forearm skin with the primary objective of assessing the safety and tolerability of this new therapeutic clinical trial number: NCT02935712). So far, the results have shown significantly increased local blood flow in the skin within 7 days of modRNA injection as well as elevated VEGFA protein concentration in cutaneous dialysate, thereby indicating VEGFA is a potential candidate for microvasculature therapy [60].

Following acute MI, ischemic stress is associated with LV deterioration, impaired cardiac function and higher ceramide levels. These elevated sphingolipid levels result from decreased ceramidase levels and are not induced by elevated sphingomyelinase activity. Further, the increased ceramides in the blood appear to be transient, as shown in a model of ischemic-reperfused myocardium in rats [60]. Thus, the pulse-like expression of mRNA encoding the enzyme acid ceramidase (AC) directly into the injured myocardium is sufficient to induce cardioprotection after MI [57]. Treatment with AC improved cardiac function, reduced LV scar size 28 days post MI and extended long-term survival. Huang et al. used modRNA delivery into mouse myocardium to evaluate the cytoprotective efficacy of insulin-like growth factor 1 (IGF1) on hypoxia-induced CM apoptosis. As expected, IGF1 secretion was observed 24 h after injection and peaked at 48 h. Note that a single dose of intramyocardially injected IGF1 post MI augmented Akt1 phosphorylation and decreased both Casp9 activity and TUNEL-positive cell levels within the border zone of infarcted mouse hearts. These changes reduced CM apoptosis and thus enhanced CM survival under hypoxic conditions [47]. The beneficial effects of the IGF1 signaling pathway in the MI model were evaluated by Zangi et al., who demonstrated that the IGF1 receptor triggers the formation of epicardial adipose tissue in the heart. Thus, the innovative approach of delivering modRNA by applying a gel comprising IGF1 receptor dominant-negative mutants to the heart surface reduced adipogenic marker expression and led to better survival for CMs and cardiac progenitors [51]. Additionally, introducing transcriptional co-activator yes-associated protein (aYAP) modRNA in the mouse heart produced promising outcomes in IR injury. Previously established for cell proliferation, aYAP effectively curtailed the innate immune inflammatory response and boosted CM survival in the damaged myocardium. This modRNA-mediated gene delivery led to reduced scarring, improved heart function and suppressed hypertrophic remodeling 4 weeks after intervention [52].

Another important aspect of cardiac repair is inducing the CM cell cycle. In this regard, delivering modRNA encoded for follistatin-like 1 (FSTL1, with glutamine substituted for asparagine in the N-glycosylation site at position 180) increased CM proliferation both in vitro and in a mouse model post MI without inducing CM hypertrophy. FSTL1 mutation of all three N-glycosilation sites present in hFSTL1 mimicked the glycosylation state of bacterially produced FSTL1 and was sufficient and essential to activate the CM cell cycle and cease cardiac remodeling post MI [53]. In another study, Magadum et al. showed modRNA-based CM cell cycle induction via upregulating pyruvate kinase muscle isoenzyme 2 (PKM2). This isoenzyme of the glycolytic enzyme pyruvate kinase can be detected in CMs during embryonic development and immediately after birth, but not during adulthood. Introducing PKM2 in CMs in vivo increased CM cell division, improved cardiac function and enhanced long-term animal survival. These results stem from PKM2 interaction with β-catenin in CM nuclei and upregulated downstream targets Cyclin D1 and C-Myc, which remove the brakes from cell cycle arrest, in addition to reduced oxidative stress damage through activation of anabolic pathways and β-catenin [61]. The study also described a unique system to achieve CM specificity by implementing archaeal ribosomal protein L7Ae in the modRNA constructs. The authors added kink-turn motif, a specific binding site for L7Ae, to the 5′UTR of PKM2 mRNA, and when the L7Ae recognized the kink-turn motif it cleaved the modRNA and hence blocked translation. Using this cell-specific system, modRNA encoding for PKM2 with kink-turn motif was co-transfected with modRNA encoding L7Ae, which included CM-specific microRNA recognition elements (miR1–1 and miR- 208a) within 3′UTR. This co-transfection prevented PKM2 expression in all cardiac cells except CMs [58, 61]. Collectively, these studies show the therapeutic potential and effectiveness of modRNA technology in cardioprotection and cardiac repair.

7. Concluding remarks and future directions

Current structural improvements that enhance modRNA stability and escalate its translational capacity, have spiked interest in modRNA for both basic research and clinical therapeutics. The innovative progress in modRNA design has facilitated rapid mass production, reduced costs and revealed the versatility of next-generation modRNA for future therapeutics. The recent success of modRNA vaccines against SARS-COV-2 has proven that modRNA can provide robust, safe and efficient gene transfer in humans and hence is considered a promising tool for treating various disorders, including heart failure [62]. However, the multifarious obstacles concerning modRNA's large size, charge, intrinsic instability and need to be administered through intracardiac injections hamper the translation of modRNA-based cardiac therapeutics to the clinic.

Significant advances in nanodelivery systems, especially in the field of LNPs, have shown the best prospects for developing modRNA-based therapies. The US Food and Drug Administration's recent approval of short interfering based patisiran to treat hereditary transthyretin amyloidosis has made LNPs an attractive potential non-toxic carrier system for modRNA delivery [63]. Despite developments in delivery systems, predictable, efficient delivery of nanoparticles to targeted tissues remains challenging. Changes in the internal and/or external charge of the nanoparticle is one key aspect of tuning tissue tropism. To address this, Cheng et al. developed a unique method of supplementing additional molecules to established LNP molar compositions in order to tune the internal charge for selective organ targeting. The resulting formulations were able to precisely target a variety of organs and enabled high levels of modRNA delivery. Although such studies have produced highly promising results for modRNA delivery in lung, spleen and liver, more work remains to be done to create minimally invasive gene delivery models for the heart [64]. Developing such delivery models would also help resolve short span gene expression with modRNA delivery. Although transient gene delivery eliminates the risk of mutagenesis caused by protein overexpression, pulse-like expression of a gene might not be enough to induce substantial cardiac regenerative changes. Thus, the innovation of minimally invasive methods to deliver cardiac genes will mitigate the need for repeated modRNA transfections/injections to maintain effective protein levels for a longer but still controlled time period. As research on modRNA formulation and delivery rapidly accumulates, we are confident that modRNA therapy will soon become reality in the field of heart failure therapeutics.

Conflict of interest

The authors declare no conflict of interest.

Author details

Lior Zangi[1,2,3], Ravinder K. Kaundal[1,4] and Keerat Kaur[1,2,3]*

1 Cardiovascular Research Center, Icahn School of Medicine at Mount Sinai, New York, NY, USA

2 Department of Genetics and Genomic Sciences, Icahn School of Medicine at Mount Sinai, New York, NY, USA

3 Black Family Stem Cell Institute, Icahn School of Medicine at Mount Sinai, New York, NY, USA

4 Department of Pharmacology and Toxicology, National Institute of Pharmaceutical Education and Research, Raebareli, Lucknow, India

*Address all correspondence to: keerat.kaur@mssm.edu

References

[1] Kajstura J, Cheng W, Reiss K, Clark WA, Sonnenblick EH, Krajewski S et al. Apoptotic and necrotic myocyte cell deaths are independent contributing variables of infarct size in rats. Lab Invest. 1996;74(1): 86-107.00

[2] Sam F, Sawyer DB, Chang DL, Eberli FR, Ngoy S, Jain M et al. Progressive left ventricular remodeling and apoptosis late after myocardial infarction in mouse heart. Am J Physiol Heart Circ Physiol. 2000;279(1):H422-8. doi:10.1152/ajpheart.2000.279.1.H422.

[3] Brocheriou V, Hagege AA, Oubenaissa A, Lambert M, Mallet VO, Duriez M et al. Cardiac functional improvement by a human Bcl-2 transgene in a mouse model of ischemia/reperfusion injury. J Gene Med. 2000;2(5):326-33. doi:10.1002/1521-2254(200009/10)2:5<326::AID-JGM133>3.0.CO;2-1.

[4] Hochhauser E, Cheporko Y, Yasovich N, Pinchas L, Offen D, Barhum Y et al. Bax deficiency reduces infarct size and improves long-term function after myocardial infarction. Cell Biochem Biophys. 2007;47(1):11-20. doi:CBB:47:1:11 [pii].10.1385/cbb:47:1:11.

[5] Chen Z, Chua CC, Ho YS, Hamdy RC, Chua BH. Overexpression of Bcl-2 attenuates apoptosis and protects against myocardial I/R injury in transgenic mice. Am J Physiol Heart Circ Physiol. 2001;280(5):H2313-20. doi:10.1152/ajpheart.2001.280.5.H2313.

[6] Huang JQ, Radinovic S, Rezaiefar P, Black SC. In vivo myocardial infarct size reduction by a caspase inhibitor administered after the onset of ischemia. Eur J Pharmacol. 2000;402(1-2):139-42. doi:S0014-2999(00)00477-5 [pii] 10.1016/s0014-2999(00)00477-5.

[7] Frangogiannis NG. Regulation of the inflammatory response in cardiac repair. Circ Res. 2012;110(1):159-73. doi:10.1161/CIRCRESAHA.111.243162 110/1/159 [pii].

[8] Frangogiannis NG. The mechanistic basis of infarct healing. Antioxid Redox Signal. 2006;8(11-12):1907-39. doi:10.1089/ars.2006.8.1907.

[9] Kaur K, Zangi L. Modified mRNA as a Therapeutic Tool for the Heart. Cardiovasc Drugs Ther. 2020;34(6):871-80. doi:10.1007/s10557-020-07051-4.

[10] Magadum A, Kaur K, Zangi L. mRNA-Based Protein Replacement Therapy for the Heart. Mol Ther. 2019;27(4):785-93. doi:10.1016/j.ymthe.2018.11.018.

[11] Zangi L, Lui KO, von Gise A, Ma Q, Ebina W, Ptaszek LM et al. Modified mRNA directs the fate of heart progenitor cells and induces vascular regeneration after myocardial infarction. Nat Biotechnol. 2013;31(10):898-907. doi:10.1038/nbt.2682.

[12] Martinez-Rucobo FW, Kohler R, van de Waterbeemd M, Heck AJ, Hemann M, Herzog F et al. Molecular Basis of Transcription-Coupled Pre-mRNA Capping. Mol Cell. 2015;58(6):1079-89. doi:10.1016/j.molcel.2015.04.004 S1097-2765(15)00260-9 [pii].

[13] Ramanathan A, Robb GB, Chan SH. mRNA capping: biological functions and applications. Nucleic Acids Res. 2016;44(16):7511-26. doi:10.1093/nar/gkw551 gkw551 [pii].

[14] Stewart M. Polyadenylation and nuclear export of mRNAs. J Biol Chem. 2019;294(9):2977-87. doi:10.1074/jbc.REV118.005594 REV118.005594 [pii].

[15] Colgan DF, Manley JL. Mechanism and regulation of mRNA

polyadenylation. Genes Dev. 1997;11(21):2755-66. doi:10.1101/gad.11.21.2755.

[16] Gao C, Wang Y. mRNA Metabolism in Cardiac Development and Disease: Life After Transcription. Physiol Rev. 2020;100(2):673-94. doi:10.1152/physrev.00007.2019.

[17] Tanji H, Ohto U, Shibata T, Taoka M, Yamauchi Y, Isobe T et al. Toll-like receptor 8 senses degradation products of single-stranded RNA. Nat Struct Mol Biol. 2015;22(2):109-15. doi:10.1038/nsmb.2943 nsmb.2943 [pii].

[18] Chen N, Xia P, Li S, Zhang T, Wang TT, Zhu J. RNA sensors of the innate immune system and their detection of pathogens. IUBMB Life. 2017;69(5):297-304. doi:10.1002/iub.1625.

[19] Liang SL, Quirk D, Zhou A. RNase L: its biological roles and regulation. IUBMB Life. 2006;58(9):508-14. doi:QW28XRNUX638M8T1 [pii] 10.1080/15216540600838232.

[20] de Haro C, Mendez R, Santoyo J. The eIF-2alpha kinases and the control of protein synthesis. FASEB J. 1996;10(12):1378-87. doi:10.1096/fasebj.10.12.8903508.

[21] Perdiguero B, Esteban M. The interferon system and vaccinia virus evasion mechanisms. J Interferon Cytokine Res. 2009;29(9):581-98. doi:10.1089/jir.2009.0073.

[22] Schlee M. Master sensors of pathogenic RNA - RIG-I like receptors. Immunobiology. 2013;218(11):1322-35. doi:10.1016/j.imbio.2013.06.007 S0171-2985(13)00120-4 [pii].

[23] Goubau D, Deddouche S, Reis e Sousa C. Cytosolic sensing of viruses. Immunity. 2013;38(5):855-69. doi:10.1016/j.immuni.2013.05.007 S1074-7613(13)00204-5 [pii].

[24] Hartmann G. Nucleic Acid Immunity. Adv Immunol. 2017;133:121-69. doi:S0065-2776(16)30052-9 [pii] 10.1016/bs.ai.2016.11.001.

[25] Kondrat J, Sultana N, Zangi L. Synthesis of Modified mRNA for Myocardial Delivery. Methods Mol Biol. 2017;1521:127-38. doi:10.1007/978-1-4939-6588-5_8.

[26] Boo SH, Kim YK. The emerging role of RNA modifications in the regulation of mRNA stability. Exp Mol Med. 2020;52(3):400-8. doi:10.1038/s12276-020-0407-z.

[27] Kariko K, Muramatsu H, Welsh FA, Ludwig J, Kato H, Akira S et al. Incorporation of pseudouridine into mRNA yields superior nonimmunogenic vector with increased translational capacity and biological stability. Mol Ther. 2008;16(11):1833-40. doi:10.1038/mt.2008.200.

[28] Kierzek E, Malgowska M, Lisowiec J, Turner DH, Gdaniec Z, Kierzek R. The contribution of pseudouridine to stabilities and structure of RNAs. Nucleic Acids Res. 2014;42(5):3492-501. doi:10.1093/nar/gkt1330.

[29] Kocmik I, Piecyk K, Rudzinska M, Niedzwiecka A, Darzynkiewicz E, Grzela R et al. Modified ARCA analogs providing enhanced translational properties of capped mRNAs. Cell Cycle. 2018;17(13):1624-36. doi:10.1080/15384101.2018.1486164.

[30] Stepinski J, Waddell C, Stolarski R, Darzynkiewicz E, Rhoads RE. Synthesis and properties of mRNAs containing the novel "anti-reverse" cap analogs 7-methyl(3'-O-methyl)GpppG and 7-methyl (3'-deoxy)GpppG. RNA. 2001;7(10):1486-95.

[31] Hadas Y, Sultana N, Youssef E, Sharkar MTK, Kaur K, Chepurko E et al. Optimizing Modified mRNA In Vitro

Synthesis Protocol for Heart Gene Therapy. Mol Ther Methods Clin Dev. 2019;14:300-5. doi:10.1016/j.omtm.2019.07.006.

[32] Asrani KH, Farelli JD, Stahley MR, Miller RL, Cheng CJ, Subramanian RR et al. Optimization of mRNA untranslated regions for improved expression of therapeutic mRNA. RNA Biol. 2018;15(6):756-62. doi:10.1080/15476286.2018.1450054.

[33] Sultana N, Hadas Y, Sharkar MTK, Kaur K, Magadum A, Kurian AA et al. Optimization of 5' Untranslated Region of Modified mRNA for Use in Cardiac or Hepatic Ischemic Injury. Mol Ther Methods Clin Dev. 2020;17:622-33. doi:10.1016/j.omtm.2020.03.019.

[34] Moore MJ. From birth to death: the complex lives of eukaryotic mRNAs. Science. 2005;309(5740):1514-8. doi:10.1126/science.1111443.

[35] Waggoner SA, Liebhaber SA. Regulation of alpha-globin mRNA stability. Exp Biol Med (Maywood). 2003;228(4):387-95. doi:10.1177/153537020322800409.

[36] Peixeiro I, Silva AL, Romao L. Control of human beta-globin mRNA stability and its impact on beta-thalassemia phenotype. Haematologica. 2011;96(6):905-13. doi:10.3324/haematol.2010.039206.

[37] Orlandini von Niessen AG, Poleganov MA, Rechner C, Plaschke A, Kranz LM, Fesser S et al. Improving mRNA-Based Therapeutic Gene Delivery by Expression-Augmenting 3' UTRs Identified by Cellular Library Screening. Mol Ther. 2019;27(4):824-36. doi:10.1016/j.ymthe.2018.12.011.

[38] Legnini I, Alles J, Karaiskos N, Ayoub S, Rajewsky N. FLAM-seq: full-length mRNA sequencing reveals principles of poly(A) tail length control. Nat Methods. 2019;16(9):879-86. doi:10.1038/s41592-019-0503-y.

[39] Sultana N, Sharkar MTK, Hadas Y, Chepurko E, Zangi L. In Vitro Synthesis of Modified RNA for Cardiac Gene Therapy. Methods Mol Biol. 2021;2158:281-94. doi:10.1007/978-1-0716-0668-1_21.

[40] Turnbull IC, Eltoukhy AA, Anderson DG, Costa KD. Lipidoid mRNA Nanoparticles for Myocardial Delivery in Rodents. Methods Mol Biol. 2017;1521:153-66. doi:10.1007/978-1-4939-6588-5_10.

[41] Turnbull IC, Eltoukhy AA, Fish KM, Nonnenmacher M, Ishikawa K, Chen J et al. Myocardial Delivery of Lipidoid Nanoparticle Carrying modRNA Induces Rapid and Transient Expression. Mol Ther. 2016;24(1):66-75. doi:10.1038/mt.2015.193.

[42] Pardi N, Tuyishime S, Muramatsu H, Kariko K, Mui BL, Tam YK et al. Expression kinetics of nucleoside-modified mRNA delivered in lipid nanoparticles to mice by various routes. J Control Release. 2015;217:345-51. doi:10.1016/j.jconrel.2015.08.007.

[43] Akinc A, Querbes W, De S, Qin J, Frank-Kamenetsky M, Jayaprakash KN et al. Targeted delivery of RNAi therapeutics with endogenous and exogenous ligand-based mechanisms. Mol Ther. 2010;18(7):1357-64. doi:10.1038/mt.2010.85.

[44] Dalby B, Cates S, Harris A, Ohki EC, Tilkins ML, Price PJ et al. Advanced transfection with Lipofectamine 2000 reagent: primary neurons, siRNA, and high-throughput applications. Methods. 2004;33(2):95-103. doi:10.1016/j.ymeth.2003.11.023.

[45] Lui KO, Zangi L, Silva EA, Bu L, Sahara M, Li RA et al. Driving vascular endothelial cell fate of human

multipotent Isl1+ heart progenitors with VEGF modified mRNA. Cell Res. 2013;23(10):1172-86. doi:10.1038/cr.2013.112.

[46] Singh RD, Hillestad ML, Livia C, Li M, Alekseev AE, Witt TA et al. M(3) RNA Drives Targeted Gene Delivery in Acute Myocardial Infarction. Tissue Eng Part A. 2019;25(1-2):145-58. doi:10.1089/ten.TEA.2017.0445.

[47] Huang CL, Leblond AL, Turner EC, Kumar AH, Martin K, Whelan D et al. Synthetic chemically modified mrna-based delivery of cytoprotective factor promotes early cardiomyocyte survival post-acute myocardial infarction. Mol Pharm. 2015;12(3):991-6. doi:10.1021/mp5006239.

[48] Rezvani Amin Z, Rahimizadeh M, Eshghi H, Dehshahri A, Ramezani M. The effect of cationic charge density change on transfection efficiency of polyethylenimine. Iran J Basic Med Sci. 2013;16(2):150-6.

[49] Kaur K, Sultana N, Hadas Y, Magadum A, Sharkar MTK, Chepurko E et al. Delivery of Modified mRNA in a Myocardial Infarction Mouse Model. J Vis Exp. 2020(160). doi:10.3791/60832.

[50] Sultana N, Magadum A, Hadas Y, Kondrat J, Singh N, Youssef E et al. Optimizing Cardiac Delivery of Modified mRNA. Mol Ther. 2017;25(6):1306-15. doi:10.1016/j.ymthe.2017.03.016.

[51] Zangi L, Oliveira MS, Ye LY, Ma Q, Sultana N, Hadas Y et al. Insulin-Like Growth Factor 1 Receptor-Dependent Pathway Drives Epicardial Adipose Tissue Formation After Myocardial Injury. Circulation. 2017;135(1):59-72. doi:10.1161/CIRCULATIONAHA.116.022064.

[52] Chen J, Ma Q, King JS, Sun Y, Xu B, Zhang X et al. aYAP modRNA reduces cardiac inflammation and hypertrophy in a murine ischemia-reperfusion model. Life Sci Alliance. 2020;3(1). doi:10.26508/lsa.201900424.

[53] Magadum A, Singh N, Kurian AA, Sharkar MTK, Chepurko E, Zangi L. Ablation of a Single N-Glycosylation Site in Human FSTL 1 Induces Cardiomyocyte Proliferation and Cardiac Regeneration. Mol Ther Nucleic Acids. 2018;13:133-43. doi:10.1016/j.omtn.2018.08.021.

[54] Zhang DX, Fryer RM, Hsu AK, Zou AP, Gross GJ, Campbell WB et al. Production and metabolism of ceramide in normal and ischemic-reperfused myocardium of rats. Basic Res Cardiol. 2001;96(3):267-74. doi:10.1007/s003950170057.

[55] Anttila V, Saraste A, Knuuti J, Jaakkola P, Hedman M, Svedlund S et al. Synthetic mRNA encoding VEGF-A in patients undergoing coronary artery bypass grafting: design of a phase 2a clinical trial. Molecular Therapy-Methods & Clinical Development. 2020;18:464-72.

[56] Carlsson L, Clarke JC, Yen C, Gregoire F, Albery T, Billger M et al. Biocompatible, Purified VEGF-A mRNA Improves Cardiac Function after Intracardiac Injection 1 Week Post-myocardial Infarction in Swine. Mol Ther Methods Clin Dev. 2018;9:330-46. doi:10.1016/j.omtm.2018.04.003.

[57] Hadas Y, Vincek AS, Youssef E, Zak MM, Chepurko E, Sultana N et al. Altering Sphingolipid Metabolism Attenuates Cell Death and Inflammatory Response After Myocardial Infarction. Circulation. 2020;141(11):916-30. doi:10.1161/CIRCULATIONAHA.119.041882.

[58] Magadum A, Kurian AA, Chepurko E, Sassi Y, Hajjar RJ, Zangi L. Specific Modified mRNA Translation System. Circulation. 2020;142(25):2485-8.

[59] Favaloro L, Diez M, Mendiz O, Janavel GV, Valdivieso L, Ratto R et al. High-dose plasmid-mediated VEGF gene transfer is safe in patients with severe ischemic heart disease (Genesis-I). A phase I, open-label, two-year follow-up trial. Catheter Cardiovasc Interv. 2013;82(6):899-906. doi:10.1002/ccd.24555.

[60] Gan LM, Lagerstrom-Fermer M, Carlsson LG, Arfvidsson C, Egnell AC, Rudvik A et al. Intradermal delivery of modified mRNA encoding VEGF-A in patients with type 2 diabetes. Nat Commun. 2019;10(1):871. doi:10.1038/s41467-019-08852-4.

[61] Magadum A, Singh N, Kurian AA, Munir I, Mehmood T, Brown K et al. Pkm2 Regulates Cardiomyocyte Cell Cycle and Promotes Cardiac Regeneration. Circulation. 2020;141(15):1249-65. doi:10.1161/CIRCULATIONAHA.119.043067.

[62] Chanda PK, Sukhovershin R, Cooke JP. mRNA-Enhanced Cell Therapy and Cardiovascular Regeneration. Cells. 2021;10(1):187.

[63] Wood H. FDA approves patisiran to treat hereditary transthyretin amyloidosis. Nat Rev Neurol. 2018;14(10):570. doi:10.1038/s41582-018-0065-0.

[64] Cheng Q, Wei T, Farbiak L, Johnson LT, Dilliard SA, Siegwart DJ. Selective organ targeting (SORT) nanoparticles for tissue-specific mRNA delivery and CRISPR-Cas gene editing. Nat Nanotechnol. 2020;15(4):313-20. doi:10.1038/s41565-020-0669-6.

Chapter 22

Possibility of the Subcutaneous Implantable Cardioverter-Defibrillator for Prevention of Sudden Cardiac Death in Patients with Arrhythmogenic Right Ventricular Cardiomyopathy

Shingo Sasaki

Abstract

The EMBLEM™ entirely subcutaneous implantable cardioverter-defibrillator (S-ICD) system (Boston Scientific, Marlborough, Massachusetts, USA) was introduced as a new alternative to the conventional transvenous implantable cardioverter-defibrillator and has been expected to reduce device-related complications, especially in young patients who require long-term lead placement. Arrhythmogenic right ventricular cardiomyopathy (ARVC) is a well-known hereditary disease recognized as a cause of sudden cardiac death (SCD) in young adults. However, the precise clinical role of S-ICD in patients with ARVC remains to be defined because of the low QRS amplitude of subcutaneous electrocardiogram (S-ECG) followed by the high incidence of inappropriate shock (IAS) delivery due to oversensing. It is well known that the sensing of S-ICD is largely dependent on the QRS/T ratio of S-ECG. The decrease in the QRS amplitude is more likely to lead to oversensing such as T wave or myopotential oversensing. In patients with ARVC, the decrease in the QRS amplitude due to degeneration of the right ventricular myocardium progresses overtime. In this chapter, we would like to discuss the usefulness of S-ICD lead repositioning for young adult patients with ARVC based on our experience of patients with IAS.

Keywords: arrhythmogenic right ventricular cardiomyopathy, subcutaneous implantable cardioverter-defibrillator, inappropriate shock, lead repositioning

1. Introduction

The EMBLEM™ entirely subcutaneous implantable cardioverter-defibrillator (S-ICD) system (Boston Scientific, Marlborough, Massachusetts, USA) has been used as a new alternative to the conventional transvenous implantable cardioverter-defibrillator (TV-ICD). Recently, the PREATORIAN study has shown that S-ICD is as useful as TV-ICD for prevention of sudden cardiac death (SCD), mainly in patients with ischemic cardiomyopathy [1]. Furthermore, the UNTOUCHED study also demonstrated that the inappropriate shock (IAS) rate in S-ICD-implanted patients with left ventricular ejection fraction (LVEF) ≤ 35% for primary prevention was non-inferior to that in transvenous ICD (TV-ICD)-implanted patients with similar programming as in the high-rate cutoff and long-delay therapy groups in the MADIT-RIT [2, 3].

Arrhythmogenic right ventricular cardiomyopathy (ARVC) is a well-known hereditary disease recognized as a cause of SCD in young adults [4]. However, the usefulness of S-ICD in patients with ARVC has not been established because of the low QRS amplitude of subcutaneous electrocardiogram (S-ECG) followed by the high incidence of IAS due to oversensing [5, 6]. We recently reported the usefulness of S-ICD lead repositioning to avoid IAS in patients with ARVC [7]. In this chapter, we will discuss the effectiveness of S-ICD lead repositioning for young adult patients with ARVC based on our clinical experience of patients with IAS.

2. Characteristics and problems of S-ICD sensing in patients with ARVC

The S-ICD uses a far-field bipolar electrocardiogram detected between two electrodes of S-ICD lead, or between one of the two electrodes and pulse-generator. This far-field bipolar electrocardiogram is called as subcutaneous electrocardiogram (S-ECG) and is used for detection and discrimination of tachyarrhythmias in current S-ICD system. The S-ECG shows lower QRS amplitude (0.3–4.0 mV) compared to intracardiac ECG, and longer QRS duration with many low frequency components. Since the basic morphology of S-ECG resembles a body surface ECG, it is easily affected by P wave and T wave, and is also easily affected by changes in the QRS complex to T wave (QRS/T) ratio during exercise. And S-ECG has a potential risk of myopotential interference (MPI) in certain periodic movements.

It has been suggested that fatal events occurring before overt structural myocardial changes in patients with ARVC may be caused by a primarily electrical mechanism as a consequence of the cross talk of genetically defective desmosomal proteins with the voltage-gated sodium channel complex, leading to reduced sodium currents and arrhythmogenic mechanisms similar to those in Brugada syndrome [8]. It has also been known that the phenotype of fatal arrhythmias in patients with ARVC is age-dependent. Older patients with advanced disease more often experience re-entrant ventricular tachycardia (VT) around a myocardial fibro-fatty scar, whereas young patients commonly experience sudden onsets of ventricular fibrillation (VF) reflecting acute electrical instability in the early phases of the disease. Furthermore, S-ICD has been reported to have fewer lead-related complications than TV-ICD [1], and is also useful in younger patients who require long-term lead placement. Therefore, S-ICD is expected to prevent SCD, especially in young patients with ARVC.

However, the precise clinical role of S-ICD in patients with ARVC remains to be defined. One reason is that S-ICD does not have a function of anti-tachycardia pacing that is expected to be highly effective in terminating scar-related re-entrant VT, which is often observed in patients with ARVC. Another reason is that morphological changes in S-ECG with age may lead to cardiac oversensing and IAS delivery. In an Italian multicenter registry, which enrolled 44 young ARVC patients undergoing S-ICD implantation (mean age of 37 years; mean LVEF of 53%; primary prevention of 59%), 6 (14%) experienced 8 IAS deliveries, consisting of 4 cardiac oversensing and 4 non-cardiac oversensing [5]. Furthermore, in a transatlantic cohort study [6], which enrolled 29 young ARVC patients undergoing S-ICD implantation (mean age of 34 years, mean LVEF of 56%, primary prevention of 59%), 6 (21%) experienced 39 IAS deliveries due to oversensing. These studies indicate a high incidence of IAS delivery in S-ICD-implanted ARVC patients, leading to a potential limitation of S-ICD use in these patients.

3. Usefulness of lead repositioning of S-ICD in patients with ARVC

The conventional S-ICD system that we are using to date was developed and evaluated in the initial study [9]. In that study, the substernal lead was placed parallel to and 1 to 2 cm to the left of the sternal midline, and the pulse generator was placed over the sixth rib between the midaxillary line and the anterior axillary line. And the distal sensing electrode was positioned adjacent to the manubriosternal junction, and the proximal sensing electrode was positioned adjacent to the xiphoid process. The final position of S-ICD system was determined by the defibrillation threshold or the effectiveness of defibrillation. Notably, the positioning of S-ICD system was guided exclusively by anatomical landmarks, thus no fluoroscopy was required.

Recently, we reported the usefulness of S-ICD lead repositioning to avoid IAS in young patients with ARVC [7]. The most important benefit of S-ICD lead repositioning is an improved S-ECG sensing due to changes in QRS amplitude of S-ECG. The sensing of S-ICD is largely dependent on QRS/T ratio of S-ECG, which is vulnerable to changes caused by physical activities or the progression of underlying heart diseases. It has been well known that the decrease in QRS amplitude of S-ECG due to degeneration of the right ventricular myocardium progresses overtime in ARVC patients. **Figure 1** shows ECG examples of a patient with ARVC in whom a decrease in QRS amplitude of surface ECG was confirmed over time. Of note, such changes in QRS amplitude were reflected more clearly in S-ECG compared with surface ECG. In such patients, S-ICD has a potential risk of IAS due to oversensing.

The SMART pass technology (SP) is a high-pass filter which enables to avoid sensing below 9 Hz and is expected to decrease IAS due to cardiac oversensing [10]. However, the decrease in QRS amplitude is more likely to lead to cardiac and

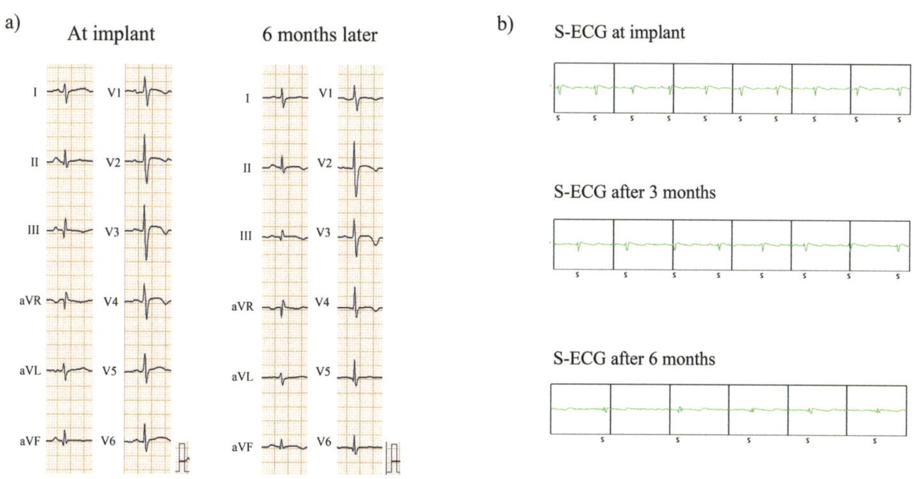

Figure 1.
Comparison of changes over time between body surface electrocardiogram and subcutaneous electrocardiogram (S-ECG). (a) Comparison of body surface ECG over time. The QRS amplitude decreases slightly over time in bipolar limb leads. (b) Comparison of S-ECG over time in the supine position. S-ECG was detected by alternate sensing vector with same detection sensitivity. The QRS amplitude of S-ECG decreases over time.

non-cardiac oversensing such as T wave or MPI, even if the SP is working properly. The SP can be set-up manually or automatically, but QRS amplitude of S-ECG is required to be higher than 0.5 mV. Furthermore, the SP is automatically terminated when there is no cardiac sensing for 10 seconds or when QRS amplitude of S-ECG decreases under 0.25 mV for 1.4 seconds or more. Therefore, there is a limitation to avoid IAS due to oversensing by SP alone in ARVC patients. For these reasons, lead repositioning of S-ICD can be a useful alternative to prevention of IAS in ARVC patients, even though the SP has been already activated.

4. Clinical practice of S-ICD lead repositioning in patients with ARVC

The potential efficacy of lead repositioning can be estimated by preoperative screening test. If two or more vectors do not pass the screening test, other sensing vectors suitable for S-ICD sensing must be searched and lead repositioning or movement of the pulse generator, or both may be required.

Here is an example of S-ICD lead repositioning. The patient was a 17-year-old man who developed VF and was resuscitated by an automated external defibrillator. He was diagnosed with ARVC based on the task force criteria [11] and underwent S-ICD implantation for secondary prevention of SCD. Alternate vector was selected for S-ICD sensing by exercise tests after S-ICD implantation, and the SP algorithm was activated. Six months later, an emergency alert was transmitted via remote monitoring to notify the occurrence of the event just before the shock delivery. A close examination immediately after the alert

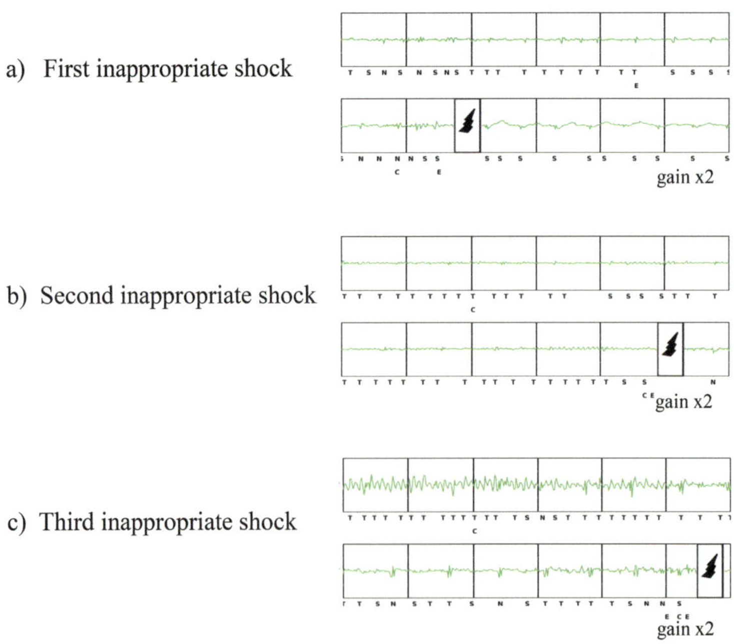

Figure 2.
Subcutaneous electrocardiogram (S-ECG) at inappropriate shock (IAS) deliveries. (a) S-ECG during the first IAS. The first IAS occurred when the patient was wiping his hair with a towel after bathing. The S-ICD was set to use the primary sensing vector at the time of IAS, and the Smart pass (SP) algorithm turned off automatically due to attenuated QRS amplitude. (b) S-ECG during the second IAS. The sensing vector was changed to alternate vector based on the results of exercise test. The IAS occurred when the patient was operating the smartphone in the left lateral position. Same as the first IAS, the SP algorithm turned off automatically due to attenuated QRS amplitude. (c) S-ECG during the third IAS. The IAS occurred when the patient was resting on the bed. The SP algorithm could not avoid IAS due to high-frequency MPI.

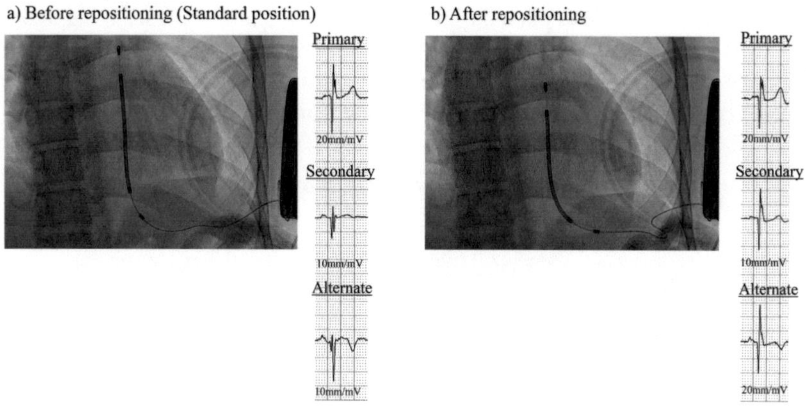

Figure 3.
Comparison of fluoroscopic images before and after lead repositioning and changes in S-ECG. The previously implanted S-ICD lead was placed at standard position based on the result of AST (a) This lead was moved to the lower left and QRS amplitude of S-ECG increased in 2 (secondary and alternate) out of 3 sensing vectors (b).

confirmed a decrease in QRS amplitude of S-ECG over time (**Figure 1**), and we changed sensing vector from the alternate vector to the primary vector. Seven months after the change of S-ICD sensing vector, the patient experienced a first IAS delivery. The S-ICD was set to use the primary sensing vector at the time of IAS, and the SP was turned off automatically due to attenuated QRS amplitude. S-ECG showed MPI that led to IAS delivery due to oversensing. After the changing the sensing vector to the alternate one, the patient had repeated IAS deliveries and eventually experienced IAS deliveries in all sensing vectors (**Figure 2**). Therefore, we performed an automated screening test (AST) on surface ECG again with a different electrode position. We performed an AST by moving the distal electrode approximately one intercostal space downward, and the proximal electrode was moved to the left, so that left ventricular electrocardiogram was more reflected on S-ECG. As a result, the QRS amplitude of S-ECG increased in 2 out of 3 sensing vectors and passed the AST. Thus, we performed repositioning of S-ICD lead under fluoroscopy (**Figure 3**). After repositioning of the S-ICD lead, the QRS amplitude of S-ECG increased and 2 (secondary and alternate sensing vectors) out of 3 vectors were suitable for S-ECG sensing, and there was no IAS for 15 months thereafter.

5. Limitation and future perspectives

As we described in the previous chapter, repositioning of the S-ICD lead to the lower left creates a new sensing vector that reflects more electrocardiograms of ventricular septum and left ventricle (**Figure 4**). Improved S-ECG sensing by the repositioning of the lead may be useful for patients not only with hereditary degenerative disease of the right ventricular myocardium such as ARVC, but also with acquired right ventricular myocardial damage such as right ventricular myocardial infarction. However, a concern in the method used in our case was that repositioned electrodes, especially the proximal electrode that was directly above or near the pectoralis major muscle, would be more vulnerable to MPI. Certainly, even after repositioning, slight MPI was observed in some sensing vectors, but it was possible to avoid MPI by selecting the optimal sensing vector based on the results of treadmill or other exercise test [12]. Furthermore, substernal tunneling method in which the distal electrode is placed on the sternum may also be useful for avoiding IAS due to MPI (**Figures 5** and **6**). More experiences and long-term follow-up may be necessary in order to establish the usefulness of the S-ICD lead repositioning in patients with ARVC. Further studies are clearly warranted.

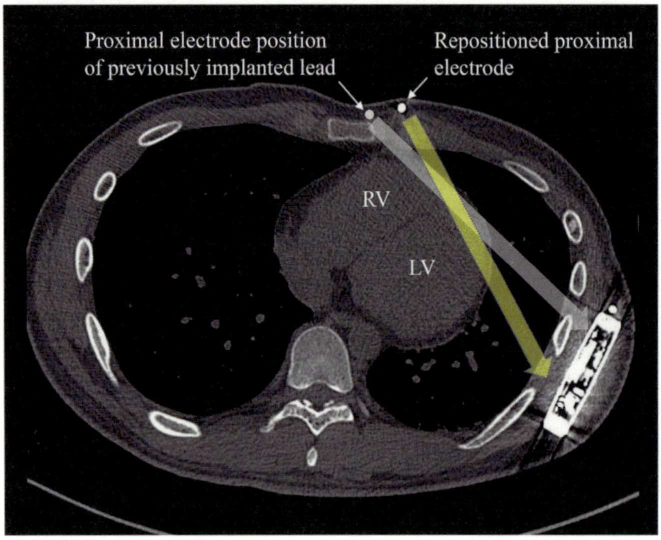

Figure 4.
Computed tomographic images after lead repositioning. It can be seen that the sensing vector between the repositioned proximal electrode and pulse generator is mediated by more left ventricular myocardium than the previously implanted proximal electrode position. The electrode position of previous implanted lead is illustrated based on previously captured CT image.

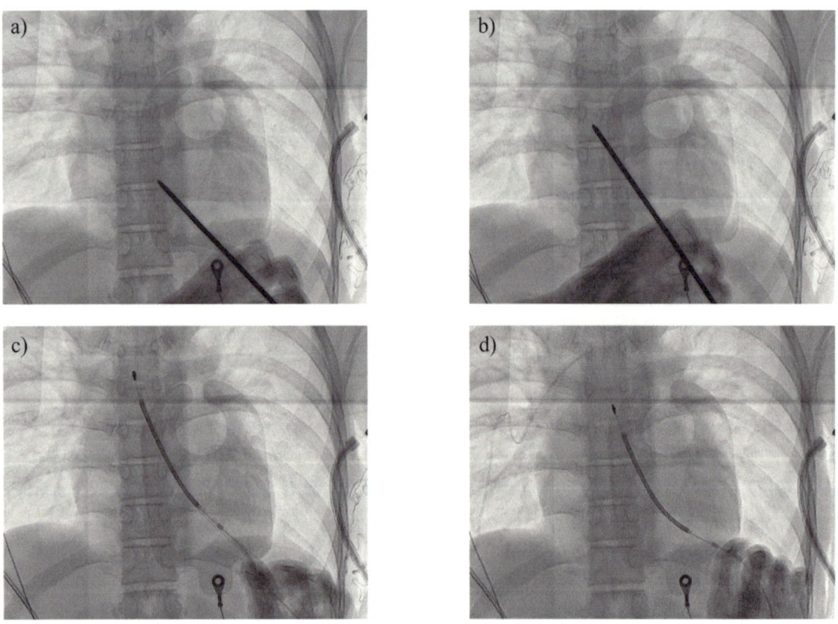

Figure 5.
Method of substernal tunneling during lead repositioning. The tunneling method is shown in the order of (a to d) At first, the tip of the insertion tool was inserted diagonally to the right, and then gradually advance it toward cranial direction (a, b) After the tunneling tool was fully inserted, the lead was inserted into the introducer sheath as much as possible with two-incision technique (c) After peeling off the sheath, the lead was pulled back and placed at the pre-planned position (d).

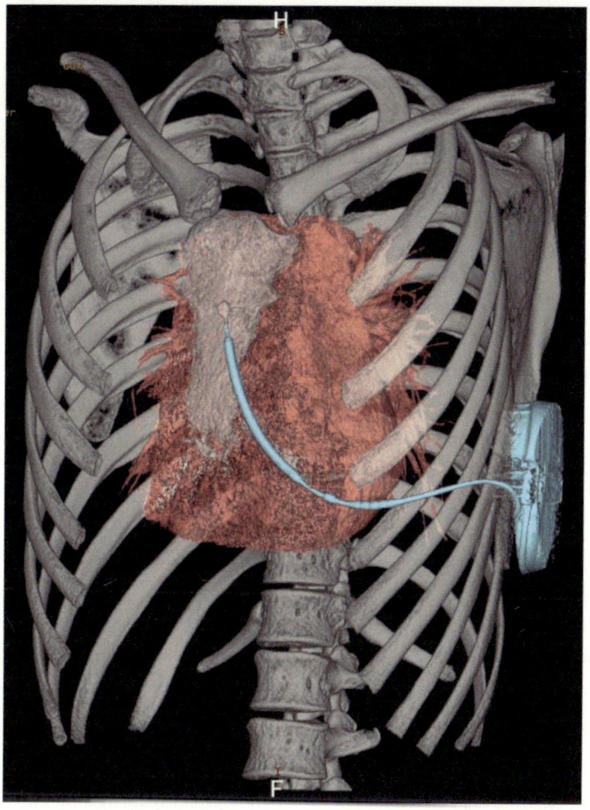

Figure 6.
The 3D computed tomographic image in the left anterior oblique position after subcutaneous implantable cardioverter-defibrillator (S-ICD) implantation.

Conflict of interest

Dr. Shingo Sasaki has received research grant supports from Medtronic Japan Co., Ltd. and Fukuda Denshi Kita-tohoku Hanbai Co., Ltd. and BIOTRONIK Japan Co., Ltd. Dr. Shingo Sasaki has received scholarship donation from Japan Lifeline Co., Ltd. and Boston Scientific Japan Co., Ltd.

Author details

Shingo Sasaki
Department of Cardiology and Nephrology, Hirosaki University Graduate School of Medicine, Hirosaki, Japan

*Address all correspondence to: sshingo@hirosaki-u.ac.jp

References

[1] Knops RE, Olde Nordkamp LRA, Delnoy PHM, Boersma LVA, Kuschyk J, El-Chami MF, Bonnemeier H, Behr ER, Brouwer TF, Kääb S, Mittal S, Quast ABE, Smeding L, van der Stuijt W, de Weger A, de Wilde KC, Bijsterveld NR, Richter S, Brouwer MA, de Groot JR, Kooiman KM, Lambiase PD, Neuzil P, Vernooy K, Alings M, Betts TR, Bracke FALE, Burke MC, de Jong JSSG, Wright DJ, Tijssen JGP, Wilde AAM; PRAETORIAN Investigators. Subcutaneous or transvenous defibrillator therapy. N Engl J Med. 2020 Aug 6;383:526-536.

[2] Gold MR, Lambiase PD, El-Chami MF, Knops RE, Aasbo JD, Bongiorni MG, Russo AM, Deharo JC, Burke MC, Dinerman J, Barr CS, Shaik N, Carter N, Stoltz T, Stein KM, Brisben AJ, Boersma LV; UNTOUCHED Investigators. Primary Results from the Understanding Outcomes with the S-ICD in Primary Prevention Patients with Low Ejection Fraction (UNTOUCHED) Trial. Circulation. 2020 Oct 19. doi: 10.1161/CIRCULATIONAHA.120.048728.

[3] Moss AJ, Schuger C, Beck CA, Brown MW, Cannom DS, Daubert JP, Estes NA 3rd, Greenberg H, Hall WJ, Huang DT, Kautzner J, Klein H, McNitt S, Olshansky B, Shoda M, Wilber D, Zareba W; MADIT-RIT Trial Investigators. Reduction in inappropriate therapy and mortality through ICD programming. N Engl J Med. 2012;367:2275-2283.

[4] Ruwald AC, Marcus F, Estes NA 3rd, Link M, McNitt S, Polonsky B, Calkins H, Towbin JA, Moss AJ, Zareba W. Association of competitive and recreational sport participation with cardiac events in patients with arrhythmogenic right ventricular cardiomyopathy: results from the North American multidisciplinary study of arrhythmogenic right ventricular cardiomyopathy. Eur Heart J. 2015;36:1735-1743.

[5] Migliore F, Viani S, Bongiorni MG, Zorzi A, Silvetti MS, Francia P, D'Onofrio A, De Franceschi P, Sala S, Donzelli S, Ricciardi G, Menardi E, Giammaria M, La Greca C, Bauce B, Rigato I, Iliceto S, Bertaglia E, Diemberger I, Corrado D. Subcutaneous implantable cardioverter defibrillator in patients with arrhythmogenic right ventricular cardiomyopathy: Results from an Italian multicenter registry. Int J Cardiol. 2019;280:74-79.

[6] Orgeron GM, Bhonsale A, Migliore F, James CA, Tichnell C, Murray B, Bertaglia E, Cadrin-Tourigny J, De Franceschi P, Crosson J, Tandri H, Corrado D, Calkins H. Subcutaneous implantable cardioverter-defibrillator in patients with arrhythmogenic right ventricular cardiomyopathy/dysplasia: a transatlantic experience. J Am Heart Assoc. 2018;7:e008782.

[7] Sasaki S, Nishizaki K, Ishida Y, Toyama Y, Hamaura S, Tomita H. Usefulness of lead repositioning to improvesubcutaneouselectrocardiogram sensing in patients with arrhythmogenic right ventricular cardiomyopathy with subcutaneous implantable cardioverter-defibrillator. Heart Rhythm Case Rep. 2020;6:786-790.

[8] Corrado D, Zorzi A, Cerrone M, Rigato I, Mongillo M, Bauce B, Delmar M. Relationship between arrhythmogenic right ventricular cardiomyopathy and brugada syndrome new insights from molecular biology and clinical implications. Circ Arrhythm Electrophysiol. 2016;9:e003631.

[9] Bardy GH, Smith WM, Hood MA, Crozier IG, Melton IC, Jordaens L, Theuns D, Park RE, Wright DJ, Connelly DT, Fynn SP, Murgatroyd FD,

Sperzel J, Neuzner J, Spitzer SG, Ardashev AV, Oduro A, Boersma L, Maass AH, Van Gelder IC, Wilde AA, van Dessel PF, Knops RE, Barr CS, Lupo P, Cappato R, Grace AA. An entirely subcutaneous implantable cardioverter-defibrillator. N Engl J Med. 2010;363(1):36-44.

[10] Theuns DAMJ, Brouwer TF, Jones PW, Allavatam V, Donnelley S, Auricchio A, Knops RE, Burke MC. Prospective blinded evaluation of a novel sensing methodology designed to reduce inappropriate shocks by the subcutaneous implantable cardioverter-defibrillator. Heart Rhythm. 2018;15:1515-1522.

[11] Marcus FI, McKenna WJ, Sherrill D, Basso C, Bauce B, Bluemke DA, Calkins H, Corrado D, Cox MG, Daubert JP, Fontaine G, Gear K, Hauer R, Nava A, Picard MH, Protonotarios N, Saffitz JE, Sanborn DM, Steinberg JS, Tandri H, Thiene G, Towbin JA, Tsatsopoulou A, Wichter T, Zareba W. Diagnosis of arrhythmogenic right ventricular cardiomyopathy/dysplasia: proposed modification of the Task Force Criteria. Eur Heart J. 2010;31:806-814.

[12] Ishida Y, Sasaki S, Toyama Y, et al. A novel screening test for inappropriate shocks due to myopotentials from the subcutaneous implantable cardioverter–defibrillator. Heart Rhythm O^2. 2020;1:27-34.